Photodynamic Therapy

Photodynamic Therapy

Editors

Kyungsu Kang
Stefano Bacci

MDPI • Basel • Beijing • Wuhan • Barcelona • Belgrade • Manchester • Tokyo • Cluj • Tianjin

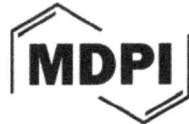

Editors
Kyungsu Kang
Korea Institute of Science and Technology
Korea

Stefano Bacci
University of Florence
Italy

Editorial Office
MDPI
St. Alban-Anlage 66
4052 Basel, Switzerland

This is a reprint of articles from the Topic published online in the open access journals *Biomedicines* (ISSN 2227-9059), *BioMed* (ISSN 2673-8430), and *Reports* (ISSN 2571-841X) (available at: https://www.mdpi.com/topics/photodynamic_therapy).

For citation purposes, cite each article independently as indicated on the article page online and as indicated below:

LastName, A.A.; LastName, B.B.; LastName, C.C. Article Title. *Journal Name* **Year**, *Volume Number*, Page Range.

ISBN 978-3-0365-5873-8 (Hbk)
ISBN 978-3-0365-5874-5 (PDF)

© 2022 by the authors. Articles in this book are Open Access and distributed under the Creative Commons Attribution (CC BY) license, which allows users to download, copy and build upon published articles, as long as the author and publisher are properly credited, which ensures maximum dissemination and a wider impact of our publications.

The book as a whole is distributed by MDPI under the terms and conditions of the Creative Commons license CC BY-NC-ND.

Contents

About the Editors . . . . **ix**

Kyungsu Kang and Stefano Bacci
Photodynamic Therapy
Reprinted from: *Biomedicines* **2022**, *10*, 2701, doi:10.3390/biomedicines10112701 . . . . **1**

Hyung Shik Kim and Dong Yun Lee
Nanomedicine in Clinical Photodynamic Therapy for the Treatment of Brain Tumors
Reprinted from: *Biomedicines* **2022**, *10*, 96, doi:10.3390/biomedicines10010096 . . . . **7**

Kohei Matsuoka, Mizuki Yamada, Mitsuo Sato and Kazuhide Sato
Near-Infrared Photoimmunotherapy for Thoracic Cancers: A Translational Perspective
Reprinted from: *Biomedicines* **2022**, *10*, 1662, doi:10.3390/biomedicines10071662 . . . . **33**

Abdulrahman A. Balhaddad, Lamia Mokeem, Sharukh S. Khajotia, Fernando L. Esteban Florez and Mary A. S. Melo
Perspectives on Light-Based Disinfection to Reduce the Risk of COVID-19 Transmission during Dental Care
Reprinted from: *BioMed* **2022**, *2*, 3, doi:10.3390/biomed2010003 . . . . **49**

Vieri Grandi, Alessandro Corsi, Nicola Pimpinelli and Stefano Bacci
Cellular Mechanisms in Acute and Chronic Wounds after PDT Therapy: An Update
Reprinted from: *Biomedicines* **2022**, *10*, 1624, doi:10.3390/biomedicines10071624 . . . . **59**

Yi-Wen Lin, Chien-Sung Tsai, Chun-Yao Huang, Yi-Ting Tsai, Chun-Ming Shih, Shing-Jong Lin, Chi-Yuan Li, Cheng-Yen Lin, Shih-Ying Sung and Feng-Yen Lin
Far-Infrared Therapy Decreases Orthotopic Allograft Transplantation Vasculopathy
Reprinted from: *Biomedicines* **2022**, *10*, 1089, doi:10.3390/biomedicines10051089 . . . . **69**

Diana Lorena Guevara Solarte, Sibylle Johanna Rau, Elmar Hellwig, Kirstin Vach and Ali Al-Ahmad
Antimicrobial Behavior and Cytotoxicity of Indocyanine Green in Combination with Visible Light and Water-Filtered Infrared A Radiation against Periodontal Bacteria and Subgingival Biofilm
Reprinted from: *Biomedicines* **2022**, *10*, 956, doi:10.3390/biomedicines10050956 . . . . **89**

Corina Elena Tisler, Radu Chifor, Mindra Eugenia Badea, Marioara Moldovan, Doina Prodan, Rahela Carpa, Stanca Cuc, Ioana Chifor and Alexandru Florin Badea
Photodynamic Therapy (PDT) in Prosthodontics: Disinfection of Human Teeth Exposed to *Streptococcus mutans* and the Effect on the Adhesion of Full Ceramic Veneers, Crowns, and Inlays: An In Vitro Study
Reprinted from: *Biomedicines* **2022**, *10*, 144, doi:10.3390/biomedicines10010144 . . . . **107**

Joseph C. Cacaccio, Farukh A. Durrani, Joseph R. Missert and Ravindra K. Pandey
Photodynamic Therapy in Combination with Doxorubicin Is Superior to Monotherapy for the Treatment of Lung Cancer
Reprinted from: *Biomedicines* **2022**, *10*, 857, doi:10.3390/biomedicines10040857 . . . . **121**

Laureline Lamy, Jacques Thomas, Agnès Leroux, Jean-François Bisson, Kari Myren, Aslak Godal, Gry Stensrud and Lina Bezdetnaya
Antitumor Effect and Induced Immune Response Following Exposure of Hexaminolevulinate and Blue Light in Combination with Checkpoint Inhibitor in an Orthotopic Model of Rat Bladder Cancer
Reprinted from: *Biomedicines* **2022**, *10*, 548, doi:10.3390/biomedicines10030548 . . . . **137**

Antonina Klimenko, Elvira E. Rodina, Denis Silachev, Maria Begun, Valentina A. Babenko, Anton S. Benditkis, Anton S. Kozlov, Alexander A. Krasnovsky, Yuri S. Khotimchenko and Vladimir L. Katanaev
Chlorin Endogenous to the North Pacific Brittle Star *Ophiura sarsii* for Photodynamic Therapy Applications in Breast Cancer and Glioblastoma Models
Reprinted from: *Biomedicines* 2022, 10, 134, doi:10.3390/biomedicines10010134 153

Viktoria Pevna, Georges Wagnières and Veronika Huntosova
Autophagy and Apoptosis Induced in U87 MG Glioblastoma Cells by Hypericin-Mediated Photodynamic Therapy Can Be Photobiomodulated with 808 nm Light
Reprinted from: *Biomedicines* 2021, 9, 1703, doi:10.3390/biomedicines9111703 167

Alex Vasilev, Roba Sofi, Stuart J. Smith, Ruman Rahman, Anja G. Teschemacher and Sergey Kasparov
Feasibility of Photodynamic Therapy for Glioblastoma with the Mitochondria-Targeted Photosensitizer Tetramethylrhodamine Methyl Ester (TMRM)
Reprinted from: *Biomedicines* 2021, 9, 1453, doi:10.3390/biomedicines9101453 185

Pei-Chi Chiang, Pei-Tzu Li, Ming-Jen Lee and Chin-Tin Chen
DNA Hypermethylation Involves in the Down-Regulation of Chloride Intracellular Channel 4 (CLIC4) Induced by Photodynamic Therapy
Reprinted from: *Biomedicines* 2021, 9, 927, doi:10.3390/biomedicines9080927 203

Carla M. Magalhães, Patricia González-Berdullas, Diana Duarte, Ana Salomé Correia, José E. Rodríguez-Borges, Nuno Vale, Joaquim C. G. Esteves da Silva and Luís Pinto da Silva
Target-Oriented Synthesis of Marine Coelenterazine Derivatives with Anticancer Activity by Applying the Heavy-Atom Effect
Reprinted from: *Biomedicines* 2021, 9, 1199, doi:10.3390/biomedicines9091199 219

Stéphane Desgranges, Petras Juzenas, Vlada Vasovic, Odrun Arna Gederaas, Mikael Lindgren, Trond Warloe, Qian Peng and Christiane Contino-Pépin
Amphiphilic Protoporphyrin IX Derivatives as New Photosensitizing Agents for the Improvement of Photodynamic Therapy
Reprinted from: *Biomedicines* 2022, 10, 423, doi:10.3390/biomedicines10020423 235

Vanya N. Mantareva, Vesselin Kussovski, Petya Orozova, Lyudmila Dimitrova, Irem Kulu, Ivan Angelov, Mahmut Durmus and Hristo Najdenski
Photodynamic Inactivation of Antibiotic-Resistant and Sensitive *Aeromonas hydrophila* with Peripheral Pd(II)- vs. Zn(II)-Phthalocyanines
Reprinted from: *Biomedicines* 2022, 10, 384, doi:10.3390/biomedicines10020384 253

Pravena Ramachandran, Boon-Keat Khor, Chong Yew Lee, Ruey-An Doong, Chern Ein Oon, Nguyen Thi Kim Thanh and Hooi Ling Lee
N-Doped Graphene Quantum Dots/Titanium Dioxide Nanocomposites: A Study of ROS-Forming Mechanisms, Cytotoxicity and Photodynamic Therapy
Reprinted from: *Biomedicines* 2022, 10, 421, doi:10.3390/biomedicines10020421 263

Jun Fang, Shanghui Gao, Rayhanul Islam, Hinata Nema, Rina Yanagibashi, Niho Yoneda, Natsumi Watanabe, Yuki Yasuda, Naoki Nuita, Jian-Rong Zhou and Kazumi Yokomizo
Styrene Maleic Acid Copolymer-Based Micellar Formation of Temoporfin (SMA@ mTHPC) Behaves as A Nanoprobe for Tumor-Targeted Photodynamic Therapy with A Superior Safety
Reprinted from: *Biomedicines* 2021, 9, 1493, doi:10.3390/biomedicines9101493 283

Kristian Espeland, Andrius Kleinauskas, Petras Juzenas, Andreas Brech, Sagar Darvekar, Vlada Vasovic, Trond Warloe, Eidi Christensen, Jørgen Jahnsen and Qian Peng
Photodynamic Effects with 5-Aminolevulinic Acid on Cytokines and Exosomes in Human Peripheral Blood Mononuclear Cells
Reprinted from: *Biomedicines* **2022**, *10*, 232, doi:10.3390/biomedicines10020232 . . . . **299**

About the Editors

Kyungsu Kang

Dr. Kyungsu Kang (Orcid number: 0000-0003-3846-7936) is a Principal Researcher at the Gangneung Institute of Natural Products, Korea Institute of Science and Technology (KIST), located in Gangwon-do, South Korea. He is also a Professor in the Division of Bio-Medical Science and Technology, KIST School, University of Science and Technology (UST), South Korea. He received his B.S. in Applied Biology and Chemistry and M.S. and Ph.D. degrees (in Agricultural Biotechnology) from the College of Agriculture and Life Science, Seoul National University, South Korea. The main research topic of Dr. Kang's laboratory is to discover bioactive natural products that can promote intestinal health and longevity. Dr. Kang and his members are interested in elucidating the biochemical and molecular mechanisms underlying the biological effects of various natural products. For this purpose, they are exploiting not only a tiny model nematode, *Caenorhabditis elegans*, but also cultured human cells and cultured human microbiota.

Stefano Bacci

Dr. Stefano Bacci (Orcid number: 0000-0002-3651-229X) is a Professor of Cytology and Histology and Developmental Biology at the University of Florence and has resided, during his training, at the Schepens Eye Research Institute, Harvard Medical School, Boston (MA), USA. His main research concerns the understanding of the cellular mechanisms involved during wound healing in relation to the type of treatment used, including relating to photodynamic therapy. He is the author of more than 100 articles within his research sector, including publications of high scientific impact. For other related information, please see the following web page: https://sciprofiles.com/profile/915428.

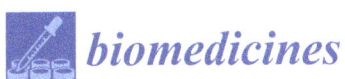

Editorial

Photodynamic Therapy

Kyungsu Kang [1,2] and Stefano Bacci [3,*]

1. Natural Product Informatics Research Center, Gangneung Institute of Natural Products, Korea Institute of Science and Technology, Gangneung 25451, Gangwon-do, Korea
2. Division of Bio-Medical Science & Technology, KIST School, University of Science and Technology (UST), Gangneung 25451, Gangwon-do, Korea
3. Research Unit of Histology and Embriology, Department of Biology, University of Florence, Viale Pieraccini 6, 50139 Florence, Italy
* Correspondence: stefano.bacci@unifi.it

Citation: Kang, K.; Bacci, S. Photodynamic Therapy. *Biomedicines* 2022, 10, 2701. https://doi.org/10.3390/biomedicines10112701

Received: 26 September 2022
Accepted: 17 October 2022
Published: 26 October 2022

Publisher's Note: MDPI stays neutral with regard to jurisdictional claims in published maps and institutional affiliations.

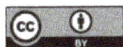

Copyright: © 2022 by the authors. Licensee MDPI, Basel, Switzerland. This article is an open access article distributed under the terms and conditions of the Creative Commons Attribution (CC BY) license (https://creativecommons.org/licenses/by/4.0/).

In 1903, Von Tappeiner and Jesionek [1] showed the efficacy of light treatment together with a photosensitizer and oxygen, which is so-called "photodynamic action". Medically, photodynamic therapy (PDT) application is now extensively used, and PDT has been exploited to treat various oncological and non-oncological human diseases.

This editorial provides an up-to-date brief review of "Photodynamic therapy" appearing in biomedicine and some recent studies related to this therapy. We summarize the various contributions highlighting new analytic approaches and updates related to photodynamic therapy. The editorial is dedicated to concise updates on general or specific arguments regarding the utility of photodynamic therapy.

Review of General Arguments

About tumors: since the rate of survival for subjects with tumors like glioblastoma multiforme (GBM) greater risk malignancy is below a year, clinical outcomes of patients with GBM who received PDT may be improved through the use of nanomedicine. The review by Kim and Lee summarizes the utility of clinical PDT applications of nanomedicine for the management of GBM (for more information, see [2]). Matsuoka et al., reviewed the role of PDT for the management of early stage malignant lung tumors. Recently, a near-infrared photoimmunotherapy (NIR-PIT) has been developed for the treatment of recurrent head and neck malignancies due to its specificity and efficacy. In this review, NIR-PIT is introduced, and its potential therapeutic utilities for thoracic cancers are elaborated (for more details, see [3]).

About SARS-CoV-2: Balhaddad et al., discuss the current efforts and limitations on utilizing biophotonic approaches to prevent the transmission of SARS-CoV-2 in dental care and provide relevant information regarding the intricacies and complexities of infection control in dental care (for more details, see [4]).

On chronic wounds: since wound healing process involves a complex interplay and organization of different cells and biomolecules and any modification with these extremely organized events may cause prolonged or excessive healing, Grandi et al., elucidated the cellular mechanisms described, upon therapy with 5-aminovuleinic acid (ALA)-PDT, in chronic wounds, that may be linked with social isolation and high costs (for more details, see [5]).

Research Articles of Specific Topics

About the studies on transplantation: Lin et al., explore the possibility of far-infrared (FIR) in preventing orthotopic allograft transplantation (OAT) using an aorta graft from PVG/Seac to ACI/NKyo rats, and human endothelial progenitor cells (EPC). The authors reported that FIR treatment decreased vasculopathy in OAT-recipient ACI/NKyo rats, as well as the immune responses mediated by the spleen and the release of serum inflammatory markers. Higher mobilization and circulating EPC levels related to vessel repair in

OAT-recipient ACI/NKyo rats were seen. In vitro studies showed that this process may be related to the blockade of the Smad2-Slug signaling axis of endothelial mesenchymal transition. The authors proposed that FIR therapy can be considered a potential strategy to mitigate chronic rejection-induced vasculopathy (for more details, see [6]).

About the studies on periodontal treatments: Solarte et al., evaluated the antimicrobial effect and cytotoxicity of PDT with indocyanine green with visible light and water-filtered infrared A in patients with chronic periodontitis. Almost all bacterial pathogens were eliminated as well as significant differences were found in the subgingival biofilms. The authors propose this photodynamic therapy as an adjuvant to periodontal treatments (see [7] for additional details).Tisler et al., assessed the effect of PDT to improve the bond strength of full ceramic restorations. Their investigation demonstrates that the bacterial number was decreased from colonized marked tooth exteriors, manifesting with a rise in the bond strength following the PDT treatment. The authors indicate that PDT treatment before the final adhesive cementation of ceramic restorations may be an optimistic strategy compared to conventional practice (for more information, see [8]).

About the studies on tumors: Cacaccio et al., studied the efficacy of PDT with a non-radioactive sensitizer (PS) in tumors derived from lung cancer patients in mice models. The in vitro and in vivo efficacy was also evaluated in combination with doxorubicin, and long-term tumor response was significantly increased. The authors propose that the iodinated PS is efficient for the treatment of lung tumors (for additional information, see [9]). Lamy et al., studied if the use of hexaminolevulinate and blue light cystoscopy in an orthotopic rat model of bladder cancer may have therapeutic efficacy by modulation of a tumor-specific immune response and measured if its delivery in combination with a checkpoint inhibitor may enhance any effects observed. Positive anti-tumor effect was related to the timing of the process with a localization of CD3+ and CD8+ cells at long term: the effect was increased when delivered in combination with intravesical anti-PD-L1 (for more information, see [10]). Klimenko et al., describe the activity of (3S,4S)-14-Ethyl-9-(hydroxymethyl)−4,8,13,18-tetramethyl-20-oxo-3-phorbinepropanoic acid (ETPA) as a crucial metabolite of the North Pacific brittle stars *Ophiura sarsii* in a mouse model of glioblastoma. Intravenous ETPA administered in addition with a targeted red laser irradiation induced strong necrotic ablation of glioblastoma. The authors propose ETPA as a natural product-based photodynamic drug (for more information, see [11]). Pevna et al., measured the efficacy of hypericin-mediated PDT in U87 MG cells human GBM cells subjected to the treatment with rotenone that influence their metabolic activity. This treatment stimulates autophagy and increases the anticancer efficacy and leads to apoptosis. This seems to decrease the damage in surrounding normal tissues when hypericin-PDT is utilized for in vivo tumor treatments (For more information, see [12]). Vasilev et al., demonstrate that tetramethylrhodamine methyl ester (TMRM), which is a fluorescent dye to evaluate mitochondrial potential, may be utilized as a photosensitizer to select GBM cells. The results show that PDT with TMRM and low-intensity green light stimulated mitochondrial damage and led to GBM cell death, but not cultured rat astrocytes. The authors propose that TMRM as a mitochondrially targeted photosensitizer may be considered for preclinical or clinical studies (for more information, see [13]). Chiang et al., attempted to make the processes associated with PDT-mediated chloride intracellular channel (CLIC4) inhibition in human melanoma A375 cells and in human breast cancer MDA-MB-231 cells clear. The findings show the increase of the release and enzymatic effects of DNA methyltransferase 1 (DNMT1), the hypermethylation in the *CLIC4* promoter region and the involvement of P53 in the higher DNMT1 release in PDT-treated cells. The authors propose that CLIC4 suppression induced by PDT is modulated by DNMT1-mediated hypermethylation and revolves around p53, which suggests a coordinated process for regulating CLIC4 release in tumorigenesis (for more information, see [14]). Magalhaes et al., assessed the heavy-atom effect (HEA) as a mechanism for anticancer activity to coelenterazine derivatives, a chemiluminescent molecule widespread in marine organisms. The study findings suggest the use of HEA facilitates these molecules to manifest readily available triplet states in a chemiluminescent reaction stimulated by a tumor marker, but the potency of the anticancer activity is determined by the tumor type. The authors propose that the utilization of the HEA to marine coelenterazine may be an optimistic strategy for the development of new tumor-selective sensitizers for light-free PDT (for more information, see [15]).

About the studies on the efficacy of photosensitizers: Desgranges et al., studied a series of amphiphilic protoporphyrin derivatives since protoporphyrin IX (PpIX), is limited in clinical PDT by relative insolubility in watery and the possibility to self-aggregate. The findings demonstrate the therapeutic potency of these new PpIX because some of them demonstrated a higher photodynamic activity compared to the parent PpIX (for more information, see [16]). Mantareva et al., present the efficacy of a new sensitizer with peripheral positions of methylpiridoxy substitution groups (pPdPc and ZnPcMe) on Gram-negative bacteria *Aeromonas hydrophila*, antibiotic-resistant and sensitive strains. The photoinactivation demonstrated a complete activity with 8 µM pPdPc for antibiotic-sensitive strain and with 5 µM ZnPcMe for both antibiotic-resistant and sensitive strains. These results suggest that the uptakes and photoinactivation efficacy of the applied phthalocyanines are not related to the drug sensitivity of both strains (for more information, see [17]). In a study by Ramachandran et al., TiO_2 NPs and TiO_2 conjugated with N-GQDs/TiO_2 NCs were synthetized via microwave-assisted synthesis and two-pot hydrothermal method, respectively. Upon the photo-activation with near-infrared (NIR) light, the nanocomposites elaborated reactive oxygen species (ROS), which caused more significant mitochondria-associated apoptotic cell death in human breast cancer MDA-MB-231 cells than in human foreskin fibroblast HS27 cells. The authors propose that titanium dioxide-based nanocomposite upon photoactivation is a possible photosensitizer for PDT against human breast cancer care (for more information, see [18]). Fang et al., produced a styrene maleic acid copolymer (SMA) micelle encapsulating temoporfin (mTHPC), which is medically a PDT drug. SMA@mTHPC, showed a pH-dependent release profile, and higher expression took place at acidic pH, indicating that marked expression of free mTHPC may take place in the weak acidic pH setting of cancers and more so during internalization into cancer cells. In vitro cytotoxicity assay indicated a smaller activity of SMA@mTHPC compared to free mTHPC; but severe side effects were observed during free mTHPC treatment to the contrary of SMA@mTHPC. The better safety profile of SMA@mTHPC was mainly because of its micelle formation and the increased permeability and retention effect-based tumor accumulation, and the tumor environment-responsive release properties. These observations indicated that SMA@mTHPC may be PDT drugs for targeted tumor treatment with a lower side effect (for more details, see [19]). Polat and Kang, reviewed natural photosensitizers and synthetic derivatives photosensitizers for antimicrobial photodynamic therapy (APDT) to control various pathogenic organisms. Regards to natural photosensitizers, many single compounds, as well as many plant extracts have been used for photosensitizers for APDT. Preclinical experimental models using a model nematode, *Caenorhabditis elegans*, wax moth, in addition to rodent model are used to evaluate the efficacy and side effects of new APDT. Various emerging technologies such as cell surface and protein engineering, photosensitizer uptake strategies, nano-delivery systems, and computational simulation are introduced in this review (for more information, see [20]). Alam et al., reported natural photosensitizers prepared from the medicinal plant *Tripterygium wilfordii* for antimicrobial photodynamic purposes. Ethanol extract (TWE) and a photosensitizer-enriched fraction contain six pheophorbide derivatives as active compounds. Cotreatment of red light (660 nm, 120 W/m^2) and natural photosensitizers (TWE) potently killed pathogenic bacteria and fungi, especially various skin pathogens in vitro. Their in vivo APDT efficacies and adverse effects were assessed using the model nematode *C. elegans* infected with *Staphylococcus aureus* and *Streptococcus pyogenes*, which are representative skin pathogens (for more information, see [21]).

About the studies on the cellular mechanisms evoked by PDT: Espeland et al., studied the effects of ALA-PDT on cytokines and exosomes of human peripheral blood mononuclear cells. The therapy appeared to lower all pro-inflammatory cytokines, indicating that the PDT may lead to a strong anti-inflammatory effect. In addition, the therapy lowered the levels of different types of exosomes, in particular the HLA-DRDPDQ exosome, which is very crucial in the rejection process of organ transplantation and autoimmune diseases. Their study suggests future therapeutic strategies of ALA-PDT for modulation of immune systems (for more details about this article see [22]).

Discussion

This research topic gives an opportunity for the meeting of experts on photodynamic therapy. The reviews proposed are clear in their content and the research articles cover new approaches and therapeutic targets that will certainly be deepened in future. In conclusion, from these studies, it emerges that through this therapy there is more hope in the clinical field for the eradication of diseases that have always pursued humanity.

Author Contributions: K.K. and S.B.: writing—review and editing, visualization, project administration. All authors have read and agreed to the published version of the manuscript.

Funding: This project received funding from intramural research grant from Korea Institute of Science Technology (KIST, 2E31881).

Acknowledgments: We acknowledge the authors of the articles referred to in this editorial for their valuable contributions and the referees for their rigorous review. We also acknowledge Eastern Zhuang for her support.

Conflicts of Interest: The authors declare no conflict of interest.

References

1. Szeimies, R.M.; Drager, J.; Abels, C.; Landthaler, M. History of photodynamic therapy in dermatology. In *Photodynamic Therapy and Fluorescence Diagnosis in Therapy*; Calzavara-Pinton, P., Rolf-Markus, S., Ortel, B., Eds.; Elsevier Science: Amsterdam, the Netherlands, 2001.
2. Kim, H.S.; Lee, D.Y. Nanomedicine in clinical photodynamic therapy for the treatment of brain tumors. *Biomedicines* **2022**, *10*, 96. [CrossRef] [PubMed]
3. Matsuoka, K.; Yamada, M.; Sato, M.; Sato, K. Near-infrared photoimmunotherapy for thoracic cancers: A translational perspective. *Biomedicines* **2022**, *10*, 1662. [CrossRef] [PubMed]
4. Balhaddad, A.A.; Mokeem, L.; Khajotia, S.S.; Florez, F.L.E.; Melo, M.A.S. Perspectives on light-based disinfection to reduce the risk of COVID-19 transmission during dental care. *BioMed* **2022**, *2*, 27–36. [CrossRef]
5. Grandi, V.; Corsi, A.; Pimpinelli, N.; Bacci, S. Cellular mechanisms in acute and chronic wounds after PDT therapy: An update. *Biomedicines* **2022**, *10*, 1624. [CrossRef]
6. Lin, Y.-W.; Tsai, C.-S.; Huang, C.-Y.; Tsai, Y.-T.; Shih, C.-M.; Lin, S.-J.; Li, C.-Y.; Lin, C.-Y.; Sung, S.-Y.; Lin, F.-Y. Far-infrared therapy decreases orthotopic allograft transplantation vasculopathy. *Biomedicines* **2022**, *10*, 1089. [CrossRef]
7. Solarte, D.L.G.; Rau, S.J.; Hellwig, E.; Vach, K.; Al-Ahmad, A. Antimicrobial behavior and cytotoxicity of indocyanine green in combination with visible light and water-filtered infrared a radiation against periodontal bacteria and subgingival biofilm. *Biomedicines* **2022**, *10*, 956. [CrossRef]
8. Tisler, C.E.; Chifor, R.; Badea, M.E.; Moldovan, M.; Prodan, D.; Carpa, R.; Cuc, S.; Chifor, I.; Badea, A.F. Photodynamic Therapy (PDT) in prosthodontics: Disinfection of human teeth exposed to *Streptococcus mutans* and the effect on the adhesion of full ceramic veneers, crowns, and inlays: An in vitro study. *Biomedicines* **2022**, *10*, 144. [CrossRef]
9. Cacaccio, J.C.; Durrani, F.A.; Missert, J.R.; Pandey, R.K. Photodynamic therapy in combination with doxorubicin is superior to monotherapy for the treatment of lung cancer. *Biomedicines* **2022**, *10*, 857. [CrossRef]
10. Lamy, L.; Thomas, J.; Leroux, A.; Bisson, J.-F.; Myren, K.; Godal, A.; Stensrud, G.; Bezdetnaya, L. Antitumor effect and induced immune response following exposure of hexaminolevulinate and blue light in combination with checkpoint inhibitor in an orthotopic model of rat bladder cancer. *Biomedicines* **2022**, *10*, 548. [CrossRef]
11. Klimenko, A.; Rodina, E.E.; Silachev, D.; Begun, M.; Babenko, V.A.; Benditkis, A.S.; Kozlov, A.S.; Krasnovsky, A.A.; Khotimchenko, Y.S.; Katanaev, V.L. Chlorin endogenous to the North Pacific brittle star *Ophiura sarsii* for photodynamic therapy applications in breast cancer and glioblastoma models. *Biomedicines* **2022**, *10*, 134. [CrossRef]
12. Pevna, V.; Wagnières, G.; Huntosova, V. Autophagy and apoptosis induced in U87 MG glioblastoma cells by hypericin-mediated photodynamic therapy can be photobiomodulated with 808 nm light. *Biomedicines* **2021**, *9*, 1703. [CrossRef] [PubMed]
13. Vasilev, A.; Sofi, R.; Smith, S.J.; Rahman, R.; Teschemacher, A.G.; Kasparov, S. Feasibility of photodynamic therapy for glioblastoma with the Mitochondria-Targeted Photosensitizer Tetramethylrhodamine Methyl Ester (TMRM). *Biomedicines* **2021**, *9*, 1453. [CrossRef] [PubMed]
14. Chiang, P.-C.; Li, P.-T.; Lee, M.-J.; Chen, C.-T. DNA hypermethylation involves in the down-regulation of Chloride Intracellular Channel 4 (CLIC4) induced by photodynamic therapy. *Biomedicines* **2021**, *9*, 927. [CrossRef] [PubMed]

15. Magalhães, C.M.; González-Berdullas, P.; Duarte, D.; Correia, A.S.; Rodríguez-Borges, J.E.; Vale, N.; Esteves da Silva, J.C.G.; Pinto da Silva, L. Target-oriented synthesis of marine coelenterazine derivatives with anticancer activity by applying the heavy-atom effect. *Biomedicines* **2021**, *9*, 1199. [CrossRef] [PubMed]
16. Desgranges, S.; Juzenas, P.; Vasovic, V.; Gederaas, O.A.; Lindgren, M.; Warloe, T.; Peng, Q.; Contino-Pépin, C. Amphiphilic protoporphyrin IX derivatives as new photosensitizing agents for the improvement of photodynamic therapy. *Biomedicines* **2022**, *10*, 423. [CrossRef]
17. Mantareva, V.N.; Kussovski, V.; Orozova, P.; Dimitrova, L.; Kulu, I.; Angelov, I.; Durmus, M.; Najdenski, H. Photodynamic inactivation of antibiotic-resistant and sensitive *Aeromonas hydrophila* with Peripheral Pd(II)- vs. Zn(II)-Phthalocyanines. *Biomedicines* **2022**, *10*, 384. [CrossRef]
18. Ramachandran, P.; Khor, B.-K.; Lee, C.Y.; Doong, R.-A.; Oon, C.E.; Thanh, N.T.K.; Lee, H.L. N-doped graphene quantum dots/titanium dioxide nanocomposites: A study of ROS-forming mechanisms, cytotoxicity and photodynamic therapy. *Biomedicines* **2022**, *10*, 421. [CrossRef]
19. Fang, J.; Gao, S.; Islam, R.; Nema, H.; Yanagibashi, R.; Yoneda, N.; Watanabe, N.; Yasuda, Y.; Nuita, N.; Zhou, J.-R.; et al. Styrene maleic acid copolymer-based micellar formation of temoporfin (SMA@ mTHPC) behaves as a nanoprobe for tumor-targeted photodynamic therapy with a superior safety. *Biomedicines* **2021**, *9*, 1493. [CrossRef]
20. Polat, E.; Kang, K. Natural photosensitizers in antimicrobial photodynamic therapy. *Biomedicines* **2021**, *9*, 584. [CrossRef]
21. Alam, S.T.; Hwang, H.; Son, J.D.; Nguyen, U.T.T.; Park, J.S.; Kwon, H.C.; Kwon, J.; Kang, K. Natural photosensitizers from *Tripterygium wilfordii* and their antimicrobial photodynamic therapeutic effects in a *Caenorhabditis elegans* model. *J. Photochem. Photobiol. B* **2021**, *218*, 112184. [CrossRef]
22. Espeland, K.; Kleinauskas, A.; Juzenas, P.; Brech, A.; Darvekar, S.; Vasovic, V.; Warloe, T.; Christensen, E.; Jahnsen, J.; Peng, Q. Photodynamic effects with 5-aminolevulinic acid on cytokines and exosomes in human peripheral blood mononuclear cells. *Biomedicines* **2022**, *10*, 232. [CrossRef] [PubMed]

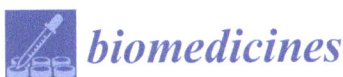

Review

Nanomedicine in Clinical Photodynamic Therapy for the Treatment of Brain Tumors

Hyung Shik Kim [1] and Dong Yun Lee [1,2,*]

1. Department of Bioengineering, College of Engineering, Hanyang University, Seoul 04763, Korea; kimhs5774@naver.com
2. Institute of Nano Science and Technology (INST), Hanyang University, Seoul 04763, Korea
* Correspondence: dongyunlee@hanyang.ac.kr; Tel.: +82-2-2220-2348

Abstract: The current treatment for malignant brain tumors includes surgical resection, radiotherapy, and chemotherapy. Nevertheless, the survival rate for patients with glioblastoma multiforme (GBM) with a high grade of malignancy is less than one year. From a clinical point of view, effective treatment of GBM is limited by several challenges. First, the anatomical complexity of the brain influences the extent of resection because a fine balance must be struck between maximal removal of malignant tissue and minimal surgical risk. Second, the central nervous system has a distinct microenvironment that is protected by the blood–brain barrier, restricting systemically delivered drugs from accessing the brain. Additionally, GBM is characterized by high intra-tumor and inter-tumor heterogeneity at cellular and histological levels. This peculiarity of GBM-constituent tissues induces different responses to therapeutic agents, leading to failure of targeted therapies. Unlike surgical resection and radiotherapy, photodynamic therapy (PDT) can treat micro-invasive areas while protecting sensitive brain regions. PDT involves photoactivation of photosensitizers (PSs) that are selectively incorporated into tumor cells. Photo-irradiation activates the PS by transfer of energy, resulting in production of reactive oxygen species to induce cell death. Clinical outcomes of PDT-treated GBM can be advanced in terms of nanomedicine. This review discusses clinical PDT applications of nanomedicine for the treatment of GBM.

Keywords: glioblastoma multiform (GBM); photodynamic therapy (PDT); photosensitizer (PS); reactive oxygen species (ROS); surgical resection; radiotherapy; chemotherapy; tumor microenvironment; blood–brain barrier (BBB); targeted therapy

1. Introduction

As photodynamic therapy (PDT) has been developed since the 1980s, many other treatment options have been improved. PDT has proven useful for many types of tumors, such as melanoma [1,2], esophageal cancer [3,4], and multidrug-resistant lung and breast cancers [5,6]. After other oncology applications, interest in PDT as a high-grade glioma treatment stems from both the nature of tumor growth and the limited effectiveness of modern therapies available to this patient population [7]. Although surgical resection, partial radiation, and chemotherapy are key treatments for intracranial brain tumors, the invasive growth patterns, particularly in the central region of the cerebrum, complicate total resection. Unlike surgical resection and radiation, PDT can treat micro-invasive areas while protecting sensitive brain areas. These advantages over conventional therapies have been reported to improve outcomes in patient populations with overall very poor survival and incidence of iatrogenic injury.

Clinical trials for brain tumors exist to date, but there are many questions about PDT and its usefulness as a standard adjuvant therapy. First, the effect of PDT alone reported in clinical trials were positive based on parallel administration of standard treatment. Variables that should be standardized across further studies include photosensitizer (PS)

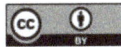

selection, injected dose, irradiation light wavelength, sensitivity of brain tumor types, and adjuvant use of chemotherapy and radiation. Furthermore, additional studies are needed to enhance the targeting of brain tumors while considering the pharmacokinetic aspects and methods of improving the quantum yield of the PS, which generates effective reactive oxygen species under light irradiation. In this regard, the rapidly developing fields of nanotechnology and nanomedicine are producing nanostructured materials that can overcome the shortcomings of delivery systems used in clinical practice. In fact, the functional presence of the blood–brain barrier (BBB) limits the delivery of drugs to the brain tumors. To overcome this limitation, many strategies for temporarily opening the BBB through physical impact such as magnetic resonance (MR)-guided focused ultrasound have been studied recently, but this raises a problem in compatibility [8]. Therefore, the use of multifunctional nanocarriers as drug delivery systems is emerging as one of the most promising strategies [9]. In general, intracellular transport of nanocarriers is mediated by the vesicular system, and three types of intracellular vesicles are involved (e.g., clathrin-mediated, caveolae-mediated and macropinocytotic vesicles) [10]. Therefore, in order to pass through these pathways, nanocarriers covalently bound with specific targeting ligands to guide the drug across the BBB to specific sites in each tumor type. The physicochemical and mechanical properties of nanocarriers differ depending on the material, size, shape (mesoporous structure, rod shape, particle), and the selected ligand. This allows customization for increased brain-targeted delivery of PS or therapeutic drugs. Although many PS nanocarriers are still in the early stages of translation, many advances have been made in recent years for functional nanomedicines based on BBB crossing.

Another advantage of nanoparticles is that they can increase the low solubility of PS, prolong blood circulation, promote targeted delivery and cellular uptake, while protecting the drug from degradation. This makes it an interesting alternative to traditional PDT because the nanostructures can enable efficient transport of PS and ameliorate the lack of anticancer activity [11]. To date, in addition to micellar self-assembly techniques for PS delivery, numerous nanoparticles, such as gold, silica, upconversion, and carbon-based particles, have been studied to increase their phototoxic properties and to increase their concentrations in tumor sites.

In this study, we classify brain tumors according to malignancy and examine the applicability of PDT for each type. We discuss the use of PDT and the properties and clinical applications of nanoparticles as potential delivery tools for PS delivery. In addition, the possibility of application to brain tumors is discussed through clinical cases of nanomedicine-based PDT.

2. Classification of Brain Tumor Grade

A brain tumor, a tumor that develops within the skull, is an abnormal mass of tissue in which cells grow and multiply out of control. Although more than 150 types of brain tumors have been reported, they are macroscopically divided into primary and metastatic groups [12]. Tumors that arise directly from the brain tissue or surrounding the brain are classified as primary brain tumors. More specifically, they are classified as either glial composed of glial cells or comparative cells that arise from brain structures containing blood vessels, nerves, and sweat glands [13]. Metastatic brain tumors, commonly considered malignant tumors, include tumors that develop elsewhere in the body, such as the lungs or breast, and travel through the bloodstream to the brain It is reported that there are more than 150,000 tumors that have metastasized to the brain each year, accounting for about 25% of cancer patients [14]. Typically, up to 40% of lung cancer patients develop metastatic brain tumors, and the survival rate of those diagnosed with this tumor is very fatal, typically taking only a few weeks from diagnosis to death. A grading system was developed by the World Health Organization (WHO) to indicate whether a tumor is malignant or benign based on histological features observed under the microscope, such as most malignant, widely invasive, rapidly growing and prone to aggressive necrosis, and rapid recurrence (Table 1) [15].

Table 1. WHO classification of brain tumor grades.

	Grade	Tumor Types	Characteristics
Low Grade	Grade I	• Craniopharyngioma • Chordomas • Ganglioglioma • Gangliocytoma • Pilocytic astrocytoma	• Possibly curable via surgery alone • Long-term survival • Least malignant (benign) • Non-infiltrative
	Grade II	• Pineocytoma • "Diffuse" astrocytoma • Pure oligodendroglioma	• Slight infiltrative • Relatively slow growing • Can recur as higher grade
High Grade	Grade III	• Anaplastic ependymoma • Anaplastic astrocytoma • Anaplastic oligodendroglioma	• Malignant • Infiltrative • Tend to recur as higher grade
	Grade IV	• Glioblastoma multiforme • Medulloblastoma • Ependymoblastoma • Pineoblastoma	• Most malignant • Rapidly growing and aggressive • Widely infiltrative • Recurrence • Tendency for necrosis

2.1. Types of Low Grade (Grade I and Grade II) Brain Tumors

2.1.1. Craniopharyngiomas

Craniopharyngiomas are a rare type of benign brain tumor and do not spread to other tissues, but they are difficult to remove because they are located deep in the brain and near critical structures such as the pituitary gland. They usually affect the function of the pituitary gland, which regulates many hormones in the body; thus, almost all patients are treated with hormone replacement therapy.

2.1.2. Chordomas

Chordomas are rare axial skeletal malignancies that most commonly occur in people between the ages of 50 and 60, accounting for less than 1% of intracranial tumors and 4% of bone tumors [16]. Because the most common locations are below the spine and at the base of the skull, they can invade adjacent bones and put lasting pressure on the surrounding nerve tissue [17]. Radiation therapy is the most practiced treatment, but radiation dose is limited because stability of important nerve structures such as the brainstem and nerves must be ensured. Therefore, highly focused radiation therapy such as carbon ion therapy and proton therapy are known as a more effective treatment method than conventional X-ray radiation [18].

2.1.3. Gangliogliomas and Gangliocytomas

Gangliogliomas, gangliocytomas, and anaplastic gliomas are rare tumors containing glial cells and relatively well-differentiated neoplastic nerve cells [19]. They usually develop in the two temporal lobes, one on each side of the brain around the ear. In this location, these tumors tend to cause epilepsy; thus, seizures can be the first sign of ganglioglioma [20]. Gangliogliomas are rare, occur primarily in young adults, and account for about 1 to 2% of all brain tumors.

2.1.4. Schwannomas

Schwannoma is a benign brain tumor that usually arises from cells involved in electrical insulation of nerve cells, and the diagnoses are high in adults between the ages of 20 and 50 years [21]. Schwannomas are also called neuromas, neurolemomas, or neurilemomas. A typical schwannoma is an auditory neuroma, which arises from the eighth cranial nerve or vestibular cochlear nerve, which lines the brain from the ear. Because schwannoma is found in the outer skin surrounding the nerve, radiation surgery is widely used as a treatment and surgery can be completed without nerve damage, except for vestibular schwannoma, which frequently causes hearing loss [22].

2.1.5. Pituitary Adenomas and Pineocytomas

Pituitary adenoma is the second most common intracranial tumor after glioma, meningioma, and schwannoma. Most pituitary adenomas are benign and grow slowly. Adenoma is the most common disease affecting the pituitary gland, and even malignant pituitary tumors rarely spread to other parts of the body [23]. Pineocytoma is a benign lesion that usually develops in the cells of the pineal gland and mainly occurs in adults [24]. They are mostly homogeneous, non-invasive, and slow growing. Most of these tumors can be successfully treated.

2.2. Types of High Grade (Grade III and Grade IV) Brain Tumors

Glioma is the most common type of adult brain tumor, accounting for 78% of malignant brain tumors [25]. They occur in supporting glial cells in the brain which are subdivided into astrocytes, oligodendrocytes, and ependymal cells. These glial tumors are discussed in the following sections [26].

2.2.1. Anaplastic Astrocytomas

Although astrocytoma can occur in many parts of the brain, it most commonly occurs in the cerebrum and is the most common type of glioma, accounting for more than half of all primary brain and spinal cord tumors [27,28]. Anaplastic astrocytoma is considered a more malignant evolutionary form of the previously lower-grade astrocytoma, with more aggressive features, including a faster growth rate and greater invasion into the brain. Histologically, it shows greater cellular abnormalities and evidence of cell proliferation (mitosis) compared to Grade II tumors. Surgical resection is not considered a complete cure for these tumors and will always need to be followed by radiation therapy and chemotherapy [29].

2.2.2. Anaplastic Oligodendrogliomas

Oligodendrogliomas are generally found in the white matter and the outer layer of the brain called the cortex but can arise anywhere in the central nervous system [30]. They are usually derived from cells that produce myelin, the insulator for nerves in the brain. Oligodendrocytes are classified into two grades, Grade II and Grade III, based on growth rate and invasiveness; the more malignant ones are called anaplastic oligodendrogliomas. The first line of treatment for anaplastic oligodendrogliomas is surgical resection, if possible. The goal of surgery is to excise tissue to determine the type of tumor and to remove as many tumors as possible without causing more symptoms in the patient [31]. Treatment after surgery can include radiation, chemotherapy, or clinical trials.

2.2.3. Glioblastoma Multiforme (GBM)

Glioblastoma multiforme (GBM) consists of several types of cells, such as astrocytes and oligodendrocytes, which are the most aggressive, malignant and common forms of neuronal supporting astrocytoma that develop within the brain. It is characterized by cells that appear histologically abnormal, proliferation, areas of dead tissue, and formation of new blood vessels [32]. GBM presents as a malignant progression in a previously present lower-grade astrocytoma in less than 10% of cases. In more than 90% of cases, it can begin as a Grade IV tumor. The standard approach to treatment in the newly diagnosed setting includes postoperative concomitant radiation therapy with temozolomide and additional adjuvant temozolomide. Unfortunately, there is no standard treatment for relapses. However, surgery, radiation therapy and chemotherapy or systemic therapy with bevacizumab are all options depending on patient circumstances [33].

3. Strategies to Improve Permeability of Nanocarrier through the Blood-Brain Barrier

One of the major limitations of treating brain tumors is the difficulty of delivering drugs to the brain. The brain is surrounded by the blood–brain barrier (BBB), a selective barrier formed by endothelial cells in the cerebral microvessels, which regulates nutrient and ion transport and protects the brain from neurotoxic molecules to maintain brain homeostasis [34]. Unfortunately, most drugs cannot cross the BBB via physiological pathways due to the extreme selectivity of the barrier, which constitutes the greatest obstacle to systemic treatment for most central nervous system (CNS) diseases. In the recent decade, many strategies have been studied, such as topical delivery, implantation of a sustained drug-release scaffold [35], nasal administration [36], ultrasound to temporarily open the BBB [37], and nanoparticle functionalization to enhance BBB penetration [38]. However, local drug delivery methods are considered highly invasive because they require procedural surgery. In addition, the intranasal route has a disadvantage in that the delivered dose varies greatly depending on the condition of the nasal mucosa. Therefore, despite the difficulties across the BBB, the most popular and well-studied delivery route remains the systemic route through the functionalization of nanoparticles.

Nanocarriers can traverse the BBB using a variety of physiological pathways, including receptor-mediated transcytosis (RMT) or adsorption-mediated transcytosis (AMT). To achieve this goal, many nanocarrier systems, such as inorganic, polymeric, or lipid-based nanoparticles, have been developed and shown to cross the BBB due to their tailored surface properties. Numerous studies have demonstrated that physically coating nanoparticles with surfactants and chemical functionalization with specific ligands is a successful strategy to enhance BBB traversing via the physiological pathways mentioned above [39,40]. The size and charge of nanoparticles are also aspects that can affect brain penetration, but if the surface functionalization is done properly, there is no significant difference in a wide size range (from 5 to 400 nm) [41]. Smaller nanoparticles can cross the BBB more easily and diffuse better through the brain, but larger nanoparticles can also cross the BBB in slightly smaller amounts when properly functionalized. On the other hand, larger particles can load a greater amount of drug but reach the brain at a lower concentration, and smaller nanoparticles cannot contain a large amount of drug but reach the brain at a higher concentration. Therefore, the key to increasing the amount of drug delivered to the brain is finding the optimal particle size and designing a nanoparticle system that fits the purpose.

4. Advantages and Clinical Application of PDT for the Treatment of Brain Tumors

4.1. PDT Mechanism and Advantages for Brain Tumor Treatment

PDT is a therapy in which treatment is implemented through photoactivation of PS present or selectively accumulated around tumor cells. Photoirradiation activates PS by energy transfer of PS with structural specificity that excites molecular oxygen to singlet or triplet states. In the singlet state, the first step through excitation, energy is converted to heat by internal conversion or emitted as fluorescence. In the triplet state of a stage capable of reacting with surrounding or tissue oxygen, energy induces cell death by generating reactive oxygen species (ROS) (Figure 1). The generated ROS reacts rapidly with macromolecules that make up cells, including unsaturated fatty acids, proteins, and cholesterol, and this reaction destroys the membranes of intracellular organelles, such as lysosomes, mitochondria, and endoplasmic reticulum, which are directly related to cell viability [42]. Therefore, PDT ultimately induces apoptosis and necrosis of tumor cells, as well as inhibits tumor cell growth by generating local ischemia due to occlusion of tumor microvessels that supply nutrients and oxygen to the tumor. Furthermore, damage-associated molecular patterns (DAMPs) and various cytokines secreted by tumor cell death activate the subsequent host immune response, providing an opportunity for combination with immunotherapy [43]. Therefore, cancer treatment through surgery, chemotherapy, radiation, immunotherapy, monoclonal antibody, and various combinations thereof are currently being applied, and the selection of each combination is determined by considering the type and stage of the disease and the patient's overall health.

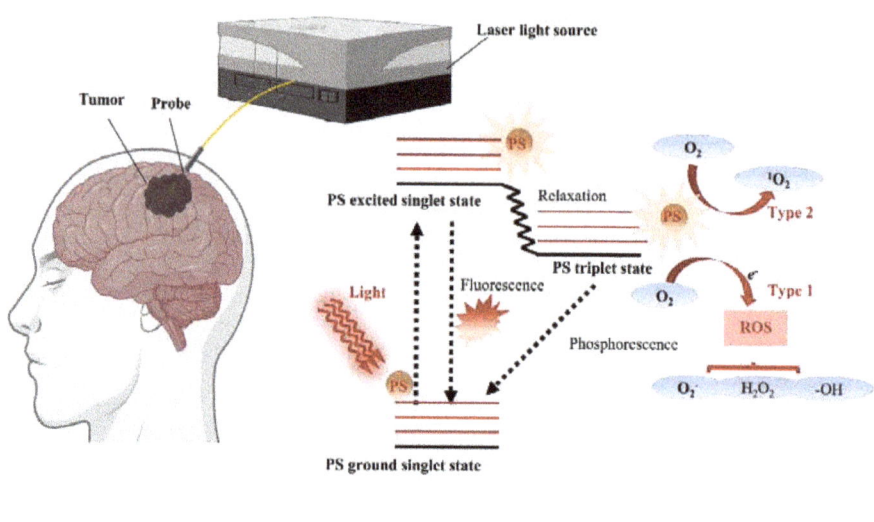

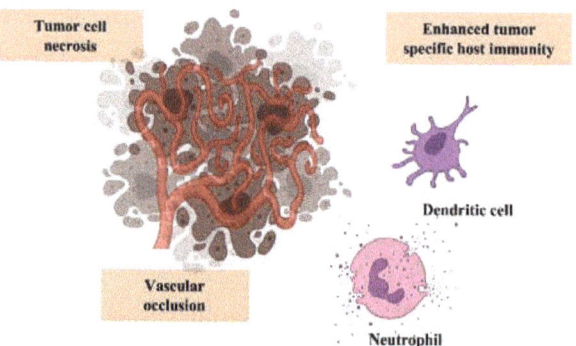

Figure 1. Schematic illustration of photodynamic therapy (PDT) for GBM treatment with energy diagram of the oxygen dependent response. If the photosensitizer (PS) in the ground singlet state is excited by the light wavelength, then the PS in the excited singlet state can convert to the excited triplet state via intersystem crossing. In the presence of molecular oxygen, the PS in the triplet state can undergo a Type 1 or Type 2 redox reaction, producing reactive oxygen species (ROS) that cause tumor cell necrosis, vascular occlusion, and tumor-specific host immunity.

A major problem with most existing cancer therapies, such as chemotherapy and radiation, is the combination of high toxicity to the patient's nonspecific cells and low specificity to cancer cells [44]. PDT is a promising alternative method for treating brain tumors, as PSs are used to target specific dysfunctional cells, and light is targeted to specific location to induce destruction of oncogenic cells [45]. Moreover, PS photodynamic activity results in release of cytotoxic ROS, such as single-molecule oxygen, based on photo-oxidation reactions that trigger many subsequent biochemical and molecular reactions [46]. Unlike surgical resection and radiotherapy, PDT can treat micro-invasive areas while protecting sensitive brain regions [47]. These advantages over current therapies can reduce the incidence of iatrogenic injury and improve outcomes in patient populations with poor survival and recurrence rates from GBM.

4.2. Clinical Trials of PDT for Brain Tumors

The therapeutic application of PDT for cancer began in the late 1970s with tests of the effects of light irradiation on hematoporphyrin derivatives (HPDs) in five patients with bladder cancer [48]. Since this initial work, more than 250 clinical trials of PDT have been conducted, with targets ranging from pre-malignant skin cancers [49–54] to peritoneal carcinomatosis [55,56], gastrointestinal cancers [57–64], lung cancers [65], and brain tumors [66,67]. Although many clinical trials of PDT for the treatment of malignant brain tumors have been conducted, most of them are phase I or II trials [66]. The heterogeneity of adjuvant therapies and tumor subtype therapies in the procedures used in clinical studies of the effects of PDT on brain tumors hampered the evaluation of the effectiveness of PDT.

In the 1990s, the PDT with PHOTOFRIN® (porfimer sodium) was evaluated at low or moderate light intensity, and in some cases, intraoperative adjuvant therapy was applied [68,69]. The above clinical trial was conducted on newly diagnosed GBM patients and recurrent GBM patients, and the results were significant. They had overall survival (OS) values of 6–9 months for newly diagnosed GBM [70] and 6–7 months for recurrent GBM [71]. Furthermore, in 2006, the researchers conducted a large phase III clinical trial (NCT00003788) with subjects with 150 newly diagnosed patients and 120 patients with recurrent glioma. At this time, the concentration of the photosensitizer was fixed at 2 mg/kg of PHOTOFRIN®, but the amount of light was varied with an average of 58 ± 17 J/cm^2. However, the results showed that the OS of newly diagnosed GBM was 7.6 months and the OS of recurrent GBM was 6.7 months, which was not improved compared to previous studies. Furthermore, a phase 1 clinical trial (NCT01682746) was initiated using step-by-step dose escalation of PHOTOFRIN® and fixed light intensity to determine the maximum safe dose for pediatric patients. Three patients with infratentorial tumors were enrolled and treated with PHOTOFRIN® at 0.5 mg/kg, and PDT did not adversely affect these patients.

In addition, PDT was applied in light dose escalation studies up to 230 J/cm^2 in phase I or II trials, resulting in OS values of 14.3 months for newly diagnosed GBM and 13.5 months for recurrent GBM [72,73]. The team conducting the clinical trial proceeded to a therapeutic condition in which light could penetrate deep enough into solid tumors to reach and kill migrating cancer cells without affecting normal cells. Therapeutic application was achieved by an i/o plane-cut laser fiber inserted into the lipid pool of the resection cavity, and the results were superior to those of other examinations at the time and comparable to the current standard of care. A phase II clinical adult trial (NCT01966809) was conducted using these conditions, but subsequent results were not reported because it aimed to reproduce the reported survival improvement and to define the antitumor activity of PHOTOFRIN®.

A total of 136 patients, including 78 patients with GBM and 58 patients with anaplastic astrocytoma who underwent tumor resection in 2005, was treated with an HPD at 5 mg/kg and then laser irradiated [73]. For newly diagnosed patients, 73% and 25% of patients with anaplastic astrocytoma and GBM survived at least 36 months, respectively, and 57% and 41% of patients with anaplastic astrocytoma and GBM, respectively, survived after repeated surgery.

Large phase III clinical trials aimed to study the efficacy and safety of 5-aminolevulinic acid (5-ALA) in combination with PDT in patients with high-grade glioma (HGG) [74,75]. 5-ALA and PHOTOFRIN® PDT, irradiated at a wavelength of 630 nm, using an implanted catheter, were performed on primary GBM patients on the day of fluorescence-guided surgery (FGS) after the patient recovered from surgery. Patients in the control group underwent traditional surgical resection, whereas patients who received PHOTOFRIN® PDT therapy received a total of 5 PDT sessions at daily intervals. Compared with conventional surgery, the mean tumor progression was delayed by 3.8 months in GBM patients treated with PDT after FGS, and the mean survival increased from 24.6 weeks to 52.8 months. 5-ALA has been reported to have fewer side effects when applied to HGG compared to PHOTOFRIN® PDT. PHOTOFRIN® has been reported to damage normal brain tissue due to vascular occlusion of the compound and concluded that it increases the risk of nerve damage and permanent defects at total applied light doses greater than 4000 J using diffuse tip fibers [76]. On the other hand, 5-ALA could be safely applied to patients in the high energy range of 4320 to 11,520 J. It was also noncytotoxic when applied systemically and did not appear to be significantly redistributed by edema volume flow around the tumor.

5. Nanotechnology for Enhanced Photodynamic Therapy

Nanotechnology generally involves development of materials with dimensions between 1 and 100 nm, a scale at which the properties of materials differ significantly from those of bulk materials and can be tailored to the desired application [77]. These new chemical and physical properties are usually derived from rapidly increasing surface-to-volume ratios and are associated with plasmonic and quantum effects. With rapidly advancing nanotechnology, nanomaterials are excellent therapeutic and diagnostic tools, and thousands of new compounds and nanostructures are developed each year for diverse applications [78]. This approach using nanotechnology could help overcome several obstacles that have prevented photodynamic therapy from attaining widespread clinical success. The nanostructures studied so far have been applied as a drug delivery platform for PDT and as a strategy to improve the efficiency of photosensitizers that generate ROS upon irradiation. Nanoparticles can be made up of a variety of components, organic and inorganic; can have a variety of shapes and sizes within the nanoscale scale and can act as photosensitizers or as energy converters [79]. Moreover, nanocarriers prevent aggregation caused by the low solubility of photosensitizers in aqueous media such as blood and bypass healthy tissues to increase tumor accumulation. In this section, we discuss cases where nanocarriers provide sufficient therapeutic efficacy and address issues such as undesirable biodistribution or rapid drug clearance from tumor areas.

5.1. Recent Advances in Preclinical Application of Nanocarriers for PDT

Although modern PDT has significantly improved the quality of life and increased overall survival of cancer patients, it is important to further improve the therapeutic effects of nanocarriers to minimize notable side effects such as hydrophobic PS and off-target side effects. In this regard, researchers have studied numerous nanocarriers such as polymers, liposomes, micelles, inorganic oxide, and novel metal nanoparticles to increase the therapeutic efficacy of photosensitizers (Table 2). First and foremost, it is important to utilize nanocarriers to efficiently deliver photosensitizers and generated singlet oxygen molecules to the target site in an optimal therapeutic range. The pharmacokinetic or pharmacodynamic characteristics of the nanocarriers should be confirmed for clinical use. Therefore, these are being studied for diagnostic as well as photodynamic/chemotherapeutic application using multifunctional nanoparticles.

5.2. Self-Assembled NP via Transformation into Amphiphilic PS-Derivatives

Second-generation PSs have a variety of functional groups including carboxyl, hydroxyl and amine groups in addition to their basic porphyrin structure, allowing hydrophobic modifications via chemical or physical approaches to form amphiphilic PS derivatives. The PS derivatives synthesized to be amphiphilic can form NPs with various nanostructures such as micelles [89,95–98], PS-drug conjugates [82,86,92,99,100], polymersomes [101], and nanogels [84,102] through self-assembly. According to the nanostructure, nanoparticles can be generally categorized into three types: 1) NPs with mixed hydrophilic and hydrophobic domains, 2) NPs with a core-shell structure, and 3) NPs with a double-layered capsule structure (Figure 2). In this respect, natural polysaccharides such as hyaluronic acid (HA) [102–105], chitosan [102,106–108], chitin, heparin [95,99,100], and fucoidan [84] have been utilized as potential photosensitizer carriers due to their biocompatibility and biodegradability. In addition, not only polymers but also hydrophobic small molecule anticancer drugs (such as doxorubicin [96], docetaxel [97,107,109,110], paclitaxel [85,93,103,111,112], camptothecin, and quercetin [113,114]) can be grafted onto PS.

Table 2. Recent advances in the preclinical development of nanopharmaceuticals to perform PDT.

Photosensitizer (PS)	Type of Nanomaterials	Tumor Type Treated	Results and Highlights	Year	Ref.
Chlorin e6 (Ce6)	Stem cell membrane-camouflaged bioinspired nanoparticles	Lung cancer	The enhanced antitumor effect of Ng/Ce6@SCV after NIR irradiation significantly inhibits primary tumor growth with fewer side effects.	2020	[80]
	Hyaluronic acid (HA)-based nanomaterials	Primary tumor and melanoma	Multifunctional nanosystem (HPR@CCP) exerted combined photodynamic and immunotherapeutic activity to amplify the therapeutic effect on primary tumors and distant metastases.	2020	[81]
	Peptide p 18-4/chlorin e6 (Ce6)-conjugated polyhedral oligomeric silsesquioxane (PPC) nanoparticles	Breast cancer cells	Cancer-targeting peptide p 18-4/chlorin e6 (Ce6)-conjugated polyhedral oligomeric silsesquioxane (PPC) nanoparticles improved the targeting ability of Ce6 to breast cancer cells to enhance PDT efficacy.	2020	[82]
	Ce6 loaded to the peroxidase-mimic metal-organic framework (MOF) MIL-100 (Ce6@MIL-100)	Breast cancer cell (4T1 cell line)	Peroxidase mimic metal-organic framework efficiently ablated tumors in microenvironment.	2020	[83]
	A fucoidan-based theranostic nanogel consisting of a fucoidan backbone, redox-responsive cleavable linker and Ce6	Human fibrosarcoma cell line (HT1080)	Fucoidan, the polymer backbone of the nanogel platform, enabled cancer targeting by P-selectin binding and enhanced the antitumor effect by inhibiting the binding of vascular endothelial growth factor.	2020	[84]
	Ligation of an anticancer cabazitaxel (CTX) drug via reactive oxygen species-activated thioketal linkage produces a dimeric TKdC prodrug, followed by co-assembly with a photosensitizer, Ce6	Human melanoma patient-derived xenograft (PDX)	Administration of psTKdC NAs followed by laser irradiation produced durable tumor regression, with tumors completely eradicated in three of six PDXs.	2020	[81]
	Light-enhanced PTX nanoparticles (Ce6/PTX2-Azo NPs) were prepared by synthesizing a hypoxia-activated self-sacrificing prodrug of paclitaxel (PTX2-Azo) and encapsulating it with a peptide copolymer decorated with the photosensitizer Ce6	The innately hypoxic microenvironment of most solid tumors	PTX2-Azo prevented premature drug leakage and realized specific release in a hypoxic tumor microenvironment, and the photosensitizer Ce6 efficiently generated singlet oxygen under light irradiation and acted as a positive amplifier to promote the release of PTX	2020	[85]
	Ce6-caspase 3 cleavable peptide (Asp-Glu-Val-Asp, DEVD)-anticancer drug monomethyl auristatin E (MMAE) conjugate, resulting in Ce6-DEVD-MMAE nanoparticles	Squamous cell carcinoma 7 (SCC7)	Light-induced therapeutic strategy based on apoptotic activation of Ce6-DEVD-MMAE nanoparticles can be used to treat solid tumors inaccessible to conventional PDT.	2019	[86]

Table 2. Cont.

Photosensitizer (PS)	Type of Nanomaterials	Tumor Type Treated	Results and Highlights	Year	Ref.
5-aminolevulinic acid (5-ALA)	Gold nanoparticles (GNP) conjugated to 5-ALA	Nonmelanoma skin cancer Subcutaneous squamous cell carcinoma (cSCC)	GNP conjugated to 5-ALA significantly enhanced the antitumor efficacy of PDT in HaCat and A431 cells	2020	[87]
	Gefitinib PLGA nanoparticles	Lung cancer	Synergistic therapeutic effects were identified by the combination of chemotherapy and photodynamic therapy	2020	[88]
Pheophorbide A (PhA)	Photoactivatable nanomicelles, which are constructed by self-assembly of poly (ethylene glycol) (PEG)-stearamine (C18) conjugate (PTS) with a ROS-sensitive thioketal linker (TL) and co-loaded with doxorubicin (DOX) and photosensitizer pheophorbide A (PhA)	Colon cancer cell line (CT-26)	The gradual elevation of local ROS levels generated by photoactivated PhA synergistically inhibited tumor growth and enhanced anti-tumor immunity by ROS-induced release of DOX.	2020	[89]
	Acid-responsive polygalactose-co-polycinnamaldehyde polyprodrug (PGGA) self-assembled with PhA	Hepatocarcinoma (HepG2)	Intravenous injection of PGCA@PA NPs strongly inhibited tumor growth of hepatocellular carcinoma with negligible side effects.	2020	[90]
	PEG-doxorubicin conjugate	Colon cancer (CT-26)	Synergistically maximized the efficacy of the combination of chemotherapy and photodynamic therapy.	2020	[91]
IR780	IR780 loaded on the prodrug micelle that consisted of camptothecin (CPT) andpolyethylene glycol (PEG) with further modification of iRGD peptide.	Glioma	The targeted prodrug system could effectively cross various barriers to reach the glioma site and greatly enhanced the antitumor effect with laser irradiation.	2020	[92]
	Poly-ε-caprolactone nanoparticles (PCL NPs) modified with LHRH peptide and loaded with IR780 and paclitaxel (PTX)	Ovarian cancer	LHRH peptide modified PCL (PCL-LHRH) NPs demonstrated increased internalization in ovarian tumor cells in vitro and selective targeting in tumor xenografts in vivo	2020	[93]
Indocyanine	Graphene oxide nanoparticle	Osteosarcoma	Nanoparticle consisting of polyethylene glycol (PEG), folic acid (FA), PS indocyanine green (ICG), and doxorubicin inhibited the proliferation and migration of osteosarcoma cells.	2020	[90]
	Self-assembled nanoparticle with indocyanine, camptothecin, RGD peptide	Human cervical carcinoma cell lines (HeLa); Human hepatoma (BEL-7402)	This facile and effective self-assembly strategy to construct nanodrugs demonstrated enhanced performance for cancer theranostics.	2018	[94]

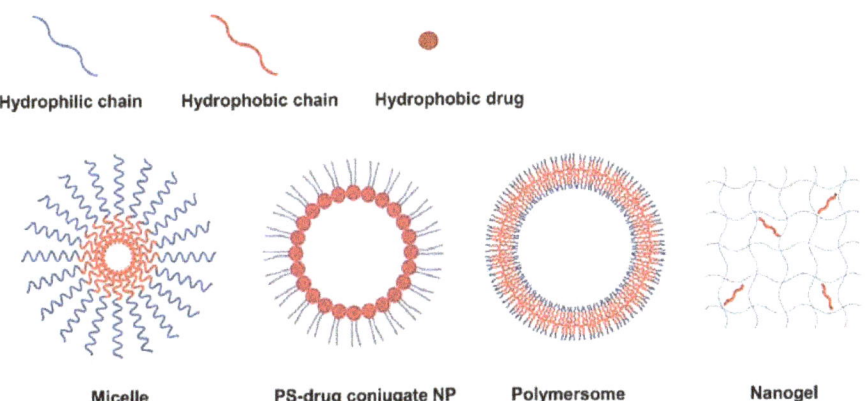

Figure 2. Representative types of NPs classified according to nanostructure.

5.2.1. Self-Assembly Methods for Amphiphilic PS Derivatives

Until recently, various approaches have been tried and developed to promote the self-assembly behavior of amphiphilic PS derivatives. In general, the dispersion method is a suitable method for an amphiphilic material having high water solubility to prepare nanoparticles with a core-shell structure [115]. The process can include mechanical agitation, mild heating or sonication. As an alternative to amphiphilic PS derivatives with low solubility in aqueous media, dialysis has been the most reported method [116,117]. On this basis, the PS derivative can be dissolved in an organic solvent such as dimethyl sulfoxide, dimethyl formamide, or methanol mixed with water and dialyzed against an aqueous solution to remove the solvent. Alternatively, the emulsion method, in which the drug is encapsulated in the oil phase of an oil-in-water emulsion, has received much attention because the drug-loading system has a high loading efficiency [118]. In general, controlled drug release was achieved with the development of dual emulsion technology via water-in-oil in water emulsions [119]. For instance, the structural design of nanocarriers using polyethylene glycolated poly(lactide-co-glycolide) (PEG-PLGA) were obtained as the most suitable approach in nanoemulsions, such as a water-in-oil-in-water evaporation process. In the hydrophilic part of the nanocarrier, cisplatin, a cell proliferation inhibitor, was placed and encapsulated by placing the hydrophobic porphyrin photosensitive dye verteporfin in the oil phase. As a result, PLGA nanocarriers were enabled to efficiently deliver hybrid cargo to cancer cells and PDT-supported enhanced apoptosis.

5.2.2. Carboxyl Group Modification of PS-Derivatives

The carboxyl modification of PS for linking to hyaluronic acid, chitosan, and heparin is mainly achieved through esterification or amidation. Esterification is used to join hydroxyl groups from PS to carboxyl groups in modifiers mediated by coupling agents or catalysts such as dicyclohexyl carbodiimide (DCC) and 4-dimethylaminopyridine (DMAP) (Figure 3a). Most carbodiimides are nonhydrophilic, limiting their application in hydrophilic systems of PS, with the exception of 1-(3-dimethylaminopropyl)-3-ethylcarbodiimide hydrochloride (EDC), which is extensively used in PS preparation. Another approach for modifying PS is to form an amide bond between the amine group of the hydrophobic material and the carboxyl group of the PS, where EDC and N-hydroxysuccinimide (NHS) are commonly used as condensing agents and catalysts, respectively (Figure 3a).

a) Carboxyl group modification of PS

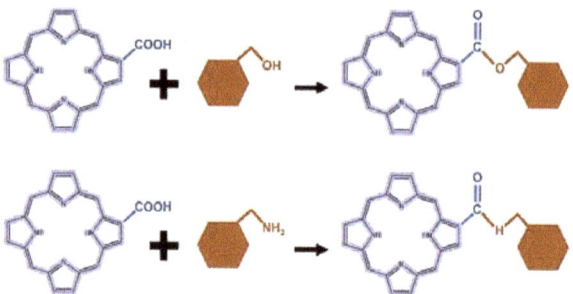

b) Hydroxyl group modification of PS

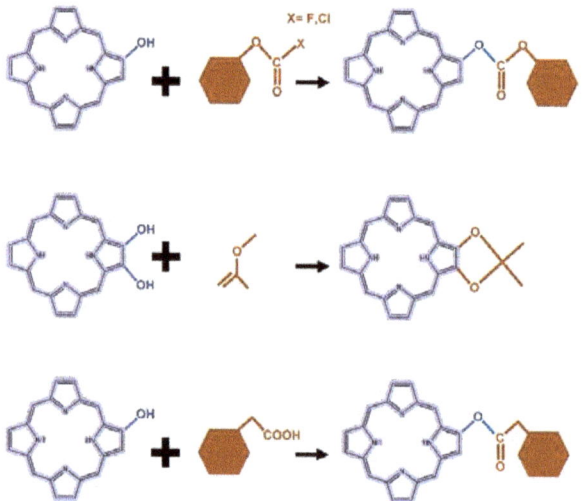

c) Amine group modification of PS

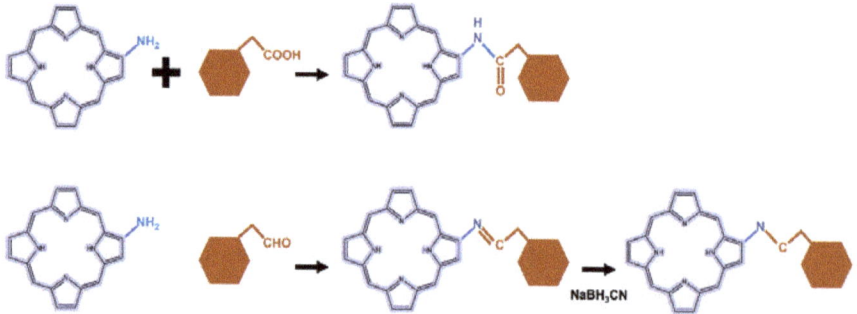

Figure 3. Representative reactions to modify the functional groups of PS-derivative based on (**a**) carboxyl, (**b**) hydroxyl, and (**c**) amine.

5.2.3. Hydroxyl Group Modification of PS-Derivatives

In the case of hydroxyl groups, there are several representative reactions such as etherification and esterification that occur in the presence of alkylating or acylating agents

(Figure 3b). As an example, light-controllable host–guest supramolecular amphiphilic complexes between azobenzene mediation porphyrin (TPP-Azo) were synthesized by esterification between TPPC6-COOH and AzoC6-OH [120]. Moreover, dextran alkyl carbonates were synthesized using various types of acylating agents such as butyl chloroformate, butyl fluoroformate, and ethyl chloroformate [121]. A cholesteryl hemisuccinate grafted hyaluronan synthesized through esterification of the carboxyl and hydroxyl groups of hemisuccinate-modified cholesteryl in the presence of DCC/DMAP has also been reported [81].

5.2.4. Amine Group Modification of PS-Derivatives

Heparin [122] and carboxymethyl chitosan [123] of the adipic acid dihydrazide(ADH)-modified polysaccharide type were rendered hydrophobic directly by conjugation of the amino group with the carboxylate moiety of PS via an amino bond in the presence of a catalyst such as EDC/NHS. Another typical strategy is a condensation reaction where the amine group of PS reacts with a carbonyl compound to form an imine intermediate and then is reduced under NaBH$_3$CN (Figure 3c). For these synthetic methods, the most important consideration is the determination of suitable solvents for both hydrophilic PS and hydrophobic molecules.

Chitosan has functional groups such as hydroxyl and amine; therefore, it can be easily modified and crosslinked with other polymers. Of particular benefit in terms of drug delivery, the amino groups of chitosan can be protonated in acidic environments, leading to pH-responsive behavior favored by acidic intracellular organelles such as endosomes and lysosomes. Therefore, chitosan-based nanoparticles have aroused great interest in the field of bio-nanomedicine, especially drug delivery. A dual reactive nanosystem comprised of indocyanine green (ICG) loaded mesoporous silica nanoparticles covered with ZnO quantum dots and coated with erlotinib-modified chitosan for synergistic photodynamic/molecular targeted therapy has been reported. The nanosystem showed a fairly distinct distribution in various nonsmall cell lung cancer models, with favorable anticancer results [124]. Moreover, biodegradable polymer nanoparticles based on chitosan that conjugate various amounts of the photosensitizer tetraphenylchlorin have been developed. These nanoparticles showed high drug loading efficiency and strong retention due to hydrophobic interactions such as π-π stacking between the aromatic photosensitizer group of the polymer and the drug. Nanoparticles have an excellent photodynamic therapeutic effect through photo-induced photochemical activation through high-dose drug delivery, and thus have a strong therapeutic effect on breast cancer cells [125].

5.2.5. Hyaluronic Acid-Modified NPs for PDT

HA is rich in functional groups including carboxyl, hydroxyl and N-acetyl groups, is ready to be transformed into a hydrophobic material, and has a negative charge that can provide a binding platform for hydrophobic macromolecules with a positive charge. Notably, its bioactivity binding to receptors upregulated in cancer cells, such as the cluster determinant 44 (CD44) receptor, the HA-mediated motility receptor (RHAMM), and the lymphatic endothelial (LYVE)-1, allows it to be used for targeted therapeutics. Therefore, HA can act as both a carrier and a target receptor, and HA-based NPs have been extensively studied in the field of drug delivery. HA-related nanosystems (AuNCs-HA) for decorating gold nanocages were developed and exhibited significant photocatalytic properties for PDT, large surface areas, and photothermal therapy (PTT) or PDT properties under near-infrared (NIR) stimulation. In vivo assays showed complete inhibition through the combination of PDT and PTT in AuNCs-HA-treated tumor cells than when each therapy was treated individually [126]. In another study, 5-ALA, Cy7.5 and anti-HER2 antibodies were conjugated to HA and mounted on a gold nanorod (GNR) surface to yield multifunctional GNR-HAALA/Cy7.5-HER2 nanoplatform. As a result, the tumor targeting by HER2 was improved, and side effects were minimized, and the combination of PDT and PTT mediated by 5-ALA and Cy7.5 effectively caused tumor regression [127].

5.3. Application of Inorganic Nanomaterials in PDT

5.3.1. Silica Nanoparticles

Although silica lacks PDT activity on its own, silica nanoparticles can be used to encapsulate PS in PDT due to the chemically inert, nontoxic, and optically transparent nature of silica [128]. In addition, it is commonly used for drug delivery in research because it is possible to functionalize chemicals to the silica through the hydroxyl groups on the silica surface (Figure 4) [129,130]. Mesoporous silica nanoparticles (MSNs) have been extensively utilized to deliver PSs, typically due to their interesting features such as large surface area and pore volume as well as high chemical stability [131–133]. One group has developed mesoporous silica-based nanoparticles to exploit continuous oxygen evolution to enhance the effectiveness of PDT treatment in hypoxic cancer environments [132]. To assemble Fe_3O_4 nanocrystals on silica nanoparticles doped with mesoporous dye, the surface was treated with 3-aminopropyltriethoxysilane and functionalized with amine groups. The oleic acid-stabilized Fe_3O_4 nanocrystals synthesized in an organic medium were reacted with the amine group of 2-bromo-2-methylpropionic acid, and the resulting Fe_3O_4 nanocrystals were assembled on the MSN surface by direct nucleophilic substitution between terminal bromine groups. The synthesized biocompatible manganese ferrite nanoparticle-immobilized mesoporous silica nanoparticles alleviated the hypoxic state of tumors with only a small number of nanoparticles and improved the treatment outcome of PDT in vivo.

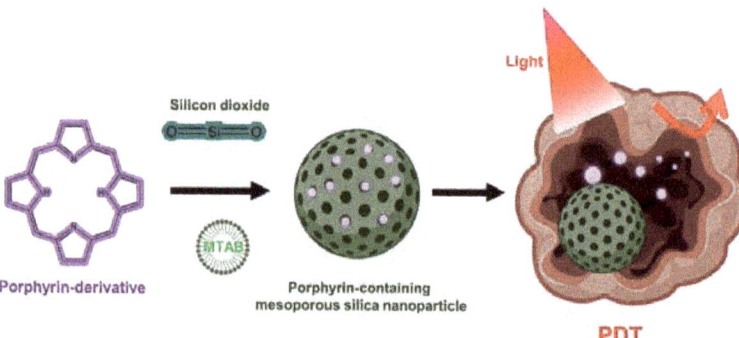

Figure 4. Porphyrin-containing mesoporous silica nanoparticles for PDT.

NIR light-reactive multifunctional nanoparticles are ferrocene-modified with ICG rods and β-cyclodextrin (β-CD) capping for cooperative chemo-dynamic/photothermal/photodynamic (CDT/PTT/PDT) NPs made of mesoporous silica [131]. As a mechanism of chemo-dynamic therapy, ferrocene released from multifunctional nanoparticles was able to efficiently kill cancer cells by converting intracellular H_2O_2 into toxic OH through a ferrocene-mediated Fenton reaction. Moreover, $^1O_2$ generated by ICG from near-infrared irradiation can kill cancer cells in cooperation with PDT. The results of in vitro experiments show that the CDT/PTT/PDT collaboration significantly amplified the inhibition rate of HeLa cells.

It was reported in one study that silica nanoparticles modified with folic acid (FA) could enhance the site-specific delivery of PS chlorin e6 (Ce6) [134]. By improving the efficiency of targeted drug delivery by FA, efficient generation of singlet oxygen at 670 nm irradiation was obtained, which improved the killing efficacy of NPs on MDA-MB-231 cells compared to free Ce6. Furthermore, a perfluoro hexane (PFH)-encapsulated MSN-based multifunctional nanoplatform using the PS ICG loaded into a polydopamine (PDA) layer and PEG-FA decoration was presented [135]. When excited with 808 nm light irradiation, it mediates the vaporization of PFH, creating bubbles for tumor ultrasound imaging and simultaneously inducing burst drug release. The PTT effect was exerted on the PDA layer, and the loaded ICG was able to generate ROS, a PDT mechanism, while providing NIR fluorescence emission.

5.3.2. Gold Nanoparticles

Gold nanoparticles have been studied for many years for effective PDT induction as well as drug carriers due to promising properties such as high surface area, facile surface modification through gold thiol chemistry, and biocompatibility. Furthermore, gold nanoparticles are being extensively studied for diagnostic applications because of their ability to tune optical scattering and absorption via physical features such as surface plasmon resonance effects [136]. Gold nanoparticles can be applied to PDT without the use of an organic PS. The first use of gold nanorods (AuNRs) alone was reported in 2014 [137]. Upon excitation with relatively long-wavelength NIR light (915 nm), gold nanorods were able to generate a singlet oxygen ($^1O_2$) and destroy B16F0 melanoma tumors in mice. Excitation of gold nanorods at a wavelength of 780 nm (λ2), at which the PTT effect can be expected after generation of $^1O_2$, increases the temperature around the tumor tissue, as confirmed by formation of heat shock protein (HSP 70) in which photon energy is converted into heat. By changing the activation wavelength band, the dominant phototherapeutic effect can be switched between PDT and PTT and a synergistic effect can be obtained. It was also possible to trace the distribution of gold nanorods in vivo through self-emitting single-photon-induced fluorescence.

The same group tested the effect of PDT by comparing different types of gold nanoshells, including nanorod-in-shell, nanocage and nanoparticle-in-shell, and demonstrated that it could completely eliminate solid tumors in mice [138]. They can modulate and switch the dominant roles of PDT and PTT by altering the activation wavelength that can excite the gold nanocage. As the most optimal conditions suggested by them, the nanocages mostly showed PDT effect when excited by 980 nm light, whereas 808 nm irradiation induced effective PTT. In vivo studies at 940 nm excitation, a wavelength band between 980 nm and 808 nm, demonstrate that gold nanoshells could induce dual-mode PDT/PTT for more efficient treatment of B16F0 melanoma tumors than that of doxorubicin, a clinically used drug.

Another group found that singlet oxygen could be produced when irradiated with a wide range of wavelengths (660–975 nm) [139]. Even under low-intensity light irradiation of 200 mW/cm^2, the highest production of $^1O_2$ was observed when a wavelength overlapped with the localized surface plasmon resonance (LSPR) peak, which is a characteristic of gold nanoparticles.

Many previous studies have demonstrated the ability of metal nanoparticles to efficiently excite PS through a single-photon excitation mechanism to generate singlet oxygen, which has been applied to typical PDT therapy [140,141]. However, one-photon excitation can cause potential photodamage to tissues adjacent to the tumor site due to the high energy provided by the comparatively short light wavelength. Therefore, two-photon excitation that precisely manipulates the therapeutic dose is preferable in this sense. To overcome this, a two-photon PDT was developed using a femtosecond laser beam capable of obtaining a high luminous flux. In one study, two-photon-induced singlet oxygen generation was observed by irradiating femtosecond laser pulses at 800 nm to aggregates of gold nanospheres and gold nanorods developed using non-agglomerated or aggregated gold nanoparticles [142]. As a result, the $^1O_2$ generation capacity in gold nanoparticle was generally enhanced by the agglomerated state and was 8.3 times higher than that of the non-agglomerated gold nanoparticles. A similar trend was observed when the agglomerated gold nanorods were used; the singlet oxygen production efficiency was improved by 1.8 times compared to the non-agglomerated gold nanorods.

With the rapid advances in nanotechnology, there are a variety of synthetic methods available to researchers to obtain gold nanoparticles with suitable structures and features for PDT applications [143]. In addition to the various physicochemical properties, the additional chemical modification potential mentioned above could improve bioavailability and usability, suggesting gold nanoparticles as a promising candidate for clinical cancer treatment.

5.3.3. Graphene Nanomaterials

Graphene-based nanomaterials, including graphene oxide (GO) and graphene quantum dots (GQD), have been widely used for cancer treatment such as anticancer drug delivery and PDT [144–146]. GO produced through oxidation process shows more favorable properties in terms of PS transport mediation due to improved water solubility and various functionalization chemistries. Characterized by abundant oxygen-containing moieties on their surface, GO nanomaterials allow further modification by many functional molecules such as targeting agents, activators and hydrophilic macromolecules, expanding biological applications and reducing toxicity [147]. Because the fluorescence quenching ability of GO nanomaterials is very high, it modulates the activity that generates ROS, further expanding the applications of PDT (Figure 5).

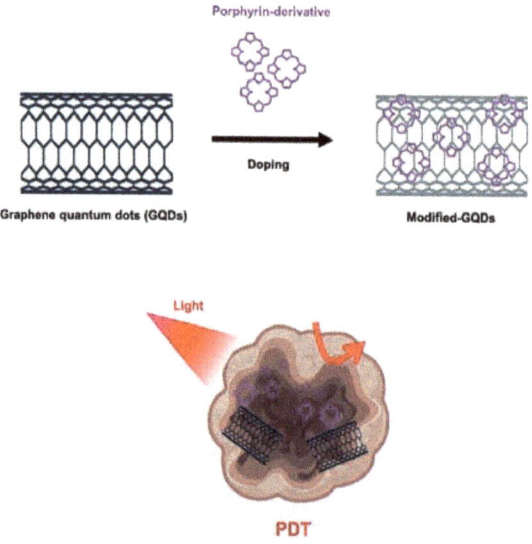

Figure 5. Graphene quantum dots (GQDs)-based nanomaterials for PDT.

Numerous studies have been conducted to achieve tumor targeting, in vivo imaging, and improved PDT effects through functionalization on the GO surface. In one study, PEG-functionalized GO was loaded with the PS 2-(1-hexyloxyethyl)-2-devinyl pyropheophorbide-alpha (HPPH) via supramolecular π-π stacking [148]. HPPH radiolabeled with ^{64}Cu enabled in vivo positron emission tomography and fluorescence imaging, resulting in improved cellular uptake of HPPH compared to free HPPH with GO-PEG-HPPH through a more aggressive endocytosis strategy. As a result, GO-PEG-HPPH exhibited enhanced phototoxicity to breast cancer cells when irradiated with light at a wavelength of 671 nm. Through in vivo experiments, mice injected with GO-PEG-HPPH showed a 16-day longer lifespan than mice treated with free HPPH. This indicates that GO-PEG-HPPH utilizing GO as a nanocarrier delivered the drug more efficiently and thereby increased long-term survival. In another study, the PS hypocrelin A (HA) and TiO_2 nanoparticles were mounted on GO surfaces to form a light-sensitive drug delivery system [149]. By loading TiO_2 onto GO, ROS could be generated upon exposure to visible light, and the ability to generate ROS was improved through a mutual sensitization mechanism in which a sensitizing effect contributed by the HA-TiO_2 stable complex. The generated ROS were able to destroy GO, indicating a potential use of this drug delivery system in clinical PDT in terms of metabolism.

In another study, PS Ce6 was conjugated to GO via a redox-responsive cleavable disulfide linker (GO-SS-Ce6) to develop a form that could be released on-demand from cancer cells at significantly higher GSH concentrations compared to normal cells. Therefore, fluorescence and ROS generation were selectively activated by redox agents such as glutathione at high concentrations in tumor cells [150]. On the other hand, in the absence of glutathione, the fluorescence of Ce6 bound to GO was largely quenched due to the FRET process, avoiding the nonspecific excitation and poor targeting ability of PS. The developed GO-SS-Ce6 complex has been proposed as an effective drug delivery vehicle with the strengths of GO's high surface area and improved chemical tethering properties.

Furthermore, GQDs doped with quantum dots in graphene could provide excellent quantum yield of singlet oxygen as a PDT agent [151]. It is known as a common method to synthesize GQDs using polythiophene as a carbon precursor using hydrothermal methods. The GQDs fabricated in the study were excited by visible light and showed photodynamic activity; their PDT effects were observed through apoptosis of HeLa cells and oncolysis of BALB/nude mice with breast cancer. On the other hand, more advanced studies showed that GQDs could be functionalized and doped with nitrogen and amino groups to show that the amino-N-GQDs exhibited excellent singlet oxygen generation capacity in the NIR region (800 nm) [152].

5.3.4. Upconversion Nanoparticles

Upconversion nanoparticles (UCNPs) are a unique class of optical nanomaterials characterized by their ability to convert low-energy NIR light into high-energy visible/ultraviolet light using a nonlinear anti-Stokes mechanism [153]. The upconversion phenomenon is based on inorganic host crystal lattices doped with trivalent lanthanide ions such as Yb^{3+}, Er^{3+}, and Tm^{3+}. UCNPs require the presence of two different dopant ions [154]. One acts as a sensitizer to absorb NIR radiation, and the other acts as an activator to emit visible light. Two frequently used rare earth ion pairs are ytterbium-thulium (Yb^{3+}-Tm^{3+}) and ytterbium-erbium (Yb^{3+}-Er^{3+}). The Yb^{3+} ions act as antennas, absorbing NIR light at about 900–1100 nm and transmitting it to the lanthanide ions, where they mutually upconvert. If this ion is Er^{3+}, green and red emission is observed, whereas if it is Tm^{3+}, the emitted light is near-ultraviolet, blue and red. In addition, the emission band of UCNP is similar to the band in which PS can be excited, which is characterized by improved ROS production efficiency [128]. In this regard, UCNP may serve as a promising carrier to overcome the limitations of PDT due to the insufficient tissue penetrating ability of short wavelengths (600–850 nm) (Figure 6).

The $NaYF_4$: Yb^{3+}/ Er^{3+}, the first UCNPs used in PDT studies, showed strong emission spectrum in the visible region around 537 and 635 nm when excited by an infrared light source of 974 nm [155]. During the silica coating procedure in the UNCP synthesis, the PS molecule merocyanine 540 (MC-540) was mounted on the nanoparticle. However, the activation wavelength of these PSs is under 700 nm, which is a range in which endogenous molecules such as hemoglobin have strong absorption, a great limitation in their use in PDT. A study successfully detected the generation of singlet oxygen mediated by UCNPs coated with MC-540 with NIR excitation by measuring the decrease in the fluorescence band of the $^1O_2$ sensor 9,10-anthracenedipropionic acid. Moreover, the first application of UCNP-mediated PDT for in vivo tumor therapy is $NaYF_4$:Yb/Er nanoparticles coated with mesoporous silica as nano-transducers and carriers of two different PSs such as MC-540 and ZnPc [156]. Another study found that UCNPs synthesized using dual PS had higher PDT efficacy than using single PS, with improved ROS production capacity and enhanced cytotoxicity. In the tumor-bearing mice, both intratumoral injection of UCNP or intravenous injection of FA and PEG-modified UCNPs (FA-PEG-UCNP) into tumor resulted in tumor growth inhibition at 980 nm excitation. In addition, the tumor-targeting ability and circulating lifespan of UCNP were improved by FA and PEG, respectively, indicating a greater PDT effect when administered intravenously.

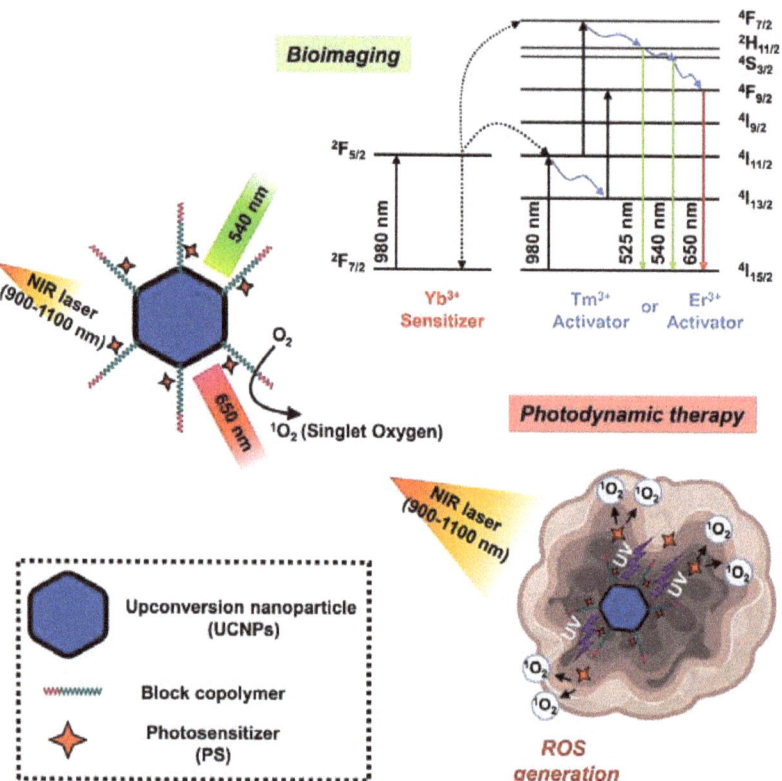

Figure 6. Schematic diagram showing the mechanism of photodynamic therapy and bioimaging through long-wavelength to short-wavelength conversion of upconversion nanoparticles (UCNPs).

One research team prepared NaYF$_4$:Er/Yb/Gd upconversion nanocrystals by doping NaYF$_4$:Yb/Er UCNP with gadolinium ions and loading them with PS drugs to use as a carrier [157]. Through a water-in-oil inverse microemulsion strategy, methylene blue (MB), a hydrophilic PS drug, was efficiently conjugated to UCNPs in a silica matrix to provide UCNP/MB nanocomposites with a particle size less than 50 nm. The obtained UCNP/MB-based PDT drug successfully generated singlet oxygen at 980 nm excitation, whereas no signal was observed with free MB solution alone or with NaYF$_4$:Er/Yb/Gd under the same conditions. Furthermore, polymer-coated NaYF$_4$:Yb/Er nanoparticles were used as transport mediators of PS Ce6 to form UCNP-Ce6 supramolecular complexes [158]. Because this UCNP-Ce6 nanosystem showed two emission bands at 550 nm and 660 nm with 980 nm irradiation, PDT performance was improved in that the 660 nm emission wavelength overlapped the absorption band of Ce6, and singlet oxygen production was increased under NIR light irradiation. In particular, there were few observations of UCNPs administered to mice after 1–2 months, demonstrating their nontoxicity to the treated animals.

Although it is common to form NaYF$_4$ crystals with a host co-doped with Yb^{3+}/Er^{3+} in UCNP-based PDT, doping NaYF$_4$ with a Yb^{3+}/Tm^{3+} couple shows a similar phenomenon. In one study, NaYF$_4$:Yb/Tm UCNPs were coated with a nanometer silica layer, which was further modified with (3-aminopropyl)triethoxysilane APTES using the Stöber method [159]. After that, the UCNPs were covalently bound to PS Ce6 via the amino group of the silica layer. A low concentration (50 µg/mL) of this UCNP-Ce6 nanocomposite was used to kill 50% of CF-7 human breast adenocarcinoma cells at a low dose (7 mW/cm^2) of 980 nm light for 10 min. Furthermore, they achieved a cell viability greater than 90% under the same conditions without light irradiation, indicating low toxicity of this UCNP-Ce6 nanosystem in the effective concentration range. Alternatively, LiYF$_4$:Tm^{3+}/Yb^{3+}-UCNPs prepared using m-THPC with PS modified with 4-(bromomethyl)benzoic acid performed better when activated with 980 nm NIR irradiation compared to conventional NaYF$_4$UCNPs. They emitted an intense blue color and produced a larger amount of singlet oxygen [124,160,161].

More recently, research on multifunctional UCNP-based nanocomposites combining image-guided PDT and multimodal therapy has been attracting attention. UCNPs coated with the PS TiO$_2$ were adopted for in vivo PDT image induction that realized complete optical switching in the UV-blue region [162]. In this work, the newly developed photoswitchable upconversion nanoparticles (PUCNPs) were not doped with Nd^{3+}. The prominent UV-blue emission of Tm^{3+} characteristic of these PUCNPs was activated at 980 nm excitation and showed excellent photoswitching properties that could be completely deactivated with 800 nm light. As a result, the Tm^{3+} emission band of 350 nm at 980 nm excitation can be well synchronized with the absorption of TiO$_2$, which could lead to ROS generation and effective PDT, while also enabling real-time tumor imaging. In contrast, only the Er^{3+} emission band at 660 nm was activated when excited with 800 nm, which made it possible to monitor emission near 650 nm in vivo to track the treatment process.

In addition to the excellent optical properties and abundant surface functions of UCNP, the energy transfer ability of UCNP to deep tissues such as brain tumors efficiently forms ROS, providing a great development for clinical application in the field of brain tumor treatment. However, due to the low upconversion of UCNPs developed with the techniques to date, the quantum yield is less than 3%, and the relatively poor biocompatibility in the physiological environment hinders biological applications. Therefore, more studies on high-efficiency UCNPs considering stability in the future should be conducted.

6. Conclusions

The field of PDT has developed rapidly and is constantly being evaluated for new technology. Molecular strategies based on the nanotechnology are being developed to increase the effectiveness and selectivity of PDT. Therefore, numerous organic and inorganic nanoparticles have been newly researched and developed for targeted delivery of photosensitizer pharmaceuticals. This review presents examples of the improved overall effectiveness of PDT cancer treatment by demonstrating that NPs can provide a solution to the important limitations of traditional PS drug delivery. However, because intracranial brain tumors arise from structurally complex and unique organs, such as those surrounded by the blood–brain barrier, compared to other tumors, it is unknown whether they can be completely eradicated using the same approach. Further questions to be explored include whether PDT can be used to treat malignant brain tumors that cannot be resected because of their location. Ongoing study of the various PDTs presented in this manuscript will determine whether advances in cancer research will alleviate morbidity and mortality from treatment of intracranial malignancies and have the potential to revolutionize the treatment of brain tumors. Therefore, while the development of new PDT technology is important, establishment of treatment standards through large-scale clinical practice should be pursued.

Author Contributions: H.S.K. and D.Y.L. drafted and edited the manuscript. All authors have read and agreed to the published version of the manuscript.

Funding: This research was funded by the National Research Foundation of Korea (NRF) funded by the Ministry of Science, ICT & Future Planning, grant number NRF-2020R1A2C3005834.

Conflicts of Interest: The authors declare no conflict of interest.

References

1. Abramova, O.B.; Kaplan, M.A.; Grin, M.A.; Yuzhakov, V.V.; Suvorov, N.V.; Mironov, A.F.; Drozhzhina, V.V.; Churikova, T.P.; Kozlovtseva, E.A.; Bandurko, L.N.; et al. Photodynamic Therapy of Melanoma B16 with Chlorin E6 Conjugated with a PSMA-Ligand. *Bull. Exp. Biol. Med.* **2021**, *171*, 468–471. [CrossRef] [PubMed]
2. Gu, X.; Zhao, S.; Shen, M.; Su, J.; Chen, X. Laser-assisted photodynamic therapy vs. conventional photodynamic therapy in non-melanoma skin cancers: Systematic review and meta-analysis of randomized controlled trials. *Photodermatol. Photoimmunol. Photomed.* **2021**, *37*, 556–558. [CrossRef] [PubMed]
3. Inoue, T.; Ishihara, R. Photodynamic Therapy for Esophageal Cancer. *Clin. Endosc.* **2021**, *54*, 494–498. [CrossRef]
4. Yano, T.; Minamide, T.; Takashima, K.; Nakajo, K.; Kadota, T.; Yoda, Y. Clinical Practice of Photodynamic Therapy Using Talaporfin Sodium for Esophageal Cancer. *J. Clin. Med.* **2021**, *10*, 2785. [CrossRef] [PubMed]
5. Shi, C.; Huang, H.; Zhou, X.; Zhang, Z.; Ma, H.; Yao, Q.; Shao, K.; Sun, W.; Du, J.; Fan, J.; et al. Reversing Multidrug Resistance by Inducing Mitochondrial Dysfunction for Enhanced Chemo-Photodynamic Therapy in Tumor. *ACS Appl. Mater. Interfaces* **2021**, *13*, 45259–45268. [CrossRef]
6. Shi, X.; Yang, X.; Liu, M.; Wang, R.; Qiu, N.; Liu, Y.; Yang, H.; Ji, J.; Zhai, G. Chondroitin sulfate-based nanoparticles for enhanced chemo-photodynamic therapy overcoming multidrug resistance and lung metastasis of breast cancer. *Carbohydr. Polym.* **2021**, *254*, 117459. [CrossRef]
7. Akimoto, J. Photodynamic Therapy for Malignant Brain Tumors. *Neurol. Med. Chir. (Tokyo)* **2016**, *56*, 151–157. [CrossRef]
8. Novell, A.; Kamimura, H.A.S.; Cafarelli, A.; Gerstenmayer, M.; Flament, J.; Valette, J.; Agou, P.; Conti, A.; Selingue, E.; Badin, R.A.; et al. A new safety index based on intrapulse monitoring of ultra-harmonic cavitation during ultrasound-induced blood-brain barrier opening procedures. *Sci. Rep.* **2020**, *10*. [CrossRef]
9. Mulvihill, J.J.E.; Cunnane, E.M.; Ross, A.M.; Duskey, J.T.; Tosi, G.; Grabrucker, A.M. Drug delivery across the blood-brain barrier: Recent advances in the use of nanocarriers. *Nanomedicine* **2020**, *15*, 205–214. [CrossRef] [PubMed]
10. Villasenor, R.; Lampe, J.; Schwaninger, M.; Collin, L. Intracellular transport and regulation of transcytosis across the blood-brain barrier. *Cell. Mol. Life Sci.* **2019**, *76*, 1081–1092. [CrossRef]
11. Zhang, Y.; Wang, B.; Zhao, R.; Zhang, Q.; Kong, X. Multifunctional nanoparticles as photosensitizer delivery carriers for enhanced photodynamic cancer therapy. *Mater. Sci. Eng. C* **2020**, *115*, 111099. [CrossRef] [PubMed]
12. Biratu, E.S.; Schwenker, F.; Ayano, Y.M.; Debelee, T.G. A Survey of Brain Tumor Segmentation and Classification Algorithms. *J. Imaging* **2021**, *7*, 179. [CrossRef]
13. Khan, M.A.; Lali, I.U.; Rehman, A.; Ishaq, M.; Sharif, M.; Saba, T.; Zahoor, S.; Akram, T. Brain tumor detection and classification: A framework of marker-based watershed algorithm and multilevel priority features selection. *Microsc. Res. Tech.* **2019**, *82*, 909–922. [CrossRef]
14. Asano, K.; Hasegawa, S.; Matsuzaka, M.; Ohkuma, H. Brain tumor-related epilepsy and risk factors for metastatic brain tumors: Analysis of 601 consecutive cases providing real-world data. *J. Neurosurg.* **2021**, *1*, 1–12. [CrossRef] [PubMed]
15. van den Bent, M.J.; Weller, M.; Wen, P.Y.; Kros, J.M.; Aldape, K.; Chang, S. A clinical perspective on the 2016 WHO brain tumor classification and routine molecular diagnostics. *Neuro-Oncology* **2017**, *19*, 614–624. [CrossRef]
16. Tauziede-Espariat, A.; Burel-Vandenbos, F.; Pedeutour, F.; Gareton, A.; Saffroy, R.; Andreiuolo, F.; Blauwblomme, T.; Dangouloff-Ros, V.; Boddaert, N.; Lechapt, E.; et al. Intracranial chondromas: A histopathologic and molecular study of three cases. *Clin. Neuropathol.* **2020**, *39*, 171–178. [CrossRef]
17. Robles, L.A.; Mundis, G.M. Chondromas of the Lumbar Spine: A Systematic Review. *Glob. Spine. J.* **2021**, *11*, 232–239. [CrossRef]
18. DeLaney, T.F.; Liebsch, N.J.; Pedlow, F.X.; Adams, J.; Weyman, E.A.; Yeap, B.Y.; Depauw, N.; Nielsen, G.P.; Harmon, D.C.; Yoon, S.S.; et al. Long-term results of Phase II study of high dose photon/proton radiotherapy in the management of spine chordomas, chondrosarcomas, and other sarcomas. *J. Surg. Oncol.* **2014**, *110*, 115–122. [CrossRef] [PubMed]
19. Pekmezci, M.; Villanueva-Meyer, J.E.; Goode, B.; Van Ziffle, J.; Onodera, C.; Grenert, J.P.; Bastian, B.C.; Chamyan, G.; Maher, O.M.; Khatib, Z.; et al. The genetic landscape of ganglioglioma. *Acta Neuropathol. Commun.* **2018**, *6*, 47. [CrossRef]
20. Sauer, A.; Blavin, J.; Lhermitte, B.; Speeg-Schatz, C. Conjunctival ganglioglioma as a feature of basal cell nevus syndrome. *J. Am. Assoc. Pediatr. Ophthalmol. Strabismus* **2011**, *15*, 387–388. [CrossRef]
21. Erickson, N.J.; Schmalz, P.G.R.; Agee, B.S.; Fort, M.; Walters, B.C.; McGrew, B.M.; Fisher, W.S. Koos Classification of Vestibular Schwannomas: A Reliability Study. *Neurosurgery* **2019**, *85*, 409–414. [CrossRef]
22. Younes, E.; Montava, M.; Bachelard-Serra, M.; Jaloux, L.; Salburgo, F.; Lavieille, J.P. Intracanalicular Vestibular Schwannomas: Initial Clinical Manifestation, Imaging Classification, and Risk Stratification for Management Proposal. *Otol. Neurotol.* **2017**, *38*, 1345–1350. [CrossRef] [PubMed]
23. Dehdashti, A.R.; Chakraborty, S. Aggressive pituitary adenomas: Is pathology the only feature of aggressiveness? *Acta Neurochir.* **2018**, *160*, 57–58. [CrossRef] [PubMed]
24. Wilson, D.A.; Awad, A.W.; Brachman, D.; Coons, S.W.; McBride, H.; Youssef, E.; Nakaji, P.; Shetter, A.G.; Smith, K.A.; Spetzler, R.F.; et al. Long-term radiosurgical control of subtotally resected adult pineocytomas. *J. Neurosurg.* **2012**, *117*, 212–217. [CrossRef] [PubMed]
25. de Groot, J.F.; Lamborn, K.R.; Chang, S.M.; Gilbert, M.R.; Cloughesy, T.F.; Aldape, K.; Yao, J.; Jackson, E.F.; Lieberman, F.; Robins, H.I.; et al. Phase II study of aflibercept in recurrent malignant glioma: A North American Brain Tumor Consortium study. *J. Clin. Oncol.* **2011**, *29*, 2689–2695. [CrossRef]

26. Quesada, A.; Prada, F.A.; Aguilera, Y.; Espinar, A.; Carmona, A.; Prada, C. Peripapillary glial cells in the chick retina: A special glial cell type expressing astrocyte, radial glia, neuron, and oligodendrocyte markers throughout development. *Glia* **2004**, *46*, 346–355. [CrossRef]
27. She, D.; Liu, J.; Xing, Z.; Zhang, Y.; Cao, D.; Zhang, Z. MR Imaging Features of Anaplastic Pleomorphic Xanthoastrocytoma Mimicking High-Grade Astrocytoma. *AJNR Am. J. Neuroradiol.* **2018**, *39*, 1446–1452. [CrossRef]
28. Jungk, C.; Reinhardt, A.; Warta, R.; Capper, D.; Deimling, A.V.; Herold-Mende, C.; Unterberg, A. Extent of Resection, MGMT Promoter Methylation Status and Tumor Location Independently Predict Progression-Free Survival in Adult Sporadic Pilocytic Astrocytoma. *Cancers* **2019**, *11*, 1072. [CrossRef]
29. Tjahjadi, M.; Arifin, M.Z.; Sobana, M.; Avianti, A.; Caropeboka, M.S.; Eka, P.A.; Agustina, H. Cystic pilomyxoid astrocytoma on suprasellar region in 7-year-old girl: Treatment and strategy. *Asian J. Neurosurg.* **2015**, *10*, 154–157. [CrossRef]
30. Figarella-Branger, D.; Mokhtari, K.; Dehais, C.; Jouvet, A.; Uro-Coste, E.; Colin, C.; Carpentier, C.; Forest, F.; Maurage, C.A.; Vignaud, J.M.; et al. Mitotic index, microvascular proliferation, and necrosis define 3 groups of 1p/19q codeleted anaplastic oligodendrogliomas associated with different genomic alterations. *Neuro-Oncology* **2014**, *16*, 1244–1254. [CrossRef]
31. Achey, R.L.; Khanna, V.; Ostrom, Q.T.; Kruchko, C.; Barnholtz-Sloan, J.S. Incidence and survival trends in oligodendrogliomas and anaplastic oligodendrogliomas in the United States from 2000 to 2013: A CBTRUS Report. *J. Neurooncol.* **2017**, *133*, 17–25. [CrossRef]
32. Ye, Z.; Price, R.L.; Liu, X.; Lin, J.; Yang, Q.; Sun, P.; Wu, A.T.; Wang, L.; Han, R.H.; Song, C.; et al. Diffusion Histology Imaging Combining Diffusion Basis Spectrum Imaging (DBSI) and Machine Learning Improves Detection and Classification of Glioblastoma Pathology. *Clin. Cancer Res.* **2020**, *26*, 5388–5399. [CrossRef]
33. Tan, A.C.; Ashley, D.M.; Lopez, G.Y.; Malinzak, M.; Friedman, H.S.; Khasraw, M. Management of glioblastoma: State of the art and future directions. *CA. Cancer J. Clin.* **2020**, *70*, 299–312. [CrossRef]
34. Achar, A.; Myers, R.; Ghosh, C. Drug Delivery Challenges in Brain Disorders across the Blood-Brain Barrier: Novel Methods and Future Considerations for Improved Therapy. *Biomedicines* **2021**, *9*, 1834. [CrossRef]
35. Chaichana, K.L.; Pinheiro, L.; Brem, H. Delivery of local therapeutics to the brain: Working toward advancing treatment for malignant gliomas. *Ther. Deliv.* **2015**, *6*, 353–369. [CrossRef] [PubMed]
36. Lochhead, J.J.; Thorne, R.G. Intranasal delivery of biologics to the central nervous system. *Adv. Drug Deliv. Rev.* **2012**, *64*, 614–628. [CrossRef]
37. Abbasi, J. Guided Ultrasound Opens Blood-Brain Barrier to Cancer Drugs. *JAMA* **2021**, *326*, 1785. [CrossRef]
38. Lombardo, S.M.; Schneider, M.; Tureli, A.E.; Gunday Tureli, N. Key for crossing the BBB with nanoparticles: The rational design. *Beilstein J. Nanotechnol.* **2020**, *11*, 866–883. [CrossRef] [PubMed]
39. Khongkow, M.; Yata, T.; Boonrungsiman, S.; Ruktanonchai, U.R.; Graham, D.; Namdeel, K. Surface modification of gold nanoparticles with neuron-targeted exosome for enhanced blood-brain barrier penetration. *Sci. Rep.* **2019**, *9*, 8278. [CrossRef] [PubMed]
40. Del Amo, L.; Cano, A.; Ettcheto, M.; Souto, E.B.; Espina, M.; Camins, A.; Garcia, M.L.; Sanchez-Lopez, E. Surface Functionalization of PLGA Nanoparticles to Increase Transport across the BBB for Alzheimer's Disease. *Appl. Sci.* **2021**, *11*, 4305. [CrossRef]
41. Jo, D.H.; Kim, J.H.; Lee, T.G.; Kim, J.H. Size, surface charge, and shape determine therapeutic effects of nanoparticles on brain and retinal diseases. *Nanomedicine* **2015**, *11*, 1603–1611. [CrossRef] [PubMed]
42. Hirschberg, H.; Berg, K.; Peng, Q. Photodynamic therapy mediated immune therapy of brain tumors. *Neuroimmunol. Neuroinflamm.* **2018**, *5*, 27. [CrossRef] [PubMed]
43. Kaneko, S.; Fujimoto, S.; Yamaguchi, H.; Yamauchi, T.; Yoshimoto, T.; Tokuda, K. Photodynamic Therapy of Malignant Gliomas. *Prog. Neurol. Surg.* **2018**, *32*, 1–13. [CrossRef]
44. Hotchkiss, K.M.; Sampson, J.H. Temozolomide treatment outcomes and immunotherapy efficacy in brain tumor. *J. Neurooncol.* **2021**, *151*, 55–62. [CrossRef]
45. Borah, B.M.; Cacaccio, J.; Durrani, F.A.; Bshara, W.; Turowski, S.G.; Spernyak, J.A.; Pandey, R.K. Sonodynamic therapy in combination with photodynamic therapy shows enhanced long-term cure of brain tumor. *Sci. Rep.* **2020**, *10*, 21791. [CrossRef]
46. Lim, C.K.; Heo, J.; Shin, S.; Jeong, K.; Seo, Y.H.; Jang, W.D.; Park, C.R.; Park, S.Y.; Kim, S.; Kwon, I.C. Nanophotosensitizers toward advanced photodynamic therapy of Cancer. *Cancer Lett.* **2013**, *334*, 176–187. [CrossRef]
47. Akimoto, J.; Haraoka, J.; Aizawa, K. Preliminary clinical report on safety and efficacy of photodynamic therapy using talaporfin sodium for malignant gliomas. *Photodiagn. Photodyn. Ther.* **2012**, *9*, 91–99. [CrossRef] [PubMed]
48. Kelly, J.F.; Snell, M.E. Hematoporphyrin derivative: A possible aid in the diagnosis and therapy of carcinoma of the bladder. *J. Urol.* **1976**, *115*, 150–151. [CrossRef]
49. Bay, C.; Vissing, A.C.; Thaysen-Petersen, D.; Lerche, C.M.; Togsverd-Bo, K.; Heydenreich, J.; Haedersdal, M. Skin reactions after photodynamic therapy are unaffected by 839 nm photobiomodulation therapy: A randomized, double-blind, placebo-controlled, clinical trial. *Lasers Surg. Med.* **2017**, *49*, 810–818. [CrossRef]
50. Dixon, A.J.; Anderson, S.J.; Mazzurco, J.D.; Steinman, H.K. Novel photodynamic therapy does not prevent new skin cancers–randomized controlled trial. *Dermatol. Surg.* **2014**, *40*, 412–419. [CrossRef]
51. Hendel, K.; Mogensen, M.; Wenande, E.; Dierickx, C.; Haedersdal, M.; Togsverd-Bo, K. Fractional 1,927 nm Thulium Laser Plus Photodynamic Therapy Compared and Combined for Photodamaged Decollete Skin: A Side-by-Side Randomized Controlled Trial. *Lasers Surg. Med.* **2020**, *52*, 44–52. [CrossRef]

52. Miola, A.C.; Ferreira, E.R.; Abbade, L.P.F.; Schmitt, J.V.; Miot, H.A. Randomized clinical trial testing the efficacy and safety of 0.5% colchicine cream versus photodynamic therapy with methyl aminolevulinate in the treatment of skin field cancerization: Study protocol. *BMC Cancer* **2018**, *18*, 340. [CrossRef]
53. Miola, A.C.; Ferreira, E.R.; Lima, T.R.R.; Schmitt, J.V.; Abbade, L.P.F.; Miot, H.A. Effectiveness and safety of 0.5% colchicine cream vs. photodynamic therapy with methyl aminolaevulinate in the treatment of actinic keratosis and skin field cancerization of the forearms: A randomized controlled trial. *Br. J. Dermatol.* **2018**, *179*, 1081–1087. [CrossRef] [PubMed]
54. Togsverd-Bo, K.; Omland, S.H.; Wulf, H.C.; Sorensen, S.S.; Haedersdal, M. Primary prevention of skin dysplasia in renal transplant recipients with photodynamic therapy: A randomized controlled trial. *Am. J. Transplant.* **2015**, *15*, 2986–2990. [CrossRef]
55. Hendren, S.K.; Hahn, S.M.; Spitz, F.R.; Bauer, T.W.; Rubin, S.C.; Zhu, T.; Glatstein, E.; Fraker, D.L. Phase II trial of debulking surgery and photodynamic therapy for disseminated intraperitoneal tumors. *Ann. Surg. Oncol.* **2001**, *8*, 65–71. [CrossRef]
56. Hahn, S.M.; Fraker, D.L.; Mick, R.; Metz, J.; Busch, T.M.; Smith, D.; Zhu, T.; Rodriguez, C.; Dimofte, A.; Spitz, F.; et al. A phase II trial of intraperitoneal photodynamic therapy for patients with peritoneal carcinomatosis and sarcomatosis. *Clin. Cancer Res.* **2006**, *12*, 2517–2525. [CrossRef] [PubMed]
57. Barr, H. Photodynamic therapy in gastrointestinal cancer: A realistic option? *Drugs Aging* **2000**, *16*, 81–86. [CrossRef]
58. Dougherty, T.J. Photodynamic therapy in gastrointestinal cancer. *Lasers Surg. Med.* **1992**, *12*, 114. [CrossRef] [PubMed]
59. Gossner, L.; Sroka, R.; Hahn, E.G.; Ell, C. Photodynamic therapy: Successful destruction of gastrointestinal cancer after oral administration of aminolevulinic acid. *Gastrointest. Endosc.* **1995**, *41*, 55–58. [CrossRef]
60. Hayata, Y.; Kato, H.; Okitsu, H.; Kawaguchi, M.; Konaka, C. Photodynamic therapy with hematoporphyrin derivative in cancer of the upper gastrointestinal tract. *Semin. Surg. Oncol.* **1985**, *1*, 1–11. [CrossRef]
61. Jin, M.L.; Yang, B.Q.; Zhang, W.; Ren, P. Evaluation of photodynamic therapy in advanced gastrointestinal cancer. *J. Clin. Laser Med. Surg.* **1991**, *9*, 45–48. [CrossRef] [PubMed]
62. Karanov, S.; Shopova, M.; Getov, H. Photodynamic therapy in gastrointestinal cancer. *Lasers Surg. Med.* **1991**, *11*, 395–398. [CrossRef] [PubMed]
63. Kubba, A.K. Role of photodynamic therapy in the management of gastrointestinal cancer. *Digestion* **1999**, *60*, 1–10. [CrossRef] [PubMed]
64. Yano, T.; Wang, K.K. Photodynamic Therapy for Gastrointestinal Cancer. *Photochem. Photobiol.* **2020**, *96*, 517–523. [CrossRef] [PubMed]
65. Hayata, Y.; Kato, H.; Konaka, C.; Hayashi, N.; Tahara, M.; Saito, T.; Ono, J. Fiberoptic bronchoscopic photoradiation in experimentally induced canine lung cancer. *Cancer* **1983**, *51*, 50–56. [CrossRef]
66. Eljamel, M.S.; Goodman, C.; Moseley, H. ALA and Photofrin fluorescence-guided resection and repetitive PDT in glioblastoma multiforme: A single centre Phase III randomised controlled trial. *Lasers Med. Sci.* **2008**, *23*, 361–367. [CrossRef]
67. Fayter, D.; Corbett, M.; Heirs, M.; Fox, D.; Eastwood, A. A systematic review of photodynamic therapy in the treatment of pre-cancerous skin conditions, Barrett's oesophagus and cancers of the biliary tract, brain, head and neck, lung, oesophagus and skin. *Health Technol. Assess.* **2010**, *14*, 1–288. [CrossRef] [PubMed]
68. Muller, P.J.; Wilson, B.C. Photodynamic therapy of malignant brain tumours. *Can. J. Neurol. Sci.* **1990**, *17*, 193–198. [CrossRef] [PubMed]
69. Perria, C.; Casu, G.; Sgaramella, E. Proposal of a protocol for the photodynamic therapy of malignant brain tumours. *J. Photochem. Photobiol. B* **1990**, *6*, 443–449. [CrossRef]
70. Muller, P.J.; Wilson, B.C. Photodynamic therapy for malignant newly diagnosed supratentorial gliomas. *J. Clin. Laser Med. Surg.* **1996**, *14*, 263–270. [CrossRef]
71. Muller, P.J.; Wilson, B.C. Photodynamic therapy for recurrent supratentorial gliomas. *Semin. Surg. Oncol.* **1995**, *11*, 346–354. [CrossRef]
72. Kaye, A.H.; Morstyn, G.; Brownbill, D. Adjuvant high-dose photoradiation therapy in the treatment of cerebral glioma: A phase 1-2 study. *J. Neurosurg.* **1987**, *67*, 500–505. [CrossRef]
73. Stylli, S.S.; Kaye, A.H.; MacGregor, L.; Howes, M.; Rajendra, P. Photodynamic therapy of high grade glioma-long term survival. *J. Clin. Neurosci.* **2005**, *12*, 389–398. [CrossRef] [PubMed]
74. Beck, T.J.; Kreth, F.W.; Beyer, W.; Mehrkens, J.H.; Obermeier, A.; Stepp, H.; Stummer, W.; Baumgartner, R. Interstitial photodynamic therapy of nonresectable malignant glioma recurrences using 5-aminolevulinic acid induced protoporphyrin IX. *Lasers Surg. Med.* **2007**, *39*, 386–393. [CrossRef] [PubMed]
75. Mahmoudi, K.; Garvey, K.L.; Bouras, A.; Cramer, G.; Stepp, H.; Jesu Raj, J.G.; Bozec, D.; Busch, T.M.; Hadjipanayis, C.G. 5-aminolevulinic acid photodynamic therapy for the treatment of high-grade gliomas. *J. Neurooncol.* **2019**, *141*, 595–607. [CrossRef]
76. Krishnamurthy, S.; Powers, S.K.; Witmer, P.; Brown, T. Optimal light dose for interstitial photodynamic therapy in treatment for malignant brain tumors. *Lasers Surg. Med.* **2000**, *27*, 224–234. [CrossRef]
77. Calixto, G.M.; Bernegossi, J.; de Freitas, L.M.; Fontana, C.R.; Chorilli, M. Nanotechnology-Based Drug Delivery Systems for Photodynamic Therapy of Cancer: A Review. *Molecules* **2016**, *21*, 342. [CrossRef] [PubMed]
78. Chizenga, E.P.; Abrahamse, H. Nanotechnology in Modern Photodynamic Therapy of Cancer: A Review of Cellular Resistance Patterns Affecting the Therapeutic Response. *Pharmaceutics* **2020**, *12*, 632. [CrossRef]

79. Garg, T.; Jain, N.K.; Rath, G.; Goyal, A.K. Nanotechnology-Based Photodynamic Therapy: Concepts, Advances, and Perspectives. *Crit. Rev. Ther. Drug Carr. Syst.* **2015**, *32*, 389–439. [CrossRef]
80. Feng, J.J.; Wang, S.Y.; Wang, Y.M.; Wang, L.P. Stem cell membrane-camouflaged bioinspired nanoparticles for targeted photodynamic therapy of lung cancer. *J. Nanopart. Res.* **2020**, *22*, 1–11. [CrossRef]
81. Yang, C.; Fu, Y.; Huang, C.; Hu, D.; Zhou, K.; Hao, Y.; Chu, B.; Yang, Y.; Qian, Z. Chlorin e6 and CRISPR-Cas9 dual-loading system with deep penetration for a synergistic tumoral photodynamic-immunotherapy. *Biomaterials* **2020**, *255*, 120194. [CrossRef]
82. Kim, Y.J.; Lee, H.I.; Kim, J.K.; Kim, C.H.; Kim, Y.J. Peptide 18-4/chlorin e6-conjugated polyhedral oligomeric silsesquioxane nanoparticles for targeted photodynamic therapy of breast cancer. *Colloids Surf. B Biointerfaces* **2020**, *189*, 110829. [CrossRef] [PubMed]
83. Sheng, S.; Liu, F.; Lin, L.; Yan, N.; Wang, Y.; Xu, C.; Tian, H.; Chen, X. Nanozyme-mediated cascade reaction based on metal-organic framework for synergetic chemo-photodynamic tumor therapy. *J. Control. Release* **2020**, *328*, 631–639. [CrossRef]
84. Cho, M.H.; Li, Y.; Lo, P.C.; Lee, H.; Choi, Y. Fucoidan-Based Theranostic Nanogel for Enhancing Imaging and Photodynamic Therapy of Cancer. *Nano-Micro Lett.* **2020**, *12*, 47. [CrossRef] [PubMed]
85. Zhou, S.Y.; Hu, X.L.; Xia, R.; Liu, S.; Pei, Q.; Chen, G.; Xie, Z.G.; Jing, X.B. A Paclitaxel Prodrug Activatable by Irradiation in a Hypoxic Microenvironment. *Angew. Chem. Int. Ed.* **2020**, *59*, 23198–23205. [CrossRef]
86. Um, W.; Park, J.; Ko, H.; Lim, S.; Yoon, H.Y.; Shim, M.K.; Lee, S.; Ko, Y.J.; Kim, M.J.; Park, J.H.; et al. Visible light-induced apoptosis activatable nanoparticles of photosensitizer-DEVD-anticancer drug conjugate for targeted cancer therapy. *Biomaterials* **2019**, *224*, 119494. [CrossRef] [PubMed]
87. Chi, Y.F.; Qin, J.J.; Li, Z.; Ge, Q.; Zeng, W.H. Enhanced anti-tumor efficacy of 5-aminolevulinic acid-gold nanoparticles-mediated photodynamic therapy in cutaneous squamous cell carcinoma cells. *Braz. J. Med. Biol. Res.* **2020**, *53*, e8457. [CrossRef]
88. Huang, C.; Chen, F.; Zhang, L.; Yang, Y.; Yang, X.; Pan, W. (99m)Tc Radiolabeled HA/TPGS-Based Curcumin-Loaded Nanoparticle for Breast Cancer Synergistic Theranostics: Design, in vitro and in vivo Evaluation. *Int. J. Nanomed.* **2020**, *15*, 2987–2998. [CrossRef]
89. Uthaman, S.; Pillarisetti, S.; Mathew, A.P.; Kim, Y.; Bae, W.K.; Huh, K.M.; Park, I.K. Long circulating photoactivable nanomicelles with tumor localized activation and ROS triggered self-accelerating drug release for enhanced locoregional chemo-photodynamic therapy. *Biomaterials* **2020**, *232*, 119702. [CrossRef]
90. Feng, Z.; Guo, J.; Liu, X.; Song, H.; Zhang, C.; Huang, P.; Dong, A.; Kong, D.; Wang, W. Cascade of reactive oxygen species generation by polyprodrug for combinational photodynamic therapy. *Biomaterials* **2020**, *255*, 120210. [CrossRef] [PubMed]
91. Kim, Y.; Uthaman, S.; Pillarisetti, S.; Noh, K.; Huh, K.M.; Park, I.K. Bioactivatable reactive oxygen species-sensitive nanoparticulate system for chemo-photodynamic therapy. *Acta Biomater.* **2020**, *108*, 273–284. [CrossRef]
92. Lu, L.; Zhao, X.J.; Fu, T.W.; Li, K.; He, Y.; Luo, Z.; Dai, L.L.; Zeng, R.; Cai, K.Y. An iRGD-conjugated prodrug micelle with blood-brain-barrier penetrability for anti-glioma therapy. *Biomaterials* **2020**, *230*, 119666. [CrossRef] [PubMed]
93. Pan, Q.Q.; Tian, J.J.; Zhu, H.H.; Hong, L.J.; Mao, Z.W.; Oliveira, J.M.; Reis, R.L.; Li, X. Tumor-Targeting Polycaprolactone Nanoparticles with Codelivery of Paclitaxel and IR780 for Combinational Therapy of Drug-Resistant Ovarian Cancer. *ACS Biomater. Sci. Eng.* **2020**, *6*, 2175–2185. [CrossRef] [PubMed]
94. Ji, C.; Gao, Q.; Dong, X.; Yin, W.; Gu, Z.; Gan, Z.; Zhao, Y.; Yin, M. A Size-Reducible Nanodrug with an Aggregation-Enhanced Photodynamic Effect for Deep Chemo-Photodynamic Therapy. *Angew. Chem. Int. Ed. Engl.* **2018**, *57*, 11384–11388. [CrossRef] [PubMed]
95. Debele, T.A.; Mekuria, S.L.; Tsai, H.C. A pH-sensitive micelle composed of heparin, phospholipids, and histidine as the carrier of photosensitizers: Application to enhance photodynamic therapy of cancer. *Int. J. Biol. Macromol.* **2017**, *98*, 125–138. [CrossRef] [PubMed]
96. Kim, D.H.; Hwang, H.S.; Na, K. Photoresponsive Micelle-Incorporated Doxorubicin for Chemo-Photodynamic Therapy to Achieve Synergistic Antitumor Effects. *Biomacromolecules* **2018**, *19*, 3301–3310. [CrossRef] [PubMed]
97. Li, R.; Shan, L.; Yao, Y.; Peng, F.; Jiang, S.; Yang, D.; Ling, G.; Zhang, P. Black phosphorus nanosheets and docetaxel micelles co-incorporated thermoreversible hydrogel for combination chemo-photodynamic therapy. *Drug Deliv. Transl. Res.* **2021**, *11*, 1133–1143. [CrossRef]
98. Wu, J.; Xia, L.; Liu, Z.; Xu, Z.; Cao, H.; Zhang, W. Fabrication of a Dual-Stimuli-Responsive Supramolecular Micelle from a Pillar[5]arene-Based Supramolecular Diblock Copolymer for Photodynamic Therapy. *Macromol. Rapid Commun.* **2019**, *40*, e1900240. [CrossRef]
99. Li, L.; Cho, H.; Kim, S.; Kang, H.C.; Huh, K.M. Polyelectrolyte nanocomplex formation of heparin-photosensitizer conjugate with polymeric scavenger for photodynamic therapy. *Carbohydr. Polym.* **2015**, *121*, 122–131. [CrossRef]
100. Wu, Y.; Li, F.; Zhang, X.; Li, Z.; Zhang, Q.; Wang, W.; Pan, D.; Zheng, X.; Gu, Z.; Zhang, H.; et al. Tumor microenvironment-responsive PEGylated heparin-pyropheophorbide-a nanoconjugates for photodynamic therapy. *Carbohydr. Polym.* **2021**, *255*, 117490. [CrossRef]
101. Wang, M.; Geilich, B.M.; Keidar, M.; Webster, T.J. Killing malignant melanoma cells with protoporphyrin IX-loaded polymersome-mediated photodynamic therapy and cold atmospheric plasma. *Int. J. Nanomed.* **2017**, *12*, 4117–4127. [CrossRef] [PubMed]
102. Pan, Y.T.; Ding, Y.F.; Han, Z.H.; Yuwen, L.; Ye, Z.; Mok, G.S.P.; Li, S.; Wang, L.H. Hyaluronic acid-based nanogels derived from multicomponent self-assembly for imaging-guided chemo-photodynamic cancer therapy. *Carbohydr. Polym.* **2021**, *268*, 118257. [CrossRef]

103. Chang, E.; Bu, J.; Ding, L.; Lou, J.W.H.; Valic, M.S.; Cheng, M.H.Y.; Rosilio, V.; Chen, J.; Zheng, G. Porphyrin-lipid stabilized paclitaxel nanoemulsion for combined photodynamic therapy and chemotherapy. *J. Nanobiotechnol.* **2021**, *19*, 154. [CrossRef]
104. Sundaram, P.; Abrahamse, H. Effective Photodynamic Therapy for Colon Cancer Cells Using Chlorin e6 Coated Hyaluronic Acid-Based Carbon Nanotubes. *Int. J. Mol. Sci.* **2020**, *21*, 4745. [CrossRef]
105. Zhou, Y.; Chang, C.; Liu, Z.; Zhao, Q.; Xu, Q.; Li, C.; Chen, Y.; Zhang, Y.; Lu, B. Hyaluronic Acid-Functionalized Hollow Mesoporous Silica Nanoparticles as pH-Sensitive Nanocarriers for Cancer Chemo-Photodynamic Therapy. *Langmuir* **2021**, *37*, 2619–2628. [CrossRef]
106. Potara, M.; Nagy-Simon, T.; Focsan, M.; Licarete, E.; Soritau, O.; Vulpoi, A.; Astilean, S. Folate-targeted Pluronic-chitosan nanocapsules loaded with IR780 for near-infrared fluorescence imaging and photothermal-photodynamic therapy of ovarian cancer. *Colloids Surf. B Biointerfaces* **2021**, *203*, 111755. [CrossRef]
107. Wang, X.; Li, S.; Liu, H. Co-delivery of chitosan nanoparticles of 5-aminolevulinic acid and shGBAS for improving photodynamic therapy efficacy in oral squamous cell carcinomas. *Photodiagn. Photodyn. Ther.* **2021**, *34*, 102218. [CrossRef]
108. Zhu, T.; Shi, L.; Ma, C.; Xu, L.; Yang, J.; Zhou, G.; Zhu, X.; Shen, L. Fluorinated chitosan-mediated intracellular catalase delivery for enhanced photodynamic therapy of oral cancer. *Biomater. Sci.* **2021**, *9*, 658–662. [CrossRef]
109. Gaio, E.; Conte, C.; Esposito, D.; Miotto, G.; Quaglia, F.; Moret, F.; Reddi, E. Co-delivery of Docetaxel and Disulfonate Tetraphenyl Chlorin in One Nanoparticle Produces Strong Synergism between Chemo- and Photodynamic Therapy in Drug-Sensitive and -Resistant Cancer Cells. *Mol. Pharm.* **2018**, *15*, 4599–4611. [CrossRef] [PubMed]
110. Li, W.; Peng, J.; Tan, L.; Wu, J.; Shi, K.; Qu, Y.; Wei, X.; Qian, Z. Mild photothermal therapy/photodynamic therapy/chemotherapy of breast cancer by Lyp-1 modified Docetaxel/IR820 Co-loaded micelles. *Biomaterials* **2016**, *106*, 119–133. [CrossRef] [PubMed]
111. Wang, D.; Zhang, S.; Zhang, T.; Wan, G.; Chen, B.; Xiong, Q.; Zhang, J.; Zhang, W.; Wang, Y. Pullulan-coated phospholipid and Pluronic F68 complex nanoparticles for carrying IR780 and paclitaxel to treat hepatocellular carcinoma by combining photothermal therapy/photodynamic therapy and chemotherapy. *Int. J. Nanomed.* **2017**, *12*, 8649–8670. [CrossRef] [PubMed]
112. Yang, X.; Shi, X.; Zhang, Y.; Xu, J.; Ji, J.; Ye, L.; Yi, F.; Zhai, G. Photo-triggered self-destructive ROS-responsive nanoparticles of high paclitaxel/chlorin e6 co-loading capacity for synergetic chemo-photodynamic therapy. *J. Control. Release* **2020**, *323*, 333–349. [CrossRef] [PubMed]
113. de Paula Rodrigues, R.; Tini, I.R.; Soares, C.P.; da Silva, N.S. Effect of photodynamic therapy supplemented with quercetin in HEp-2 cells. *Cell Biol. Int.* **2014**, *38*, 716–722. [CrossRef]
114. Thakur, N.S.; Mandal, N.; Patel, G.; Kirar, S.; Reddy, Y.N.; Kushwah, V.; Jain, S.; Kalia, Y.N.; Bhaumik, J.; Banerjee, U.C. Co-administration of zinc phthalocyanine and quercetin via hybrid nanoparticles for augmented photodynamic therapy. *Nanomedicine* **2021**, *33*, 102368. [CrossRef]
115. He, J.; Huang, X.; Li, Y.C.; Liu, Y.; Babu, T.; Aronova, M.A.; Wang, S.; Lu, Z.; Chen, X.; Nie, Z. Self-assembly of amphiphilic plasmonic micelle-like nanoparticles in selective solvents. *J. Am. Chem. Soc.* **2013**, *135*, 7974–7984. [CrossRef]
116. Huntosova, V.; Datta, S.; Lenkavska, L.; Macajova, M.; Bilcik, B.; Kundekova, B.; Cavarga, I.; Kronek, J.; Jutkova, A.; Miskovsky, P.; et al. Alkyl Chain Length in Poly(2-oxazoline)-Based Amphiphilic Gradient Copolymers Regulates the Delivery of Hydrophobic Molecules: A Case of the Biodistribution and the Photodynamic Activity of the Photosensitizer Hypericin. *Biomacromolecules* **2021**, *22*, 4199–4216. [CrossRef]
117. Li, H.; Yu, Z.; Wang, S.; Long, X.; Zhang, L.M.; Zhu, Z.; Yang, L. Photosensitizer-encapsulated amphiphilic chitosan derivative micelles: Photoactivity and enhancement of phototoxicity against human pancreatic cancer cells. *J. Photochem. Photobiol. B Biol.* **2015**, *142*, 212–219. [CrossRef]
118. Bazylinska, U.; Kulbacka, J.; Chodaczek, G. Nanoemulsion Structural Design in Co-Encapsulation of Hybrid Multifunctional Agents: Influence of the Smart PLGA Polymers on the Nanosystem-Enhanced Delivery and Electro-Photodynamic Treatment. *Pharmaceutics* **2019**, *11*, 405. [CrossRef]
119. Malacarne, M.C.; Banfi, S.; Rugiero, M.; Caruso, E. Drug delivery systems for the photodynamic application of two photosensitizers belonging to the porphyrin family. *Photochem. Photobiol. Sci.* **2021**, *20*, 1011–1025. [CrossRef]
120. Xu, L.; Zhang, W.; Cai, H.; Liu, F.; Wang, Y.; Gao, Y.; Zhang, W. Photocontrollable release and enhancement of photodynamic therapy based on host-guest supramolecular amphiphiles. *J. Mater. Chem. B* **2015**, *3*, 7417–7426. [CrossRef] [PubMed]
121. Elschner, T.; Wondraczek, H.; Heinze, T. Syntheses and detailed structure characterization of dextran carbonates. *Carbohydr. Polym.* **2013**, *93*, 216–223. [CrossRef]
122. Yang, X.; Cai, X.; Yu, A.; Xi, Y.; Zhai, G. Redox-sensitive self-assembled nanoparticles based on alpha-tocopherol succinate-modified heparin for intracellular delivery of paclitaxel. *J. Colloid Interface Sci.* **2017**, *496*, 311–326. [CrossRef]
123. Jena, S.K.; Sangamwar, A.T. Polymeric micelles of amphiphilic graft copolymer of alpha-tocopherol succinate-g-carboxymethyl chitosan for tamoxifen delivery: Synthesis, characterization and in vivo pharmacokinetic study. *Carbohydr. Polym.* **2016**, *151*, 1162–1174. [CrossRef]
124. Wang, Y.H.; Song, S.Y.; Zhang, S.T.; Zhang, H.J. Stimuli-responsive nanotheranostics based on lanthanide-doped upconversion nanoparticles for cancer imaging and therapy: Current advances and future challenges. *Nano Today* **2019**, *25*, 38–67. [CrossRef]
125. Pandya, A.D.; Overbye, A.; Sahariah, P.; Gaware, V.S.; Hogset, H.; Masson, M.; Hogset, A.; Maelandsmo, G.M.; Skotland, T.; Sandvig, K.; et al. Drug-Loaded Photosensitizer-Chitosan Nanoparticles for Combinatorial Chemo- and Photodynamic-Therapy of Cancer. *Biomacromolecules* **2020**, *21*, 1489–1498. [CrossRef]

126. Xu, X.; Chong, Y.; Liu, X.; Fu, H.; Yu, C.; Huang, J.; Zhang, Z. Multifunctional nanotheranostic gold nanocages for photoacoustic imaging guided radio/photodynamic/photothermal synergistic therapy. *Acta Biomater.* **2019**, *84*, 328–338. [CrossRef] [PubMed]
127. Xu, W.; Qian, J.; Hou, G.; Wang, Y.; Wang, J.; Sun, T.; Ji, L.; Suo, A.; Yao, Y. A dual-targeted hyaluronic acid-gold nanorod platform with triple-stimuli responsiveness for photodynamic/photothermal therapy of breast cancer. *Acta Biomater.* **2019**, *83*, 400–413. [CrossRef]
128. Krajczewski, J.; Rucinska, K.; Townley, H.E.; Kudelski, A. Role of various nanoparticles in photodynamic therapy and detection methods of singlet oxygen. *Photodiagn. Photodyn. Ther.* **2019**, *26*, 162–178. [CrossRef] [PubMed]
129. Kundu, M.; Sadhukhan, P.; Ghosh, N.; Ghosh, S.; Chatterjee, S.; Das, J.; Brahmachari, G.; Sil, P.C. In vivo therapeutic evaluation of a novel bis-lawsone derivative against tumor following delivery using mesoporous silica nanoparticle based redox-responsive drug delivery system. *Mater. Sci. Eng. C* **2021**, *126*. [CrossRef] [PubMed]
130. Chen, H.; Kuang, Y.; Liu, R.; Chen, Z.Y.; Jiang, B.B.; Sun, Z.G.; Chen, X.Q.; Li, C. Dual-pH-sensitive mesoporous silica nanoparticle-based drug delivery system for tumor-triggered intracellular drug release. *J. Mater. Sci.* **2018**, *53*, 10653–10665. [CrossRef]
131. Han, R.L.; Wu, S.; Yan, Y.Y.; Chen, W.; Tang, K.Q. Construction of ferrocene modified and indocyanine green loaded multifunctional mesoporous silica nanoparticle for simultaneous chemodynamic/photothermal/photodynamic therapy. *Mater. Today Commun.* **2021**, *26*, 101842. [CrossRef]
132. Kim, J.; Cho, H.R.; Jeon, H.; Kim, D.; Song, C.; Lee, N.; Choi, S.H.; Hyeon, T. Continuous O-2-Evolving MnFe2O4 Nanoparticle-Anchored Mesoporous Silica Nanoparticles for Efficient Photodynamic Therapy in Hypoxic Cancer. *J. Am. Chem. Soc.* **2017**, *139*, 10992–10995. [CrossRef]
133. Sun, J.; Fan, Y.; Zhang, P.; Zhang, X.; Zhou, Q.; Zhao, J.; Ren, L.Q. Self-enriched mesoporous silica nanoparticle composite membrane with remarkable photodynamic antimicrobial performances. *J. Colloid Interfaces Sci.* **2020**, *559*, 197–205. [CrossRef]
134. Bharathiraja, S.; Moorthy, M.S.; Manivasagan, P.; Seo, H.; Lee, K.D.; Oh, J. Chlorin e6 conjugated silica nanoparticles for targeted and effective photodynamic therapy. *Photodiagn. Photodyn. Ther.* **2017**, *19*, 212–220. [CrossRef]
135. Huang, C.L.; Zhang, Z.M.; Guo, Q.; Zhang, L.; Fan, F.; Qin, Y.; Wang, H.; Zhou, S.; Ou, W.B.Y.; Sun, H.F.; et al. A Dual-Model Imaging Theragnostic System Based on Mesoporous Silica Nanoparticles for Enhanced Cancer Phototherapy. *Adv. Healthc. Mater.* **2019**, *8*, e1900840. [CrossRef]
136. Dey, P.; Blakey, I.; Stone, N. Diagnostic prospects and preclinical development of optical technologies using gold nanostructure contrast agents to boost endogenous tissue contrast. *Chem. Sci.* **2020**, *11*, 8671–8685. [CrossRef] [PubMed]
137. Vankayala, R.; Huang, Y.K.; Kalluru, P.; Chiang, C.S.; Hwang, K.C. First Demonstration of Gold Nanorods-Mediated Photodynamic Therapeutic Destruction of Tumors via Near Infra-Red Light Activation. *Small* **2014**, *10*, 1612–1622. [CrossRef] [PubMed]
138. Vankayala, R.; Lin, C.C.; Kalluru, P.; Chiang, C.S.; Hwang, K.C. Gold nanoshells-mediated bimodal photodynamic and photothermal cancer treatment using ultra-low doses of near infra-red light. *Biomaterials* **2014**, *35*, 5527–5538. [CrossRef] [PubMed]
139. Lv, J.L.; Zhang, X.; Li, N.N.; Wang, B.J.; He, S.L. Absorption-dependent generation of singlet oxygen from gold bipyramids excited under low power density. *RSC Adv.* **2015**, *5*, 81897–81904. [CrossRef]
140. Vankayala, R.; Sagadevan, A.; Vijayaraghavan, P.; Kuo, C.L.; Hwang, K.C. Metal Nanoparticles Sensitize the Formation of Singlet Oxygen. *Angew. Chem. Int. Ed.* **2011**, *50*, 10640–10644. [CrossRef]
141. Pasparakis, G. Light-Induced Generation of Singlet Oxygen by Naked Gold Nanoparticles and its Implications to Cancer Cell Phototherapy. *Small* **2013**, *9*, 4130–4134. [CrossRef]
142. Jiang, C.F.; Zhao, T.T.; Yuan, P.Y.; Gao, N.Y.; Pan, Y.L.; Guan, Z.P.; Zhou, N.; Xu, Q.H. Two-Photon Induced Photoluminescence and Singlet Oxygen Generation from Aggregated Gold Nanoparticles. *ACS Appl. Mater. Interfaces* **2013**, *5*, 4972–4977. [CrossRef]
143. Pakravan, A.; Salehi, R.; Mahkam, M. Comparison study on the effect of gold nanoparticles shape in the forms of star, hallow, cage, rods, and Si -Au and Fe -Au core-shell on photothermal cancer treatment. *Photodiagn. Photodyn. Ther.* **2021**, *33*, 102144. [CrossRef]
144. Shih, C.Y.; Huang, W.L.; Chiang, I.T.; Su, W.C.; Teng, H.S. Biocompatible hole scavenger-assisted graphene oxide dots for photodynamic cancer therapy. *Nanoscale* **2021**, *13*, 8431–8441. [CrossRef]
145. Mangalath, S.; Babu, P.S.S.; Nair, R.R.; Manu, P.M.; Krishna, S.; Nair, S.A.; Joseph, J. Graphene Quantum Dots Decorated with Boron Dipyrromethene Dye Derivatives for Photodynamic Therapy. *ACS Appl. Nano Mater.* **2021**, *4*, 4162–4171. [CrossRef]
146. Roeinfard, M.; Zahedifar, M.; Darroudi, M.; Zak, A.K.; Sadeghi, E. Preparation and characterization of selenium-decorated graphene quantum dots with high afterglow for application in photodynamic therapy. *Luminescence* **2020**, *35*, 891–896. [CrossRef] [PubMed]
147. Yi, L.Y.; Zhang, Y.N.; Shi, X.Q.; Du, X.Y.; Wang, X.Y.; Yu, A.H.; Zhai, G.X. Recent progress of functionalised graphene oxide in cancer therapy. *J. Drug Target.* **2019**, *27*, 125–144. [CrossRef] [PubMed]
148. Rong, P.F.; Yang, K.; Srivastan, A.; Kiesewetter, D.O.; Yue, X.Y.; Wang, F.; Nie, L.M.; Bhirde, A.; Wang, Z.; Liu, Z.; et al. Photosensitizer Loaded Nano-Graphene for Multimodality Imaging Guided Tumor Photodynamic Therapy. *Theranostics* **2014**, *4*, 229–239. [CrossRef] [PubMed]
149. Ding, Y.; Zhou, L.; Chen, X.; Wu, Q.; Song, Z.Y.; Wei, S.H.; Zhou, J.H.; Shen, J. Mutual sensitization mechanism and self-degradation property of drug delivery system for in vitro photodynamic therapy. *Int. J. Pharmaceut.* **2016**, *498*, 335–346. [CrossRef]

150. Cho, Y.; Choi, Y. Graphene oxide-photosensitizer conjugate as a redox-responsive theranostic agent. *Chem. Commun.* **2012**, *48*, 9912–9914. [CrossRef]
151. Ge, J.C.; Lan, M.H.; Zhou, B.J.; Liu, W.M.; Guo, L.; Wang, H.; Jia, Q.Y.; Niu, G.L.; Huang, X.; Zhou, H.Y.; et al. A graphene quantum dot photodynamic therapy agent with high singlet oxygen generation. *Nat. Commun.* **2014**, *5*, 1–8. [CrossRef]
152. Kuo, W.S.; Shao, Y.T.; Huang, K.S.; Chou, T.M.; Yang, C.H. Antimicrobial Amino-Functionalized Nitrogen-Doped Graphene Quantum Dots for Eliminating Multidrug-Resistant Species in Dual-Modality Photodynamic Therapy and Bioimaging under Two-Photon Excitation. *ACS Appl. Mater. Interfaces* **2018**, *10*, 14438–14446. [CrossRef] [PubMed]
153. Fang, W.K.; Wei, Y.C. Upconversion nanoparticle as a theranostic agent for tumor imaging and therapy. *J. Innov. Opt. Health Sci.* **2016**, *9*, 1630006. [CrossRef]
154. Hamblin, M.R. Upconversion in photodynamic therapy: Plumbing the depths. *Dalton Trans.* **2018**, *47*, 8571–8580. [CrossRef]
155. Zhang, P.; Steelant, W.; Kumar, M.; Scholfield, M. Versatile photosensitizers for photodynamic therapy at infrared excitation. *J. Am. Chem. Soc.* **2007**, *129*, 4526–4527. [CrossRef]
156. Idris, N.M.; Gnanasammandhan, M.K.; Zhang, J.; Ho, P.C.; Mahendran, R.; Zhang, Y. In vivo photodynamic therapy using upconversion nanoparticles as remote-controlled nanotransducers. *Nat. Med.* **2012**, *18*, 1580–1585. [CrossRef] [PubMed]
157. Chen, F.; Zhang, S.J.; Bu, W.B.; Chen, Y.; Xiao, Q.F.; Liu, J.A.; Xing, H.Y.; Zhou, L.P.; Peng, W.J.; Shi, J.L. A Uniform Sub-50 nm-Sized Magnetic/Upconversion Fluorescent Bimodal Imaging Agent Capable of Generating Singlet Oxygen by Using a 980 nm Laser. *Chem. Eur. J.* **2012**, *18*, 7082–7090. [CrossRef]
158. Wang, C.; Tao, H.Q.; Cheng, L.; Liu, Z. Near-infrared light induced in vivo photodynamic therapy of cancer based on upconversion nanoparticles. *Biomaterials* **2011**, *32*, 6145–6154. [CrossRef]
159. Dou, Q.Q.; Teng, C.P.; Ye, E.Y.; Loh, X.J. Effective near-infrared photodynamic therapy assisted by upconversion nanoparticles conjugated with photosensitizers. *Int. J. Nanomed.* **2015**, *10*, 419–432. [CrossRef]
160. Yu, Q.; Rodriguez, E.M.; Naccache, R.; Forgione, P.; Lamoureux, G.; Sanz-Rodriguez, F.; Scheglmann, D.; Capobianco, J.A. Chemical modification of temoporfin—A second generation photosensitizer activated using upconverting nanoparticles for singlet oxygen generation. *Chem. Commun.* **2014**, *50*, 12150–12153. [CrossRef]
161. Li, K.M.; Hong, E.L.; Wang, B.; Wang, Z.Y.; Zhang, L.W.; Hu, R.X.; Wang, B.Q. Advances in the application of upconversion nanoparticles for detecting and treating cancers. *Photodiagn. Photodyn. Ther.* **2019**, *25*, 177–192. [CrossRef] [PubMed]
162. Zuo, J.; Tu, L.; Li, Q.; Feng, Y.; Que, I.; Zhang, Y.; Liu, X.; Xue, B.; Cruz, L.J.; Chang, Y.; et al. Near Infrared Light Sensitive Ultraviolet-Blue Nanophotoswitch for Imaging-Guided "Off-On" Therapy. *ACS Nano* **2018**, *12*, 3217–3225. [CrossRef] [PubMed]

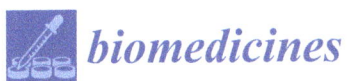

Review

Near-Infrared Photoimmunotherapy for Thoracic Cancers: A Translational Perspective

Kohei Matsuoka [1], Mizuki Yamada [1], Mitsuo Sato [1] and Kazuhide Sato [2,3,4,*]

[1] Department of Integrated Health Sciences, Nagoya University Graduate School of Medicine, 1-1-20, Daiko, Higashi-ku, Nagoya 461-8673, Japan; matsuoka.kouhei.h4@f.mail.nagoya-u.ac.jp (K.M.); yamada.mizuki.s3@s.mail.nagoya-u.ac.jp (M.Y.); msato@met.nagoya-u.ac.jp (M.S.)

[2] Respiratory Medicine, Nagoya University Graduate School of Medicine, Tsurumai-cho 65, Chikusa-ku, Nagoya 466-8550, Japan

[3] B3 Unit, Advanced Analytical and Diagnostic Imaging Center (AADIC)/Medical Engineering Unit (MEU), Nagoya University Institute for Advanced Research, Nagoya University, Tsurumai-cho 65, Showa-ku, Nagoya 466-8550, Japan

[4] FOREST-Souhatsu, CREST, JST, Goban-cho 7, Chiyoda-ku, Tokyo 102-0076, Japan

* Correspondence: k-sato@med.nagoya-u.ac.jp; Tel.: +81-052-744-2167

Abstract: The conventional treatment of thoracic tumors includes surgery, anticancer drugs, radiation, and cancer immunotherapy. Light therapy for thoracic tumors has long been used as an alternative; conventional light therapy also called photodynamic therapy (PDT) has been used mainly for early-stage lung cancer. Recently, near-infrared photoimmunotherapy (NIR-PIT), which is a completely different concept from conventional PDT, has been developed and approved in Japan for the treatment of recurrent and previously treated head and neck cancer because of its specificity and effectiveness. NIR-PIT can apply to any target by changing to different antigens. In recent years, it has become clear that various specific and promising targets are highly expressed in thoracic tumors. In combination with these various specific targets, NIR-PIT is expected to be an ideal therapeutic approach for thoracic tumors. Additionally, techniques are being developed to further develop NIR-PIT for clinical practice. In this review, NIR-PIT is introduced, and its potential therapeutic applications for thoracic cancers are described.

Keywords: near-infrared photoimmunotherapy; NIR-PIT; phototherapy; thoracic tumor; lung cancer; target antigens

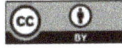

1. Introduction

Thoracic tumors, including lung cancer and malignant pleural mesothelioma (MPM), are the most lethal cancers worldwide [1,2]. To overcome thoracic cancer, NIR-PIT may be an ideal treatment and can lead to significant improvements in treatment outcomes. There are four conventional treatments for cancer: surgery, radiation therapy, chemotherapy, and immunotherapy. However, these existing treatments injure not only cancer cells but also the surrounding normal cells, tissues, and organs. In particular, these treatments may impact the vital organs such as the liver, the heart and the thoracic aorta, and bone marrow. The highly specific and effective NIR-PIT can overcome this problem because of its combined and multidisciplinary approach. In addition, NIR-light used in NIR-PIT is transmitted easily through the tissue filled by air. NIR light with a wavelength range of 650–900 nm is not readily absorbed by water or hemoglobin, and penetration through the tissue is maximal [3–6]. Therefore, the NIR wavelength of 690 nm used in NIR-PIT is thought to be a suitable wavelength for human therapy and is not toxic to the body.

Historically, thoracic tumors have been treated with light. The first bronchoscopic PDT was carried out in a patient with early central lung cancer by Hyata et al. with encouraging results. Since then about 1000 cases of ECLC have received PDT [7]. Additionally, O.J.

Balchum and colleagues used PDT to treat patients with lung cancer. All of these studies showed promising responses in early-stage patients, so PDT was recommended for patients with early-stage cancers that were inoperable, due to other complications [8]. However, PDT, which is mediated ROS, can damage not only target cancer cells but also normal cells. On the other hand, NIR-PIT is highly specific and effective as a result of its combined and multidisciplinary approach.

In this review, we describe the potential application of NIR-PIT for thoracic cancer and discuss this perspective in detail.

2. Summary

NIR-PIT is an ultra-specific and effective cancer photoimmunotherapy method that can be used to treat cancers throughout the body. NIR-PIT utilizes an antibody-photon absorbent conjugate of IRDye700DX (IR700), a near-infrared water-soluble silicon phthalocyanine derivative, and an mAb that targets surface antigens expressed on cancer cells [9,10]. Irradiation of the targeted tumor site with near-infrared light (approximately 690 nm) activates the conjugates (Figure 1①,②), induces aggregation of antibody and antigen proteins, and causes cell death (Figure 1③). This two-step targeted selection (antibody and light) provides a double level of specificity, which is not found in conventional cancer treatments.

The mechanism of NIR-PIT was elucidated after the launch of the first phase III study [10]. Specifically, when the conjugates were irradiated with near-infrared (NIR) light in the presence of sufficient electron donors, the hydrophilic side chains of the IR700 molecule (silanol) dissociated through a photochemical ligand reaction, and the remaining structure, including the antibody, rapidly became hydrophobic and aggregated. At that time, the antibody binding the surface antigen on the cell membrane of the tumor also aggregated, forcing cells to break. Fluorescence imaging could track where the conjugates were distributed and how well mAb-IR700 conjugates reacted, and the increase in IR700-fluorescence indicated that the mAb-IR700 was well connected to the target, while the decrease could confirm the photochemical reactions caused by NIR light irradiation and correlated with the treatment effect. The development of NIR-PIT was interdisciplinary, involving biology, physics, and chemistry, making use of the advantages of each discipline.

The unique feature that makes IR700 useful and valuable is its hydrophilicity. It never permeates the lipid bilayers of cell membranes and does not change the pharmacokinetics of mAbs in vivo, unlike hydrophobic photosensitizers in conventional photo-based cancer therapies such as PDT. In addition, mAb-IR700 conjugates mainly bind to the membrane of targeted tumor cells after intravenous injection and destroy the cell membrane with NIR light. Moreover, it was elucidated that reactive oxidative species (ROS) were not included in the main mechanism for NIR-PIT, since the cell death reaction in NIR-PIT proceeded even after the cell function was stopped at 4 °C, and the inhibition of cell death was not sufficiently effective even when oxidative stress inhibitors (free radical scavengers) were added. Moreover, the mass spectrometric analysis revealed that photochemical reaction is the trigger of the cell death induced by NIR-PIT [11]. The pharmacodynamics of the photosensitizer and pharmacokinetics of the conjugates in vivo are completely different between traditional PDT and NIR-PIT, which makes NIR-PIT a new photo-based modality [10].

NIR-PIT not only causes physical destruction of cells during NIR irradiation, but also induces secondary immunogenic cell death (ICD) due to damage-associated molecular patterns (DAMPs), and the release of entities such as adenosine triphosphate (ATP), calreticulin (CRT), and high mobility group box 1 (HMGB1) [12]. ICD has also been reported to occur with other radiotherapies, chemotherapy, and PDT, but these treatments themselves have a certain degree of toxicity to immune cells. NIR-PIT especially benefits from ICD [13–15], because this immunogenic cell death is not limited to the irradiated tumor but also has an effect on tumors elsewhere and on metastatic tumors. This combination of NIR-PIT and immune checkpoint inhibitors is currently being tested in phase II trials worldwide, but these do not include thoracic cancer (https://rakuten-med.com/us/pipeline/ accessed on 9 July 2022).

3. SUPR Effect

Cancer treatment with drugs has been considered an inappropriate therapy in vivo largely because of difficulties in drug retention in affected areas, such as vascular heterogeneity and high interstitial pressure [16,17]. Tumor tissue has increased permeability and retention of nanoparticles due to vascular abundance and lack of lymphoid tissue, referred to as the EPR effect. Conventional anti-cancer nanopharmaceuticals aim to take advantage of this effect to accumulate in tumors [18–20]. Although the EPR effect improves drug delivery to tumors compared to normal tissue, the effect is not significant and only low concentrations of nanodrugs reach and accumulate in tumors. The best-known nanopharmaceuticals are liposomal formulations such as Doxil and DaunoXome, both of which are as effective as small molecule formulations, but require more frequent administration and are impractical [21,22].

NIR PIT helps deliver nano-sized drugs desired to stay in the tumor; NIR-PIT is a very specific therapy that ruptures only the cancer cells labeled with the conjugate. Administered intravenously into the body as a drug, mAb-IR700 reacts from the vascular periphery to bind to target cells and specifically destroy them. The rapid rupture of surrounding cancer cells causes 10~20 times the EPR effect of vasodilation, increased blood flow, decreased blood flow velocity in the tumor, and increased vascular permeability, called super permeabilization and retention (SUPR) [23,24]. In other words, NIR-PIT can contribute to direct therapy and enhanced delivery of nanodrugs.

4. The Versatile Targets: EGFR, HER2, CD44, and CEA

NIR-PIT can be used to change the treatment pathway by creating mAb-IR700 using antibodies that target different ligands. As an entry point of research, it is simple to apply targets that have already been used in clinical practice (Table 1).

Table 1. Candidate targets for thoracic cancer.

	Target Antigens
Versatile targets	EGFR
	CD44
	CEA
	HER2
	GPR87
	PDPN
	MSLN
Exploring targets	GPR87
	DLL3
	CD26
	CDH
	TROP2
	XAGE1
Immune targets	CD25
	PD-L1
	CTLA4

4.1. EGFR

Epidermal growth factor receptor (EGFR) is a transmembrane tyrosine kinase receptor belonging to the erythroblastosis oncogene B (ErbB) family [25]. EGFR overexpression is associated with poor prognosis in several tumor types, including thoracic cancer [26]. Physiologically, EGFR regulates epithelial tissue development and homeostasis. EGFR mutation and/or overexpression has been observed in several human cancers, and EGFR-targeted therapy has become a routine part of the treatment of several cancers. EGFR is considered a suitable target for early clinical trials of NIR-PIT. Several studies have confirmed the therapeutic efficacy of NIR-PIT targeting EGFR in in vivo models of several types of cancer, including lung cancer [27–35]. Cetuximab-IR700, a chimeric IgG1 monoclonal antibody against EGFR, was approved under certain conditions, such as limiting its use to HNSCC and was the first EGFR-targeted NIR-PIT drug to be registered for clinical use in Japan in 2020 [36]. For 30 patients enrolled in Phase 2 of the clinical practice (RM-1929) for NIR-PIT against recurrent HNSCC with Cetuximab-IR700, the median OS was 9.30 months (95% CI 5.16–16.92 months). Unconfirmed ORR was achieved in 13 (43.3%, 95% CI 25.46%–62.57%) patients, with 4 (13%) patients achieving CR and 9 (30.0%) patients demonstrating PR. Disease control was observed in 24 (80%, 95% CI 61.43%–92.29%) patients [37]. Theoretically, EGFR-targeted NIR-PIT is applied to any type of cancer in which EGFR is overexpressed, and clinical trials are expected to progress in thoracic tumors.

4.2. HER2

HER2 is a membrane tyrosine kinase receptor and, together with EGFR, is a member of the ErbB family [25]. When overexpression of HER2 occurs, it forms homodimers or heterodimers with other ErbB family receptors; thus, activating oncogenic downstream signals that promote cell proliferation, survival, and angiogenesis [38]. Several antibody drugs, including trastuzumab, pertuzumab, and trastuzumab emtansine (T-DM1), have been approved by the FDA for the treatment of breast cancer, with HER2 positivity rates of 15–20% [39]. In addition, trastuzumab and fam-trastuzumab deruxtecan-nxki have already been approved by the FDA for the treatment of gastric cancer, where approximately 20% of cases are HER2 positive. These have been applied as mAbs in NIR-PIT; NIR-PIT with trastuzumab-IR700 showed valid results in a pleural dissemination model with HER2-expressing NSCLC cells and a lung metastasis model with HER2-expressing 3T3 cells [40–42]. In addition, it has been reported that chemo drugs, especially cisplatin-resistant (SBC-3/CDDP) cell lines upregulate HER2 expression. NIR-PIT against HER2 is effective also against tumors in patients who have already become resistant to chemotherapy [43].

4.3. CD44

CD44, a non-kinase transmembrane glycoprotein, regulates intercellular adhesion and epithelial–mesenchymal transition in normal cells. At the same time, it is a marker for the identification of cancer stem cells (CSCs), as CD44 increases tumor development and progression. Various types of cancer, including lung cancer, express CD44, which has been shown to be a poor prognostic factor [44–46]. Therefore, CD44 is an important approach for antibody therapeutics to eliminate CSCs [47]. In NIR-PIT targeting CD44 positive oral squamous cell carcinoma and breast cancer in a mouse model, tumor progression was significantly inhibited and survival was prolonged [48,49]. Additionally, in immunocompetent mouse models, the effect was further enhanced combined with immune activation using type 1 cytokine or immune checkpoint inhibitors [50–52].

4.4. CEA

Carcinoembryonic antigen (CEA), a glycoprotein involved in cell adhesion, is highly expressed in many epithelial cells of tumors, including lung adenocarcinomas. It has already been used as a tumor marker for various cancers, and its expression level has been associated with the prognosis of patients with colorectal cancer [53–55]. NIR-PIT targeting CEA significantly inhibited tumor progression without side effects in xenograft models of gastric cancer and orthotopic pancreatic tumor models [56,57]. In pancreatic cancer, the use of NIR-PIT as an adjunct to surgery to treat residual pancreatic cancer in a patient-derived orthotopic xenograft model also was found to improve overall survival [58,59].

CEA is also expressed in normal cells, mostly derived from surface cells of the colon, which are released into the intestinal tract and excreted in the stool [56]. Therefore, even if stray NIR light irradiated to the chest reaches normal colonic tissue, it is suggested that the side effects are very minimal. Thus, CEA is a promising target for the treatment of thoracic cancer.

5. Exploring Other Targets to Detect More Specific and Effective Markers for Lung NIR-PIT: PDPN, MSLN, GPR87, and DLL3

5.1. PDPN

Podoplanin (PDPN) is a type I transmembrane glycoprotein expressed in lymphatic endothelial cells, type I alveolar epithelial cells, and glomerular podocytes. Antibodies against PDPN (D2-40) have long been used as specific pathological diagnostic markers to confirm the presence of MPM [60,61]. PDPN has been reported to be expressed in various tumors, including MPMs [62,63]. NIR-PIT, which targets PDPN with NZ-1 antibody, is a promising target against MPM and exhibits tumor-suppressive effects in both xenograft and orthotopic MPM models [64]. It has also been shown to be effective in an orthotopic mouse model of pleural disseminated lung cancer [65].

5.2. MSLN

Mesothelin (MSLN) is a cell surface glycoprotein and a tumor differentiation marker expressed in multiple tumors, including lung cancer and MPM [66]. The association between MSLN overexpression and poor survival in MPM has not been consistently reported [67,68]. However, in MPM, MSLN is known to be associated with epithelial–mesenchymal transition (EMT) and binding to mucin 16 (MUC16/CA125), which is associated with cancer progression and aggressiveness [69,70]. MSLN is highly expressed in tumors, while its expression in normal cells is limited, making it a promising biomarker and therapeutic target [71,72]. NIR-PIT targeting MSLN was effective in a mouse xenograft model [73]. Thus, NIR-PIT targeting MSLN holds good potential for the treatment of tumors expressing mesothelin.

5.3. GPR87

GPR87 is a G-protein receptor that is highly expressed specifically in both lung cancer and MPM and is rarely expressed in normal cells [74,75]. GPR87 is a poor prognostic factor [75–77]. NIR-PIT targeting GPR87 produced a therapeutic effect in a mouse model with transplanted cell lines of lung adenocarcinoma, SCLC, and MPM [78]. GPR87 may be an ideal target for treating thoracic tumors.

5.4. DLL3

Delta-like protein 3 (DLL3) is a ligand for the Notch receptor and a promising therapeutic target molecule for small cell lung cancer (SCLC) and other neuroendocrine tumors [79,80]. Its expression is rarely observed in normal tissues. Rovalpituzumab, a DLL3-targeted antibody drug, has already been used in human clinical trials [81]. NIR-PIT targeting DLL3 with rovalpituzumab in an SCLC xenograft model has shown significant anti-tumor effects, suggesting that DLL3 is a promising target [82].

5.5. CD26

CD26 is a type II transmembrane protein that recognizes chemokines with the penultimate proline or alanine and cleaves the NH2-terminal dipeptide [83,84]. Immunohistochemical analysis has shown that CD26 is highly expressed in MPM cells, indicating its pro-carcinogenic function and relevance as a prognostic marker [85]. Promising results have also been obtained with antibody therapy targeting CD26 in phase I clinical trials [86]. It is expected that NIR-PIT will be indicated for MPM.

5.6. CDH3

CDH3 is a calcium-dependent adhesion molecule and a member of the cadherin superfamily [87]. It is overexpressed in advanced lung adenocarcinoma and has been reported to be associated with poor prognosis and EGFR-TKI resistance [88,89].

5.7. TROP2

Trophoblast surface antigen 2 (Trop2) is a widely expressed transmembrane glycoprotein and a member of the epithelial cell adhesion molecule (EpCAM) family [90]. It is highly expressed in a variety of epithelial tumors, including NSCLC, and has been reported to be associated with prognosis and as a potential new therapeutic target [91,92].

5.8. XAGE1

XAGE1 is a member of the cancer/testis (CT) antigen family expressed in a variety of cancers including NSCLC and in testicular germ cells [93]. CT antigens are widely expressed in cancers but rarely in normal cells and are highly immunogenic, making them promising targets for immunotherapies such as cancer vaccines and NIR PIT [94–96].

6. Immunogenic Targets to Detect More Specific and Effective Markers for Lung NIR-PIT: CD25, PD-L1, CTLA4

Although the tumor microenvironment(TME) is rich in T cells and natural killer (NK) cells that can recognize cancer cells, the presence of immunosuppressive cells such as regulatory T cells (Tregs) in the vicinity acts as a mechanism to evade their cytotoxic function [97]. Immune checkpoint (ICP) molecules are also known to inhibit anti-tumor immune reactions. The regulation of immunosuppressive cells or ICP in the tumor microenvironment is an important step for enhancing anticancer immune responses. Spatiotemporal decrease in Tregs or modulating ICP could augment anti-tumor immune reactions and inhibit tumor growth. Therefore, immunosuppressed cells within the TME are a promising target for NIR-PIT cancer therapy.

6.1. CD25

CD25 is the undisputed IL-2 receptor mainly expressed on activated Tregs but not on naive T cells, and NIR-PIT targeting this receptor has been developed to manipulate the cellular environment of the tumor microenvironment [98].

Tregs are highly immunosuppressive, and a higher proportion of Tregs in tumor-infiltrating lymphocytes (TILs) is associated with a poorer prognosis; in HNSCC, the degree of Treg infiltration in the TME correlated with prognosis [99,100]. Systemic administration of simple anti-CD25-IgG has been reported to deplete peripheral Tregs [98] and may also induce autoimmune adverse events such as cytokine storms. However, NIR-PIT can selectively reduce only Tregs in the TME without removing local effector T cells or Tregs present in other organs by precise irradiation.

NIR-PIT targeting CD25 caused necrotic cell death in CD25-expressing helper T cell lines in vitro and had no effect on cancer cells. However, in an in vivo syngeneic mouse model, it induced regression of the treated tumors with rapid activation of CD8+ T cells and NK cells infiltrating the tumors and activation of antigen-presenting cells. CD25-targeted NIR-PIT selectively depleted Tregs from TME, resulting in activation of effector cells and upregulation of anti-tumor immunity. Furthermore, CD8+ T cell and NK cell activation and antitumor effects were also observed in non-irradiated, distant, non-treated tumors (abscopal effect) [97]. Local CD25-targeted NIR-PIT may be a safer alternative to systemic Treg depletion because it depletes Tregs only at the tumor site where the NIR light is irradiated. The effect of Treg depletion by NIR-PIT lasted for 3–4 days, followed by gradual repopulation of Tregs, reaching the pre-treatment number of Tregs approximately 6 days after treatment [97]. If the tumor recurs, NIR-PIT can be repeated, and repeated depletion of Treg cells by CD25-targeted NIR-PIT can prolong tumor control and survival. Combination NIR-PIT dramatically improved the CR rate in a syngeneic mouse model [101].

6.2. PD-L1

Programmed death ligand 1 (PD-L1) is an immune checkpoint that binds to PD-1 (CD279) on T cells to reduce immune response cytokines and induce immune tolerance in tumor cells [102,103]. It is overexpressed in many cancer cells, including lung cancer, and is associated with poor prognosis by inhibiting T-cell immune responses [104].

NIR-PIT against PD-L1 is effective even when tumor PD-L1 expression is low and is suitable for tumors in a variety of patients, regardless of the type or organ. It is also therapeutically effective against tumors in remote areas that are not directly irradiated, even though NIR-PIT causes minimal side effects in areas that are not irradiated. In addition, in the inflammation of tumor cells caused by photocytotoxicity, cytokines such as INF-γ can promote the expression of PD-L1 and activate PD-L1 in treated tumor cells. Therefore, NIR-PIT targeting PD-L1 provides additional benefits from repeated PD-L1-targeted therapy.

NIR-PIT with antibodies against PD-L1 significantly inhibited tumor growth and prolonged survival in xenograft models by activating CD8+ T cells and NK cells in the tumor microenvironment by promoting PD-L1 positive cell rupture and inhibiting tumor immunosuppressive pathways [105,106].

6.3. CTLA4

Cytotoxic T-lymphocyte antigen-4 (CTLA4) is an immune checkpoint protein expressed on regulatory T (Treg) cells and activated T cells that downregulate T cell activation and suppress anti-tumor immune responses in response to T cell receptor engagement [107–109]. Local depletion of CTLA4 expressing cells by NIR-PIT promotes the activation and infiltration of CD8+ T cells in the tumor microenvironment and prolonged survival in vivo [110] with observation of CD8+ T cell activation and infiltration. Additionally, the same as CD25, combination NIR-PIT dramatically improves the CR rate in syngeneic mouse models [111].

7. NIR Light Irradiating Devices

NIR light significantly attenuates through deep and hard tissues by depending on the light penetration limit. Additionally, NIR-PIT against immunogenic targets in the normal lung tissue can cause an acute respiratory distress syndrome (ARDS)-like reaction, although it has already been proven that the one against the target of tumor antigen, such as HER2, does not adversely affect normal tissue. The precise irradiation and evaluation of NIR light irradiation are required. For this reason, an optical fiber diffuser in the form of a flexible cylindrical optical fiber was proposed [112–117]. The optical fibers are utilized through the bronchoscope to deliver NIR-light to key areas. This bronchoscope technique can be navigated with a 3D navigation system from CT images beforehand to guide the fiber precisely to the tumor in the lung. With these techniques, damage to the normal lung fields could be minimized. In addition, an implantable wireless NIR light-emitting diode has been developed that can be implanted once and used for irradiation several times [118]. Treatment with a single dose of high-energy NIR light can injure even normal tissues; however, multiple doses at the recommended energy of 500 mW/cm2 (at 690 nm) or less can produce anti-tumor effects. By combining this with an endoscope or catheter, it is possible to deliver light locally within the body without burns or other injuries [119–122].

8. Imaging Modality

Visualization of the NIR-PIT irradiation site and monitoring of the treatment effect at that site in real time or immediately after treatment are important to determine if accurate treatment is being achieved and if additional treatment is needed.

Fluorescence imaging of the IR700 can confirm the distribution of antibody–photo-absorber conjugates, and the NIR laser light irradiation causes the IR700 to photobleach; thus, reducing fluorescence during treatment. In the preclinical setting, the fluorescence wavelength of the IR700 (720 nm) could be measured, but a new, dedicated measurement device would have to be installed to handle it in the clinical setting. In addition, preclinically, bioluminescence imaging using luciferase can be used to evaluate the therapeutic effect of NIR-PIT after treatment, but clinical implementation is not possible [123].

Taking advantage of the broad emission spectrum of IR700, a clinically approved camera designed to detect indocyanine green, typically at 830 nm, was proposed for use during NIR-PIT, the distribution of previous IR700, and the progression of photochemical reactions can be monitored in real time and would allow optimization of NIR light irradiation during NIR-PIT [124,125]. In addition, there have been attempts to evaluate treatment efficacy by assessing the SUPR effect with the administration of indocyanine green (ICG) particles. Previous studies have shown that dynamic fluorescence imaging with ICG shows increased signal intensity in tumors after NIR-PIT treatment; significantly higher ICG intensity was demonstrated from NIR-PIT-treated tumors as early as 20 min after ICG injection [126], indicating the possibility of using SUPR effect assessment by ICG imaging to evaluate the acute cytotoxic effects of NIR-PIT [124,125,127]. Magnetic resonance imaging (MRI) imaging using gadofosveset also showed gradual signal enhancement up to 30 min in NIR-PIT-treated tumors, suggesting that it may be a useful imaging biomarker for detecting treatment changes after NIR-PIT [128].

Tumors require excess glucose due to the Warburg effect, which dramatically increases the rate of glucose uptake [129,130]. ^{18}F-fluorodeoxyglucose positron emission tomography (^{18}F-FDG PET) has been used to exploit this, for example, for tumor detection [131–133]. ^{18}FDG-PET is useful as a rapid response marker of therapeutic response, as glucose metabolism in treated tumors was greatly reduced early after NIR-PIT [134].

9. Perspective on ADCs (Antibody–Drug Conjugates)

The mAb carriers used in ADCs, which aim to reduce the impact of toxic chemical cancer drugs on normal tissues, always have inherent off-target toxicity. Even very small amounts of mAb–drug conjugates reaching epitopes in normal cells are considered to be highly toxic; therefore, lowering the therapeutic index. The application of ADCs in NIR-PIT studies has been reported to enhance the antitumor effect of the T-DM1-IR700 conjugate and the transport of NIR light-sensitive drug-releasing antibodies by the SUPR effect [135–137]. The mAb used in this conjugate was the first to reach clinical implementation, and the IR700 added to the ADC caused the SUPR effect, which is an inherent nanoparticle accumulation enhancement phenomenon occurring after NIR-PIT, to accumulate the antibody carrier in the tumor area, followed by NIR light-triggered release to expose the drug only to a specific area. The fluorescence signal evaluation confirmed the accumulation of the antibody carrier and the released anticancer drug in the tumor area, indicating an additional antitumor effect of the anticancer drug. The active and potent agent is produced only at the irradiated site, whereas the non-irradiated, non-targeted mAb–dye conjugate is essentially non-toxic. Therefore, they can be used to treat cancer as a secondary effect of each other with reduced toxicity, without compromising specificity or their respective advantages [105].

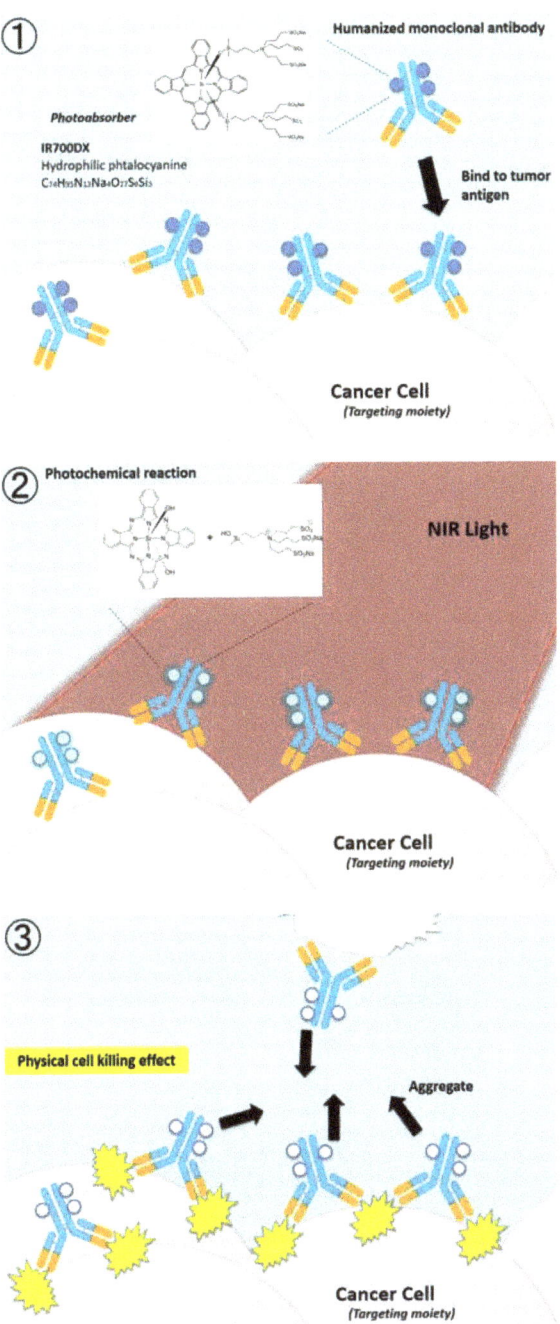

Figure 1. Schematic representation of near-infrared photoimmunotherapy. The conjugates, consisting of humanized monoclonal antibody and photo absorber IR700DX, can target specific cancer cell antigens. Once NIR-light irradiates, the targeting cancer cells are ruptured.

10. Conclusions

NIR-PIT overcomes the side effects that used to be a problem with anticancer drugs and photodynamic therapy, and has achieved a new, ultra-specific, multidisciplinary therapy that can approach cancer treatment directly and immunologically at the cancer site. Not only that, it has the potential to be widely applicable to any type of cancer by replacing antibodies.

NIR-PIT for thoracic cancer was not realistic because of the difficulty of external irradiation due to the surrounding ribs and the concern about ARDS symptoms caused by the ICD associated with the treatment. Recently, the development of uniform irradiation methods and modalities that enable rapid monitoring of treatment effects has made it possible to provide appropriate and effective treatment to localized thoracic tumors. NIR-PIT is a very promising treatment candidate for thoracic cancer.

Author Contributions: K.M., M.Y. and K.S. performed the literature search and discussed the review. M.S. checked and advised on the review. K.M., M.Y. and K.S. wrote the manuscript. All authors have read and agreed to the published version of the manuscript.

Funding: This research was supported by the Program for Developing Next-generation Researchers (Japan Science and Technology Agency), KAKEN (18K15923, 21K07217)(JSPS), CREST (JPMJCR19H2, JST), and FOREST-Souhatsu (JPMJFR2017, JST). Funders only provided financial support and had no role in the study design, data collection, data analysis, interpretation, and writing of the report.

Institutional Review Board Statement: Not applicable.

Informed Consent Statement: Not applicable.

Data Availability Statement: Not applicable.

Conflicts of Interest: The authors declare no conflict of interest.

Abbreviations

PDT: photodynamic therapy; NIR-PIT, near-infrared photoimmunotherapy; MPM, malignant pleural mesothelioma; IR700, IRDye700DX; NIR, near-infrared; ROS, reactive oxygen spicies;L-NaAA, l-sodium ascorbate; ICD, immunogenic cell death; DAMPs, damage-associated molecular patterns; ATP, adenosine triphosphate; CRT, calreticulin; HMGB1, high mobility group box 1; SUPR, super permeabilization and retention; EGFR, epidermal growth factor receptor; ErbB, erythroblastosis oncogene B; HNSCC, squamous cell carcinoma of the head and neck; CSCs, cancer stem cells; CEA, Carcinoembryonic antigen; T-DM1, trastuzumab emtansine; PDPN, Podoplanin; EMT, epithelial–mesenchymal transition; MUC16, mucin 16; DLL3, Delta-like protein 3; SCLC, small cell lung cancer; Trop2, Trophoblast surface antigen 2; EpCAM, epithelial cell adhesion molecule; CT antigen, cancer/testis antigen; NK cells, natural killer cells; PD-L1, Programmed death ligand 1; CTLA4, Cytotoxic T-lymphocyte antigen-4; ADCs, antibody–drug conjugates.

References

1. Sung, H.; Ferlay, J.; Siegel, R.L.; Laversanne, M.; Soerjomataram, I.; Jemal, A.; Bray, F. Global Cancer Statistics 2020: GLOBOCAN Estimates of Incidence and Mortality Worldwide for 36 Cancers in 185 Countries. *CA. Cancer J. Clin.* **2021**, *71*, 209–249. [CrossRef] [PubMed]
2. Bibby, A.C.; Tsim, S.; Kanellakis, N.; Ball, H.; Talbot, D.C.; Blyth, K.G.; Maskell, N.A.; Psallidas, I. Malignant Pleural Mesothelioma: An Update on Investigation, Diagnosis and Treatment. *Eur. Respir. Rev.* **2016**, *25*, 472–486. [CrossRef] [PubMed]
3. Ash, C.; Dubec, M.; Donne, K.; Bashford, T. Effect of Wavelength and Beam Width on Penetration in Light-Tissue Interaction Using Computational Methods. *Lasers Med. Sci.* **2017**, *32*, 1909. [CrossRef] [PubMed]
4. Ripoll, J.; Weissleder, R.; Ntziachristos, V. Would Near-Infrared Fluorescence Signals Propagate through Large Human Organs for Clinical Studies?–Errata. *Opt. Lett.* **2002**, *27*, 1652. [CrossRef]
5. Zhang, M.; Qin, X.; Xu, W.; Wang, Y.; Song, Y.; Garg, S.; Luan, Y. Engineering of a Dual-Modal Phototherapeutic Nanoplatform for Single NIR Laser-Triggered Tumor Therapy. *J. Colloid Interface Sci.* **2021**, *594*, 493–501. [CrossRef] [PubMed]
6. Zhou, Y.; Ren, X.; Hou, Z.; Wang, N.; Jiang, Y.; Luan, Y. Engineering a Photosensitizer Nanoplatform for Amplified Photodynamic Immunotherapy via Tumor Microenvironment Modulation. *Nanoscale Horiz.* **2021**, *6*, 120–131. [CrossRef]

7. Moghissi, K.; Dixon, K. Update on the Current Indications, Practice and Results of Photodynamic Therapy (PDT) in Early Central Lung Cancer (ECLC). *Photodiagnosis Photodyn. Ther.* **2008**, *5*, 10–18. [CrossRef]
8. Balchum, O.J.; Doiron, D.R.; Huth, G.C. Photoradiation Therapy of Endobronchial Lung Cancers Employing the Photodynamic Action of Hematoporphyrin Derivative. *Lasers Surg. Med.* **1984**, *4*, 13–30. [CrossRef]
9. Kobayashi, H.; Choyke, P.L. Near-Infrared Photoimmunotherapy of Cancer. *Acc. Chem. Res.* **2019**, *52*, 2332–2339. [CrossRef]
10. Sato, K.; Ando, K.; Okuyama, S.; Moriguchi, S.; Ogura, T.; Totoki, S.; Hanaoka, H.; Nagaya, T.; Kokawa, R.; Takakura, H.; et al. Photoinduced Ligand Release from a Silicon Phthalocyanine Dye Conjugated with Monoclonal Antibodies: A Mechanism of Cancer Cell Cytotoxicity after Near-Infrared Photoimmunotherapy. *ACS Cent. Sci.* **2018**, *4*, acscentsci.8b00565. [CrossRef]
11. Kato, T.; Okada, R.; Goto, Y.; Furusawa, A.; Inagaki, F.; Wakiyama, H.; Furumoto, H.; Daar, D.; Turkbey, B.; Choyke, P.L.; et al. Electron Donors Rather Than Reactive Oxygen Species Needed for Therapeutic Photochemical Reaction of Near-Infrared Photoimmunotherapy. *ACS Pharmacol. Transl. Sci.* **2021**, *4*, 1689–1701. [CrossRef] [PubMed]
12. Ogawa, M.; Tomita, Y.; Nakamura, Y.; Lee, M.-J.; Lee, S.; Tomita, S.; Nagaya, T.; Sato, K.; Yamauchi, T.; Iwai, H.; et al. Immunogenic Cancer Cell Death Selectively Induced by near Infrared Photoimmunotherapy Initiates Host Tumor Immunity. *Oncotarget* **2017**, *8*, 10425–10436. [CrossRef] [PubMed]
13. Buytaert, E.; Dewaele, M.; Agostinis, P. Molecular Effectors of Multiple Cell Death Pathways Initiated by Photodynamic Therapy. *Biochim. Biophys. Acta Rev. Cancer* **2007**, *1776*, 86–107. [CrossRef] [PubMed]
14. Vanpouille-Box, C.; Alard, A.; Aryankalayil, M.J.; Sarfraz, Y.; Diamond, J.M.; Schneider, R.J.; Inghirami, G.; Coleman, C.N.; Formenti, S.C.; Demaria, S. DNA Exonuclease Trex1 Regulates Radiotherapy-Induced Tumour Immunogenicity. *Nat. Commun.* **2017**, *8*, 15618. [CrossRef]
15. Kroemer, G.; Galluzzi, L.; Kepp, O.; Zitvogel, L. Immunogenic Cell Death in Cancer Therapy. *Annu. Rev. Immunol.* **2013**, *31*, 51–72. [CrossRef]
16. Minchinton, A.I.; Tannock, I.F.; AI, M.; IF, T. Drug Penetration in Solid Tumours. *Nat. Rev. Cancer* **2006**, *6*, 583–592. [CrossRef]
17. Hambley, T.W. Is Anticancer Drug Development Heading in the Right Direction? *Cancer Res.* **2009**, *69*, 1259–1262. [CrossRef]
18. Peer, D.; Karp, J.M.; Hong, S.; Farokhzad, O.C.; Margalit, R.; Langer, R. Nanocarriers as an Emerging Platform for Cancer Therapy. *Nat. Nanotechnol.* **2007**, *2*, 751–760. [CrossRef]
19. Maeda, H. Tumor-Selective Delivery of Macromolecular Drugs via the EPR Effect: Background and Future Prospects. *Bioconjug. Chem.* **2010**, *21*, 797–802. [CrossRef]
20. Maeda, H.; Matsumura, Y. EPR Effect Based Drug Design and Clinical Outlook for Enhanced Cancer Chemotherapy. *Adv. Drug Deliv. Rev.* **2011**, *63*, 129–130. [CrossRef]
21. Forssen, E.A.; Coulter, D.M.; Proffitt, R.T. Selective in Vivo Localization of Daunorubicin Small Unilamellar Vesicles in Solid Tumors. *Cancer Res.* **1992**, *52*, 3255–3261. [PubMed]
22. Presant, C.A.; Scolaro, M.; Kennedy, P.; Blayney, D.W.; Flanagan, B.; Lisak, J.; Presant, J. Liposomal Daunorubicin Treatment of HIV-Associated Kaposi's Sarcoma. *Lancet* **1993**, *341*, 1242–1243. [CrossRef]
23. Sano, K.; Nakajima, T.; Choyke, P.L.; Kobayashi, H. Markedly Enhanced Permeability and Retention Effects Induced by Photo-Immunotherapy of Tumors. *ACS Nano* **2012**, *7*, 717–724. [CrossRef] [PubMed]
24. Kobayashi, H.; Choyke, P.L. Super Enhanced Permeability and Retention (SUPR) Effects in Tumors Following near Infrared Photoimmunotherapy. *Nanoscale* **2016**, *8*, 12504–12509. [CrossRef]
25. Roskoski, R. The ErbB/HER Family of Protein-Tyrosine Kinases and Cancer. *Pharmacol. Res.* **2014**, *79*, 34–74. [CrossRef]
26. Nicholson, R.; Gee, J.M.; Harper, M. EGFR and Cancer Prognosis. *Eur. J. Cancer* **2001**, *37*, 9–15. [CrossRef]
27. Nagaya, T.; Okuyama, S.; Ogata, F.; Maruoka, Y.; Knapp, D.W.; Karagiannis, S.N.; Fazekas-Singer, J.; Choyke, P.L.; LeBlanc, A.K.; Jensen-Jarolim, E.; et al. Near Infrared Photoimmunotherapy Targeting Bladder Cancer with a Canine Anti-Epidermal Growth Factor Receptor (EGFR) Antibody. *Oncotarget* **2018**, *9*, 19026–19038. [CrossRef]
28. Nagaya, T.; Sato, K.; Harada, T.; Nakamura, Y.; Choyke, P.L.; Kobayashi, H. Near Infrared Photoimmunotherapy Targeting EGFR Positive Triple Negative Breast Cancer: Optimizing the Conjugate-Light Regimen. *PLoS ONE* **2015**, *10*, e0136829. [CrossRef]
29. Siddiqui, M.R.; Railkar, R.; Sanford, T.; Crooks, D.R.; Eckhaus, M.A.; Haines, D.; Choyke, P.L.; Kobayashi, H.; Agarwal, P.K. Targeting Epidermal Growth Factor Receptor (EGFR) and Human Epidermal Growth Factor Receptor 2 (HER2) Expressing Bladder Cancer Using Combination Photoimmunotherapy (PIT). *Sci. Rep.* **2019**, *9*, 2084. [CrossRef]
30. Mitsunaga, M.; Ogawa, M.; Kosaka, N.; Rosenblum, L.T.; Choyke, P.L.; Kobayashi, H. Cancer Cell-Selective in Vivo near Infrared Photoimmunotherapy Targeting Specific Membrane Molecules. *Nat. Med.* **2011**, *17*, 1685–1691. [CrossRef]
31. Nakajima, T.; Sato, K.; Hanaoka, H.; Watanabe, R.; Harada, T.; Choyke, P.L.; Kobayashi, H. The Effects of Conjugate and Light Dose on Photo-Immunotherapy Induced Cytotoxicity. *BMC Cancer* **2014**, *14*, 389. [CrossRef] [PubMed]
32. Sato, K.; Nakajima, T.; Choyke, P.L.; Kobayashi, H. Selective Cell Elimination in Vitro and in Vivo from Tissues and Tumors Using Antibodies Conjugated with a near Infrared Phthalocyanine. *RSC Adv.* **2015**, *5*, 25105–25114. [CrossRef] [PubMed]
33. Sato, K.; Watanabe, R.; Hanaoka, H.; Harada, T.; Nakajima, T.; Kim, I.; Paik, C.H.; Choyke, P.L.; Kobayashi, H. Photoimmunotherapy: Comparative Effectiveness of Two Monoclonal Antibodies Targeting the Epidermal Growth Factor Receptor. *Mol. Oncol.* **2014**, *8*, 620–632. [CrossRef] [PubMed]
34. Burley, T.A.; Mączyńska, J.; Shah, A.; Szopa, W.; Harrington, K.J.; Boult, J.K.R.; Mrozek-Wilczkiewicz, A.; Vinci, M.; Bamber, J.C.; Kaspera, W.; et al. Near-Infrared Photoimmunotherapy Targeting EGFR-Shedding New Light on Glioblastoma Treatment. *Int. J. Cancer* **2018**, *142*, 2363–2374. [CrossRef]

35. Nakamura, Y.; Ohler, Z.W.; Householder, D.; Nagaya, T.; Sato, K.; Okuyama, S.; Ogata, F.; Daar, D.; Hoa, T.; Choyke, P.L.; et al. Near Infrared Photoimmunotherapy in a Transgenic Mouse Model of Spontaneous Epidermal Growth Factor Receptor (EGFR)-Expressing Lung Cancer. *Mol. Cancer Ther.* **2017**, *16*, 408–414. [CrossRef]
36. Rakuten Medical, Inc. Study of RM-1929 and Photoimmunotherapy in Patients with Recurrent Head and Neck Cancer. Available online: https://clinicaltrials.gov/ct2/show/NCT02422979 (accessed on 9 July 2022).
37. Cognetti, D.M.; Johnson, J.M.; Curry, J.M.; Kochuparambil, S.T.; McDonald, D.; Mott, F.; Fidler, M.J.; Stenson, K.; Vasan, N.R.; Razaq, M.A.; et al. Phase 1/2a, Open-Label, Multicenter Study of RM-1929 Photoimmunotherapy in Patients with Locoregional, Recurrent Head and Neck Squamous Cell Carcinoma. *Head Neck* **2021**, *43*, 3875–3887. [CrossRef]
38. Meric-Bernstam, F.; Johnson, A.M.; Dumbrava, E.E.I.; Raghav, K.; Balaji, K.; Bhatt, M.; Murthy, R.K.; Rodon, J.; Piha-Paul, S.A. Advances in HER2-Targeted Therapy: Novel Agents and Opportunities Beyond Breast and Gastric Cancer. *Clin. Cancer Res.* **2019**, *25*, 2033–2041. [CrossRef]
39. Krishnamurti, U.; Silverman, J.F. HER2 in Breast Cancer. *Adv. Anat. Pathol.* **2014**, *21*, 100–107. [CrossRef]
40. Sato, K.; Nagaya, T.; Choyke, P.L.; Kobayashi, H. Near Infrared Photoimmunotherapy in the Treatment of Pleural Disseminated NSCLC: Preclinical Experience. *Theranostics* **2015**, *5*, 698–709. [CrossRef]
41. Sato, K.; Nagaya, T.; Mitsunaga, M.; Choyke, P.L.; Kobayashi, H. Near Infrared Photoimmunotherapy for Lung Metastases. *Cancer Lett.* **2015**, *365*, 112–121. [CrossRef]
42. Sato, K.; Nagaya, T.; Nakamura, Y.; Harada, T.; Choyke, P.L.; Kobayashi, H. Near Infrared Photoimmunotherapy Prevents Lung Cancer Metastases in a Murine Model. *Oncotarget* **2015**, *6*, 19747–19758. [CrossRef] [PubMed]
43. Takahashi, K.; Taki, S.; Yasui, H.; Nishinaga, Y.; Isobe, Y.; Matsui, T.; Shimizu, M.; Koike, C.; Sato, K. HER2 Targeting Near-infrared Photoimmunotherapy for a CDDP-resistant Small-cell Lung Cancer. *Cancer Med.* **2021**, *10*, 8808–8819. [CrossRef] [PubMed]
44. Chen, C.; Zhao, S.; Karnad, A.; Freeman, J.W. The Biology and Role of CD44 in Cancer Progression: Therapeutic Implications. *J. Hematol. Oncol.* **2018**, *11*, 64. [CrossRef] [PubMed]
45. Zhao, S.; He, J.L.; Qiu, Z.X.; Chen, N.Y.; Luo, Z.; Chen, B.J.; Li, W.M. Prognostic Value of CD44 Variant Exon 6 Expression in Non-Small Cell Lung Cancer: A Meta-Analysis. *Asian Pacific J. Cancer Prev.* **2014**, *15*, 6761–6766. [CrossRef]
46. Zöller, M. CD44: Can a Cancer-Initiating Cell Profit from an Abundantly Expressed Molecule? *Nat. Rev. Cancer* **2011**, *11*, 254–267. [CrossRef]
47. Yan, Y.; Zuo, X.; Wei, D. Concise Review: Emerging Role of CD44 in Cancer Stem Cells: A Promising Biomarker and Therapeutic Target. *Stem Cells Transl. Med.* **2015**, *4*, 1033–1043. [CrossRef]
48. Nagaya, T.; Nakamura, Y.; Okuyama, S.; Ogata, F.; Maruoka, Y.; Choyke, P.L.; Allen, C.; Kobayashi, H. Syngeneic Mouse Models of Oral Cancer Are Effectively Targeted by Anti-CD44-Based NIR-PIT. *Mol. Cancer Res.* **2017**, *15*, 1667–1677. [CrossRef]
49. Jin, J.; Krishnamachary, B.; Mironchik, Y.; Kobayashi, H.; Bhujwalla, Z.M. Phototheranostics of CD44-Positive Cell Populations in Triple Negative Breast Cancer. *Sci. Rep.* **2016**, *6*, 27871. [CrossRef]
50. Maruoka, Y.; Furusawa, A.; Okada, R.; Inagaki, F.; Wakiyama, H.; Kato, T.; Nagaya, T.; Choyke, P.L.; Kobayashi, H. Interleukin-15 after Near-Infrared Photoimmunotherapy (NIR-PIT) Enhances T Cell Response against Syngeneic Mouse Tumors. *Cancers* **2020**, *12*, 2575. [CrossRef]
51. Nagaya, T.; Friedman, J.; Maruoka, Y.; Ogata, F.; Okuyama, S.; Clavijo, P.E.; Choyke, P.L.; Allen, C.; Kobayashi, H. Host Immunity Following Near-Infrared Photoimmunotherapy Is Enhanced with PD-1 Checkpoint Blockade to Eradicate Established Antigenic Tumors. *Cancer Immunol. Res.* **2019**, *7*, 401–413. [CrossRef]
52. Maruoka, Y.; Furusawa, A.; Okada, R.; Inagaki, F.; Fujimura, D.; Wakiyama, H.; Kato, T.; Nagaya, T.; Choyke, P.L.; Kobayashi, H. Near-Infrared Photoimmunotherapy Combined with CTLA4 Checkpoint Blockade in Syngeneic Mouse Cancer Models. *Vaccines* **2020**, *8*, 528. [CrossRef] [PubMed]
53. Campos-da-Paz, M.; Dórea, J.G.; Galdino, A.S.; Lacava, Z.G.M.; de Fatima Menezes Almeida Santos, M. Carcinoembryonic Antigen (CEA) and Hepatic Metastasis in Colorectal Cancer: Update on Biomarker for Clinical and Biotechnological Approaches. *Recent Pat. Biotechnol.* **2018**, *12*, 269–279. [CrossRef] [PubMed]
54. Grunnet, M.; Sorensen, J.B.B. Carcinoembryonic Antigen (CEA) as Tumor Marker in Lung Cancer. *Lung Cancer* **2012**, *76*, 138–143. [CrossRef]
55. Hammarström, S. The Carcinoembryonic Antigen (CEA) Family: Structures, Suggested Functions and Expression in Normal and Malignant Tissues. *Semin. Cancer Biol.* **1999**, *9*, 67–81. [CrossRef] [PubMed]
56. Shirasu, N.; Yamada, H.; Shibaguchi, H.; Kuroki, M.M.; Kuroki, M.M. Potent and Specific Antitumor Effect of CEA-Targeted Photoimmunotherapy. *Int. J. Cancer* **2014**, *135*, 2697–2710. [CrossRef] [PubMed]
57. Maawy, A.A.; Hiroshima, Y.; Zhang, Y.; Heim, R.; Makings, L.; Garcia-Guzman, M.; Luiken, G.A.; Kobayashi, H.; Hoffman, R.M.; Bouvet, M. Near Infra-Red Photoimmunotherapy with Anti-CEA-IR700 Results in Extensive Tumor Lysis and a Significant Decrease in Tumor Burden in Orthotopic Mouse Models of Pancreatic Cancer. *PLoS ONE* **2015**, *10*, e0121989. [CrossRef]
58. Hiroshima, Y.; Maawy, A.; Zhang, Y.; Guzman, M.G.; Heim, R.; Makings, L.; Luiken, G.A.; Kobayashi, H.; Tanaka, K.; Endo, I.; et al. Photoimmunotherapy Inhibits Tumor Recurrence After Surgical Resection on a Pancreatic Cancer Patient-Derived Orthotopic Xenograft (PDOX) Nude Mouse Model. *Ann. Surg. Oncol.* **2015**, *22*, 1469–1474. [CrossRef]

59. Maawy, A.A.; Hiroshima, Y.; Zhang, Y.; Garcia-Guzman, M.; Luiken, G.A.; Kobayashi, H.; Hoffman, R.M.; Bouvet, M. Photoimmunotherapy Lowers Recurrence after Pancreatic Cancer Surgery in Orthotopic Nude Mouse Models. *J. Surg. Res.* **2015**, *197*, 5–11. [CrossRef]
60. Quintanilla, M.; Montero-Montero, L.; Renart, J.; Martín-Villar, E. Podoplanin in Inflammation and Cancer. *Int. J. Mol. Sci.* **2019**, *20*, 707. [CrossRef]
61. Schacht, V.; Ramirez, M.I.; Hong, Y.-K.K.; Hirakawa, S.; Feng, D.; Harvey, N.; Williams, M.; Dvorak, A.M.; Dvorak, H.F.; Oliver, G.; et al. T1α/Podoplanin Deficiency Disrupts Normal Lymphatic Vasculature Formation and Causes Lymphedema. *EMBO J.* **2003**, *22*, 3546–3556. [CrossRef]
62. Wicki, A.; Lehembre, F.; Wick, N.; Hantusch, B.; Kerjaschki, D.; Christofori, G. Tumor Invasion in the Absence of Epithelial-Mesenchymal Transition: Podoplanin-Mediated Remodeling of the Actin Cytoskeleton. *Cancer Cell* **2006**, *9*, 261–272. [CrossRef] [PubMed]
63. Wicki, A.; Christofori, G. The Potential Role of Podoplanin in Tumour Invasion. *Br. J. Cancer* **2007**, *96*, 1–5. [CrossRef] [PubMed]
64. Nishinaga, Y.; Sato, K.; Yasui, H.; Taki, S.; Takahashi, K.; Shimizu, M.; Endo, R.; Koike, C.; Kuramoto, N.; Nakamura, S.; et al. Targeted Phototherapy for Malignant Pleural Mesothelioma: Near-Infrared Photoimmunotherapy Targeting Podoplanin. *Cells* **2020**, *9*, 1019. [CrossRef] [PubMed]
65. Yasui, H.; Nishinaga, Y.; Taki, S.; Takahashi, K.; Isobe, Y.; Sato, K. Near Infrared Photoimmunotherapy for Mouse Models of Pleural Dissemination. *J. Vis. Exp.* **2021**, *2021*, e61593. [CrossRef]
66. Ordóñez, N.G. Application of Mesothelin Immunostaining in Tumor Diagnosis. *Am. J. Surg. Pathol.* **2003**, *27*, 1418–1428. [CrossRef]
67. Vizcaya, D.; Farahmand, B.; Walter, A.O.; Kneip, C.; Jöhrens, K.; Tukiainen, P.; Schmitz, A.A. Prognosis of Patients with Malignant Mesothelioma by Expression of Programmed Cell Death 1 Ligand 1 and Mesothelin in a Contemporary Cohort in Finland. *Cancer Treat. Res. Commun.* **2020**, *25*, 100260. [CrossRef]
68. Feng, F.; Zhang, H.; Zhang, Y.; Wang, H. Level of Mesothelin Expression Can Indicate the Prognosis of Malignant Pleural Mesothelioma. *Transl. Cancer Res.* **2020**, *9*, 7479–7485. [CrossRef]
69. He, X.; Wang, L.; Riedel, H.; Wang, K.; Yang, Y.; Dinu, C.Z.; Rojanasakul, Y. Mesothelin Promotes Epithelial-to-Mesenchymal Transition and Tumorigenicity of Human Lung Cancer and Mesothelioma Cells. *Mol. Cancer* **2017**, *16*, 63. [CrossRef]
70. Kaneko, O.; Gong, L.; Zhang, J.; Hansen, J.K.; Hassan, R.; Lee, B.; Ho, M. A Binding Domain on Mesothelin for CA125/MUC16. *J. Biol. Chem.* **2009**, *284*, 3739–3749. [CrossRef]
71. Weidemann, S.; Gagelmann, P.; Gorbokon, N.; Lennartz, M.; Menz, A.; Luebke, A.M.; Kluth, M.; Hube-Magg, C.; Blessin, N.C.; Fraune, C.; et al. Mesothelin Expression in Human Tumors: A Tissue Microarray Study on 12,679 Tumors. *Biomedicines* **2021**, *9*, 397. [CrossRef]
72. Yeo, D.; Castelletti, L.; van Zandwijk, N.; Rasko, J.E.J. Hitting the Bull's-Eye: Mesothelin's Role as a Biomarker and Therapeutic Target for Malignant Pleural Mesothelioma. *Cancers* **2021**, *13*, 3932. [CrossRef] [PubMed]
73. Nagaya, T.; Nakamura, Y.; Sato, K.; Zhang, Y.-F.; Ni, M.; Choyke, P.L.; Ho, M.; Kobayashi, H. Near Infrared Photoimmunotherapy with an Anti-Mesothelin Antibody. *Oncotarget* **2016**, *7*, 23361–23369. [CrossRef] [PubMed]
74. Cohen, A.S.; Khalil, F.K.; Welsh, E.A.; Schabath, M.B.; Enkemann, S.A.; Davis, A.; Zhou, J.-M.; Boulware, D.C.; Kim, J.; Haura, E.B.; et al. Cell-Surface Marker Discovery for Lung Cancer. *Oncotarget* **2017**, *8*, 113373–113402. [CrossRef]
75. Gugger, M.; White, R.; Song, S.; Waser, B.; Cescato, R.; Rivière, P.; Reubi, J.C. GPR87 Is an Overexpressed G-Protein Coupled Receptor in Squamous Cell Carcinoma of the Lung. *Dis. Markers* **2008**, *24*, 41–50. [CrossRef]
76. Nii, K.; Tokunaga, Y.; Liu, D.; Zhang, X.; Nakano, J.; Ishikawa, S.; Kakehi, Y.; Haba, R.; Yokomise, H. Overexpression of G Protein-Coupled Receptor 87 Correlates with Poorer Tumor Differentiation and Higher Tumor Proliferation in Non-Small-Cell Lung Cancer. *Mol. Clin. Oncol.* **2014**, *2*, 539–544. [CrossRef] [PubMed]
77. Wang, L.; Zhou, W.; Zhong, Y.; Huo, Y.; Fan, P.; Zhan, S.; Xiao, J.; Jin, X.; Gou, S.; Yin, T.; et al. Overexpression of G Protein-Coupled Receptor GPR87 Promotes Pancreatic Cancer Aggressiveness and Activates NF-KB Signaling Pathway. *Mol. Cancer* **2017**, *16*, 61. [CrossRef]
78. Yasui, H.; Nishinaga, Y.; Taki, S.; Takahashi, K.; Isobe, Y.; Shimizu, M.; Koike, C.; Taki, T.; Sakamoto, A.; Katsumi, K.; et al. Near-Infrared Photoimmunotherapy Targeting GPR87: Development of a Humanised Anti-GPR87 MAb and Therapeutic Efficacy on a Lung Cancer Mouse Model. *EBioMedicine* **2021**, *67*, 103372. [CrossRef]
79. Katoh, M.; Katoh, M. Precision Medicine for Human Cancers with Notch Signaling Dysregulation (Review). *Int. J. Mol. Med.* **2020**, *45*, 279–297. [CrossRef]
80. Owen, D.H.; Giffin, M.J.; Bailis, J.M.; Smit, M.-A.D.; Carbone, D.P.; He, K. DLL3: An Emerging Target in Small Cell Lung Cancer. *J. Hematol. Oncol.* **2019**, *12*, 61. [CrossRef]
81. Rudin, C.M.; Pietanza, M.C.; Bauer, T.M.; Ready, N.; Morgensztern, D.; Glisson, B.S.; Byers, L.A.; Johnson, M.L.; Burris, H.A.; Robert, F.; et al. Rovalpituzumab Tesirine, a DLL3-Targeted Antibody-Drug Conjugate, in Recurrent Small-Cell Lung Cancer: A First-in-Human, First-in-Class, Open-Label, Phase 1 Study. *Lancet Oncol.* **2017**, *18*, 42–51. [CrossRef]
82. Isobe, Y.; Sato, K.; Nishinaga, Y.; Takahashi, K.; Taki, S.; Yasui, H.; Shimizu, M.; Endo, R.; Koike, C.; Kuramoto, N.; et al. Near Infrared Photoimmunotherapy Targeting DLL3 for Small Cell Lung Cancer. *EBioMedicine* **2020**, *52*, 102632. [CrossRef] [PubMed]
83. De Zutter, A.; Van Damme, J.; Struyf, S. The Role of Post-Translational Modifications of Chemokines by CD26 in Cancer. *Cancers* **2021**, *13*, 4247. [CrossRef]

84. Enz, N.; Vliegen, G.; De Meester, I.; Jungraithmayr, W. CD26/DPP4—A Potential Biomarker and Target for Cancer Therapy. *Pharmacol. Ther.* **2019**, *198*, 135–159. [CrossRef] [PubMed]
85. Inamoto, T.; Yamada, T.; Ohnuma, K.; Kina, S.; Takahashi, N.; Yamochi, T.; Inamoto, S.; Katsuoka, Y.; Hosono, O.; Tanaka, H.; et al. Humanized Anti-CD26 Monoclonal Antibody as a Treatment for Malignant Mesothelioma Tumors. *Clin. Cancer Res.* **2007**, *13*, 4191–4200. [CrossRef]
86. Angevin, E.; Isambert, N.; Trillet-Lenoir, V.; You, B.; Alexandre, J.; Zalcman, G.; Vielh, P.; Farace, F.; Valleix, F.; Podoll, T.; et al. First-in-Human Phase 1 of YS110, a Monoclonal Antibody Directed against CD26 in Advanced CD26-Expressing Cancers. *Br. J. Cancer* **2017**, *116*, 1126–1134. [CrossRef] [PubMed]
87. Sheng, Q.; D'Alessio, J.A.; Menezes, D.L.; Karim, C.; Tang, Y.; Tam, A.; Clark, S.; Ying, C.; Connor, A.; Mansfield, K.G.; et al. PCA062, a P-Cadherin Targeting Antibody–Drug Conjugate, Displays Potent Antitumor Activity against P-Cadherin–Expressing Malignancies. *Mol. Cancer Ther.* **2021**, *20*, 1270–1282. [CrossRef] [PubMed]
88. Hsiao, T.F.; Wang, C.L.; Wu, Y.C.; Feng, H.P.; Chiu, Y.C.; Lin, H.Y.; Liu, K.J.; Chang, G.C.; Chien, K.Y.; Yu, J.S.; et al. Integrative Omics Analysis Reveals Soluble Cadherin-3 as a Survival Predictor and an Early Monitoring Marker of EGFR Tyrosine Kinase Inhibitor Therapy in Lung Cancer. *Clin. Cancer Res.* **2020**, *26*, 3220–3229. [CrossRef]
89. Imai, S.; Kobayashi, M.; Takasaki, C.; Ishibashi, H.; Okubo, K. High Expression of P-Cadherin Is Significantly Associated with Poor Prognosis in Patients with Non-Small-Cell Lung Cancer. *Lung Cancer* **2018**, *118*, 13–19. [CrossRef]
90. Lenárt, S.; Lenárt, P.; Šmarda, J.; Remšík, J.; Souček, K.; Beneš, P. Trop2: Jack of All Trades, Master of None. *Cancers* **2020**, *12*, 3328. [CrossRef]
91. Zeng, P.; Chen, M.B.; Zhou, L.N.; Tang, M.; Liu, C.Y.; Lu, P.H. Impact of TROP2 Expression on Prognosis in Solid Tumors: A Systematic Review and Meta-Analysis. *Sci. Rep.* **2016**, *6*, 33658. [CrossRef]
92. Ahmed, Y.; Berenguer-Pina, J.J.; Mahgoub, T. The Rise of the TROP2-Targeting Agents in NSCLC: New Options on the Horizon. *Oncology* **2021**, *99*, 673–680. [CrossRef] [PubMed]
93. Scanlan, M.J.; Gure, A.O.; Jungbluth, A.A.; Old, L.J.; Chen, Y.T. Cancer/Testis Antigens: An Expanding Family of Targets for Cancer Immunotherapy. *Immunol. Rev.* **2002**, *188*, 22–32. [CrossRef] [PubMed]
94. Sakai, Y.; Kurose, K.; Sakaeda, K.; Abo, H.; Atarashi, Y.; Ide, N.; Sato, T.; Kanda, E.; Fukuda, M.; Oga, T.; et al. A Novel Automated Immunoassay for Serum NY-ESO-1 and XAGE1 Antibodies in Combinatory Prediction of Response to Anti-Programmed Cell Death-1 Therapy in Non-Small-Cell Lung Cancer. *Clin. Chim. Acta* **2021**, *519*, 51–59. [CrossRef] [PubMed]
95. Ohue, Y.; Kurose, K.; Mizote, Y.; Matsumoto, H.; Nishio, Y.; Isobe, M.; Fukuda, M.; Uenaka, A.; Oka, M.; Nakayama, E. Prolongation of Overall Survival in Advanced Lung Adenocarcinoma Patients with the XAGE1 (GAGED2a) Antibody. *Clin. Cancer Res.* **2014**, *20*, 5052–5063. [CrossRef]
96. Nakagawa, K.; Noguchi, Y.; Uenaka, A.; Sato, S.; Okumura, H.; Tanaka, M.; Shimono, M.; Eldib, A.M.A.; Ono, T.; Ohara, N.; et al. XAGE-1 Expression in Non–Small Cell Lung Cancer and Antibody Response in Patients. *Clin. Cancer Res.* **2005**, *11*, 5496–5503. [CrossRef]
97. Sato, K.; Sato, N.; Xu, B.; Nakamura, Y.; Nagaya, T.; Choyke, P.L.; Hasegawa, Y.; Kobayashi, H. Spatially Selective Depletion of Tumor-Associated Regulatory T Cells with near-Infrared Photoimmunotherapy. *Sci. Transl. Med.* **2016**, *8*, 352.ra110. [CrossRef]
98. Spolski, R.; Li, P.; Leonard, W.J. Biology and Regulation of IL-2: From Molecular Mechanisms to Human Therapy. *Nat. Rev. Immunol.* **2018**, *18*, 648–659. [CrossRef]
99. Lu, J.; Chen, X.M.; Huang, H.R.; Zhao, F.P.; Wang, F.; Liu, X.; Li, X.P. Detailed Analysis of Inflammatory Cell Infiltration and the Prognostic Impact on Nasopharyngeal Carcinoma. *Head Neck* **2018**, *40*, 1245–1253. [CrossRef]
100. Zou, W. Regulatory T Cells, Tumour Immunity and Immunotherapy. *Nat. Rev. Immunol.* **2006**, *6*, 295–307. [CrossRef]
101. Maruoka, Y.; Furusawa, A.; Okada, R.; Inagaki, F.; Fujimura, D.; Wakiyama, H.; Kato, T.; Nagaya, T.; Choyke, P.L.; Kobayashi, H.; et al. Combined CD44- and CD25-Targeted Near-Infrared Photoimmunotherapy Selectively Kills Cancer and Regulatory T Cells in Syngeneic Mouse Cancer Models. *Cancer Immunol.* **2020**, *8*, 345–355. [CrossRef]
102. Sharpe, A.H.; Wherry, E.J.; Ahmed, R.; Freeman, G.J. The Function of Programmed Cell Death 1 and Its Ligands in Regulating Autoimmunity and Infection. *Nat. Immunol.* **2007**, *8*, 239–245. [CrossRef] [PubMed]
103. Patel, S.P.; Kurzrock, R. PD-L1 Expression as a Predictive Biomarker in Cancer Immunotherapy. *Mol. Cancer Ther.* **2015**, *14*, 847–856. [CrossRef] [PubMed]
104. Pardoll, D.M. The Blockade of Immune Checkpoints in Cancer Immunotherapy. *Nat. Rev. Cancer* **2012**, *12*, 252–264. [CrossRef] [PubMed]
105. Taki, S.; Matsuoka, K.; Nishinaga, Y.; Takahashi, K.; Yasui, H.; Koike, C.; Shimizu, M.; Sato, M.; Sato, K. Spatiotemporal Depletion of Tumor-Associated Immune Checkpoint PD-L1 with near-Infrared Photoimmunotherapy Promotes Antitumor Immunity. *J. Immunother. Cancer* **2021**, *9*, e003036. [CrossRef] [PubMed]
106. Nagaya, T.; Nakamura, Y.; Sato, K.; Harada, T.; Choyke, P.L.; Hodge, J.W.; Schlom, J.; Kobayashi, H. Near Infrared Photoimmunotherapy with Avelumab, an Anti-Programmed Death-Ligand 1 (PD-L1) Antibody. *Oncotarget* **2017**, *8*, 8807–8817. [CrossRef]
107. Buchbinder, E.I.; Desai, A. CTLA-4 and PD-1 Pathways. *Am. J. Clin. Oncol.* **2016**, *39*, 98–106. [CrossRef]
108. Rowshanravan, B.; Halliday, N.; Sansom, D.M. CTLA-4: A Moving Target in Immunotherapy. *Blood* **2018**, *131*, 58–67. [CrossRef]
109. Walker, L.S.K.; Sansom, D.M. The Emerging Role of CTLA4 as a Cell-Extrinsic Regulator of T Cell Responses. *Nat. Rev. Immunol.* **2011**, *11*, 852–863. [CrossRef]

110. Okada, R.; Kato, T.; Furusawa, A.; Inagaki, F.; Wakiyama, H.; Choyke, P.L.; Kobayashi, H. Local Depletion of Immune Checkpoint Ligand CTLA4 Expressing Cells in Tumor Beds Enhances Antitumor Host Immunity. *Adv. Ther.* **2021**, *4*, 2000269. [CrossRef]
111. Kato, T.; Okada, R.; Furusawa, A.; Inagaki, F.; Wakiyama, H.; Furumoto, H.; Okuyama, S.; Fukushima, H.; Choyke, P.L.; Kobayashi, H. Simultaneously Combined Cancer Cell- and CTLA4-Targeted NIR-PIT Causes a Synergistic Treatment Effect in Syngeneic Mouse Models. *Mol. Cancer Ther.* **2021**, *20*, 2262–2273. [CrossRef]
112. Hirata, H.; Kuwatani, M.; Nakajima, K.; Kodama, Y.; Yoshikawa, Y.; Ogawa, M.; Sakamoto, N. Near-Infrared Photoimmunotherapy (NIR-PIT) on Cholangiocarcinoma Using a Novel Catheter Device with Light Emitting Diodes. *Cancer Sci.* **2021**, *112*, 828–838. [CrossRef] [PubMed]
113. Sato, K.; Watanabe, R.; Hanaoka, H.; Nakajima, T.; Choyke, P.L.; Kobayashi, H. Comparative Effectiveness of Light Emitting Diodes (LEDs) and Lasers in near Infrared Photoimmunotherapy. *Oncotarget* **2016**, *7*, 14324–14335. [CrossRef] [PubMed]
114. Okuyama, S.; Nagaya, T.; Sato, K.; Ogata, F.; Maruoka, Y.; Choyke, P.L.; Kobayashi, H. Interstitial Near-Infrared Photoimmunotherapy: Effective Treatment Areas and Light Doses Needed for Use with Fiber Optic Diffusers. *Oncotarget* **2018**, *9*, 11159–11169. [CrossRef] [PubMed]
115. Okada, R.; Furusawa, A.; Inagaki, F.; Wakiyama, H.; Kato, T.; Okuyama, S.; Furumoto, H.; Fukushima, H.; Choyke, P.L.; Kobayashi, H.; et al. Endoscopic Near-Infrared Photoimmunotherapy in an Orthotopic Head and Neck Cancer Model. *Cancer Sci.* **2021**, *112*, 3041–3049. [CrossRef]
116. Zhong, W.; Celli, J.P.; Rizvi, I.; Mai, Z.; Spring, B.Q.; Yun, S.H.; Hasan, T. In Vivo High-Resolution Fluorescence Microendoscopy for Ovarian Cancer Detection and Treatment Monitoring. *Br. J. Cancer* **2009**, *101*, 2015–2022. [CrossRef]
117. Henderson, T.A.; Morries, L.D.; TA, H.; LD, M.; Henderson, T.A.; Morries, L.D. Near-Infrared Photonic Energy Penetration: Can Infrared Phototherapy Effectively Reach the Human Brain? *Neuropsychiatr. Dis. Treat.* **2015**, *11*, 2191–2208. [CrossRef]
118. Nakajima, K.; Kimura, T.; Takakura, H.; Yoshikawa, Y.; Kameda, A.; Shindo, T.; Sato, K.; Kobayashi, H.; Ogawa, M. Implantable Wireless Powered Light Emitting Diode (LED) for near-Infrared Photoimmunotherapy: Device Development and Experimental Assessment in Vitro and in Vivo. *Oncotarget* **2018**, *9*, 20048–20057. [CrossRef]
119. Ogata, F.; Nagaya, T.; Nakamura, Y.; Sato, K.; Okuyama, S.; Maruoka, Y.; Choyke, P.L.; Kobayashi, H.; Ogata, F.; Nagaya, T.; et al. Near-Infrared Photoimmunotherapy: A Comparison of Light Dosing Schedules. *Oncotarget* **2017**, *8*, 35069–35075. [CrossRef]
120. Matsuoka, K.; Sato, M.; Sato, K. Hurdles for the Wide Implementation of Photoimmunotherapy. *Immunotherapy* **2021**, *13*, 1427–1438. [CrossRef]
121. Okuyama, S.; Nagaya, T.; Ogata, F.; Maruoka, Y.; Sato, K.; Nakamura, Y.; Choyke, P.L.; Kobayashi, H. Avoiding Thermal Injury during Near-Infrared Photoimmunotherapy (NIR-PIT): The Importance of NIR Light Power Density. *Oncotarget* **2017**, *8*, 113194–113201. [CrossRef]
122. Furumoto, H.; Kato, T.; Wakiyama, H.; Furusawa, A.; Choyke, P.L.; Kobayashi, H. Endoscopic Applications of Near-Infrared Photoimmunotherapy (NIR-PIT) in Cancers of the Digestive and Respiratory Tracts. *Biomedicines* **2022**, *10*, 846. [CrossRef] [PubMed]
123. Maruoka, Y.; Nagaya, T.; Nakamura, Y.; Sato, K.; Ogata, F.; Okuyama, S.; Choyke, P.L.; Kobayashi, H. Evaluation of Early Therapeutic Effects after Near-Infrared Photoimmunotherapy (NIR-PIT) Using Luciferase-Luciferin Photon-Counting and Fluorescence Imaging. *Mol. Pharm.* **2017**, *14*, 4628–4635. [CrossRef] [PubMed]
124. Inagaki, F.F.; Fujimura, D.; Furusawa, A.; Okada, R.; Wakiyama, H.; Kato, T.; Choyke, P.L.; Kobayashi, H. Fluorescence Imaging of Tumor-Accumulating Antibody-IR700 Conjugates Prior to Near-Infrared Photoimmunotherapy (NIR-PIT) Using a Commercially Available Camera Designed for Indocyanine Green. *Mol. Pharm.* **2021**, *18*, 1238–1246. [CrossRef] [PubMed]
125. Okuyama, S.; Fujimura, D.; Inagaki, F.; Okada, R.; Maruoka, Y.; Wakiyama, H.; Kato, T.; Furusawa, A.; Choyke, P.L.; Kobayashi, H. Real-Time IR700 Fluorescence Imaging During Near-Infrared Photoimmunotherapy Using a Clinically-Approved Camera for Indocyanine Green. *Cancer Diagn. Progn.* **2021**, *1*, 29–34. [CrossRef]
126. Ali, T.; Nakajima, T.; Sano, K.; Sato, K.; Choyke, P.L.; Kobayashi, H. Dynamic Fluorescent Imaging with Indocyanine Green for Monitoring the Therapeutic Effects of Photoimmunotherapy. *Contrast Media Mol. Imaging* **2014**, *9*, 276–282. [CrossRef]
127. Inagaki, F.F.; Fujimura, D.; Furusawa, A.; Okada, R.; Wakiyama, H.; Kato, T.; Choyke, P.L.; Kobayashi, H. Diagnostic Imaging in Near-infrared Photoimmunotherapy Using a Commercially Available Camera for Indocyanine Green. *Cancer Sci.* **2021**, *112*, 1326–1330. [CrossRef]
128. Nakamura, Y.; Bernardo, M.; Nagaya, T.; Sato, K.; Harada, T.; Choyke, P.L.; Kobayashi, H. MR Imaging Biomarkers for Evaluating Therapeutic Effects Shortly after near Infrared Photoimmunotherapy. *Oncotarget* **2016**, *7*, 17354. [CrossRef]
129. Vaupel, P.; Multhoff, G. Revisiting the Warburg Effect: Historical Dogma versus Current Understanding. *J. Physiol.* **2021**, *599*, 1745–1757.
130. Vaupel, P.; Schmidberger, H.; Mayer, A. The Warburg Effect: Essential Part of Metabolic Reprogramming and Central Contributor to Cancer Progression. *Int. J. Radiat. Biol.* **2019**, *95*, 912–919. [CrossRef]
131. Van der Vos, C.S.; Koopman, D.; Rijnsdorp, S.; Arends, A.J.; Boellaard, R.; van Dalen, J.A.; Lubberink, M.; Willemsen, A.T.M.; Visser, E.P. Quantification, Improvement, and Harmonization of Small Lesion Detection with State-of-the-Art PET. *Eur. J. Nucl. Med. Mol. Imaging* **2017**, *44*, 4–16. [CrossRef]
132. Aarntzen, E.H.J.G.; Heijmen, L.; Oyen, W.J.G. 18F-FDG PET/CT in Local Ablative Therapies: A Systematic Review. *J. Nucl. Med.* **2018**, *59*, 551–556. [CrossRef] [PubMed]

133. Zhang, X.; Higuchi, T.; Achmad, A.; Bhattarai, A.; Tomonaga, H.; Thu, H.N.; Yamaguchi, A.; Hirasawa, H.; Taketomi-Takahashi, A.; Tsushima, Y. Can 18F-Fluorodeoxyglucose Positron Emission Tomography Predict the Response to Radioactive Iodine Therapy in Metastatic Differentiated Thyroid Carcinoma? *Eur. J. Hybrid Imaging* **2018**, *2*, 22. [CrossRef]
134. Sano, K.; Mitsunaga, M.; Nakajima, T.; Choyke, P.L.; Kobayashi, H. Acute Cytotoxic Effects of Photoimmunotherapy Assessed by 18F-FDG PET. *J. Nucl. Med.* **2013**, *54*, 770–775. [CrossRef] [PubMed]
135. Ito, K.; Mitsunaga, M.; Nishimura, T.; Saruta, M.; Iwamoto, T.; Kobayashi, H.; Tajiri, H. Near-Infrared Photochemoimmunotherapy by Photoactivatable Bifunctional Antibody–Drug Conjugates Targeting Human Epidermal Growth Factor Receptor 2 Positive Cancer. *Bioconjug. Chem.* **2017**, *28*, 1458. [CrossRef] [PubMed]
136. Nani, R.R.; Gorka, A.P.; Nagaya, T.; Yamamoto, T.; Ivanic, J.; Kobayashi, H.; Schnermann, M.J. In Vivo Activation of Duocarmycin-Antibody Conjugates by Near-Infrared Light. *ACS Cent. Sci.* **2017**, *3*, 329–337. [CrossRef]
137. Nagaya, T.; Gorka, A.P.; Nani, R.R.; Okuyama, S.; Ogata, F.; Maruoka, Y.; Choyke, P.L.; Schnermann, M.J.; Kobayashi, H. Molecularly Targeted Cancer Combination Therapy with Near-Infrared Photoimmunotherapy and Near-Infrared Photorelease with Duocarmycin–Antibody Conjugate. *Mol. Cancer Ther.* **2018**, *17*, 661–670. [CrossRef] [PubMed]

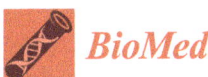

Review

Perspectives on Light-Based Disinfection to Reduce the Risk of COVID-19 Transmission during Dental Care

Abdulrahman A. Balhaddad [1,2], Lamia Mokeem [1], Sharukh S. Khajotia [3], Fernando L. Esteban Florez [3] and Mary A. S. Melo [1,4,*]

[1] Dental Biomedical Sciences, University of Maryland School of Dentistry, Baltimore, MD 21201, USA; aabalhaddad@umaryland.edu (A.A.B.); lsmokeem@umaryland.edu (L.M.)
[2] Department of Restorative Dental Sciences, College of Dentistry, Imam Abdulrahman Bin Faisal University, Dammam 31441, Saudi Arabia
[3] Department of Restorative Sciences, Division of Dental Biomaterials, College of Dentistry, The University of Oklahoma Health Sciences Center, Oklahoma City, OK 73117, USA; sharukh-khajotia@ouhsc.edu (S.S.K.); fernando-Esteban-Florez@ouhsc.edu (F.L.E.F.)
[4] Division of Operative Dentistry, Department of General Dentistry, University of Maryland Dental School, Baltimore, MD 21201, USA
* Correspondence: mmelo@umaryland.edu

Abstract: Severe Acute Respiratory Syndrome 2 (SARS-CoV-2) is a positive-sense single-stranded RNA coronavirus capable of causing potentially lethal pneumonia-like infectious diseases in mammals and birds. The main mechanisms by which SARS-CoV-2 spreads include airborne transmission (aerosols and droplets) and the direct exposure of tissues (conjunctival, nasal, and oral mucosa) to contaminated fluids. The aerosol formation is universal in dentistry due to the use of rotary instruments (handpieces), ultrasonic scalers, and air–water syringes. Several layers of infection control should protect key stakeholders such as dentists, dental staff, and patients. These include the utilization of personal protective equipment, high-volume evacuation systems, pre-procedural mouthwashes, rubber dam, and more recently, antimicrobial photodynamic therapy and intra-oral visible light irradiation. These non-specific light-based approaches are relatively simple, inexpensive, and effective against viruses, bacteria, and fungi. Therefore, the present perspective review discusses the current efforts and limitations on utilizing biophotonic approaches as adjunct infection control methods to prevent the transmission of SARS-CoV-2 in dental settings. In addition, the present perspective review may positively impact subsequent developments in the field, as it offers relevant information regarding the intricacies and complexities of infection control in dental settings.

Keywords: photodynamic therapy; coronavirus; low-level light therapy; photochemotherapy

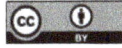

1. Introduction

Coronaviruses are a large family of viruses that include the Middle East Respiratory Syndrome (MERS-CoV), Severe Acute Respiratory Syndrome (SARS-CoV), and Severe Acute Respiratory Syndrome 2 (SARS-CoV-2), which is responsible for the ongoing coronavirus disease (COVID-19) pandemic. These are known to cause infectious respiratory diseases in birds and mammals that range from the common cold to more severe and potentially lethal pneumonia-like diseases. SARS-CoV-2, a positive-sense single-stranded RNA virus, was transferred from bats (original host) and pangolins (intermediate host) to humans in wet markets in Wuhan [1]. According to Chinese health authorities, COVID-19 is clinically translated in patients in the form of flu-like symptoms, including fever (low to mild), runny nose, sputum production, abnormal CT scans of the lungs (opaque glass), and respiratory dysfunction [2]. Even though SARS-CoV-2 incubation times are restricted to between 5 and 6 days, 14 days of quarantine are typically recommended to individuals with suspected COVID-19 exposure, [3] as recent reports indicate that infected patients may continuously shed significant SARS-CoV-2 quanta (viral dose required to cause infection).

The highly contagious characteristics of SARS-CoV-2, its airborne transmission mechanisms, the occurrence of asymptomatic [4] and/or super-spreaders associated with intense intercontinental air travel have significantly favored the exponential spread of this virus amongst humans. These combined factors resulted in global proportions (5) characterized by unprecedented occupational challenges for healthcare workers, including physicians, nurses, dentists, and staff members. Such an event has overwhelmed the healthcare system of numerous countries and was shown to affect people independently of their socioeconomic status, gender, color, or age [5]. Despite the concerning mortality rates previously reported (2–15%), most cases are associated with mild symptoms that do not require any medical intervention or emergency care. However, in severe cases, affected patients display life-threatening conditions, such as dyspnea, acute respiratory distress syndrome (ARDS), acute cardiac injury, acute hepatic injury, acute kidney injury, and multi-organ failure. [6]

SARS-CoV-2 is transmitted via aerosols (<50 μm) and droplets (>50 μm) [7] formed during breathing, speaking, sneezing, and coughing [8,9]. Generated aerosols have been shown to remain suspended in air (still or turbulent) for long periods while maintaining their infectious nature for up to 3 h [10]. The settling of aerosols with potential pathogenic behavior on surfaces (polymeric, ceramic, or metallic) is also of concern for health care settings because contaminated surfaces may act as transmission sources [11].

Once a significant amount of virus has been inhaled by the host, primary viral replication occurs at the upper and lower respiratory tracts. [7] According to Ni et al., the Angiotensin Convertase Enzyme 2 (ACE2), which is a homolog of the angiotensin-converting enzyme (ACE), mediates SARS-CoV-2 infection by allowing the viral spike glycoprotein (two-part protein; S1—primary attachment, S2—viral infusion) to specifically bind to host cells' membrane receptors. After initial attachment, virus' and host cells' membranes fuse, and viral RNA is then released into the cytoplasm, thereby establishing the COVID-19 infection. Even though varying levels of ACE2 expression have been found in different tissues and organs, recent studies have demonstrated that lungs display the highest levels of ACE2 expression in the human body. Other studies have found that SARS-CoV-2 display binding affinities to ACE2 10 to 20 times higher than those previously reported for SARS-CoV-1 [12], which indicates a multifactorial process (aerosol transmission, ACE2 expression, and affinity) by which SARS-CoV-2 preferentially attacks the lungs [13].

ACE2 has important and broad biological functionalities in negating the renin–angiotensin system's role (RAS) in numerous diseases, such as hypertension, myocardial infarction, and heart failure. In addition, ACE2 has also been identified in multiple sites within the oral cavity, including the tongue, gingival tissues, and buccal mucosa, which indicates that the oral cavity could work as a port of entry for SARS-CoV-2. [14]

2. SARS-CoV-2 Transmission in Dental Settings

Even though the current scientific evidence is not conclusive in demonstrating the transmission of SARS-CoV-2 in dental settings due to routine dental procedures (e.g., prophylaxis, cavity preparation, and ultrasonic scaling), it has been shown that SARS-CoV-2 is present in saliva. According to recent studies, SARS-CoV-2 is transferred from the respiratory tract to the oral cavity via liquid droplets and blood from gingival cervical fluids or salivary glands [15]. Despite this knowledge gap, it is well known that aerosol generation is ubiquitous in dentistry, which is considered critical for transmitting SARS-CoV-2 [16]. Previous reports have indicated that the amount of aerosol generated is procedure-specific. The amount of aerosols in dental prophylaxis, cavity preparation, root planing and scaling is dependent on the type of handpiece used (low- and high-speed rotary instruments, ultrasonic scalers, and air/water syringes) (Figure 1). The hands-on nature and limited field of view characteristic in dentistry practice obligate both dentists and dental assistants to work nearby (almost face-to-face) to the source where aerosols with potential pathogenic behavior are generated (e.g., the oral cavity).

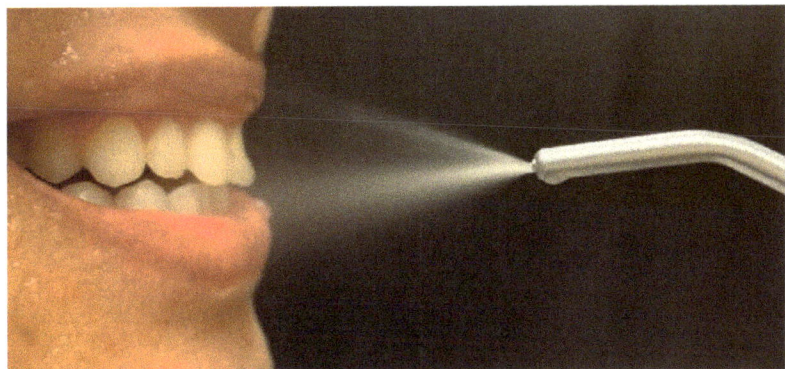

Figure 1. Aerosols generated by air–water syringes hit the hard and soft oral tissues, causing contaminated aerosols, which could be a source of transmitted infection.

In this critical scenario, several manuscripts have indicated that dental settings are particularly susceptible to transmitting different types of microorganisms, including bacteria, fungi, and viruses (Figure 2). In addition, other viruses (noroviruses, rabies, hepatitis B and C, human papillomavirus, Epstein–Barr, herpes simplex, HIV, etc.) [17,18] are present in the oral cavity. These can be efficiently transmitted during dental procedures because aerosols typically get in touch with saliva, dental plaque, and blood [19]. Therefore, based on the context presented and considering the intrinsic characteristics of SARS-CoV-2's and its transmission mechanisms, it is possible to affirm that the oral cavity is a potential source for the transmission of SARS-CoV-2. In a recent report conducted among 2195 dentists in the United States, approximately 0.9% of them were tested positive for SARS-CoV-2 [20]. As aerosols are associated with higher risks for SARS-CoV-2 transmission, many dental organizations have released new infection control protocols in dental settings [21,22].

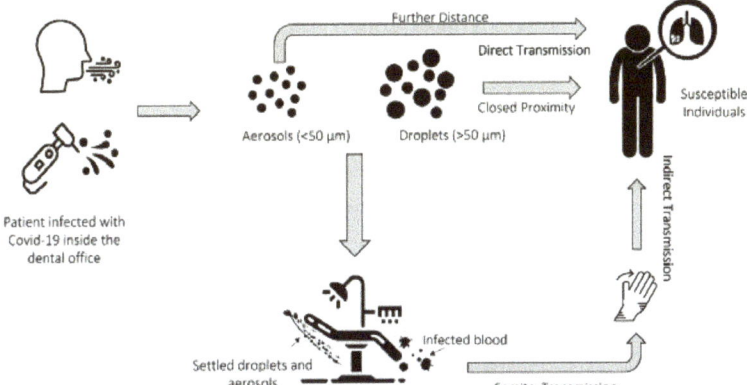

Figure 2. Infectious diseases, including COVID-19, can be directly or indirectly transmitted.

3. Infection Control in Dental Settings

Oral care providers must be familiar with SARS-CoV-2 transmission routes in dental settings. Recently proposed approaches are implementing remote screening procedures (Zoom, Skype, and FaceTime) before the dental visit (24) and limiting the number of key stakeholders in the building to allow for social distancing and the maintenance of fundamental clinical skills operations. It is also essential to frequently disinfect surfaces in clinical (dental chair, cabinets, floors, etc.) and non-clinical areas (restrooms, chairs, sofas, front desk, etc.) that are directly or indirectly exposed to aerosols generated during routine clinical care. Besides, oral care providers should recognize patients with suspected exposure to SARS-CoV-2 or those displaying symptoms of COVID-19 and refer them for further testing and potential treatment, as necessary [23]. To prevent any physical contact with patients during screening procedures and before granting them access to the building, it is advisable that the dental staff use free-hand forehead thermometers to measure patients' temperatures. However, even though laser-based thermometers offer the advantage of a contactless screening procedure, some reports have indicated that these devices cannot accurately determine patients' temperatures when the weather is cold [24]. Consequently, repeated temperature measurements in non-clinical areas (e.g., waiting room) are necessary before executing any dental procedure [25].

Based on the highly infectious nature of SARS-CoV-2, its transmission routes, and the clinical practice of dentistry, which generates large volumes of aerosols with potential pathogenic behavior, it is recommended that three levels of protective measures (primary, secondary, and tertiary) be used [19]. The primary protection level is intended to create a physical barrier that protects the operator and the supporting staff and includes disposable gloves, gowns, surgical masks, N95 masks, goggles, and face shields. Secondary protection involves using disposable isolation clothing over primary protection to further prevent the operator's exposure and shield staff from exposure to highly contagious organic contaminants. Finally, the tertiary level of protection is based on the utilization of containment clothing (also known as Haz-suits) and P95 respirators to fully isolate the operator and supporting staff when a COVID-19 positive patient must be admitted into the dental clinics for emergency dental care [19].

Recent reports have suggested using high-volume saliva evacuators, aerosol containment devices, and four-hand techniques to minimize aerosols' generation with pathogenic behavior in dentistry [26,27]. Despite this critical scenario, elective dental procedures are being conducted in many countries without proper mitigation strategies and independently of the risks of the transmission of SARS-CoV-2. According to Samaranayake, Reid, and Evans (33), dental dams' intraoral utilization can efficiently control approximately 70% of all airborne particles generated during routine dental treatment. Therefore, it should be used as a mechanism to diminish the transmission of SARS-CoV-2 in dental settings. Anti-retraction handpieces are another critical layer of protection in clinical dentistry. These prevent the backflow of liquids containing microorganisms commonly found in the oral cavity into the handpiece's tubbings [28] and has been shown to decrease the potential for hepatitis B transmission. Detailed guidelines for the safe treatment of patients in dental offices during the COVID-19 pandemics can be accessed at the Centers for Disease Control and Prevention (CDC) [22].

4. Preprocedural Disinfection to Prevent the Spreading of SARS-CoV-2

The use of antiseptic mouth rinses before dental procedures has been shown to reduce the microbial load inside the oral cavity, thereby diminishing the risk for the transmission of infectious diseases in dental settings. Chlorhexidine, the most commonly used mouth rinse in dentistry, was demonstrated not to be effective against SARS-CoV-2 [9,29]. However, ongoing investigations have shown possibilities of contributions to reduce viral load. One study has shown that using 0.12% chlorhexidine as a mouth rinse could suppress the activity of SARS-CoV-2 inside the oral cavity for 2 h [30]. Another study has indicated that combining ethanol with chlorhexidine increases the chances for the inactivation of SARS-CoV-2 [31]. Another recently tested approach involved the utilization of povidone-iodine (PVP-I) as a rinse to inactivate SARS-CoV-2 [32,33].

The efficacy of hydrogen peroxide-containing mouth rinses has also been tested, and reported results have demonstrated that these materials only displayed limited inactivation levels against SARS-CoV-2 [33,34]. Therefore, it can be concluded that different mouth rinses display varying inactivation levels against SARS-CoV-2 and that their utilization should not be focused on preventing SARS-CoV-2 transmission in dental settings. Further investigations are necessary to elucidate the mechanisms of action by which these materials may exert unintended antiviral actions against SARS-CoV-2 and determine whether their long-term utilization may increase the risks associated with developing multi-drug resistant bacteria in the oral cavity. In this context, non-specific, broad range, and inexpensive disinfection strategies must be developed, investigated, and validated to mitigate the potential for transmitting infectious diseases in dental settings.

5. Current Trends in Light-Based Oral Disinfection

The use of antimicrobial photodynamic therapy (aPDT) to disinfect dental tissues (soft and hard) has been reported in previous studies [35,36]. aPDT has been shown to effectively reduce oral cariogenic bacteria's viability and those implicated in gingivitis, periodontitis, peri-implantitis, and root canal infections [37]. In this technique, a photosensitizer is typically used in combination with a specific wavelength to generate large quantities of different reactive oxygen species (ROS) such as singlet and triplet oxygen [38]. and These highly oxidative and short-lived species can oxidize, in a non-specific manner, the membranes of numerous microorganisms present in the oral cavity [39]. aPDT is a minimally invasive and ultraconservative technique with several advantages compared to traditional antibiotic disinfection approaches, including its broad-spectrum efficacy against bacteria, fungi, and viruses and its implementation is fast and inexpensive [40,41]. Several studies have also demonstrated that the long-term utilization of aPDT does not induce the development of resistant bacteria because its mechanism of action does not depend on a structure or metabolic pathway [42]. The vast majority of studies investigating the efficacy of aPDT against oral microorganisms have focused on specific target sites such as teeth, periodontal tissues, root canals, or alveolar bones. However, a few reports are available regarding the use of aPDT as a disinfecting approach for the entire oral cavity [43]. In the disinfection approach, the patient is asked to rinse his/her mouth with a photosensitizer's solution, and then, a light irradiation is used to activate the photosensitizer and disinfect the oral cavity (Figure 3).

In 2012, Araujo et al. investigated the efficacy of aPDT to promote oral cavity disinfection in a pilot clinical trial for the first time in dentistry [44]. In that study, participants were instructed not to use any antibiotics or be subjected to professional dental hygiene before the study. Participants fasted for 12 h before collecting saliva samples (before aPDT). After baseline saliva collection, participants were required to swish the curcumin photosensitizer for 5 min forcefully. After that, a visible wavelength (457 nm ± 15 nm) emitted from a light-emitting diode (LED, 67 mW/cm^2) was used to irradiate the oral cavity for 5 min (20.1 J/cm^2). Participants in the control group swished the photosensitizer for 5 min, but the light was not used. Immediately after the intervention (aPDT), saliva samples were collected to assess the presence and quantity of common oral microorganisms. Results reported lower microbial loads in participants treated with aPDT than those observed in the control group.

Even though all participants in the aPDT group have had microbial loads lower than baseline levels, 50% of those participants displayed microbial reductions higher than 80%. However, in the control group, most participants (>50%) did not show any reduction in the observed microbial load. In combination, the findings reported by Araujo et al. in 2012 indicate that aPDT has a solid potential to be used as an adjunct preprocedural disinfection technique to diminish the transmission of airborne infectious diseases. However, despite these promising results, the study cited did not investigate the efficacy of protocols proposed in controlling the oral microbial load 30 to 60 min after the intervention. Such determination is critically important in today's day and age because most dental procedures last for almost an hour and generate large quantities of aerosols with pathogenic behavior [44]. Based on a substantial amount of promising results, [43] the research group led by Dr. Bagnato in Brazil advances the clinical investigation on the efficacy of aPDT approaches to prevent oral infections by conducting a two-arm-randomized clinical trial.

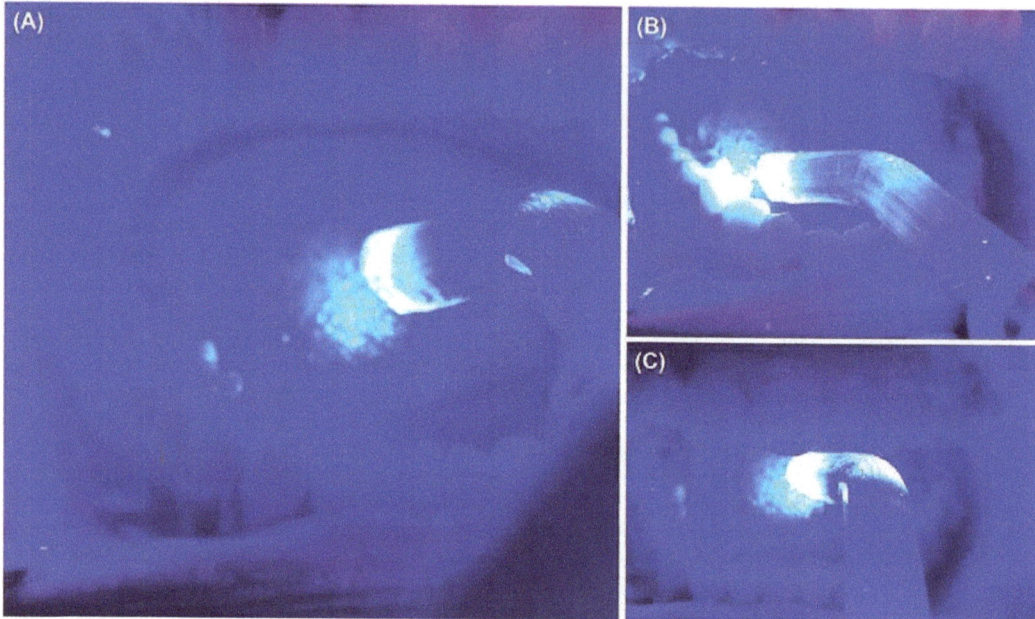

Figure 3. Antimicrobial blue light therapy (aBLT) is a possible alternative way to control COVID-19 transmission during dental care. Patients are asked to rinse their mouth with a photosensitizer-containing solution. Then, the entire oral cavity is irradiated with light in a specific wavelength to activate the photosensitizer (**A**). aBLT can also be applied to other areas at risk of infection or to be treated which can also be disinfected in this intended approach (**B**,**C**).

Leite et al. [43] conducted a study under similar conditions but with higher clinical relevancy because saliva collections took place before disinfection, immediately after aPDT, and 1 and 2 h after that [43]. In that study, participants were then divided into three groups (aPDT, light irradiation only, and curcumin only) and were asked to use 20 mL of curcumin (30 mg/L) for 5 min, followed by visible light irradiation (455 nm ± 15 nm) of the oral cavity for 5 min ($\cong$200 J/cm^2). Time-dependent (immediate, 1 h and 2 h after aPDT) analysis of results demonstrated that aPDT could exert significant and sustainable microbial load reductions in the order of 1-log (90%) compared to baseline values. These promising results were not observed in groups subjected to either light irradiation or curcumin alone, thereby underscoring the necessity to combine light irradiation with a photosensitizer to promote ROS and the consequent death of oral microorganisms. These are critical results because most routine dental visits are usually restricted to a couple of hours. Therefore, determining aPDT's long-term efficacy to disinfect the oral cavity is of fundamental importance to diminish the chances of transmitting infectious diseases in dental settings (Box 1) [43].

Box 1. Summary of the clinical studies concerning the use of antimicrobial photodynamic therapy (aPDT) to disinfect the oral cavity prior to dental procedures.

- The most frequently used photosensitizer to disinfect the oral cavity is curcumin at the following concentrations: 25 mg/L; 30 mg/L; 100 mg/L; 1 g/L, and 1.5 g/L.
- Typical doses of energy used include 20.1 J/cm^2, 85 J/cm^2, 100 J/cm^2 and 200 J/cm^2.
- Concentration-dependent mechanism (higher concentration = higher reductions).
- High curcumin concentrations were found to exert long-term (24 h) effects.
- Future studies should consider different photosensitizers and energy doses.
- aPDT disinfection approaches cited should be investigated against SARS-CoV-2.

In 2016, Panhóca et al. tested the efficacy of aPDT mediated by visible light and curcumin combined or not to sodium dodecyl sulfate (surfactant with known antibacterial properties) as an oral decontamination approach for patients with fixed orthodontic appliances. In that study, participants were randomly distributed into four groups: aPDT (curcumin (1 g/L) + light irradiation (450 nm ± 10 nm)), PDT (curcumin (1 g/L)+ sodium dodecyl sulfate (SDS, 0.1%)) + light irradiation (450 nm ± 10 nm)), light irradiation alone (450 nm ± 10 nm), and 0.12% chlorhexidine gluconate (CHX) [45]. Participants were then requested to forcefully swish the photosensitizer solution with and without the surfactant for 2 min. The intraoral irradiation was then performed for 5 min, with a dose of energy of approximately 100 J/cm^2. Participants in the group subjected to CHX forcefully swished the solution for 30 s.

In all groups, saliva collection occurred immediately after swishing (curcumin alone, curcumin + surfactant or 5% DMSO in water), and immediately after the aPDT. The observed microbial load reductions indicated that the tested protocols established a decreasing efficacy order by which the investigated treatments could be rank-ordered in terms of their antimicrobial potential, as follows: CHX > aPDT + SDS > aPDT > light only. The reported results not only confirm that aPDT can reduce the oral microbial load in orthodontic patients with fixed appliances but have also indicated that surfactants such as SDS may be used in combination to improve the efficacy of aPDT. Therefore, additional studies should be conducted to expand the parameters tested and investigate the effectiveness of light-based approaches against SARS-CoV-2. In addition, it is recommended that follow-up studies consider collecting saliva after 1 and 2 h to explore the intervention's sustainability.

The previous study concerning the use of PDT for oral cavity disinfection was conducted among 50 healthy participants. Visible light (either 450 nm ± 10 nm or 630 nm ± 10 nm) emitted from LED light sources were used to irradiate either curcumin (25 and 100 mg/L) or Photogem (25 and 100 µg/L) [46]. Saliva collection was performed immediately following aPDT and 24 h after. Even though aPDT mediated by curcumin (25 mg/mL) and blue light was shown to reduce the microbial load by 1-log immediately after the intervention, a similar trend could not be observed after 24 h. However, when the aPDT was mediated by curcumin at higher concentrations (100 mg/mL), the immediate microbial load reduction of 1-log was observed after the intervention and maintained for up to 24 h, suggesting a concentration-dependent mechanism, by which sustainability may be achieved through biophotonic approaches. For Photogem, both concentrations tested (25 and 100 µg/mL) immediately induced significant microbial reductions (1-log and 1.5-log, respectively). Furthermore, the results at 24 h indicated microbial loads similar to baseline levels and those on control groups.

In combination, aPDT mediated by curcumin (100 mg/mL) and blue light irradiation may exert microbial load reductions that last for up to 24 h, which indicates that these techniques could be used to significantly decrease the microbial load in the oral cavity when lengthy procedures (orthognathic surgeries, facial reconstruction, and full mouth rehabilitation) are to be performed. On the other hand, aPDT mediated by Photogem and red light irradiation could be efficiently used to significantly decrease the oral cavity's microbial load for short periods. Additional studies are made necessary to further explore the long-term efficacy of Photogem against the oral cavity microbial load [46].

The current scientific evidence on biophotonic techniques suggests that aPDT can be safely and effectively used as adjunct preprocedural disinfection protocols to decrease the microbial load in the oral cavity and potentially reduce the spreading of highly infectious viral diseases in dental settings [47]. Despite these indications, it is crucial to understand previous reports' limitations when using published results (from in vitro, in situ, and in vivo studies) to prove safety and clinical efficacy. The significant restriction relies on reducing oral bacteria, and no reports are available to substantiate the efficacy of biophotonics techniques against SARS-CoV-2. Even though it has been documented that aPDT is effective against several oral and respiratory viruses, including herpes simplex and oral human papilloma, the effect of aPDT against SARS-CoV-2 in saliva has not been established to date.

Therefore, studies should be conducted using similar experimental designs to address the viral load and viability of SARS-CoV-2 in saliva following aPDT protocols. Indocyanine green (ICG) irradiated by a diode laser was found helpful in inactivating herpes simplex types 1 and 2 isolated from the oral cavity in two studies [48,49]. In addition, several studies have reported that ultraviolet irradiation can efficiently inactivate different types of coronaviruses [50].

6. Perspective and Future Outlook

Based on the reported evidence, light-based approaches to disinfect the oral cavity before regular dental exams or treatments are promising but not thoroughly investigated. Studies on the efficacy of aPDT in reducing SARS-CoV-2 levels in the oral cavity and suspended in saliva are lacking. Some points should be considered when designing future clinical trials in this area. Optimum dosimetry (wavelength, power intensity, time, continuous, pulsed, etc.), photosensitizer type and concentration, pre-irradiation time, and the use of surfactants are some of the relevant parameters. For intra-oral applications, it is crucial to determine the effect of influencing factors, such as the position of the light source concerning the oral cavity, irradiation angle (to control non-linear scattering and reflection phenomena), and distance light tip-target area, to name a few. Light-based disinfection approaches that seek to reduce viral and bacterial load can help prevent transmission during dental care, but must be placed in a broader oral health context, recognizing that a single approach using light is insufficient to address the need to prevent the spreading of SARS-CoV-2 in dental settings.

Author Contributions: A.A.B., L.M., S.S.K., F.L.E.F. and M.A.S.M. contributed to the design and the writing of the manuscript. S.S.K., F.L.E.F. and M.A.S.M. contributed to the critical review of the manuscript. All authors have read and agreed to the published version of the manuscript.

Funding: This research received no external funding.

Institutional Review Board Statement: Not applicable.

Informed Consent Statement: Not applicable.

Data Availability Statement: Not applicable.

Acknowledgments: A.A.B. acknowledges the scholarship during his Ph.D. studies from the Imam Abdulrahman bin Faisal University, Dammam, Saudi Arabia, and the Saudi Arabian Cultural Mission.

Conflicts of Interest: The authors declare no conflict of interest.

References

1. Zhu, H.; Wei, L.; Niu, P. The Novel Coronavirus Outbreak in Wuhan, China. *Glob. Health Res. Policy* **2020**, *5*, 6. [CrossRef]
2. Song, F.; Shi, N.; Shan, F.; Zhang, Z.; Shen, J.; Lu, H.; Ling, Y.; Jiang, Y.; Shi, Y. Emerging 2019 Novel Coronavirus (2019-NCoV) Pneumonia. *Radiology* **2020**, *295*, 210–217. [CrossRef]
3. Backer, J.A.; Klinkenberg, D.; Wallinga, J. Incubation Period of 2019 Novel Coronavirus (2019-NCoV) Infections among Travellers from Wuhan, China, 20-28 January 2020. *Eurosurveillance* **2020**, *25*, 2000062. [CrossRef] [PubMed]

4. Li, Q.; Guan, X.; Wu, P.; Wang, X.; Zhou, L.; Tong, Y.; Ren, R.; Leung, K.S.M.; Lau, E.H.Y.; Wong, J.Y.; et al. Early Transmission Dynamics in Wuhan, China, of Novel Coronavirus-Infected Pneumonia. *N. Engl. J. Med.* **2020**, *382*, 1199–1207. [CrossRef]
5. Sohrabi, C.; Alsafi, Z.; O'Neill, N.; Khan, M.; Kerwan, A.; Al-Jabir, A.; Iosifidis, C.; Agha, R. World Health Organization Declares Global Emergency: A Review of the 2019 Novel Coronavirus (COVID-19). *Int. J. Surg.* **2020**, *76*, 71–76. [CrossRef]
6. Zaim, S.; Chong, J.H.; Sankaranarayanan, V.; Harky, A. COVID-19 and Multiorgan Response. *Curr. Probl. Cardiol.* **2020**, *45*, 100618. [CrossRef] [PubMed]
7. Subbarao, K.; Mahanty, S. Respiratory Virus Infections: Understanding COVID-19. *Immunity* **2020**, *52*, 905–909. [CrossRef] [PubMed]
8. Chen, J. Pathogenicity and Transmissibility of 2019-NCoV-A Quick Overview and Comparison with Other Emerging Viruses. *Microbes Infect.* **2020**, *22*, 69–71. [CrossRef]
9. Kampf, G.; Todt, D.; Pfaender, S.; Steinmann, E. Persistence of Coronaviruses on Inanimate Surfaces and Their Inactivation with Biocidal Agents. *J. Hosp. Infect.* **2020**, *104*, 246–251. [CrossRef]
10. Harrel, S.K.; Molinari, J. Aerosols and Splatter in Dentistry: A Brief Review of the Literature and Infection Control Implications. *J. Am. Dent. Assoc.* **2004**, *135*, 429–437. [CrossRef]
11. Chia, P.Y.; Coleman, K.K.; Tan, Y.K.; Ong, S.W.X.; Gum, M.; Lau, S.K.; Lim, X.F.; Lim, A.S.; Sutjipto, S.; Lee, P.H.; et al. Detection of Air and Surface Contamination by SARS-CoV-2 in Hospital Rooms of Infected Patients. *Nat. Commun.* **2020**, *11*, 2800. [CrossRef] [PubMed]
12. Wrapp, D.; Wang, N.; Corbett, K.S.; Goldsmith, J.A.; Hsieh, C.-L.; Abiona, O.; Graham, B.S.; McLellan, J.S. Cryo-EM Structure of the 2019-NCoV Spike in the Prefusion Conformation. *Science* **2020**, *367*, 1260–1263. [CrossRef]
13. Hamming, I.; Timens, W.; Bulthuis, M.L.C.; Lely, A.T.; Navis, G.J.; van Goor, H. Tissue Distribution of ACE2 Protein, the Functional Receptor for SARS Coronavirus. A First Step in Understanding SARS Pathogenesis. *J. Pathol.* **2004**, *203*, 631–637. [CrossRef]
14. Xu, H.; Zhong, L.; Deng, J.; Peng, J.; Dan, H.; Zeng, X.; Li, T.; Chen, Q. High Expression of ACE2 Receptor of 2019-NCoV on the Epithelial Cells of Oral Mucosa. *Int. J. Oral Sci.* **2020**, *12*, 8. [CrossRef]
15. Sabino-Silva, R.; Jardim, A.C.G.; Siqueira, W.L. Coronavirus COVID-19 Impacts to Dentistry and Potential Salivary Diagnosis. *Clin. Oral Investig.* **2020**, *24*, 1619–1621. [CrossRef]
16. Banakar, M.; Bagheri Lankarani, K.; Jafarpour, D.; Moayedi, S.; Banakar, M.H.; MohammadSadeghi, A. COVID-19 Transmission Risk and Protective Protocols in Dentistry: A Systematic Review. *BMC Oral Health* **2020**, *20*, 275. [CrossRef]
17. Hindson, J. COVID-19: Faecal-Oral Transmission? *Nat. Rev. Gastroenterol. Hepatol.* **2020**, *17*, 259. [CrossRef]
18. De Graaf, M.; Beck, R.; Caccio, S.M.; Duim, B.; Fraaij, P.L.; Le Guyader, F.S.; Lecuit, M.; Le Pendu, J.; de Wit, E.; Schultsz, C. Sustained Fecal-Oral Human-to-Human Transmission Following a Zoonotic Event. *Curr. Opin. Virol.* **2017**, *22*, 1–6. [CrossRef] [PubMed]
19. Peng, X.; Xu, X.; Li, Y.; Cheng, L.; Zhou, X.; Ren, B. Transmission Routes of 2019-NCoV and Controls in Dental Practice. *Int. J. Oral Sci.* **2020**, *12*, 9. [CrossRef]
20. Estrich, C.G.; Mikkelsen, M.; Morrissey, R.; Geisinger, M.L.; Ioannidou, E.; Vujicic, M.; Araujo, M.W.B. Estimating COVID-19 Prevalence and Infection Control Practices among US Dentists. *J. Am. Dent. Assoc.* **2020**, *151*, 815–824. [CrossRef] [PubMed]
21. American Dental Association. ADA Interim Guidance for Minimizing Risk of COVID-19 Transmission Risk when Treating Dental Emergencies. Available online: https://www.ada.org/publications/ada-news/2020/april/ada-releases-interim-guidance-on-minimizing-covid-19-transmission-risk-when-treating-emergencies (accessed on 1 April 2020).
22. Centers for Disease and Prevention. Guidance for Dental Settings: Interim Infection Prevention and Control Guidance for Dental Settings during the Coronavirus Disease (COVID-19) Pandemic. Available online: Https://Www.Cdc.Gov/Coronavirus/2019-Ncov/Hcp/Dental-Settings.Html (accessed on 29 June 2020).
23. World Health Organization. Clinical Management of Severe Acute Respiratory Infection When Novel Coronavirus (2019-NCoV) Infection Is Suspected: Interim Guidance. 2020. Available online: https://Www.Who.Int/Publications-Detail/Clinical-Management-of-Severe-Acute-Respiratory-InfecTion-When-Novel-Coronavirus-(Ncov)-Infection-Is-Suspected (accessed on 17 February 2020).
24. Dzien, C.; Halder, W.; Winner, H.; Lechleitner, M. Covid-19 Screening: Are Forehead Temperature Measurements during Cold Outdoor Temperatures Really Helpful? *Wien. Klin. Wochenschr.* **2021**, *133*, 331–335. [CrossRef] [PubMed]
25. Hsiao, S.-H.; Chen, T.-C.; Chien, H.-C.; Yang, C.-J.; Chen, Y.-H. Measurement of Body Temperature to Prevent Pandemic COVID-19 in Hospitals in Taiwan: Repeated Measurement Is Necessary. *J. Hosp. Infect.* **2020**, *105*, 360–361. [CrossRef]
26. Bescos, R.; Casas-Agustench, P.; Belfield, L.; Brookes, Z.; Gabaldón, T. Coronavirus Disease 2019 (COVID-19): Emerging and Future Challenges for Dental and Oral Medicine. *J. Dent. Res.* **2020**, *99*, 1113. [CrossRef]
27. Samaranayake, L.P.; Peiris, M. Severe Acute Respiratory Syndrome and Dentistry: A Retrospective View. *J. Am. Dent. Assoc.* **2004**, *135*, 1292–1302. [CrossRef] [PubMed]
28. Hu, T.; Li, G.; Zuo, Y.; Zhou, X. Risk of Hepatitis B Virus Transmission via Dental Handpieces and Evaluation of an Anti-Suction Device for Prevention of Transmission. *Infect. Control. Hosp. Epidemiol.* **2007**, *28*, 80–82. [CrossRef]
29. Fehr, A.R.; Perlman, S. Coronaviruses: An Overview of Their Replication and Pathogenesis. *Methods Mol. Biol.* **2015**, *1282*, 1–23. [CrossRef]
30. Yoon, J.G.; Yoon, J.; Song, J.Y.; Yoon, S.-Y.; Lim, C.S.; Seong, H.; Noh, J.Y.; Cheong, H.J.; Kim, W.J. Clinical Significance of a High SARS-CoV-2 Viral Load in the Saliva. *J. Korean Med. Sci.* **2020**, *35*, e195. [CrossRef] [PubMed]

31. Kelly, N.; Nic Íomhair, A.; McKenna, G. Can Oral Rinses Play a Role in Preventing Transmission of Covid 19 Infection? *Evid. Based Dent.* **2020**, *21*, 42–43. [CrossRef]
32. Bidra, A.S.; Pelletier, J.S.; Westover, J.B.; Frank, S.; Brown, S.M.; Tessema, B. Rapid In-Vitro Inactivation of Severe Acute Respiratory Syndrome Coronavirus 2 (SARS-CoV-2) Using Povidone-Iodine Oral Antiseptic Rinse. *J. Prosthodont.* **2020**, *29*, 529–533. [CrossRef]
33. Bidra, A.S.; Pelletier, J.S.; Westover, J.B.; Frank, S.; Brown, S.M.; Tessema, B. Comparison of In Vitro Inactivation of SARS CoV-2 with Hydrogen Peroxide and Povidone-Iodine Oral Antiseptic Rinses. *J Prosthodont* **2020**, *29*, 599–603. [CrossRef]
34. Gottsauner, M.J.; Michaelides, I.; Schmidt, B.; Scholz, K.J.; Buchalla, W.; Widbiller, M.; Hitzenbichler, F.; Ettl, T.; Reichert, T.E.; Bohr, C.; et al. A Prospective Clinical Pilot Study on the Effects of a Hydrogen Peroxide Mouthrinse on the Intraoral Viral Load of SARS-CoV-2. *Clin. Oral Investig.* **2020**, *24*, 3707–3713. [CrossRef]
35. Melo, M.a.S.; Rolim, J.P.M.L.; Passos, V.F.; Lima, R.A.; Zanin, I.C.J.; Codes, B.M.; Rocha, S.S.; Rodrigues, L.K.A. Photodynamic Antimicrobial Chemotherapy and Ultraconservative Caries Removal Linked for Management of Deep Caries Lesions. *Photodiagn. Photodyn. Ther.* **2015**, *12*, 581–586. [CrossRef]
36. Melo, M.A.S. Photodynamic Antimicrobial Chemotherapy as a Strategy for Dental Caries: Building a More Conservative Therapy in Restorative Dentistry. *Photomed. Laser Surg.* **2014**, *32*, 589–591. [CrossRef]
37. Balhaddad, A.A.; Garcia, I.M.; Ibrahim, M.S.; Rolim, J.P.M.L.; Gomes, E.A.B.; Martinho, F.C.; Collares, F.M.; Xu, H.; Melo, M.A.S. Prospects on Nano-Based Platforms for Antimicrobial Photodynamic Therapy Against Oral Biofilms. *Photobiomodul. Photomed. Laser Surg.* **2020**, *38*, 481–496. [CrossRef]
38. Rolim, J.P.M.L.; de-Melo, M.A.S.; Guedes, S.F.; Albuquerque-Filho, F.B.; de Souza, J.R.; Nogueira, N.A.P.; Zanin, I.C.J.; Rodrigues, L.K.A. The Antimicrobial Activity of Photodynamic Therapy against Streptococcus Mutans Using Different Photosensitizers. *J. Photochem. Photobiol. B* **2012**, *106*, 40–46. [CrossRef]
39. Balhaddad, A.A.; AlQranei, M.S.; Ibrahim, M.S.; Weir, M.D.; Martinho, F.C.; Xu, H.H.K.; Melo, M.A.S. Light Energy Dose and Photosensitizer Concentration Are Determinants of Effective Photo-Killing against Caries-Related Biofilms. *Int. J. Mol. Sci.* **2020**, *21*, 7612. [CrossRef] [PubMed]
40. Alfirdous, R.A.; Garcia, I.M.; Balhaddad, A.A.; Collares, F.M.; Martinho, F.C.; Melo, M.A.S. Advancing Photodynamic Therapy for Endodontic Disinfection with Nanoparticles: Present Evidence and Upcoming Approaches. *Appl. Sci.* **2021**, *11*, 4759. [CrossRef]
41. Balhaddad, A.A.; Xia, Y.; Lan, Y.; Mokeem, L.; Ibrahim, M.S.; Weir, M.D.; Xu, H.H.K.; Melo, M.A.S. Magnetic-Responsive Photosensitizer Nanoplatform for Optimized Inactivation of Dental Caries-Related Biofilms: Technology Development and Proof of Principle. *ACS Nano* **2021**, *15*, 19888–19904. [CrossRef] [PubMed]
42. Teófilo, M.Í.S.; de Carvalho Russi, T.M.A.Z.; de Barros Silva, P.G.; Balhaddad, A.A.; Melo, M.A.S.; Rolim, J.P.M.L. The Impact of Photosensitizers Selection on Bactericidal Efficacy of PDT against Cariogenic Biofilms: A Systematic Review and Meta-Analysis. *Photodiagn. Photodyn. Ther.* **2020**, *33*, 102046. [CrossRef]
43. Leite, D.P.V.; Paolillo, F.R.; Parmesano, T.N.; Fontana, C.R.; Bagnato, V.S. Effects of Photodynamic Therapy with Blue Light and Curcumin as Mouth Rinse for Oral Disinfection: A Randomized Controlled Trial. *Photomed. Laser Surg.* **2014**, *32*, 627–632. [CrossRef] [PubMed]
44. Araújo, N.C.; Fontana, C.R.; Gerbi, M.E.M.; Bagnato, V.S. Overall-Mouth Disinfection by Photodynamic Therapy Using Curcumin. *Photomed. Laser Surg.* **2012**, *30*, 96–101. [CrossRef]
45. Panhóca, V.H.; Esteban Florez, F.L.; Corrêa, T.Q.; Paolillo, F.R.; de Souza, C.W.O.; Bagnato, V.S. Oral Decontamination of Orthodontic Patients Using Photodynamic Therapy Mediated by Blue-Light Irradiation and Curcumin Associated with Sodium Dodecyl Sulfate. *Photomed. Laser Surg.* **2016**, *34*, 411–417. [CrossRef] [PubMed]
46. Ricci Donato, H.A.; Pratavieira, S.; Grecco, C.; Brugnera-Júnior, A.; Bagnato, V.S.; Kurachi, C. Clinical Comparison of Two Photosensitizers for Oral Cavity Decontamination. *Photomed. Laser Surg.* **2017**, *35*, 105–110. [CrossRef] [PubMed]
47. Kellesarian, S.V.; Qayyum, F.; de Freitas, P.C.; Akram, Z.; Javed, F. Is Antimicrobial Photodynamic Therapy a Useful Therapeutic Protocol for Oral Decontamination? A Systematic Review and Meta-Analysis. *Photodiagn. Photodyn. Ther.* **2017**, *20*, 55–61. [CrossRef] [PubMed]
48. Namvar, M.A.; Vahedi, M.; Abdolsamadi, H.-R.; Mirzaei, A.; Mohammadi, Y.; Azizi Jalilian, F. Effect of Photodynamic Therapy by 810 and 940 Nm Diode Laser on Herpes Simplex Virus 1: An in Vitro Study. *Photodiagn. Photodyn. Ther.* **2019**, *25*, 87–91. [CrossRef]
49. Jin, J.; Zhang, Y.; Zhiyue, L. Successful Treatment of Oral Human Papilloma by Local Injection 5-Aminolevulinic Acid-Mediated Photodynamic Therapy: A Case Report. *Photodiagn. Photodyn. Ther.* **2019**, *26*, 134–136. [CrossRef]
50. Heßling, M.; Hönes, K.; Vatter, P.; Lingenfelder, C. Ultraviolet Irradiation Doses for Coronavirus Inactivation—Review and Analysis of Coronavirus Photoinactivation Studies. *GMS Hyg. Infect. Control.* **2020**, *15*, Doc08. [CrossRef]

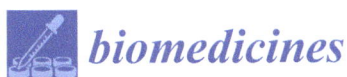

Review

Cellular Mechanisms in Acute and Chronic Wounds after PDT Therapy: An Update

Vieri Grandi [1,2], Alessandro Corsi [3], Nicola Pimpinelli [1] and Stefano Bacci [4,*]

1. Department of Health Sciences, Division of Dermatology, University of Florence, 50100 Florence, Italy; vieri.grandi@unifi.it (V.G.); pimpi@unifi.it (N.P.)
2. Guy's and ST Thomas'NHS Foundation Trust, St John's Institute of Dermatology, London SE17EP, UK
3. Simple Unit of Vulnology, S. Raffaele Hospital, 20100 Milan, Italy; corsi.alessandro@hsr.it
4. Research Unit of Histology and Embriology, Department of Biology, University of Florence, 50100 Florence, Italy
* Correspondence: stefano.bacci@unifi.it

Abstract: PDT is a two-stage treatment that combines light energy with a photosensitizer designed to destroy cancerous and precancerous cells after light activation. Photosensitizers are activated by a specific wavelength of light energy, usually from a laser. The photosensitizer is nontoxic until it is activated by light. However, after light activation, the photosensitizer becomes toxic to the targeted tissue. Among sensitizers, the topical use of ALA, a natural precursor of protoporphyrin IX, a precursor of the heme group, and a powerful photosensitizing agent, represents a turning point for PDT in the dermatological field, as it easily absorbable by the skin. Wound healing requires a complex interaction and coordination of different cells and molecules. Any alteration in these highly coordinated events can lead to either delayed or excessive healing. The goal of this review is to elucidate the cellular mechanisms involved, upon treatment with ALA-PDT, in chronic wounds, which are often associated with social isolation and high costs in terms of care.

Keywords: 5-aminolevulinic acid (ALA); angiogenesis; acute wounds; cellular infiltrate; chronic wounds; mast cells; photodynamic therapy; nerves; neurons; wound healing

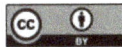

1. The Photodynamic Therapy

In 1903, Von Tappeiner, in collaboration with Jesionek, demonstrated the therapeutic action of light combined with a photosensitizer and oxygen, and coined the term "Photodynamic action" [1]. Since that time, many researchers have experimentally verified the veracity of the efficacy on different biological structures. In medicine, the use of PDT is now widely documented and well-codified for the treatment of oncological and non-oncological diseases. In dermatology, the use varies from oncological pathologies such as basal cell carcinoma, squamous cell carcinoma, actinic and non-oncologic keratoses, bacterial, fungal, viral, immunological or inflammatory infections, to the treatment of chronic wounds, and finally, cosmetology for photorejuvenation [2–5]. PDT is based on the cytotoxic action of some hyperactive oxygen species (i.e., a type of unstable oxygen molecule that easily reacts with other molecules in a cell; a build-up of reactive oxygen species in cells may cause damage to DNA, RNA, and proteins, and potentially induce cell death [6]), especially singlet oxygen, but also superoxide anions and hydroxyl radicals, generated by the transfer of energy and/or electrons from the photoexcited oxygen sensitizer. Three important mechanisms are responsible for the efficacy of PDT: (1) direct death, or inflammation, of tumor cells, (2) damage to tumor vessels, (3) immunological response associated with the stimulation of leukocytes and release of interleukins and other cytokines, growth factors, complement components, acute phase proteins, and other immunoregulators [2–5]. In wound healing, recent studies show the efficacy of PDT for its antibacterial activity, in attacking the biofilm, and in remodeling the extracellular matrix by activating MMPs, thus inducing changes in the collagen of the extracellular matrix for the tissue healing process. In addition, PDT induces cellular changes, which is the phenomenon observed during the course of tissue repair [2–5].

2. Photosensitizers

PDT is a treatment that uses a photosensitizer (administered topically or systemically), light (which interacts with the substance in question), and oxygen to cause selective cell death by necrosis or apoptosis of the cells "atypically" sensitized, in which the photosensitizer or its precursor—administered topically or intravenously—accumulate selectively.

In summary, the photodynamic effect (through photophysical, photochemical, and photobiological mechanisms) is mediated by the generation of ROS, a process that depends on the intracellular interactions of the photosensitizer with light and oxygen [2–5].

The topical use of ALA (Figure 1A), a natural precursor of protoporphyrin IX (Figure 1B) and, in turn, a precursor of the heme group and a powerful photosensitizing agent, represents an important turning point in the dermatological field, as it is easily absorbable by the skin [4,5,7–10]. At the cellular level, the pro-drug, once transformed into protoporphyrin IX, causes the production of reactive oxygen species, which induce cell death in target cells. The presence of ROS in the immediate vicinity of cellular and subcellular membranes (in particular the mitochondrial ridges) allows the release of cytochrome C, with consequent activation of the caspase cascade, which ultimately leads to the intrinsic apoptotic phenomenon. The effect is enhanced by the degeneration of small vessels via a photodynamic mechanism, and by the triggering of an inflammatory reaction [5–9]. The concentration of 5-ALA usually depends on the mode of treatment, but the range is between 2–40% systematically, and 30–50 mg/cm2 topically. It is usually applied for less than 4 h, and it reaches peak accumulation between 3 and 8 h [4,5,7–10].

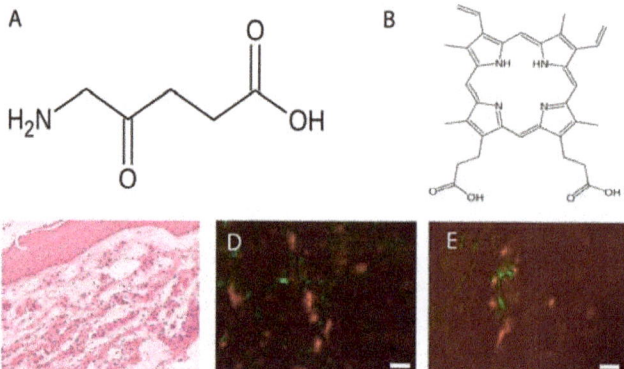

Figure 1. (**A**) Fvasconcellos (own work): Structural diagram of aminolevulinic acid. Created using ACD/ChemSketch 10.0 and Inkscape. This image of *a simple structural formula* is **ineligible for copyright** and, therefore, is in the **public domain**, because it contains no original authorship. (**B**) Fvasconcellos (own work): Skeletal formula of protoporphyrin IX. Created using ACD/ChemSketch 10.0 and Inkscape. The copyright holder of this work has released it into the public domain. This standard applies worldwide. In some countries this may not be legally possible. I grant anyone the right to use this work for any purpose, without any conditions, unless such conditions are required by law. (**C**) Chronic wound: Increased thickness of the epidermis and richness of cellular infiltrate. Hematoxylin Eosin, Light microscopy, scale bar = 10 microns. (**D**) Colocalization between MCs (stained with avidin, in red) and fibroblasts (stained with HSP47, in green) in PDT-treated chronic wounds. Fluorescence microscopy, scale bar =10 microns (see Table 1 for others information). (**E**) Colocalization between MCs (stained with avidin, in red) and DCs (stained with MHC class II, in green) in PDT-treated chronic wounds. Fluorescence microscopy, scale bar =10 microns (see Table 1 for others information).

Table 1. Reagents used to stain inflammatory cells.

Substances	Target	References
HSP 47 (Antibody)	Fibroblasts	[11]
Avidin (Egg white protein linking biotin)	MCs	[12]
MHC class II (Antibody)	Dendritic cells	[13]

3. Wound Healing

Wound healing makes organisms resilient to injuries, allowing survival [14]. This process involves the interaction of various elements, such as soluble mediators (such as cytokines and factors growth), the extracellular matrix, vessels, and various other cell types. The physiological process underlying tissue repair is traditionally divided into four phases: coagulation, inflammatory, proliferative, and maturation [15–22].

Coagulation phase: An initial process occurs during the inflammatory phase of hemostasis, with temporary vasoconstriction caused by release of vasoactive substances by damaged cells, followed by hemorrhage and subsequent platelet aggregation. The platelets, as well as being involved in clot formation, are also important producers of cytokines used in the activation of leukocytes and macrophages. With the aggregation process of the platelets, a biochemical cascade is then activated, in which dozens of factors are involved that lead to formation of an insoluble fibrin network [15–22].

Inflammatory phase: The initial vasoconstriction process is followed by vasodilation mediated by substances such as histamine and serotonin secreted by MCs [23–25]. This leads to increased blood flow in the area of the wound that determines an initial process of migration (diapedesis) of elements of blood corpuscles, such as neutrophil granulocytes, initially, and macrophages, subsequently. There is also increased plasma exudation in the interstitium. The exudate leads to a swelling of the area bordering the wound, the formation of which contributes to local acidosis [15–22]. The migration of leukocytes allows phagocytosis activity at the level of the lesion against pathogenic bacteria and damaged cells. In addition to phagocytosis, leukocytes are responsible for the production and secretion of numerous cytokines and growth factors essential for starting the subsequent phases of the healing process [15–22].

Proliferative phase: The proliferative phase leads to the formation granulation tissue. During this stage, the fibroblasts play a central role, as they are responsible for the production of precursors of collagen, elastin, and other molecules fundamental to the constitution of the extracellular matrix, and are also implicated in the regulation of migration and proliferation of the cellular protagonists involved in the re-epithelialization process and neo-angiogenesis [15–22]. A fundamental role is also played by macrophages and MCs, which provide a continuous supply of growth factors necessary to stimulate angiogenesis. The mechanism of neo-angiogenesis is operated by the endothelial cells of the delimiting vessels at the lesion site, which, undergoing numerous mitotic cycles, give rise to new vessels capable of supplying trophic substances to the granulation tissue forming at the wound. At the epidermal level, on the other hand, the keratinocytes arranged at the edges of the lesion divide and begin to migrate towards the center of the injured site until the two edges rejoin, at which there is inhibition contact [15–22]. Once an abundant collagen matrix has been deposited in the wound, the fibroblasts stop producing collagen and the granulation tissue is replaced by a scar.

Maturation phase: The remodeling of a wound can take up to 1 year. In humans, this phenomenon is characterized by two single processes, wound contraction and collagen restoration, where myofibroblasts allow contraction of the wound, with the formation of a scar both in children and adults [15–22]. During this process, the tensile strength increases, reaching approximately 80% that of unwounded skin, and is in relation to collagen crosslinking by lysyl oxidase [15–22].

4. PDT and Wound Healing

The mechanisms that lead to wound healing upon PDT treatment are not fully understood; however, one of the main reasons is represented by apoptosis, caused by damage to the cellular and mitochondrial membranes, enzymatic inactivation and arrest of cellular respiration processes, and the release of cytochrome C, leading to the activation of the caspase cascade. It has also been observed that PDT modulates the production of MMPs, cytokines, and growth factors by fibroblasts and keratinocytes, substances that can accelerate wound healing [26–28]. In particular, when the process of remodeling is required, MMPs are expressed and activated, and their contribution is related to collagen degradation and extracellular matrix remodeling [26–28].

Some authors have histologically assessed wounds treated with PDT: Mills et al. showed an improvement in matrix deposition in excision wounds [26], and Corsi et al., showed an increase in the thickness of the epidermis (demonstrated by the different location of the basal membrane), as well as that linked to the response of the inflammatory infiltrate [29,30]. An early onset of wound re-epithelialization after PDT has been described by studies in animal models, with the presence of young fibroblasts, fibrin, and granulation tissue [31].

Regarding the inflammatory process that develops [16,22], the occurrence of the following have been observed: the degranulation of MCs and neutrophil granulocytes [23–25,29,30], the formation of oxygen radicals, and the release of lysosomal enzymes and chemotactic agents. The release of antigens of dead cells, in the presence of inflammatory cytokines, determines the activation of skin DCs, which, after the presentation of these antigens to T lymphocytes in the district lymph nodes, stimulates a specific immune response [32].

Occurring simultaneously with the described cellular events, after PDT treatment, lipids are produced, as well as pro-inflammatory cytokines, such as IL-1β and IL-8, demonstrating that therapy has a significant effect on the immune system [26–28]. Moreover, since a balance between the synthesis and degradation of extracellular matrix is required, it is evident that PDT modulates the production of TGF-β [32], the isoforms of which are involved in the deposition of collagen fibers [26–28].

5. Chronic Wounds

Wounds that do not heal within 6/8 weeks are considered chronic [33–37]. Numerous factors prevent wound healing. Among local factors, it is necessary to acknowledge the presence of foreign bodies, tissue maceration, ischemia, infection, and tissue hypoxia. Among the systemic factors, advanced age, malnutrition, diabetes, and renal disease are, without doubt, factors of primary importance. In addition, reduction in the secretion of tissue growth factors, the decompensation between the proteolytic enzymes and their inhibitors, and the presence of senescent cells in the microenvironment seem to be particularly important in the pathogenesis of chronic wounds [33–37].

Chronic venous ulcers are associated with an extremely high psychosocial burden in terms of morbidity, loss of productivity, functional disability, and emotional distress, causing depression and social isolation. The difficulty, or even the impossibility, of treating these types of wounds leads to high costs, in terms of care, for the various communities [33–37].

In general, the processes involved in chronic wound healing are similar to those in acute wound healing, but their persistence leads to abundant granulation tissue and possibly fibrosis, scar contraction, and/or loss of function. Undoubtedly, MMPs, which can damage granulation tissue, are the most actively involved. During wound healing, cells in the injured area are induced by local mediators to secrete MMPs responsible of epithelization and proliferation. The dysregulation of MMPs is strongly associated with chronic wounds. In particular, increased expression of MMP-9 delays ulcer repair in diabetic patients via the activation of the ERK/AP1 signaling pathway [15,16,21,22].

Prolonged inflammation in chronic wounds [38] is mainly mediated by MCs, neutrophils, and DCs (including macrophages), which are attracted to the injured site, where they release pro-inflammatory and repair cytokines, and hydrolytic enzymes, which remove necrotic tissue, clean the wound, and prevent and resolve infection [16,21,24,32,38–40]. T cells take part in maintaining the pro-inflammatory profile of non-healing skin injuries [32]. Immune cells communicate with keratinocytes through the secretion of various signaling molecules. However, the contribution of these latter cells to the formation of a chronic wound is not fully understood [14].

6. PDT and Chronic Wounds

6.1. The Response of Cellular Infiltrate

Among the multiple properties of PDT, there is evidence of a strong cellular infiltrate response in the treated chronic wound (Figure 1C).

Moreover, in recent studies, it was found that, after PDT therapy in chronic wounds, there is a significant increase in certain inflammatory cells, such as TNF alfa+ MCs, T regs, plasmacytoid dendritic cells, MHCII positive dermal DCs [32], and macrophages [40], as well as an overall expression of TGF beta, which directly correlates with wound's volume reduction [32]. TGF beta seems to exert activities in early phases of wound healing, where it possibly promotes an epithelial–mesenchymal transition, allowing the migration of keratinocytes from the borders towards the wound's bed [41]. Finally, intercellular correlations between plasmacytoid dendritic cells and T reg have been found, confirming the fact that certain DC subsets are highly specialized in inducing regulatory T cell differentiation and, in some tissues, the local microenvironment plays a role in driving DCs towards a tolerogenic response [42,43].

Since TGF beta is also able to induce the differentiation of myofibroblasts as part of the other processes also seen in wound healing [44], in some studies [29,30], it has been reported that PDT-treated chronic wounds show an abundance of fibroblasts (Figure 1D) compared to controls and untreated wounds, providing evidence that one of the mechanisms of this therapy might be the alteration of inflammatory processes, presumably via the activation of the enzymatic systems produced by the target cells stimulated by PDT, leading to an eventual healing of the chronic wound. Since the secretion activity of fibroblasts (i.e., extracellular matrix) is stimulated by other factors present in the wound microenvironment, such as histamine by MCs [45,46], the close distances of these cells to fibroblasts (Figure 1D) and the expression of FGF in their granules, in PDT-treated wounds [30], confirms this hypothesis. Therefore, after PDT therapy, we can conclude that MCs may send signals for the recruitment and differentiation of fibroblasts, and these latter cells are involved in the healing process of chronic wounds.

Indeed, signals produced by MCs may, in turn, be delivered directly to other cellular types, such as dermal DCs (Figure 1E) [47,48], which are also directly involved in wound healing [49,50].

It has been established that, upon PDT therapy, MCs increase in number and undergo degranulation [22,29,30,32]. The origin of the increase in MC number is probably related to its response to the microenvironment, including the migration of other cells, the differentiation or influx of precursors, and their eventual transformation in MCs [24]. The time needed for the influx and differentiation of circulating precursors to MCs is not known exactly. Probably, MCs are not only recruited, but have to be activated to secrete in response to PDT treatment. The vessels of the papillary dermis appear to be an important site of cell infiltration and clustering upon therapy; consequently, it is presumable that endothelial cells, along with the recruitment of pericytes [51], can regulate the recruitment of MCs at this location [52].

6.2. Neuroimmunomodulation

In healing wounds, the activity of immune system is certainly modulated by the nervous system [53–55], and delayed wound healing is observed in animal models after surgical resection of cutaneous nerves [54,55]. Sensory neurons possess several means of detecting the presence of noxious or harmful stimuli: (1) cytokine receptors, such as IL-1β and TNFα, recognize the factors secreted by immune cells (e.g., IL-1β, TNFα, nerve growth factor), which activates MAP kinases and other signaling mechanisms to increase membrane excitability; (2) distress signal receptors, including TRP channels, P2X channels, and DAMPs, recognize exogenous signals from the environment (e.g., heat, acidity, chemicals) and signals endogenous hazards released during trauma or tissue injury (for example, ATP or uric acid) [56]. Studies have demonstrated that the stimulation of dorsal roots induces cutaneous vasodilation and enhancement of inflammatory processes [56], consisting of (a) chemotaxis and subsequent activation of neutrophils, macrophages, and lymphocytes at the site of injury; (b) degranulation of MCs; (c) an increase in blood flow, which also allows easier recruitment of inflammatory leukocytes; and (d) dendritic cell activation and subsequent T helper cell differentiation [32,38,57].

These observations clearly suggest that innervation and neuromediators play a pivotal physiological role in wound healing. Interactions between nerves and other cells involved in wound healing, such as MCs, are crucial in the healing process [24,56,58], and MCs are commonly observed in chronic wound samples [29–31]. An example of this functional relationship comes from a recent study [59], which investigated, in ALA-PDT-treated chronic wounds, MC interaction with neuronal cells containing neurotransmitters involved in wound healing processes, such as CGRP, NGF, NKA, NPY, SP, PGP 9.5, and VIP [53,54].

The results of this study [59] demonstrate that, in chronic wounds treated with ALA-PDT, there is an increase in neuronal populations containing mediators involved in wound healing, as well as that relating to the percentage of MCs containing NGF and VIP.

Since NGF and VIP stimulate MC degranulation [57,58], this last fact relates to an increase in the degranulation index of MCs after PDT treatment, as previously shown [29,30], and is probably related to nerve stimulation. Therefore, the effects of ALA-PDT therapy on chronic wounds, at least in this model, may probably be due to neuronal activation; therefore, nervous fibers can activate various cellular types during wound healing, including MCs [57,58].

The fact that MCs exhibit numerous interactions with nerve fibers [57,58], and that the VIP and NGF content in their granules increases [59] after treatment, is interesting. Keeping this in mind, at least in our model, it can be assumed that MC activity after therapy (i.e., their degranulation), probably due to a receptor [60], increases the release of NGF and VIP, which are able to interact with neurons and nerve fibers of the dermis, thus obtaining an improvement. The activation of nerve fibers could, in turn, be related to other phenomena, such as the increased secretion of extracellular matrix by fibroblasts, as has been observed previously [29,30], as well as increases in TGF beta levels [32] and the response of cellular infiltrates [29,30]. Of course, since these results derive from a single pilot study, further studies are needed to elucidate a direct correlation between clinic wound healing improvement and increased of local neuropeptides expression after ALA-PDT.

6.3. Future Perspective

Among neuronal mediators, particular attention should be directed towards nitric oxide, a neuromodulator involved in the control of vascular tone and blood pressure [61]. For example, iNOs is upregulated under stress conditions; in fact, in the presence of inflammatory cytokines and other agents (antigens of pathogens, apoptotic bodies, etc.), the expression of this enzyme increases, underlining its possible role in the inflammatory phase of wound healing, in which it could guarantee vasodilation and antibacterial activity. In our study [62], a strong response of iNOs following photodynamic therapy was reported, denoting how the latter actively participates in the improvement of the clinical condition of the wound. Experiments are underway in the laboratory to obtain further elucidation regarding this observation.

7. Current Limitations

All that has been presented in this review takes on great significance if we consider that photodynamic therapy is relatively young and, therefore, new indications for its use can be discovered in the future. As regards the effects of cellular mechanisms induced by photodynamic therapy on chronic wounds, the description of these events undoubtedly suffers from a certain immaturity, as the same chronic wounds still represent unresolved problems [63,64]. The cellular mechanisms still need to be tested before arriving at any official therapies. Certainly, the involvement of the nervous system and its interactions with the immune system must be looked at carefully and understood more fully, as they can be the key to the resolution of this type of wound if subjected to such therapy.

Author Contributions: S.B. (conceptualization), A.C., V.G. (methodology), N.P. (supervision). All authors have read and agreed to the published version of the manuscript.

Funding: This research received no external funding.

Institutional Review Board Statement: Not applicable.

Informed Consent Statement: Not applicable.

Data Availability Statement: Not applicable.

Acknowledgments: This paper is devoted to the memory of Pietro Cappugi, who passed away on 17 June 2019, this research was launched and strongly promoted by him.

Conflicts of Interest: The authors declare no conflict of interest.

Abbreviations

Acronym	Denomination
PDT	Photodynamic therapy
ROS	Reactive Oxygen Species
ALA	5-aminolevulinic acid
Matrix Metalloproteinases	MMPs
MCs	Mast Cells
Interleukin	IL
TGF	Transforming growth factor
ERK/AP1	ERK-associated changes of AP1
DCs	Dendritic cells
TNF	Tumor necrosis factor
BDCA	Blood dendritic cell antigen
HSP	Heat shock protein
FGF	Fibroblast growth factor
UEA	Ulex Europaeus Agglutinin
NGF	Nerve Growth Factor
MAP	Mitogen-activated protein
TRP	Transient receptor potential channel
P2X	ATP-gated P2X receptor cation channel family
DAMP	Damp-associated molecular pattern receptors
ATP	Adenosine triphosphate
CGRP	Calcitonin Gene Related Peptide
NKA	Neurokinin A
NPY	Neuropeptide Y
SP	Substance P
PGP 9.5	Protein Gene Product 9.5
VIP	Vasoactive intestinal peptide
iNOs	Inducible isoform of nitric oxide synthase

References

1. Szeimies, R.M.; Drager, J.; Abels, C.; Landthaler, M. History of photodynamic therapy in dermatology. In *Photodynamic Therapy and Fluorescence Diagnosis in Therapy*; Calzavara-Pinton, P., Rolf-Markus, S., Ortel, B., Eds.; Elsevier Science: Amsterdam, The Netherlands, 2001; Volume 2, pp. 3–15.

2. Tampa, M.; Sarbu, M.; Matei, C.; Mitran, C.; Mitran, M.; Caruntu, C.; Georgescu, S. Photodynamic therapy: A hot topic in dermato-oncology. *Oncol. Lett.* **2019**, *17*, 4085–4093. [CrossRef]
3. Niculescu, A.G.; Grumezescu, A.M. Photodynamic Therapy—An up-to-date review. *Appl. Sci.* **2021**, *11*, 3626. [CrossRef]
4. Kwiatkowski, S.; Knap, B.; Przystupski, D.; Saczko, J.; Kedzierska, E.; Knap-Czop, K.; Kotlinska, J.; Michel, O.; Kotowski, K.; Kulbacka, J. Photodynamic therapy—mechanisms, photosensitizers and combinations. *Biomed. Pharm.* **2018**, *106*, 1098–1107. [CrossRef]
5. Grandi, V.; Sessa, M.; Pisano, L.; Rossi, R.; Galvan, A.; Gattai, R.; Mori, M.; Tiradritti, L.; Bacci, S.; Zuccati, G.; et al. Photodynamic therapy with topical photosensitizers in mucosal and semimucosal areas: Review from a dermatologic perspective. *Photodiagnosis Photodyn. Ther.* **2018**, *23*, 119–131. [CrossRef]
6. National Cancer Institute. Available online: https://www.cancer.gov/publications/dictionaries/cancer-terms/def/reactive-oxygen-species (accessed on 28 June 2022).
7. Donnelly, R.F.; McCarron, P.A.; Woolfson, A.D. Derivatives of 5-aminolevulinic acid for photodynamic therapy. *Perspect. Med. Chem.* **2007**, *1*, 49–63. [CrossRef]
8. Wang, B.C.; Fu, C.; Qin, L.; Zeng, X.Y.; Liu, Q. Photodynamic therapy with methyl-5-aminolevulinate for basal cell carcinoma: A systematic review and meta-analysis. *Photodiagnosis Photodyn. Ther.* **2020**, *29*, 101667–101679. [CrossRef]
9. Tedesco, A.; Jesus, P. Low level energy photodynamic therapy for skin processes and regeneration. In *Photomedicine. Advances in Clinical Practice*; Yohey, T., Ed.; Intech Open: London, UK, 2017.
10. Lecci, P.P.; Corsi, A.; Cappugi, P.P.; Bacci, S. La terapia fotodinamica nel trattamento delle lesioni cutanee croniche. In *Evidenze Cliniche e Pratica Sperimentale*; Aracne Editrice: Rome, Italy, 2013; pp. 1–64.
11. Goodpaster, T.; Legesse-Miller, A.; Hameed, M.R.; Aisner, S.C.; Randolph-Habecker, J.; Coller, H.A. An immunohistochemical method for identifying fibroblasts in formalin-fixed, paraffin-embedded tissue. *J. Histochem. Cytochem.* **2008**, *56*, 347–358. [CrossRef]
12. Bergstresser, P.R.; Tigelaar, R.E.; Tharp, M.D. Conjugated avidin identifies cutaneous rodent and human mast cells. *J. Investig. Derm.* **1984**, *83*, 214–218. [CrossRef]
13. ten Broeke, T.; Wubbolts, R.; Stoorvogel, W. MHC class II antigen presentation by dendritic cells regulated through endosomal sorting. *Cold Spring Harb. Perspect. Biol.* **2013**, *5*, a016873. [CrossRef]
14. Bacci, S.; Bani, D. The epidermis in microgravity and unloading conditions and their effects on wound healing. *Front. Bioeng. Biotechnol.* **2022**, *10*, 666434. [CrossRef]
15. Martin, P.; Nunan, R. Cellular and molecular mechanisms of repair in acute and chronic wound healing. *Br. J. Derm.* **2015**, *173*, 370–378. [CrossRef]
16. Gonzalez, A.C.; Costa, T.F.; Andrade, Z.A.; Medrado, A.R. Wound healing—A literature review. *An. Bras. Dermatol.* **2016**, *91*, 614–620. [CrossRef] [PubMed]
17. Sorg, H.; Tilkorn, D.J.; Hager, S.; Hauser, J.; Mirastschijski, U. Skin wound healing: An update on the current knowledge and concepts. *Eur. Surg. Res.* **2017**, *58*, 81–94. [CrossRef] [PubMed]
18. Cañedo-Dorantes, L.; Cañedo-Ayala, M. Skin acute wound healing: A comprehensive review. *Int. J. Inflam* **2019**, *2019*, 3706315–3706329. [CrossRef] [PubMed]
19. Visha, M.G.; Karunagaran, M. A review on wound healing. *Int. J. Clin. Correl.* **2019**, *3*, 50–59.
20. Tottoli, E.M.; Dorati, R.; Genta, I.; Chiesa, E.; Pisani, S.; Conti, B. Skin wound healing process and new emerging technologies for skin wound care and regeneration. *Pharmaceutics* **2020**, *12*, 735. [CrossRef]
21. Wilkinson, H.N.; Hardman, M.J. Wound healing: Cellular mechanisms and pathological outcomes. *Open Biol.* **2020**, *10*, 200223–200236. [CrossRef]
22. Raziyeva, K.; Kim, Y.; Zharkinbekov, Z.; Kassymbek, K.; Jimi, S.; Saparov, A. Immunology of acute and chronic wound healing. *Biomolecules* **2021**, *11*, 700. [CrossRef]
23. Douahiher, J.; Succar, J.; Lancerotto, L.; Gurish, M.F.; Orgill, D.P.; Hamilton, M.J.; Krilis, S.A.; Stevens, R.L. Development of mast cells and importance of their tryptase and chymase serine proteases in inflammation and wound healing. *Adv. Immunol.* **2014**, *122*, 211–252.
24. Bacci, S. Fine regulation during wound healing by mast cells, a physiological role not yet clarified. *Int. J. Mol. Sci.* **2022**, *23*, 1820. [CrossRef]
25. Zhang, Z.; Kurashima, Y. Two sides of the coin: Mast cells as a key regulator of allergy and acute/chronic inflammation. *Cells* **2021**, *10*, 1615. [CrossRef]
26. Nesi-Reis, V.; Lera-Nonose, S.V.; Oyama, J.; Ramos-Milaré, Á.; Demarchi, I.; Alessi-Aristides, S.; Vieira-Teixeira, J.J.; Verzignassi Silveira, T.G.; Campana-Lonardoni, M.V. Contribution of photodynamic therapy in wound healing: A systematic review. *Photodiagnosis Photodyn. Ther.* **2018**, *30*, 294–305. [CrossRef]
27. Oyama, J.; Ramos-Milaré, Á.; Lera-Nonose, S.V.; Nesi-Reis, V.; Demarchi, I.; Alessi-Aristides, S.; Vieira-Teixeira, J.J.; Verzignassi Silveira, T.G.; Campana-Lonardoni, M.V. Photodynamic therapy in wound healing in vivo, a systematic review. *Photodiagnosis Photodyn. Ther.* **2020**, *10*, 101682. [CrossRef]
28. Reginato, E.; Wolf, P.; Hamblin, M.R. Immune response after photodynamic therapy increases anti-cancer and anti-bacterial effects. *World J. Immunol.* **2014**, *4*, 1–11. [CrossRef]

29. Corsi, A.; Lecci, P.P.; Bacci, S.; Cappugi, P. Chronic wounds treated with photodynamic therapy: Analysis of cellular response and preliminary results. *Acta Vulnol.* **2013**, *11*, 23–33.
30. Corsi, A.; Lecci, P.P.; Bacci, S.; Cappugi, P.; Pimpinelli, N. Early activation of fibroblasts during PDT treatment in leg ulcers. *G Ital. Derm. Venereol.* **2016**, *151*, 223–229.
31. Yang, Z.; Hu, X.; Zhou, L.; He, Y.; Zhang, X.; Yang, J.; Ju, Z.; Liou, Y.C.; Shen, H.M.; Luo, G.; et al. Photodynamic therapy accelerates skin wound healing through promoting re-epithelialization. *Burn. Trauma* **2021**, *9*, tkab008. [CrossRef]
32. Grandi, V.; Bacci, S.; Corsi, A.; Sessa, M.; Puliti, E.; Murciano, N.; Scavone, F.; Cappugi, P.; Pimpinelli, N. ALA-PDT exerts beneficial effects on chronic venous ulcers by inducing changes in inflammatory microenvironment, especially through increased TGF-beta release: A pilot clinical and translational study. *Photodiagnosis Photodyn. Ther.* **2018**, *21*, 252–256. [CrossRef]
33. Harding, K.G.; Morris, H.L.; Patel, G.K. Healing chronic wounds. *Br. Med. J.* **2002**, *324*, 160–163. [CrossRef]
34. Toporcer, T.; Lakyová, L.; Radonak, J. Venous ulcer-present view on aetiology, diagnostics and therapy. *Cas. Lek. Ceskych* **2008**, *147*, 199–205.
35. Han, G.; Ceilley, R. Chronic wound healing: A review of current management and treatments. *Adv. Ther.* **2017**, *34*, 599–610. [CrossRef] [PubMed]
36. Sen, C.K. Human wounds and its burden: An updated compendium of estimates. *Adv. Wound Care* **2019**, *8*, 39–48. [CrossRef] [PubMed]
37. Kyaw, B.M.; Järbrink, K.; Martinengo, L.; Car, J.; Harding, K.; Schmidtchen, A. Need for improved definition of chronic wounds in clinical studies. *Acta Derm. Venereol.* **2018**, *12*, 157–158. [CrossRef] [PubMed]
38. Zhao, R.; Liang, H.; Clarke, E.; Jackson, C.; Xue, M. Inflammation in chronic wounds. *Int. J. Mol. Sci.* **2016**, *17*, 2085. [CrossRef]
39. Komi, D.E.A.; Khomtchouk, K.; Santa Maria, P.L. A review of the contribution of mast cells in wound healing: Involved molecular and cellular mechanisms. *Clin. Rev. Allergy Immunol.* **2020**, *58*, 298–312. [CrossRef]
40. Yang, T.; Tan, Y.; Zhang, W.; Yang, W.; Luo, J.; Chen, L.; Liu, H.; Yang, G.; Lei, X. Effects of ALA-PDT on the healing of mouse skin wounds infected with *Pseudomonas aeruginosa* and its related mechanisms. *Front. Cell Dev. Biol.* **2020**, *8*, 585132. [CrossRef]
41. Haensel, D.; Dai, X. Epithelial-to-mesenchymal transition in cutaneous wound healing: Where we are and where we are heading. *Dev. Dyn* **2018**, *247*, 473–480. [CrossRef]
42. Kushwah, R.; Hu, J. Role of dendritic cells in the induction of regulatory T cells. *Cell Biosci.* **2011**, *1*, 20. [CrossRef]
43. Murciano, N.; University of Florence, Florence, Italy. Personal communication, 2016.
44. Frangogiannis, N. Transforming growth factor-β in tissue fibrosis. *J. Exp. Med.* **2020**, *217*, e20190103. [CrossRef]
45. Krystel-Whittemore, M.; Dileepan, K.N.; Wood, J.G. Mast cell: A multi-functional master cell. *Front. Immunol.* **2016**, *6*, 620. [CrossRef]
46. Khorsandi, K.; Fekrazad, R.; Hamblin, M.R. Low-dose photodynamic therapy effect on closure of scratch wounds of normal and diabetic fibroblast cells: An in vitro study. *J. Biophotonics* **2021**, *14*, e202100005. [CrossRef] [PubMed]
47. Bacci, S.; Pimpinelli, N.; Romagnoli, P. Contacts between mast cells and dendritic cells in the human skin. *Ital. J. Anat. Embryol.* **2010**, *11*, 25–30.
48. Gri, G.; Frossi, B.; D'Inca, F.; Danelli, L.; Betto, E.; Mion, F.; Sibilano, R.; Pucillo, C. Mast cell: An emerging partner in immune interaction. *Front. Immunol.* **2012**, *25*, 120. [CrossRef] [PubMed]
49. Bacci, S.; Defraia, B.; Cinci, L.; Calosi, L.; Guasti, D.; Pieri, L.; Lotti, V.; Bonelli, A.; Romagnoli, P. Immunohistochemical analysis of dendritic cells in skin lesions: Correlations with survival time. *Forensic Sci. Int.* **2014**, *244*, 179–185. [CrossRef]
50. Brazil, J.C.; Quiros, M.; Nusrat, A.; Parkos, C.A. Innate immune cell-epithelial crosstalk during wound repair. *J. Clin. Investig.* **2019**, *129*, 2983–2993. [CrossRef]
51. Yamazaki, T.; Mukouyama, Y.S. Tissue specific origin, development, and pathological perspectives of pericytes. *Front. Cardiovasc. Med.* **2018**, *27*, 78. [CrossRef]
52. Gaber, M.A.; Seliet, I.A.; Ehsan, N.A.; Megahed, M.A. Mast cells and angiogenesis in wound healing. *Anal. Quant. Cytopathol. Histpathol.* **2014**, *36*, 32–40.
53. Steinmann, L. Elaborate interactions between the immune and nervous system. *Nat. Immunol.* **2004**, *5*, 575–581. [CrossRef]
54. Ashrafi, M.; Baguneid, M.; Bayat, A. The role of neuromediators and innervation in cutaneous wound healing. *Acta Derm. Venereol.* **2016**, *96*, 587–594. [CrossRef]
55. Laverdet, B.; Danigo, A.; Girard, D.; Magy, L.; Demiot, C.; Desmoulière, A. Skin innervation: Important roles during normal and pathological cutaneous repair. *Histol. Histopathol.* **2015**, *30*, 875–892. [CrossRef]
56. Chiu, I.M.; von Hehn, C.A.; Woolf, C.J. Neurogenic inflammation and the peripheral nervous system in host defense and immunopathology. *Nat. Neurosci.* **2012**, *15*, 1063–1067. [CrossRef]
57. Siiskonen, H.; Harvima, I. Mast cells and sensory nerves contribute to neurogenic inflammation and pruritus in chronic skin inflammation. *Front. Cell Neurosci.* **2019**, *13*, 422. [CrossRef] [PubMed]
58. Forsythe, P. Mast cells in neuroimmune interactions. *Trends Neurosci.* **2019**, *42*, 43–55. [CrossRef] [PubMed]
59. Grandi, V.; Paroli, G.; Puliti, E.; Bacci, S.; Pimpinelli, N. Single ALA-PDT irradiation induces increase in mast cells degranulation and neuropeptide acute response in chronic venous ulcers: A pilot study. *Photodiagnosis Photodyn. Ther.* **2021**, *34*, 102222. [CrossRef]
60. Streilein, J.V.; Alard, P.; Nizzeki, H. A new concept of skin-associated lymphoid tissue (SALT): UVB light impaired cutaneous immunity reveal a preminent role for cutaneous nerves. *Kejo J. Med.* **1999**, *48*, 22–27. [CrossRef]

61. Lee, M.; Rey, K.; Besler, K.; Wang, C.; Choy, J. Immunobiology of nitric oxide and regulation of inducible nitric oxide synthase. *Results Probl. Cell Differ.* **2017**, *62*, 181–207. [CrossRef] [PubMed]
62. Rossi, F. Neuroimmunomodulation in Chronic Wounds Healing after Treatment with Photodynamic Therapy: The Role of iNOs. Bachelor's Thesis, University of Florence, Florence, Italy, 11 November 2021.
63. Bacci, S. Cellular mechanisms and therapies in wound healing: Looking toward the future. *Biomedicines* **2021**, *9*, 1611. [CrossRef]
64. Sun, Y.; Ogawa, R.; Xiao, B.H.; Feng, Y.X.; Wu, Y.; Chen, L.H.; Gao, X.H.; Chen, H.D. Antimicrobial photodynamic therapy in skin wound healing: A systematic review of animal studies. *Int. Wound J.* **2020**, *17*, 285–299. [CrossRef]

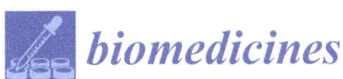

Article

Far-Infrared Therapy Decreases Orthotopic Allograft Transplantation Vasculopathy

Yi-Wen Lin [1,2,†], Chien-Sung Tsai [2,3,4,†], Chun-Yao Huang [2,5,6], Yi-Ting Tsai [3], Chun-Ming Shih [2,5,6], Shing-Jong Lin [2,5,6], Chi-Yuan Li [7,8], Cheng-Yen Lin [9], Shih-Ying Sung [3] and Feng-Yen Lin [2,5,6,*]

1. Institute of Oral Biology, National Yang Ming Chiao Tung University, Taipei 112, Taiwan; ywlin@nycu.edu.tw
2. Taipei Heart Institute, Taipei Medical University, Taipei 110, Taiwan; sung1500@mail.ndmctsgh.edu.tw (C.-S.T.); cyhuang@tmu.edu.tw (C.-Y.H.); cmshih53@tmu.edu.tw (C.-M.S.); sjlin@tmu.edu.tw (S.-J.L.)
3. Division of Cardiovascular Surgery, Tri-Service General Hospital, National Defense Medical Center, Taipei 110, Taiwan; cvsallen@mail.ndmctsgh.edu.tw (Y.-T.T.); molecule1983@gmail.com (S.-Y.S.)
4. Department and Graduate Institute of Pharmacology, National Defense Medical Center, Taipei 114, Taiwan
5. Division of Cardiology and Cardiovascular Research Center, Taipei Medical University Hospital, Taipei 110, Taiwan
6. Departments of Internal Medicine, College of Medicine, School of Medicine, Taipei Medical University, Taipei 110, Taiwan
7. Department of Anesthesiology, China Medical University Hospital, Taichung 404, Taiwan; cyli168@gmail.com
8. Graduate Institute of Clinical Medical Science, China Medical University, Taichung 404, Taiwan
9. Healthcare Information and Management Department, Ming Chuan University, Taoyuan 333, Taiwan; chengyan@mail.mcu.edu.tw
* Correspondence: g870905@tmu.edu.tw; Tel.: +886-28-791-0329
† These authors contributed equally to this paper.

Abstract: Orthotopic allograft transplantation (OAT) is a major strategy for solid heart and kidney failure. However, the recipient's immunity-induced chronic rejection induces OAT vasculopathy that results in donor organ failure. With the exception of immunosuppressive agents, there are currently no specific means to inhibit the occurrence of OAT vasculopathy. On the other hand, far-infrared (FIR) therapy uses low-power electromagnetic waves given by FIR, with a wavelength of 3–25 µm, to improve human physiological functions. Previous studies have shown that FIR therapy can effectively inhibit inflammation. It has also been widely used in adjuvant therapy for various clinical diseases, especially cardiovascular diseases, in recent years. Thus, we used this study to explore the feasibility of FIR in preventing OAT vasculopathy. In this study, the model of transplantation of an aorta graft from PVG/Seac rat to ACI/NKyo rat, and in vitro model of human endothelial progenitor cells (EPCs) was used. In this report, we presented that FIR therapy decreased the serious of vasculopathy in OAT-recipient ACI/NKyo rats via inhibiting proliferation of smooth muscle cells, accumulation of collagen, and infiltration of fibroblast in the vessel wall; humoral and cell-mediated immune responses were decreased in the spleen. The production of inflammatory proteins/cytokines also decreased in the plasma. Additionally, FIR therapy presented higher mobilization and circulating EPC levels associated with vessel repair in OAT-recipient ACI/NKyo rats. In vitro studies demonstrated that the underlying mechanisms of FIR therapy inhibiting OAT vasculopathy may be associated with the inhibition of the Smad2-Slug axis endothelial mesenchymal transition (EndoMT). Thus, FIR therapy may be the strategy to prevent chronic rejection-induced vasculopathy.

Keywords: orthotopic allograft transplantation; far-infrared (FIR) therapy; endothelial progenitor cells; endothelial mesenchymal transition

1. Introduction

Infrared light is invisible, with a wavelength between 0.75 and 1000 µm, and far-infrared (FIR) is infrared light with a wavelength >3 µm. FIR therapy uses low-power electromagnetic waves with a wavelength of 3–25 μm to improve human physiological functions. Compared to thermal radiation therapy with 0.75–1.5 μm infrared radiation, the extremely low-power electromagnetic waves provided by FIR therapy do not easily cause tissue damage. FIR therapy has been widely used in adjuvant therapy for various clinical diseases in recent years, since an increasing number of studies have shown that it can effectively control the occurrence of inflammation. Results from previous clinical studies suggest that FIR therapy can be used to increase cardiopulmonary exercise tolerance [1,2], improve patency and flow in arteriovenous fistulas in patients with hemodialysis [3] and reduce the probability of re-occlusion within one year after percutaneous transluminal angioplasties [4]. Animal studies have also shown that FIR therapy can increase the expression of heme oxygenase-1 in testes after ischemic injury [5], increase the biological effects of skin microcirculation [6], promote sciatic nerve repair in neuropathy [7], promote ischemia-induced angiogenesis, and restore high glucose-suppressed endothelial progenitor cell (EPC) functions [8]. Previous findings have shown the effectiveness of FIR therapy in the treatment of systemic diseases, including cardiovascular diseases, diabetes mellitus, tissue ischemia, malfunction of native arteriovenous fistulas and prosthetic arteriovenous grafts, chronic pain, and chronic fatigue syndrome [9].

Orthotopic allograft organ transplantation (OAT) have been the major treatment strategy for sever solid organ failure. Given that the presently offered professional approaches can efficiently regulate severe rejection, it has substantially increased the patients' short-term survival rate after transplanted surgery. Nevertheless, the chronic rejection mainly affects the patient's long-lasting survival rate.

The alloimmune system attacks the endothelium and epithelium of donor graft, causes diffuse graft damage and results in vasculopathy. This process is called chronic rejection [10]. Arteries, as well as micro vessels, which cause the parenchyma to be replaced by fibrosis, reveal hyperplasia of the vascular intima that raise narrowing and occlusion of the vessels in the transplanted graft [11]. Arterial fibrosis constrains the blood flow, resulting in graft ischemia and failure in patients after organ transplantation [12]. Therefore, OAT vasculopathy results from chronic rejection is a critical issue after organ transplantation.

The immune capacity produced by the systemic immunity is one of the major factors affecting life span of donor graft. The recipient's immune system recognizes the transplanted organ as an invader, and attempts to exclude it. The appropriate regulation of the immune capacity is crucial for the life span of the transplanted graft, and is also helpful for the recipient. Immunosuppressive therapy is widely used for patients undergoing organ transplantation. Its purpose is to control and regulate damage to the graft by the systemic immune response. Initial immunosuppressive induction and maintenance immunosuppressive therapies are included in immunosuppressive therapy. Initial immunosuppressive induction therapy provides powerful immunosuppressive effects at the hospitalization. Indeed, the success or failure of maintenance immunosuppressive therapy is a major factor in determining patient survival that may regulate chronic rejection. Mycophenolic acids (MPAs), corticosteroids, and calcineurin inhibitors (CNIs) are commonly used drugs for maintenance immunosuppressive therapy [13]. Additionally, mammalian targets of rapamycin inhibitors (mTORi), azathioprine, IL-2 receptor antagonist, monoclonal antibodies, and polyclonal antibodies can also be used in solid organ transplant patients [13,14]. Although multiple drugs are available for the control of immune-related rejection in patients receiving solid organ transplantation, clinicians are still unable to completely and effectively control the progress of chronic rejection and avoid the occurrence of OAT vasculopathy. Therefore, under the current framework of medical treatment, it is necessary to actively search for better preventive strategies for OAT vasculopathy.

FIR therapy is a non-invasive, cheap, and safe procedure that should be easily accepted by patients. Previous studies have shown that FIR therapy has a significant curative effect on inflammatory vascular diseases. Therefore, we aimed to explore the feasibility of FIR therapy for OAT-induced vasculopathy in patients undergoing organ transplantation. In this study, we transplanted the aorta from PVG/Seac rats into the ACI/NKyo rats and compared the severity after 90 days of OAT with and without FIR therapy in animals. We also analyzed the effects of FIR therapy on chronic rejection in animals and investigated the possible mechanisms of FIR therapy on OAT-induced vasculopathy. We hope that the results may increase the suitability of FIR therapy in the adjuvant strategy of prevention in OAT-induced vasculopathy.

2. Materials and Methods

2.1. Equipment

The FIR therapy device was purchased from WS Far IR Medical Technology Co., Ltd. (Model: TY-101F, Taipei, Taiwan) which provides a far infrared wavelength of 3–25 μm and power intensity of 4.95–20 mW/cm^2 at a distance of 20 cm. Following the user manual instructions, FIR therapy was administered directly to the backs of the animals or EPCs at a distance of 20 cm.

2.2. Animal Study

2.2.1. Authorization of Animal Study

All animals were managed according to the methods accredited by the institutional animal care committee of Taipei Medical University (certification no. LAC-2020-0047). Speculative procedures and animal treatment complied with the "Guide for the Care and Use of Laboratory Animals" published by the U.S. National Institutes of Health (NIH Publication No. 85-23, revised 1996).

2.2.2. Orthotopic Aortic Transplantation

Since OAT model of PVG/Seac rat-to-ACI/NKyo rat displays vasculopathy that is presented in the previous reference [15,16], therefore this model was used in this study. The 8-week-old and 250–300 g body weight (BW) male ACI/NKyo rats (NBRP rat no. 0001; recipient rats) and PVG/Seac rats (NBRP rat no. 0080; donor rats) were used in this experiment.

2.2.3. Animal Grouping

Total 20 rats were randomly divided into four groups, fed a normal rodent chow diet (scientific diet) and kept in microisolator cages on a 12 h day/night cycle. Group 1 consisted of sham-operated ACI/NKyo rats. Group 2 included OAT-recipient ACI/NKyo rats. Group 3 included OAT-recipient and low-intensity FIR therapy (4.95–8.26 mW/cm^2) ACI/NKyo rats, and treatment beginning the day after surgery. Group 4 included OAT- recipient and high-intensity FIR therapy (11.7–19.5 mW/cm^2) ACI/NKyo rats, and treatment beginning the day after surgery. All FIR therapies were performed once daily for 40 min during the experimental period. The transplanted thoracic aortas of rats were removed at day 90 of the experiment.

2.2.4. Biochemical Measurements and Enzyme-Linked Immunosorbent Assays

Plasma levels of creatinine, blood urea nitrogen (BUN), aspartate aminotransferase (AST), alanine transaminase (ALT), lactic dehydrogenase (LDH), and blood sugar were analyzed using a SPOTCHEMTM chemistry system (SP-4410; Arkray, Shanghai, China). C-reactive protein (CRP; Abcam Inc., Cambridge, MA, USA), transforming growth factor β1 (TGF-β1; Abcam Inc., Cambridge, MA, USA), High mobility group box 1 (HMGB1; LifeSpan Biosciences Inc., Seattle, WA, USA), stromal cell-derived factor 1α (SDF-1α; R&D Systems Inc., Minneapolis, MN, USA), interleukin-2 (IL-2; Abcam Inc., Cambridge, MA, USA), and interferon-γ (INF-γ; Abcam Inc., Cambridge, MA, USA) were determined by enzyme-linked immunosorbent assay (ELISA).

2.2.5. Morphological Analysis

After the animals were sacrificed on the 90th experimental day, the transplanted donor aortas spleens were harvested. Tissues were fixed, embedded in paraffin, and cross-sectioned for immunohistochemistry and hematoxylin and eosin (H&E) staining. The spleens were weighed before fixation. Aortas were also stained with Masson's trichrome and picrosirius red. Immunohistochemical staining of aortas was performed using anti-S100A4 antibody (Cell Signaling Technologies, Danvers, MA, USA) and α-smooth muscle actin antibody (αSMA; Santa Cruz Biotechnology, Dallas, TX, USA) and the spleen was performed using anti-CD138 antibody (Invitrogen, Thermo Fisher Scientific Co., Carlsbad, CA, USA) and anti-CD4, anti-CD8, anti-CD11b, and anti-CD20 antibodies, (Abcam, Cambridge, MA, USA). A light microscope was used to observe the slides.

2.2.6. Flow Cytometry

A flow cytometer was used to analyzed the circulating smooth muscle progenitor cells (SMPCs) and EPCs in rats. Rat blood was incubated with Cy5-conjugated anti-CD34 (Bioss Antibodies, Woburn, MA, USA), Alexa Fluor 488-conjugated anti-CD133 (Novus Biologicals, Centennial, CO, USA), phycoerythrin (PE)-conjugated anti-vascular endothelial growth factor (VEGF; Novus Biologicals, Centennial, CO, USA), and PE-conjugated anti-αSMA (Abcam Inc., Cambridge, MA, USA) antibodies. Isotype IgG was used as a control (Becton Dickinson, Franklin Lakes, NJ, USA). Circulating EPCs were gated using $CD133^+/CD34^+/VEGF^+$ staining in originate from the monocytic cell. Circulating SMPCs were gated using $CD133^+/\alpha SMA^+/CD34^-$ staining.

2.3. In Vitro Study

2.3.1. Cultivation of Human EPCs and FIR Therapy

Human EPCs were cultured from the total MNCs extracted from the peripheral blood. The protocol was described in a previous report [17]. EPC characterization was performed as previously described. When FIR therapy was required for EPCs, we placed the FIR device in the incubator. We maintained constant humidity and CO_2 and monitored the temperature with a thermometer (37 °C).

2.3.2. Tubing Formation Assay

In vitro tube formation assays were performed on EPCs to assess the neovasculogenic capacity, which is believed to be important for endothelial function. Human EPCs were treated with recombinant human tumor necrosis factor alpha (TNF-α for 24 h, and FIR therapy was performed simultaneously every 8 h (3 times in 24 h). After the treatment of EPCs was completed, an angiogenesis assay kit (Chemicon, Billerica, MA, USA) was used to investigate the capability of tube formation [18].

2.3.3. Cellular Senescence Assay

Senescence is the negative factor that limits the function of EPCs [19], therefore it was investigated using a cellular senescence assay. The detail protocol was demonstrated in our previous report [20].

2.3.4. Migration Assay (Wound-Healing Assay)

The migration assay was used to study the migratory capacity of EPCs, which is associated with vasculogenesis. The detail protocol was demonstrated in our previous report [20].

2.3.5. Real-Time Quantitative Polymerase Chain Reactions

Quantitative real-time polymerase chain reaction (qPCR) were performed. Glyceraldehyde 3-phosphate dehydrogenase was used as an endogenous control to normalize differences in mRNA expression. The primers are listed in Table 1.

2.3.6. Western Blotting Analysis

The total and nuclear proteins were extracted, and then subjected to sodium dodecyl sulfate-polyacrylamide gel electrophoresis (SDS-PAGE) of Western blotting. Mouse anti-vascular endothelial (VE)-cadherin (Millipore Co., Billerica, MA, USA), rabbit anti-von Willebrand factor (vWF)(Millipore Co., Billerica, MA, USA), mouse anti-αSMA (Sigma-Aldrich, Cambridge, MA, USA), anti-vimentin (Sigma-Aldrich, Cambridge, MA, USA), mouse anti-β-actin (Santa Cruz Biotechnology, Santa Cruz, CA, USA), rabbit anti-phosphorylated Smad2 (Cell Signaling Technology, Danvers, MA, USA), anti-total Smad2/3 (Cell Signaling Technology, Danvers, MA, USA), anti-Snail (Cell Signaling Technology, Danvers, MA, USA), anti-Slug (Cell Signaling Technology, Danvers, MA, USA), and anti-lamin A/C (Cell Signaling Technology, Danvers, MA, USA) antibodies were used. Immunodetection consisted of exposure to an Imaging System of ChemiDoc-ItTM (UVP, Upland, CA, USA).

Table 1. The primer sequence for real-time RCR.

Gene	Forward Primer	Reverse Primer
vWF	5′-GGC TGC AGT ATG TCA AGG TGG-3′	5′-AGA GCC ATT GGT GCA GTG CAG-3′
VE-cadherin	5′-AGA CAA TGG GAT GCC AAG TCB-3′	5′-AAG ATG AGC AGG GTG ATC ACT G-3′
αSMA	5′-CTA TCA GGG GGC ACC ACT ATG-3′	5′-CCG ATC CAG ACA GAG TAT TTG CG-3′
vimentin	5′-AGG CAA AGC AGG AGT CCA CTG A-3′	5′-ATC TGG CGT TCC AGG GAC TCAT -3′
GAPDH	5′-TGC CCC CTC TGC TGA TGC C-3′	5′-CCT CCG ACG CCT GCT TCA CCA C-3′

vWF, von Willebrand factor; αSMA, alpha smooth muscle cell actin; GAPDH, glyceraldehyde 3-phosphate dehydrogenase.

2.4. Statistical Analyses

Values are expressed as mean ± SD. The non-parametric ANOVA, followed by the Kruskal–Wallis test was used to statistical analyses. Results with a $p < 0.05$ were considered statistically significant.

3. Results

3.1. FIR Therapy Affected the Inflammation-Related Proteins Expression, Not the Biochemical Characteristics, in OAT ACI/NKyo Rats

Biochemical analyses and ELISA were performed to evaluate the effects of FIR therapy in OAT ACI/NKyo rats. The data were showed in Table 2, the body weight, BUN, creatinine, ALT, and AST did not differ between control and experimental groups during the study period. HMGB1 and LDH are associated with antibody-mediated and chronic rejection [21,22]. Significantly, increased the levels of HMGB1 and LDH in OAT ACI/NKyo rats. The data showed that OAT increased LDH (baseline: 750.8 ± 37.3; OAT: 1166.2 ± 111.5 IU/L) and HMGB1 (baseline: 3.2 ± 0.5 ng/mL; OAT: 127.5 ± 89.5 ng/mL) levels. Even with low intensity of FIR therapy, compare to the pre-OAT group (737.6 ± 26.6 IU/L) the level of LDH was still higher (1001.0 ± 142.0 IU/L). In contrast, the increased LDH level was controlled upon therapy with high-intensity FIR in the OAT + FIR group (823.7 ± 57.4 IU/L). Low and high intensity of FIR therapy also decreased the plasma levels of HMGB1 (low intensity of FIR therapy group: 36.5 ± 19.8 ng/mL; high intensity of FIR therapy group: 35.0 ± 10.9 ng/mL) compared to that in the non-FIR therapy group (127.5 ± 89.5 ng/mL) in OAT ACI/NKyo rats. These results indicated that FIR therapy might decrease rejection-mediated tissue damage in OAT ACI/NKyo rats.

3.2. FIR Therapy Decreases Vascular Damage and Accumulation of Collagen in OAT ACI/NKyo Rats

Figure 1 demonstrated the H&E staining of the harvested thoracic aortas. Vasculopathy has actually been linked in the morbid collagen accumulation [23]. Therefore, Masson's trichrome and picrosirius red staining were used to analyze the collagen phenomena. In fact, no vasculopathy were observed in PVG/Seac rats' aortas by H&E staining, and intact visualization of the collagen was performed using Masson's trichrome staining. Additionally, picrosirius red staining showed that thoracic aortas from naïve PVG/Seac rats had thick collagen fibers that presented weak orange to red signal. Additionally, fine collagen fibers were equally distributed (yellow to green) in the vessel walls. Compared to the naïve PVG/Seac rat group, thoracic aortas from recipient OAT ACI/NKyo rats showed vascular integrity damage, blurred elastin laminae, and calcified plaques accumulation after 90 days of OAT. Interestingly, a slightly vascular integrity damage and calcified plaques (vasculopathy) was observed, although slight neointimal formation still existed in OAT ACI/Nkyo rats receiving low-intensity FIR therapy. Furthermore, high-intensity FIR therapy may significantly maintain greater vascular integrity and lower OAT vasculopathy in ACI/Nkyo rats than in non-FIR therapy OAT ACI/Nkyo rats. These results imply that FIR therapy might prevent OAT vasculopathy and promote the integrity of the aortic vessel wall in OAT ACI/Nkyo rats.

Table 2. Comparison of biochemical parameters in experimental ACI/NKyo rats ($n = 5$).

	Sham Control		OAT		OAT+FIR Low Intensity		OAT+FIR High Intensity	
	baseline	90 days	baseline	90 days	baseline	90 days	baseline	90 days
Body weight (g)	256.8 ± 12.8	340.2 ± 9.5	270.8 ± 10.8	341.6 ± 10.7	258.4 ± 7.6	345.8 ± 4.4	266.2 ± 16.4	346.0 ± 13.5
BUN (mg/dL)	26.5 ± 1.4	29.6 ± 2.4	30.4 ± 2.4	29.6 ± 1.7	28.7 ± 3.1	29.7 ± 2.3	30.5 ± 2.9	33.7 ± 2.3
Creatinine (mg/dL)	0.4 ± 0.1	0.6 ± 0.1	0.6 ± 0.1	0.5 ± 0.2	0.5 ± 0.1	0.6 ± 0.1	0.6 ± 0.2	0.4 ± 0.2
ALT (IU/L)	26.3 ± 1.6	26.0 ± 1.8	27.7 ± 1.8	28.8 ± 1.2	26.7 ± 1.1	28.0 ± 1.6	26.2 ± 0.9	26.4 ± 1.8
AST (IU/L)	34.4 ± 1.3	33.8 ± 1.3	34.4 ± 1.8	34.6 ± 1.4	33.9 ± 1.2	32.6 ± 1.7	35.2 ± 2.5	34.5 ± 1.7
LDH (IU/L)	786.6 ± 37.8	732.7 ± 20.3	750.8 ± 37.3	1166.2 ± 111.5 [ab]	737.6 ± 26.6	1001.0 ± 142.0 [ab]	757.1 ± 30.5	823.7 ± 57.4 [c]
HMGB1 (ng/mL)	3.3 ± 0.7	3.4 ± 0.5	3.2 ± 0.5	127.5 ± 89.5 [ab]	2.4 ± 0.9	36.5 ± 19.8 [abc]	2.5 + 0.5	35.0 ± 10.9 [abc]

FIR, far-infrared ray; BW, body weight; OAT, orthotopic aortic transplantation; BUN, blood urea nitrogen; ALT, alanine transaminase; AST, aspartate transaminase; LDH, lactic dehydrompared. HMGB1, high mobility group box 1 protein. [a] $p < 0.05$ compared with baseline of the same group; [b] $p < 0.05$ compared with sham control ACI/NKyo (non-OAT) group at the same time point; [c] $p < 0.05$ compared with OAT (PVG/Seac to ACI/NKyo) group at the same time point.

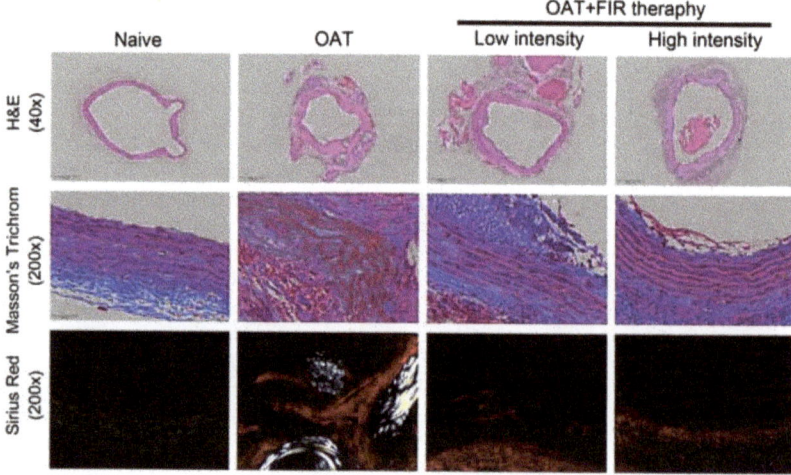

Figure 1. FIR therapy reduced allograft vasculopathy in OAT-recipient ACI/Nkyo rats. (upper column) Thoracic aortas from donor PVG/Seac rats stained with hematoxylin and eosin. The arrows indicate internal elastic lamina and arrowheads indicate calcified lesions. The images are 40× magnified. (middle column) The integrity of collagen fibers of thoracic aorta cross-sections was observed using Masson's trichome staining. (lower column) Histopathological features and collagen accumulation of thoracic aorta cross-sections were observed using picrosirius red staining. The slides were observed via light microscopy and polarized light microscopy, respectively (200× magnification).

3.3. Reduced Proliferation of SMCs and Fibroblasts in the Aortic Wall of FIR Therapy-Administered OAT ACI/Nkyo Rats

Smooth muscle cells (SMCs) and fibroblasts proliferation play important roles in allograft vasculopathy. Immunohistochemical staining was used to analyze the effects of FR therapy on SMCs and fibroblast activities. Antibodies against αSMA and S1000A4 on aortic sections were used, and the results are presented in Figure 2. Compared to the PVG/Seac thoracic aorta sections from the naïve group, the sections from the OAT aCI/NKyo rats presented a significant accumulation of fibroblasts and SMCs in the hyperplastic area on the luminal surface at day 90 after transplantation. However, SMCs and fibroblasts accumulated less in the vessel wall in both the low- and high-intensity FIR therapy groups. The efficacy of FIR therapy in inhibiting SMCs and fibroblast proliferation was positively correlated with FIR intensity. These results indicate that minimal inflammation occurred in the aortic wall of the FIR therapy groups, which may have resulted in reduced adaptive immune reaction-related SMCs and fibroblast infiltration.

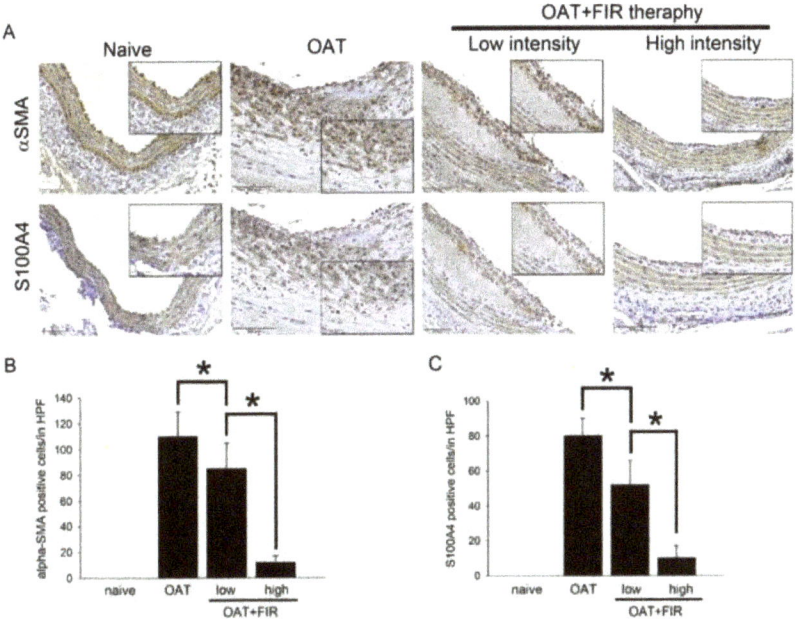

Figure 2. Administration of FIR therapy is effective against SMC and fibroblast activity in OAT-induced chronic allograft vasculopathy. (**A**) Immunohistochemistry to assess proliferated SMCs (αSMA) and fibroblasts (S100A4) in rat thoracic aortas from donor PVG/Seac rats. The lumen is uppermost in all sections; the images are 200× magnified. Similar regions are shown as enlarged images (400× magnification) in the black corners. The brown signal indicates αSMA- and S100A4-positive cells. (**B,C**) The quantification of cells in high power field (HPF) is displayed in (**B,C**). The graphs demonstrate the accumulation of cells in the aortas of rats. The results are expressed as the mean ± SD. * $p < 0.05$ was taken into consideration statistically considerable.

3.4. FIR Therapy Reduced Immune Responses in OAT ACI/NKyo Rats

Spleen weight was positively correlated with the rejection-related immune response. The spleens of experimental animals were weighed. As shown in Figure 3A, the average weight of the spleen of naive ACI/NKyo rats was 6.5 ± 0.7 g/g BW. The spleens of the OAT ACI/NKyo rats were significantly heavier than those of the naïve ACI/NKyo rats (approximately 20.8 ± 1.8 g/g BW). However, administration of FIR therapy may inhibit the spleen hypertrophy induced by immune response (11.1 ± 0.9 g/g BW in low intensity FIR therapy group and 7.1 ± 0.8 g/g BW in high intensity FIR therapy group). Additionally, the spleens were studied by immunohistochemistry to demonstrate the severity of chronic rejection. CD11b[+] macrophage is an antigen-presenting cell, that trigger adaptive responses [24]. In Figure 3B, macrophages were merely presented in the splenic periarterial lymphatic sheath (PALS) and germinal center (GC) of naive ACI/NKyo rats. In the non-FIR therapy group after OAT, a lot of macrophages was observed in the PALS and GC. In contrast, OAT with FIR therapy significantly inhibited the macrophages accumulation in splenic GC and

PALS. The $CD8^+$ killer T cells and $CD4^+$ helper T cells regulate cell-mediated immunity. In Figure 3C, the accumulation of helper T cells can be observed in the splenic GC and PALS in naïve ACI/NKyo rats. Additionally, an increased accumulation of helper T cells was presented in the splenic GC and PALS in the OAT without FIR therapy group, in contrast which decreased upon FIR therapy. Similarly, $CD8^+$ killer T cells also infiltrated the splenic PALS in the OAT ACI/NKyo rats without FIR therapy, which was twisted by FIR therapy. $CD20^+$ B cells regulate humoral immune responses and it can produce antibodies after differentiate into $CD138^+$ plasma cells. In Figure 3D, $CD20^+$ cells predominantly clustered in the GC and mantle zone and fewer $CD138^+$ cells were presented in the splenic GC, venous sinuses, and mantle zone in naïve group. ACI/NKyo rats with only OAT demonstrated with a lot of $CD20^+$ cells in the mantle zone and GC, as well as $CD138^+$ cells were presented in the splenic venous sinuses. In OAT ACI/NKyo rats, high-intensity FIR therapy resulted in a decreased accumulation of CD20 positive B cells in the GC and mantle zone. Plasma cells were slightly increased, which was observed in the venous sinuses, GC, and mantle zone in OAT ACI/NKyo rats without FIR therapy. FIR therapy may decrease plasma cell accumulation in OAT ACI/NKyo rats. Based on these results, we predicted that FIR therapy might maintain low levels of cell-mediated and humoral immune responses in OAT ACI/NKyo rats.

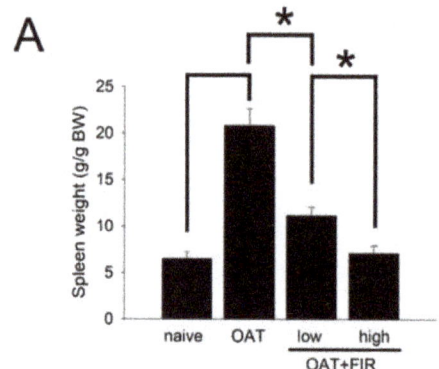

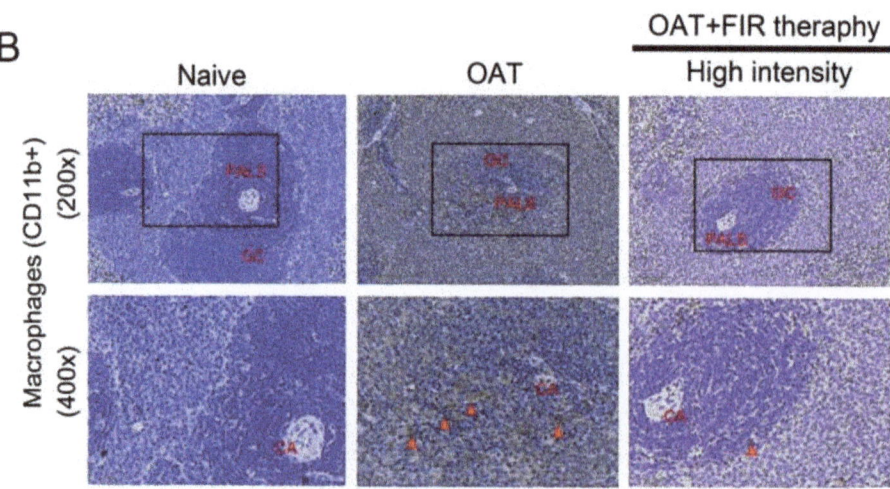

Figure 3. *Cont.*

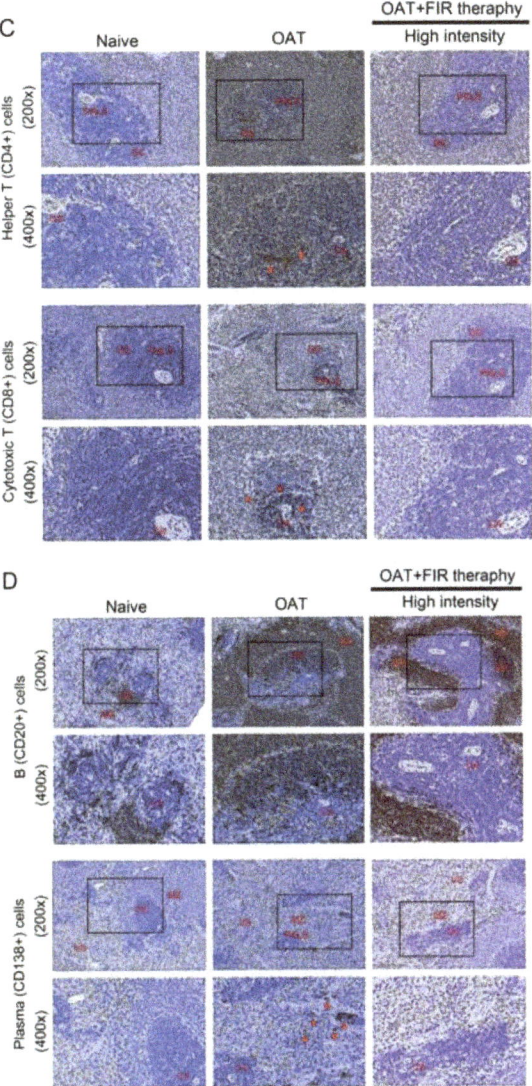

Figure 3. FIR therapy decreased splenic T lymphocytes, plasma cells, B lymphocytes, and macrophages activation in the OAT-ACI/NKyo rats. (**A**) The spleens were dissected from experimental rats after they were sacrificed. The weight of the spleen was analyzed and presented in a bar graph in g/g BW. The results are expressed as the mean ± SD. * $p < 0.05$ was taken into consideration statistically considerable. (**B**) Immunohistochemistry was used to analyze the accumulation of splenic CD11b$^+$ macrophages in the OAT-recipient ACI/NKyo rats (CA, central artery; PALS, periarterial lymphatic sheath; GC, germinal center;). The red triangle arrow heads are CD11b$^+$ macrophages. The images in the column are 200× and 400× magnification, respectively. (**C**) Immunohistochemistry was used to analyze accumulation of splenic CD8$^+$ cytotoxic T cells and CD4$^+$ helper T cells in the recipient rats. The images are presented in 200× and 400× magnification. The CD4$^+$ and CD8$^+$ cells are indicated by red arrow heads. (**D**) The splenic CD20$^+$ B cells and CD138$^+$ plasma cells accumulation in the OAT-recipient rats (MZ, mantle zone and VS, venous sinuses). The images in the column are 200× and 400× magnification, respectively. The red triangle arrow heads indicate CD138$^+$ cells. The cell nuclei were counted with hematoxylin.

3.5. FIR Therapy Lower Cytokines and Inflammation-Related Proteins Production in OAT ACI/NKyo Rats

The inflammation-related proteins and cytokines in OAT ACI/NKyo rats are shown in Table 3. CRP is an indicator of inflammation and tissue damage [25]; however, the levels were not significantly different between the baseline and 90 days of OAT in all experimental groups. Additionally, EPC function is related to the occurrence of OAT-induced vasculopathy [26]. However, SDF-1α is involved in the homing and recruitment of EPCs, and TNF-α and TGF-β1 negatively regulate EPC function [27] following OAT. Therefore, we also analyzed whether FIR therapy regulates plasma SDF-1α, TNF-α, and TGF-β1 levels, which are associated with the mechanisms of OAT in ACI/NKyo rats (the results are presented in Table 3). OAT induced an increase in SDF-1α in ACI/NKyo rats, with or without FIR therapy, indicating that FIR therapy did not increase SDF-1α production. OAT resulted in a significant TNF-α (243.8 ± 65.2 pg/mL) and TGF-β1 (418.4 ± 102.6 ng/mL) increase at day 90 compared to that of the sham control group (61.6 ± 9.8 pg/mL for TNF-α and 52.5 ± 10.8 ng/mL for TGF-β1). OAT with FIR therapy groups (both low- and high-intensity FIR) also demonstrated lower plasma TNF-α and TGF-β1 levels. Interferon-gamma (IFN-γ) mediates transplant vasculopathy through $CD8^+$ or $CD4^+$ T lymphocyte-associated injury in vascular endothelial cells. Furthermore, cytokines, such as IL-2, cause a reversible insult to the endothelium at the time of transplantation [28]. Low- and high-intensity FIR therapy may significantly decrease IFN-γ production, and high-intensity FIR therapy may significantly lower interleukin-12 (IL-12) secretion in ACI/NKyo rats after OAT compared to the non-FIR therapy group. Moreover, IFN-γ and IL-12 expression almost reached basal levels in high-intensity FIR therapy OAT ACI/NKyo rats. Based on these results, we predicted that FIR therapy might regulate alloimmunity and nonimmunity factors in appropriate situations.

Table 3. Comparison of OAT vasculopathy-related factors in ACI/NKyo rats ($n = 5$).

	Sham Control		OAT		OAT+FIR Low Intensity		OAT+FIR High Intensity	
Proteins	baseline	90 days	baseline	90 days	baseline	90 days	baseline	90 days
CRP (mg/dL)	30.9 ± 6.1	33.5 ± 14.6	33.6 ± 12.5	39.4 ± 8.5	32.6 ± 6.7	32.0 ± 11.7	33.9 ± 13.1	27.9 ± 10.5
SDF-1α (pg/mL)	180.5 ± 42.4	192.2 ± 41.1	200.7 ± 50.8	376.8 ± 103.2 [ab]	169.1 ± 63.9	367.2 ± 81.5 [ab]	259.3 ± 95.5	444.2 ± 106.9 [ab]
TNF-α (pg/mL)	68.2 ± 11.4	61.6 ± 9.8	59.0 ± 9.3	243.8 ± 65.2 [ab]	62.0 ± 7.0	110.9 ± 44.2 [abc]	70.1 ± 10.8	113.2 ± 47.7 [c]
TGF-β1 (ng/mL)	50.6 ± 11.2	52.5 ± 10.8	46.6 ± 13.3	418.4 ± 102.6 [ab]	41.6 ± 16.9	155.1 ± 54.9 [abc]	39.0 ± 7.3	136.3 ± 54.6 [abc]
INF-γ (pg/mL)	2.9 ± 0.8	2.9 ± 0.7	3.5 ± 1.0	23.2 ± 7.5 [ab]	3.5 ± 1.3	15.5 ± 3.8 [abc]	3.3 ± 1.5	4.7 ± 1.4 [bc]
IL-12 (pg/mL)	195.5 ± 38.9	181.6 ± 32.1	202.5 ± 34.7	404.6 ± 88.7 [ab]	176.7 ± 58.8	327.6 ± 60.3 [ab]	191.3 ± 45.4	187.7 ± 49.9 [c]

FIR, far-infrared ray; OAT, orthotopic aortic transplantation; CRP, C-reactive protein; TNF-α, tumor necrosis factor-alpha; SDF-1α, stromal cell-derived factor 1 alpha; INF-γ, interferon gama; IL-12, interleukin 12; TGF-β1, transforming growth factor- beta 1; Values are represented as mean ± SD. [a] $p < 0.05$ compared with baseline of the same group; [b] $p < 0.05$ compared with sham control ACI/NKyo (non-OAT) group at the same time point; [c] $p < 0.05$ compared with OAT (PVG/Seac to ACI/NKyo) group at the same time point.

3.6. FIR Therapy Mobilized Circulating EPCs, Not SMPCs, in OAT ACI/NKyo Rats

EPCs play critical roles in the repair of damaged vessels [29]. SDF-1α may trigger the mobilization of circulating EPCs [30]. Additionally, TGF-1β and IFN-γ may command T cell function and may induce endothelial-mesenchymal transition (endo-MT) in the progression of OAT-induced vasculopathy [31,32]. As shown in Table 3, performed the FIR therapy resulted in decreased TGF-1β and INF-γ production in OAT- recipient ACI/NKyo rats. Therefore, following OAT surgery, the population of circulating $CD133^+/CD34^+/VEGF^+$ EPCs and $CD133^+/\alpha SMA^+/CD34^-$ SMPCs was analyzed. The results demonstrated significantly increase in EPCs in ACI/NKyo rats compared to naive /non-OAT ACI/NKyo rats on the 30th day after OAT, and it was maintained until on the 90th day after OAT (Figure 4A). On 60th day after OAT, the low- and high-intensity FIR therapy groups increased the EPCs in circulation compared to the non-FIR therapy. However, high-intensity FIR therapy continued to maintain a significantly higher number of circulating EPCs on the 90th day after OAT compared to non-FIR therapy group. Moreover, SMPCs initiate atherosclerosis. However, flow cytometry showed that the circulating SMPCs was not related to FIR therapy (Figure 4B). These results indicate that FIR therapy might promote increased mobilization of early circulating EPCs compared to non-FIR therapy in OAT-recipient ACI/NKyo rats.

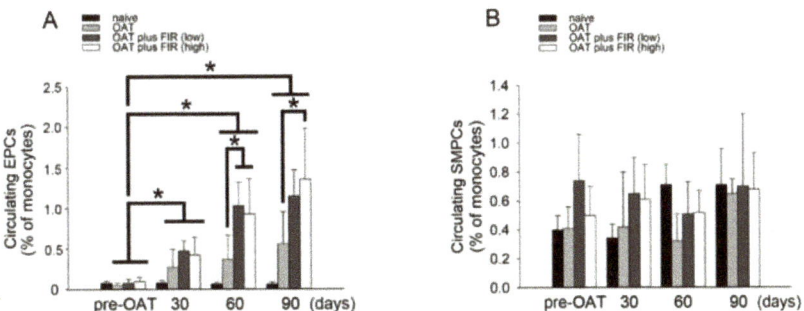

Figure 4. FIR therapy promotes EPCs mobilization in OAT-recipient ACI/NKyo rats. (**A**) CD133$^+$/VEGF$^+$/CD34$^+$ cells (defined as EPCs) mobilization at day 30–90 following OAT in ACI/NKyo rats were analyzed by flow cytometry. (**B**) CD133$^+$/αSMA$^+$/CD34$^-$ cells (defined as SMPCs) mobilization at day 30–90 following OAT in ACI/NKyo rats were studied. Quantification of EPCs (left) and SMPCs (right) in OAT-recipient rats (black bar, naive rats; light gray bar, OAT only rats; dark gray bar, OAT rats with low intensity of FIR therapy; white bar, OAT rats with high intensity of FIR therapy). All results are expressed as the mean ± SD (n = 5). * p < 0.05 was taken into consideration statistically considerable.

3.7. FIR Treatment That Regulates the Functions of EPCs May Mediate OAT Vasculopathy

As the EPCs senescence and function are associated with the OAT vasculopathy [26], we studied the effects of FIR treatment on the activity of EPCs, including tube formation capability, intracellular β-galactosidase activity, and cellular migratory performance. As shown in Figure 4A and Table 3, FIR therapy increased the differentiation of mononuclear cells into circulating EPCs in ACI/NKyo rats, and also decreased the plasma level of the cytokine TNF-α in OAT ACI/NKyo. We hypothesized that FIR therapy decreases plasma TNF-α levels and is associated with increased EPC function and activity. Figure 5 shows the results of the in vitro study. After 24 h of treatment with 2 or 10 ng/mL TNF-α, the tube-forming phenomena of EPCs was significantly decreased compared to that of the control (2 ng/mL TNF-α group: 56.4 ± 10.2% of the control; 10 ng/mL TNF-α group: 15.4 ± 9.7% of the control). In contrast, in the group of FIR treatment, the tube-forming phenomena was significantly increased (2 ng/mL TNF-α with FIR treatment group: 85.7 ± 10.3% of the control; 10 ng/mL TNF-α with FIR treatment group: 72.4 ± 9.4% of the control) compared with that of the 2 or 10 ng/mL TNF-α groups (Figure 5A). Additionally, Figure 5B shows that compared to the control group, senescence increased following TNF-α treatment (2 ng/mL TNF-α group: 54.2 ± 7.8% of the control; 10 ng/mL TNF-α group: 89.4 ± 7.5% of the control). However, compared to the FIR-treated groups, FIR treatment significantly inhibited the presentation of β-galactosidase-positive EPCs under TNF-α stimulation (2 ng/mL TNF-α with FIR treatment group: 8.1 ± 2.5% of the control; 10 ng/mL TNF-α with FIR treatment group: 10.5 ± 4.2% of the control). In addition, a migration assay was performed to study the effect of FIR treatment on TNF-α-treated EPCs. The EPCs were then cultured in the presence of TNF-α and FIR treatment, and images were taken 8 h after wounding. Significantly, 10 ng/mL TNF-α decreased the wound closure rate (10.5 ± 7.8%) compared to that in the control group (85.6 ± 7.4%), whereas FIR treatment significantly reversed the decline (79.5 ± 8.1%) (Figure 5C). FIR treatment increased the tube formation capability of naive EPCs but had no significant effect on β-galactosidase activity and migration activity of naive EPCs. These results indicate that FIR treatment might effectively promote these functions and prevented EPC senescence.

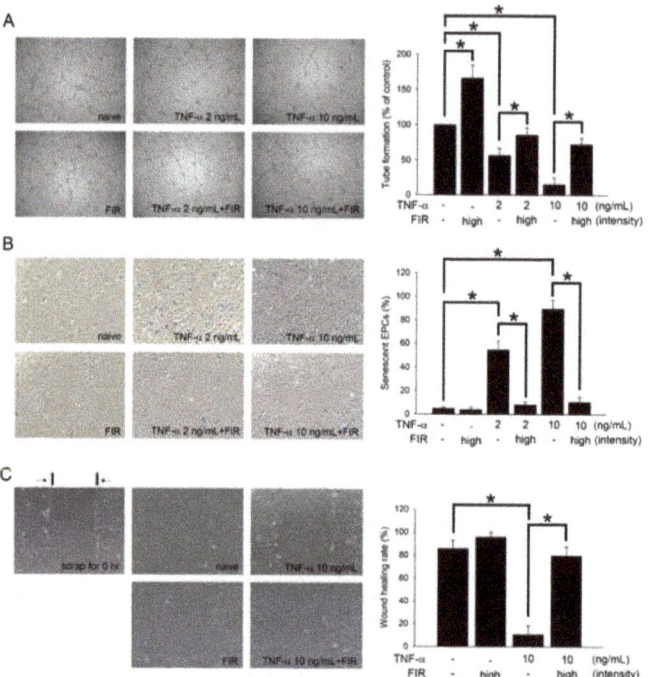

Figure 5. FIR treatment promotes the functions of human EPCs. (**A**) EPCs were stimulated with 2 or 10 ng/mL TNF-α for 24 h with or without high intensity of FIR treatment. An in vitro angiogenesis assay was used to investigate the effect of FIR therapy on EPC neovascularization. Representative photos of in vitro angiogenesis are shown. The graph shows the quantification of tube formation by TNF-α-treated EPCs following FIR treatment. (**B**) After treating EPCs with TNF-α and high intensity of FIR for 24 h, cell senescence was analyzed; the diagram shows the quantification of senescent EPCs. (**C**) A migration assay was performed to analyze the effect of FIR on TNF-α-treated EPCs. The 10 ng/mL of TNF-α were treated to EPCs, and adhered to 24 h of FIR treatment before injury scratching. Photos were taken after 8 h of injuring. Counted the migrated EPCs at the denuded location according to the black baseline under 100× high-power field. All data are expressed as the mean ± SD of three independent experiments and as the percentage of the control. * $p < 0.05$ was taken into consideration statistically considerable.

3.8. FIR Treatment Regulates the EndoMT of EPCs and May Mediate OAT Vasculopathy

As the endothelial to mesenchymal transition (EndoMT) of EPCs is associated with the process of OAT vasculopathy [33], Table 3 presents that OAT increased the plasma TGF-β1 level and reversed by FIR therapy in ACI/NKyo rats. Therefore, we hypothesized that FIR therapy may decrease plasma TGF-β1-induced EndoMT associated with OAT. We investigated the effects of FIR treatment on the EndoMT of EPCs, including the expression of related factors (vWF, VE-cadherin, αSMA, and vimentin). As shown in Figure 6A, treatment with 2 or 10 μg/mL TGF-β1 for 5 days decreased the expression of vWF mRNA and VE-cadherin mRNA compared to the control (naive group). Therapy with high-intensity FIR could reverse the decline in expression of vWF mRNA and VE-cadherin mRNA in TGF-β1 culture. In contrast, TGF-β1 significantly increased αSMA mRNA and vimentin mRNA expression, which was significantly prevented by FIR treatment (Figure 6B). Additionally, Western blot analysis demonstrated that FIR treatment increased vWF and VE-cadherin expression but reversed αSMA and vimentin expression in TGF-β1-treated EPCs (Figure 6C). Smad2 phosphorylation is associated with EndoMT. Therefore, Western blotting was performed to explore the effects of FIR therapy on Smad2 expression in TGF-β1-induced EPCs. Figure 6D presented that high-intensity FIR therapy decreased Smad2 phosphorylation in TGF-β1-treated EPCs. Transcription factors, such as Snail and Slug, positively regulate the markers expression of EndoMT [34] and mediate the loss of cellular adhesion in endothelial cells [35]. Therefore, we investigated the effect of FIR treatment on the activation of Snail and Slug. In Figure 6E, TGF-β1 increased the activation of Snail and Slug, and FIR treatment inhibited the nuclear translocation of Slug. However, FIR treatment did not affect the activation of Snail in TGF-β1-stimulated EPCs. According to these results, we conclude that high-intensity FIR can effectively and stably inhibit EndoMT by controlling the phosphorylation of Smad2 and activation of Slug transcription factors in EPCs; however, the role of other signaling pathways that were not analyzed in this study cannot be neglected.

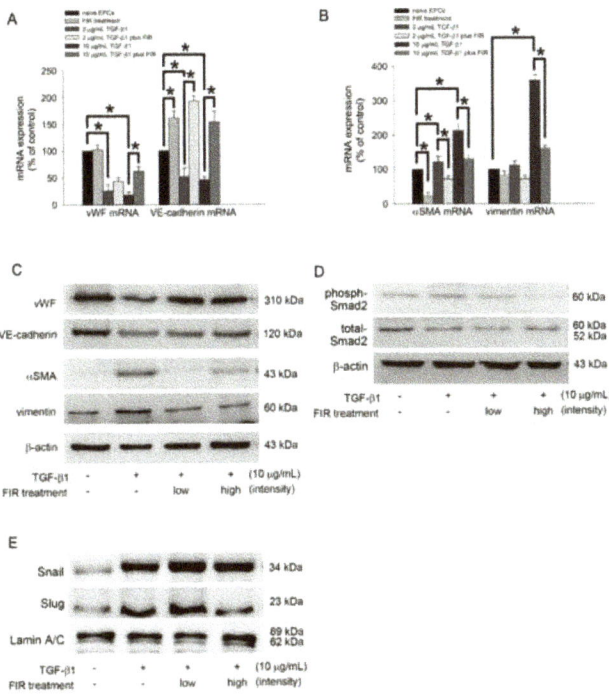

Figure 6. FIR treatment regulates TGF-β1-induced EndoMT via Smad- and Slug-dependent pathways. (**A,B**) Human EPCs were exposed to 2 or 10 μg/mL recombinant human TGF-β1 for 5 days with high intensity or without FIR treatment. The α-SMA, VE-cadherin, vWF, and vimentin mRNA expression were evaluated using reverse transcription and qPCR analysis. The expression of related mRNA expression is normalized to the expression of GAPDH mRNA, is presented as a bar graph. All data are expressed as the mean ± SD of five independent experiments and as the percentage of the control. * $p < 0.05$ was taken into consideration statistically considerable. (**C,D**) Human EPCs were exposed to 10 μg/mL TGF-β1 for 5 days with low intensity, high intensity or without FIR treatment. The total protein expression of the vWF, VE-cadherin, α-SMA, vimentin, and phosphorylated Smad2 were identified by Western blot analysis. β-actin and total-Smad2 were used as loading controls. (**E**) Human EPCs were treated with 10 μg/mL TGF-β1 in the presence or absence of FIR treatment for 5 days. Total nuclear lysates were purified, and the levels of Snail and Slug were analyzed using Western blotting; lamin A/C was used as a loading control.

4. Discussion

There are many ways to implement FIR therapy in clinical practice [6,36,37], and they always provide thermal and non-thermal effects to increase blood flow [38,39], maintain endothelial function, lower blood pressure [40,41], and regulate nerve function [42,43]. Compared to the other diseases, FIR therapy, has a significant impact on cardiovascular diseases. Ikeda et al. showed that FIR therapy can increase endothelial nitric oxide synthase (eNOS) mRNA expression, eNOS protein production, and nitric oxide (NO) levels in cardiomyopathy and heart failure [44], which may be related to the pathway of increasing Ca^{2+}/calmodulin-dependent protein kinase (CaMKII)-mediated eNOS phosphorylation [45]. Increasing eNOS activity and NO content can effectively improve vascular endothelial and cardiac function, increase cardiopulmonary exercise tolerance [1,2], and inhibit platelet aggregation and smooth muscle cell migration/proliferation [46]. Additionally, FIR therapy reduces plasma levels of lipid peroxidation and 8-epi-prostaglandin $F_{2\alpha}$ [47]. The 8-epi-prostaglandin $F_{2\alpha}$ causes systemic oxidative stress and subsequently induces atherosclerosis and congenital heart failure. NO production can be increased by reducing 8-epi-prostaglandin $F_{2\alpha}$ levels and its oxidative stress [48]. This may also be the mechanism by which FIR therapy improves vascular endothelial cell function and prevents the occurrence of cardiovascular diseases. EPC differentiation and mobilization in OAT rats is one of the factors that determines vasculopathy [26]. Additionally, eNOS activity and NO production can modify the differentiation and mobilization of EPCs [49]. In the present study, we found that FIR therapy increased the functions of EPCs, including migration and tube formation capacity, in OAT rats. Although we did not currently analyze the effect of FIR therapy on NO activity in rats after OAT, based on the results of a previous study conducted by our group which found that FIR therapy reduced oxidative stress and upregulated NO bioavailability in streptozotocine-induced diabetic mice [8], we speculate that the vasculopathy prevented by FIR therapy may be related to the regulation of NO activity.

In this experiment, we performed FIR therapy with an FIR emitter, consisting of electrified ceramic plates, and irradiated 20 cm from the skin for 40 min for each cycle. FIR therapy provides low energy to steadily increase the skin temperature. We cannot rule out thermal effects and an effect on the occurrence of OATV in animals following increased skin temperature. However, we controlled the temperature of the incubator and experimented with cells at 37 °C in an in vitro study. Therefore, we can speculate that the effects of FIR therapy on cells and tissues are due to its nonthermal effects. Previous reports have demonstrated that miRNAs are involved in the development of the cardiovascular system [50] and regulate the occurrence of cardiovascular diseases and function of vascular endothelial cells [50–52]. Plasma miRNAs, such as miRNA-1, miRNA-17, miRNA-21, miRNA-92a, miRNA-126, miRNA-133, and miRNA-145, have been considered as markers of cardiovascular diseases [51,53] and indicators to estimate the course of acute myocardial infarction [54]. In addition, the functions of EPCs, including proliferation, migration, senescence, apoptosis, mobilization, and differentiation, are regulated by many miRNAs [55]. Therefore, we speculate that FIR therapy may modulate the function of EPCs by altering the expression of miRNAs under pathological conditions to avoid vasculopathy in patients with OAT. We are analyzing the possible effects of FIR on the expression of miRNAs in EPC, and thus to understand the possible roles of miRNAs in the process of FIR treatment of OAT.

The incident of chronic rejection after OAT refer to the manufacturing of anti-bodies versus donor-specific leukocyte antigens (HLA) by the recipient [56]. Donor antigen-presenting cells existing in the tissue, such as the MHC fragments on the surface of dendritic cells, will absolutely be recognized by the T cells in the recipient, which subsequently induces the cellular immune response. On top of that, antigen fragments from donor provided externally to the recipient's antigen-presenting cells are acknowledged by the T cells in recipient [12]. This procedure is the major initiator of the immune response for chronic rejection [57]. The release of IFN-γ from activated T cells will continue to activate B cells and macrophages, and additionally amplify the endothelial cells in the graft to express cellular adhesion molecules. SMCs are also proliferation [58] and secret extracellular matrix proteins resulting from simultaneous activation. Concomitantly, anti-HLA antibodies are produced by activated B cells, which promote vasculopathy in the donor graft. In this study, we clearly observed that the concentration of IFN-γ in the plasma of OAT rats treated with FIR therapy was significantly reduced, and the infiltration of SMCs in the donor aorta was significantly inhibited compared with that in the group without FIR therapy. Immunohistochemical staining also showed that FIR therapy reduced T and B cell activity in the spleen. We are the first group to publish on FIR therapy for the suppression of chronic rejection after OAT. In addition to the clinical use of immunosuppressive and immunomodulatory agents to control autoimmune diseases or chronic rejection, the adjunctive use of FIR therapy may be a way to make traditional treatments more effective.

EPCs play an important role associated with the process of OAT vasculopathy [59]. Endo-MT, which describes the procedure where ECs differentiate into fibroblasts and also SMCs [60,61]. TGF-β1 regulates the development of fibrosis [61,62]. EPCs advertise healing and also repair of harmed endothelium [63] also keep vascular endothelial function [64]. However, current researchers have actually discovered that EPCs in the patient underwent heart transplantation are associated with the formation of vasculopathy [57,64,65]. EPCs from the recipient adhere to the vessel wall of the transplanted organ and begin EndoMT, leading to alloimmune responses following OAT [65]. Alloimmune responses can result in serious EPCs EndoMT and subsequent accumulation of SMCs and fibroblasts [65,66], leading to an excessive accumulation of extracellular matrix and neointimal formation [64]. Our research results show that FIR therapy can reduce the levels of cytokines in the plasma that induce cell-mediated and humoral immune responses, such as IL-12 and INF-γ, and reduce the attack on donor grafts after T cell and B cell activation in OAT ACI/NKyo rats. The incidence of OAT vasculopathy was reduced by reducing TGF-β-induced EndoMT via the Smad2-Slug-axis signaling pathway. Based on these results, we believe that FIR therapy might have the potential to be used more widely in the treatment of diseases related to immune system abnormalities or impaired EPCs function.

5. Conclusions

We conclude the results of this study with a scheme diagram (Figure 7). The animal study of OAT-induced vasculopathy in ACI/NKyo rats revealed that FIR therapy could prevent vasculopathy via anti-immune responses and anti-inflammatory mechanisms. In contrast, FIR therapy could increase the number of circulating EPCs in OAT ACI/NKyo rats. In vitro experiments have also confirmed that FIR can reduce the negative effects (such as EndoMT and senescence) of cytokines (such as TNF-α, TGF-β1, and INF-γ) on EPCs and increase their activity. These mechanisms are associated with the occurrence of OAT vasculopathy. Thus, this study might provide new insights into the preventive strategy of using FIR therapy to treat chronic rejection-induced vasculopathy.

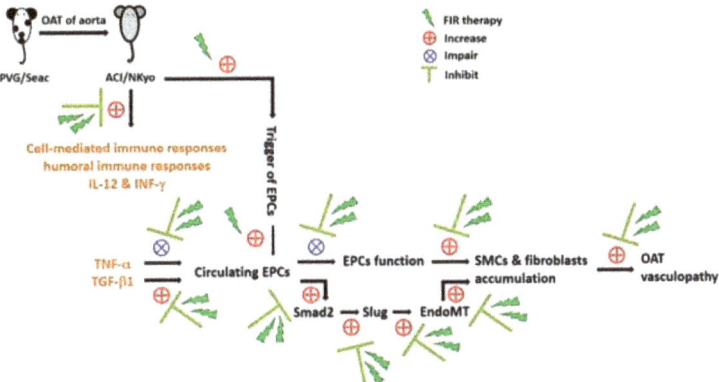

Figure 7. FIR therapy may effectively regulate chronic rejection-induced vasculopathy in OAT rats. Therapy of FIR reduced T and B lymphocytes, plasma cells, and macrophage activation in the spleens

of the OAT-recipient ACI/NKyo rats. Lowered the progression of vasculopathy in OAT-recipient ACI/NKyo rats occurred by the inhibition of cell-mediated and humoral immune responses, prevention of cytokines-induced disfunction and EndoMT in EPCs, decrease in collagen damage and pathological accumulation, and proliferation and infiltration of SMCs and fibroblasts in the vessel wall of OAT-recipient ACI/NKyo rats. Therefore, the results highlight the therapeutic roles of FIR and provides a more effective adjuvant therapeutic route in vasculopathy.

Author Contributions: Y.-W.L., C.-S.T. and F.-Y.L. conceived of the project, designed and performed experiments, and analyzed the data. C.-Y.H., Y.-T.T., S.-J.L., C.-Y.L. (Chi-Yuan Li) and S.-Y.S. contributed with regard to reagents/materials/analysis tools/consultant. C.-M.S. and C.-Y.L. (Cheng-Yen Lin) contributed to the statistical analyses. This manuscript was written by Y.-W.L. and F.-Y.L. All authors have read and agreed to the published version of the manuscript.

Funding: This work was supported by Medical Affairs Bureau Ministry of National Defense and Tri-service General Hospital (MAB-D-111003 and TSGH-C01-110014), Ministry of Science and Technology (MOST 110-2320-B-038-032-MY3 and MOST 110-2314-B-016-038-MY3) and Taipei Medical University Hospital (111TMUH-MOST-16) in Taiwan.

Institutional Review Board Statement: All animals were handled according to the protocols authorized by the institutional animal care committee of the Taipei Medical University (certification no. LAC-2020-0047).

Informed Consent Statement: Not applicable.

Data Availability Statement: The data presented in this study are available on request from the corresponding author.

Acknowledgments: We thank Tze-Liang Yang for excellent technical assistance.

Conflicts of Interest: The authors declare no conflict of interest.

References

1. Sobajima, M.; Nozawa, T.; Ihori, H.; Shida, T.; Ohori, T.; Suzuki, T.; Matsuki, A.; Yasumura, S.; Inoue, H. Repeated sauna therapy improves myocardial perfusion in patients with chronically occluded coronary artery-related ische-mia. *Int. J. Cardiol.* **2013**, *167*, 237–243. [CrossRef] [PubMed]
2. Ohori, T.; Nozawa, T.; Ihori, H.; Shida, T.; Sobajima, M.; Matsuki, A.; Yasumura, S.; Inoue, H. Effect of repeated sauna treatment on exercise tolerance and endothelial function in patients with chronic heart failure. *Am. J. Cardiol.* **2012**, *109*, 100–104. [CrossRef] [PubMed]
3. Lin, C.C.; Chang, C.F.; Lai, M.Y.; Chen, T.W.; Lee, P.C.; Yang, W.C. Far-infrared therapy: A novel treatment to im-prove access blood flow and unassisted patency of arteriovenous fistula in hemodialysis patients. *J. Am. Soc. Nephrol.* **2007**, *18*, 985–992. [CrossRef] [PubMed]
4. Lai, C.C.; Fang, H.C.; Mar, G.Y.; Liou, J.C.; Tseng, C.J.; Liu, C.P. Post-angioplasty far infrared radiation therapy improves 1-year angioplasty-free hemodialysis access patency of recurrent obstructive lesions. *Eur. J. Vasc. Endovasc. Surg.* **2013**, *46*, 726–732. [CrossRef]
5. Tu, Y.P.; Chen, S.C.; Liu, Y.H.; Chen, C.F.; Hour, T.C. Postconditioning with far-infrared irradiation increases heme oxygenase-1 expression and protects against ischemia/reperfusion injury in rat testis. *Life Sci.* **2013**, *92*, 35–41. [CrossRef]
6. Yu, S.Y.; Chiu, J.H.; Yang, S.D.; Hsu, Y.C.; Lui, W.Y.; Wu, C.W. Biological effect of far-infrared therapy on increas-ing skin microcirculation in rats. *Photodermatol. Photoimmunol. Photomed.* **2006**, *22*, 78–86. [CrossRef]
7. Chen, T.Y.; Yang, Y.C.; Sha, Y.N.; Chou, J.R.; Liu, B.S. Far-Infrared Therapy Promotes Nerve Repair following End-to-End Neurorrhaphy in Rat Models of Sciatic Nerve Injury. *Evid. Based Complement. Altern. Med.* **2015**, *2015*, 207245. [CrossRef]
8. Huang, P.H.; Chen, J.W.; Lin, C.P.; Chen, Y.H.; Wang, C.H.; Leu, H.B.; Lin, S.J. Far infra-red therapy promotes is-chemia-induced angiogenesis in diabetic mice and restores high glucose-suppressed endothelial progenitor cell functions. *Cardiovasc. Diabetol.* **2012**, *11*, 99. [CrossRef]
9. Shui, S.; Wang, X.; Chiang, J.Y.; Zheng, L. Far-infrared therapy for cardiovascular, autoimmune, and other chronic health problems: A systematic review. *Exp. Biol. Med.* **2015**, *240*, 1257–1265. [CrossRef]
10. Lund, L.H.; Edwards, L.B.; Kucheryavaya, A.Y.; Dipchand, A.I.; Benden, C.; Christie, J.D.; Dobbels, F.; Kirk, R.; Rahmel, A.O.; Yusen, R.D.; et al. The Registry of the International Society for Heart and Lung Transplantation: Thir-tieth Official Adult Heart Transplant Report–2013; focus theme: Age. *J. Heart Lung Transplant.* **2013**, *32*, 951–964. [CrossRef]
11. Costello, J.P.; Mohanakumar, T.; Nath, D.S. Mechanisms of chronic cardiac allograft rejection. *Tex. Heart Inst. J.* **2013**, *40*, 395–399. [PubMed]
12. Nath, D.S.; Basha, H.I.; Mohanakumar, T. Antihuman leukocyte antigen antibody-induced autoimmunity: Role in chronic rejection. *Curr. Opin. Organ Transplant.* **2010**, *15*, 16–20. [CrossRef] [PubMed]

13. Holt, C.D. Overview of Immunosuppressive Therapy in Solid Organ Transplantation. *Anesthesiol. Clin.* **2017**, *35*, 365–380. [CrossRef] [PubMed]
14. Jasiak, N.M.; Park, J.M. Immunosuppression in Solid-Organ Transplantation: Essentials and Practical Tips. *Crit. Care Nurs. Q.* **2016**, *39*, 227–240. [CrossRef]
15. Poston, R.S.; Billingham, M.; Hoyt, E.G.; Pollard, J.; Shorthouse, R.; Morris, R.E.; Robbins, R.C. Rapamycin reverses chronic graft vascular disease in a novel cardiac allograft model. *Circulation* **1999**, *100*, 67–74. [CrossRef]
16. Bedi, D.S.; Riella, L.V.; Tullius, S.G.; Chandraker, A. Animal models of chronic allograft injury: Contributions and limitations to understanding the mechanism of long-term graft dysfunction. *Transplantation* **2010**, *90*, 935–944. [CrossRef]
17. Chen, Y.H.; Lin, S.J.; Lin, F.Y.; Wu, T.C.; Tsao, C.R.; Huang, P.H.; Liu, P.L.; Chen, Y.L.; Chen, J.W. High glucose impairs early and late endothelial progenitor cells by modifying nitric oxide-related but not oxidative stress-mediated mechanisms. *Diabetes* **2007**, *56*, 1559–1568. [CrossRef]
18. Chen, J.Z.; Zhu, J.H.; Wang, X.X.; Xie, X.D.; Sun, J.; Shang, Y.P.; Guo, X.G.; Dai, H.M.; Hu, S.J. Effects of homocys-teine on number and activity of endothelial progenitor cells from peripheral blood. *J. Mol. Cell. Cardiol.* **2004**, *36*, 233–239. [CrossRef]
19. Goldstein, S. Replicative senescence: The human fibroblast comes of age. *Science* **1990**, *249*, 1129–1133. [CrossRef]
20. Lin, F.Y.; Shih, C.M.; Huang, C.Y.; Tsai, Y.T.; Loh, S.H.; Li, C.Y.; Lin, C.Y.; Lin, Y.W.; Tsai, C.S. Dipeptidyl Pepti-dase-4 Inhibitor Decreases Allograft Vasculopathy Via Regulating the Functions of Endothelial Progenitor Cells in Normoglycemic Rats. *Cardiovasc. Drugs Ther.* **2021**, *35*, 1111–1127.
21. Zou, H.; Yang, Y.; Gao, M.; Zhang, B.; Ming, B.; Sun, Y.; Chen, H.; Tang, X.; Chen, Z.; Xiong, P.; et al. HMGB1 is involved in chronic rejection of cardiac allograft via promoting inflammatory-like mDCs. *Am. J. Transplant.* **2014**, *14*, 1765–1777. [CrossRef] [PubMed]
22. Khan, T.T.; Mirza, A.B.; Zahid, R.; Haleem, A.; Al Hussaini, H.; Al Sulaiman, M.; Mousa, D. Antibody-mediated rejection: Importance of lactate dehydrogenase and neutrophilia in early diagnosis. *Saudi J. Kidney Dis. Transplant.* **2011**, *22*, 525–530.
23. Kato, G.J.; Hebbel, R.P.; Steinberg, M.H.; Gladwin, M.T. Vasculopathy in sickle cell disease: Biology, pathophysi-ology, genetics, translational medicine, and new research directions. *Am. J. Hematol.* **2009**, *84*, 618–625. [CrossRef] [PubMed]
24. Rua, R.; McGavern, D.B. Elucidation of monocyte/macrophage dynamics and function by intravital imaging. *J. Leukoc. Biol.* **2015**, *98*, 319–332. [CrossRef]
25. Sproston, N.R.; Ashworth, J.J. Role of C-Reactive Protein at Sites of Inflammation and Infection. *Front. Immunol.* **2018**, *9*, 754. [CrossRef]
26. Fadini, G.P.; Sartore, S.; Albiero, M.; Baesso, I.; Murphy, E.; Menegolo, M.; Grego, F.; Vigili de Kreutzenberg, S.; Tiengo, A.; Agostini, C.; et al. Number and function of endothelial progenitor cells as a marker of severity for dia-betic vasculopathy. *Arterioscler. Thromb. Vasc. Biol.* **2006**, *26*, 2140–2146. [CrossRef]
27. Pintavorn, P.; Ballermann, B.J. TGF-beta and the endothelium during immune injury. *Kidney Int.* **1997**, *51*, 1401–1412. [CrossRef]
28. Weis, M.; Wildhirt, S.M.; Schulze, C.; Pehlivanli, S.; Fraunberger, P.; Meiser, B.M.; von Scheidt, W. Modulation of coronary vasomotor tone by cytokines in cardiac transplant recipients. *Transplantation* **1999**, *68*, 1263–1267. [CrossRef]
29. Del Papa, N.; Pignataro, F. The Role of Endothelial Progenitors in the Repair of Vascular Damage in Systemic Sclerosis. *Front. Immunol.* **2018**, *9*, 1383. [CrossRef]
30. Tilling, L.; Chowienczyk, P.; Clapp, B. Progenitors in motion: Mechanisms of mobilization of endothelial progen-itor cells. *Br. J. Clin. Pharmacol.* **2009**, *68*, 484–492. [CrossRef]
31. Oh, S.A.; Li, M.O. TGF-beta: Guardian of T cell function. *J. Immunol.* **2013**, *191*, 3973–3979. [CrossRef] [PubMed]
32. Knight, R.J.; Liu, H.; Fishman, E.; Reis, E.D. Cold ischemic injury, aortic allograft vasculopathy, and pro-inflammatory cytokine expression. *J. Surg. Res.* **2003**, *113*, 201–207. [CrossRef]
33. Kovacic, J.C.; Dimmeler, S.; Harvey, R.P.; Finkel, T.; Aikawa, E.; Krenning, G.; Baker, A.H. Endothelial to Mesen-chymal Transition in Cardiovascular Disease: JACC State-of-the-Art Review. *J. Am. Coll. Cardiol.* **2019**, *73*, 190–209. [CrossRef] [PubMed]
34. Mahmoud, M.M.; Serbanovic-Canic, J.; Feng, S.; Souilhol, C.; Xing, R.; Hsiao, S.; Mammoto, A.; Chen, J.; Ariaans, M.; Francis, S.E.; et al. Shear stress induces endothelial-to-mesenchymal transition via the transcription factor Snail. *Sci. Rep.* **2017**, *7*, 3375. [CrossRef] [PubMed]
35. Platel, V.; Faure, S.; Corre, I.; Clere, N. Endothelial-to-Mesenchymal Transition (EndoMT): Roles in Tumorigene-sis, Metastatic Extravasation and Therapy Resistance. *J. Oncol.* **2019**, *2019*, 8361945. [CrossRef] [PubMed]
36. Tei, C. Waon therapy: Soothing warmth therapy. *J. Cardiol.* **2007**, *49*, 301–304. [PubMed]
37. Tei, C.; Horikiri, Y.; Park, J.C.; Jeong, J.W.; Chang, K.S.; Toyama, Y.; Tanaka, N. Acute hemodynamic improve-ment by thermal vasodilation in congestive heart failure. *Circulation* **1995**, *91*, 2582–2590. [CrossRef]
38. Akasaki, Y.; Miyata, M.; Eto, H.; Shirasawa, T.; Hamada, N.; Ikeda, Y.; Biro, S.; Otsuji, Y.; Tei, C. Repeated thermal therapy up-regulates endothelial nitric oxide synthase and augments angiogenesis in a mouse model of hindlimb ischemia. *Circ. J.* **2006**, *70*, 463–470. [CrossRef]
39. Ise, N.; Katsuura, T.; Kikuchi, Y.; Miwa, E. Effect of far-infrared radiation on forearm skin blood flow. *Ann. Physiol. Anthropol.* **1987**, *6*, 31–32. [CrossRef]
40. Kihara, T.; Biro, S.; Imamura, M.; Yoshifuku, S.; Takasaki, K.; Ikeda, Y.; Otuji, Y.; Minagoe, S.; Toyama, Y.; Tei, C. Repeated sauna treatment improves vascular endothelial and cardiac function in patients with chronic heart failure. *J. Am. Coll. Cardiol.* **2002**, *39*, 754–759. [CrossRef]

41. Ryotokuji, K.; Ishimaru, K.; Kihara, K.; Namiki, Y.; Hozumi, N. Effect of pinpoint plantar long-wavelength infra-red light irradiation on subcutaneous temperature and stress markers. *Laser Ther.* **2013**, *22*, 93–102. [CrossRef] [PubMed]
42. Su, L.H.; Wu, K.D.; Lee, L.S.; Wang, H.; Liu, C.F. Effects of far infrared acupoint stimulation on autonomic activ-ity and quality of life in hemodialysis patients. *Am. J. Chin. Med.* **2009**, *37*, 215–226. [CrossRef] [PubMed]
43. Oosterveld, F.G.; Rasker, J.J.; Floors, M.; Landkroon, R.; van Rennes, B.; Zwijnenberg, J.; van de Laar, M.A.; Koel, G.J. Infrared sauna in patients with rheumatoid arthritis and ankylosing spondylitis. A pilot study showing good tolerance, short-term improvement of pain and stiffness, and a trend towards long-term beneficial effects. *Clin. Rheumatol.* **2009**, *28*, 29–34. [CrossRef] [PubMed]
44. Ikeda, Y.; Biro, S.; Kamogawa, Y.; Yoshifuku, S.; Eto, H.; Orihara, K.; Yu, B.; Kihara, T.; Miyata, M.; Hamasaki, S.; et al. Repeated sauna therapy increases arterial endothelial nitric oxide synthase expression and nitric oxide pro-duction in cardiomyopathic hamsters. *Circ. J.* **2005**, *69*, 722–729. [CrossRef]
45. Park, J.H.; Lee, S.; Cho, D.H.; Park, Y.M.; Kang, D.H.; Jo, I. Far-infrared radiation acutely increases nitric oxide production by increasing Ca(2+) mobilization and Ca(2+)/calmodulin-dependent protein kinase II-mediated phos-phorylation of endothelial nitric oxide synthase at serine 1179. *Biochem. Biophys. Res. Commun.* **2013**, *436*, 601–606. [CrossRef]
46. Anggard, E. Nitric oxide: Mediator, murderer, and medicine. *Lancet* **1994**, *343*, 1199–1206. [CrossRef]
47. Patrono, C.; FitzGerald, G.A. Isoprostanes: Potential markers of oxidant stress in atherothrombotic disease. *Arterioscler. Thromb. Vasc. Biol.* **1997**, *17*, 2309–2315. [CrossRef]
48. Malek, A.M.; Izumo, S.; Alper, S.L. Modulation by pathophysiological stimuli of the shear stress-induced up-regulation of endothelial nitric oxide synthase expression in endothelial cells. *Neurosurgery* **1999**, *45*, 334–344, discussion 344–335. [CrossRef]
49. Aicher, A.; Heeschen, C.; Mildner-Rihm, C.; Urbich, C.; Ihling, C.; Technau-Ihling, K.; Zeiher, A.M.; Dimmeler, S. Essential role of endothelial nitric oxide synthase for mobilization of stem and progenitor cells. *Nat. Med.* **2003**, *9*, 1370–1376. [CrossRef]
50. Kuehbacher, A.; Urbich, C.; Zeiher, A.M.; Dimmeler, S. Role of Dicer and Drosha for endothelial microRNA expression and angiogenesis. *Circ. Res.* **2007**, *101*, 59–68. [CrossRef]
51. Weber, M.; Baker, M.B.; Moore, J.P.; Searles, C.D. MiR-21 is induced in endothelial cells by shear stress and mod-ulates apoptosis and eNOS activity. *Biochem. Biophys. Res. Commun.* **2010**, *393*, 643–648. [CrossRef] [PubMed]
52. Ni, C.W.; Qiu, H.; Jo, H. MicroRNA-663 upregulated by oscillatory shear stress plays a role in inflammatory re-sponse of endothelial cells. *Am. J. Physiol. Heart Circ. Physiol.* **2011**, *300*, H1762–H1769. [CrossRef] [PubMed]
53. Di Stefano, V.; Zaccagnini, G.; Capogrossi, M.C.; Martelli, F. microRNAs as peripheral blood biomarkers of cardiovascular disease. *Vascul. Pharmacol.* **2011**, *55*, 111–118. [CrossRef] [PubMed]
54. Li, C.; Pei, F.; Zhu, X.; Duan, D.D.; Zeng, C. Circulating microRNAs as novel and sensitive biomarkers of acute myocardial Infarction. *Clin. Biochem.* **2012**, *45*, 727–732. [CrossRef]
55. Qu, K.; Wang, Z.; Lin, X.L.; Zhang, K.; He, X.L.; Zhang, H. MicroRNAs: Key regulators of endothelial progenitor cell functions. *Clin. Chim. Acta* **2015**, *448*, 65–73. [CrossRef]
56. Kaczmarek, I.; Deutsch, M.A.; Kauke, T.; Beiras-Fernandez, A.; Schmoeckel, M.; Vicol, C.; Sodian, R.; Reichart, B.; Spannagl, M.; Ueberfuhr, P. Donor-specific HLA alloantibodies: Long-term impact on cardiac allograft vasculopathy and mortality after heart transplant. *Exp. Clin. Transplant.* **2008**, *6*, 229–235.
57. Weiss, M.J.; Madsen, J.C.; Rosengard, B.R.; Allan, J.S. Mechanisms of chronic rejection in cardiothoracic trans-plantation. *Front. Biosci.* **2008**, *13*, 2980–2988. [CrossRef]
58. Benatti, R.D.; Taylor, D.O. Evolving concepts and treatment strategies for cardiac allograft vasculopathy. *Curr. Treat. Options Cardiovasc. Med.* **2014**, *16*, 278. [CrossRef]
59. Skoric, B.; Cikes, M.; Ljubas Macek, J.; Baricevic, Z.; Skorak, I.; Gasparovic, H.; Biocina, B.; Milicic, D. Cardiac al-lograft vasculopathy: Diagnosis, therapy, and prognosis. *Croat. Med. J.* **2014**, *55*, 562–576. [CrossRef]
60. Borthwick, L.A.; Parker, S.M.; Brougham, K.A.; Johnson, G.E.; Gorowiec, M.R.; Ward, C.; Lordan, J.L.; Corris, P.A.; Kirby, J.A.; Fisher, A.J. Epithelial to mesenchymal transition (EMT) and airway remodelling after human lung transplantation. *Thorax* **2009**, *64*, 770–777. [CrossRef]
61. Chen, P.Y.; Qin, L.; Barnes, C.; Charisse, K.; Yi, T.; Zhang, X.; Ali, R.; Medina, P.P.; Yu, J.; Slack, F.J.; et al. FGF reg-ulates TGF-beta signaling and endothelial-to-mesenchymal transition via control of let-7 miRNA expression. *Cell Rep.* **2012**, *2*, 1684–1696. [CrossRef] [PubMed]
62. Piera-Velazquez, S.; Jimenez, S.A. Molecular mechanisms of endothelial to mesenchymal cell transition (En-doMT) in experimen-tally induced fibrotic diseases. *Fibrogenes. Tissue Repair* **2012**, *5*, S7. [CrossRef] [PubMed]
63. D'Alessandro, D.A.; Kajstura, J.; Hosoda, T.; Gatti, A.; Bello, R.; Mosna, F.; Bardelli, S.; Zheng, H.; D'Amario, D.; Padin-Iruegas, M.E.; et al. Progenitor cells from the explanted heart generate immunocompatible myocardium within the transplanted donor heart. *Circ. Res.* **2009**, *105*, 1128–1140. [CrossRef] [PubMed]
64. Hillebrands, J.L.; Klatter, F.A.; Rozing, J. Origin of vascular smooth muscle cells and the role of circulating stem cells in transplant arteriosclerosis. *Arterioscler. Thromb. Vasc. Biol.* **2003**, *23*, 380–387. [CrossRef]

65. Sathya, C.J.; Sheshgiri, R.; Prodger, J.; Tumiati, L.; Delgado, D.; Ross, H.J.; Rao, V. Correlation between circulating endothelial progenitor cell function and allograft rejection in heart transplant patients. *Transpl. Int.* **2010**, *23*, 641–648. [CrossRef] [PubMed]
66. Simper, D.; Wang, S.; Deb, A.; Holmes, D.; McGregor, C.; Frantz, R.; Kushwaha, S.S.; Caplice, N.M. Endothelial progenitor cells are decreased in blood of cardiac allograft patients with vasculopathy and endothelial cells of non-cardiac origin are enriched in transplant atherosclerosis. *Circulation* **2003**, *108*, 143–149. [CrossRef]

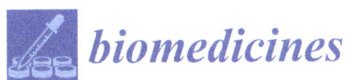

Article

Antimicrobial Behavior and Cytotoxicity of Indocyanine Green in Combination with Visible Light and Water-Filtered Infrared A Radiation against Periodontal Bacteria and Subgingival Biofilm

Diana Lorena Guevara Solarte [1,†], Sibylle Johanna Rau [1,†], Elmar Hellwig [1], Kirstin Vach [2] and Ali Al-Ahmad [1,*]

1 Department of Operative Dentistry and Periodontology, Medical Center of the University of Freiburg, Faculty of Medicine, University of Freiburg, Hugstetter Strasse 55, 79106 Freiburg, Germany; diana.lorena.guevara.solarte@uniklinik-freiburg.de (D.L.G.S.); sibylle.rau@uniklinik-freiburg.de (S.J.R.); elmar.hellwig@uniklinik-freiburg.de (E.H.)

2 Institute of Medical Biometry and Statistics, Faculty of Medicine and Medical Center, University of Freiburg, Stefan-Meier-Str. 26, 79104 Freiburg, Germany; kv@imbi.uni-freiburg.de

* Correspondence: ali.al-ahmad@uniklinik-freiburg.de; Tel.: +49-761-270-48940

† These authors contributed equally to this work.

Abstract: The widespread increase of antibiotic resistance highlights the need for alternative treatments such as antimicrobial photodynamic therapy (aPDT). This study aimed to evaluate the antimicrobial behavior and cytotoxicity of aPDT with indocyanine green (ICG) in combination with visible light (Vis) and water-filtered infrared A (wIRA). Representative periodontal bacteria (*Parvimonas micra, Atopobium riame, Slackia exigua, Actinomyces naeslundii, Porphyromonas gingivalis, Fusobacterium nucleatum, Aggregatibacter actinomycetemcomitans,* and *Prevotella nigrescens*) and subgingival in situ biofilms from periodontal patients were treated with aPDT for 5 min. ICG was used at different concentrations (50–500 µg/mL) and the number of viable cells was determined in colony forming units (CFU). Untreated negative controls and 0.2% chlorhexidine as a positive control were also prepared. The cytotoxicity test on human keratinocytes in vitro was analyzed with the AlamarBlue assay after 5, 10, and 20 min, with four ICG concentrations, and at two temperatures (room temperature and 37 °C). The tested periodontal pathogens treated with aPDT were eliminated in a range between 1.2 and 6.7 $\log_{10}$ CFU, except for *A. naeslundii*, which was killed at a lower range. The subgingival biofilm treated with aPDT expressed significant differences to the untreated controls except for at 300 µg/mL ICG concentration. The cytotoxicity was directly related to the concentration of ICG and irradiation time. These observations raise questions concerning the use of this specific aPDT as an adjuvant to periodontal treatments due to its possible toxicity towards human gingival cells.

Keywords: indocyanine green; photodynamic therapy; cytotoxicity; water filter infrared A; periodontal biofilm

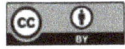

1. Introduction

According to the World Health Organization (WHO), bacteria represent the fourth leading global cause of death [1]. In addition, antimicrobial resistance is on the list of the top 10 global public health problems, as it negatively impacts healthcare systems and national economies, increases the cost of prolonged hospital stays, and negatively affects patient productivity [2].

In dentistry, antibiotics are among the most frequently prescribed treatments. According to the World Dental Federation, depending on the country, around 10% of the antibiotic prescriptions are made in the dental practice. In some cases, these are unnecessary and increase the risk of antibiotic resistance developing [3]. Therefore, finding an antimicrobial therapy with the ability to engage multiple molecular microbial targets and, thereby, make resistance unlikely is of tremendous importance. One such therapy is antimicrobial photodynamic therapy (aPDT) [4].

The principle of photodynamic therapy (PDT) was accidentally discovered in 1900 when the medical student Oscar Raab observed the inactivation of *Paramecium caudatum* under exposition to the dyes acridine or eosin in combination with sunlight, and this discovery was later applied to treat skin carcinomas [5,6]. Since then, this method has been widely used to control other diseases [7]. However, it was not until the early 1990s that the interest in aPDT increased due to the emergence of antibiotic-resistant infections [4,7]. Since then, many photosensitizers (PS) have been developed with a potential use against cancer, infections, and other diseases [8]. In general, an aPDT results from a combination of three components, namely, the PS which is a non-toxic molecule per se, molecular oxygen, and a light with an appropriate spectral range [4,7], with the final production of reactive oxygen species (ROS) [7,9]. The entire cycle can be repeated and one PS molecule is able to produce many molecules of $^1O_2$ before its destruction [7], affecting various molecular targets such proteins, lipids, and nucleic acids [4,7]. The ROS triggered by aPDT produce an oxidative degradation of the biofilm structure, making this therapy more effective and, therefore, inhibiting the acquisition of resistance [9]. As aPDT is applied locally, the risk of adverse systemic effects is also minimized [10].

In the last 20 years, new classes of PS have been optimized, developed, and tested. The main types are phenothiazium, porphyrin, chlorin, phthalocyanine, xanthene, fullerene, phenalenone, riboflavin, curcumin derivatives [7,8], and cyanines. The latter include the water-soluble and negative charged polymethine dye indocyanine green (ICG) [11], approved by the United States Food and Drug Administration (FDA) [11,12] and primarily used clinically to treat tumors and acne [11]. ICG is the "gold standard" for the application of fluorophores in vivo [13], and their absorption is near the infrared region of the spectrum [14]. Unlike other PSs, ICG has a photo-oxidative effect combined with a photothermic effect [15]. The good activity of ICG in combination with a near-infrared laser has already been described in anti-tumor therapy [16,17]. ICG also has low toxicity due to its absorption in the liver and bile ducts, rather than in the intestinal mucosa [15], good tolerance, and rapid decay also in the presence of mild liver disease [17].

As outlined previously, there is a clear need in the dental field for an alternative treatment to conventional antibiotic therapy. Therefore, ICG could be a good option for the treatment of oral infectious diseases, primarily those involving an anaerobic compound, such as periodontal diseases [18] or infections of endodontic origin [19], among others, since oxygen supply is not required to unfold its activity [18].

In an attempt to improve the use of ICG in dental practice, researchers have mostly used ICG in combination with diode lasers and against planktonic bacteria [10,20,21]. The effects of ICG in combination with diode lasers against oral biofilm bacteria have been tested less frequently, despite yielding positive results [22,23]. Clinical randomized trials were also conducted in patients with chronic periodontitis treated with ICG and diode laser without adverse effects, and this aPDT could increase the effectiveness of the non-surgical periodontal therapy [24]. However, the antimicrobial activity of ICG in combination with other sources of light has been less extensively studied, except for Nikinmaa et al. [25], who tested ICG in combination with LED-light on healthy volunteers and described a decrease in plaque formation bacteria and an anti-inflammatory and anti-proteolytic effect [25].

Interestingly, another source of light has also been used for aPDT. This is the broadband light with visible-light (Vis) in combination with water-filtered infrared A (wIRA) wavelengths. This light offers additional advantages such as flexibility in use with different PSs, portability, affordability [26,27], increase in tissue oxygen partial pressure, higher perfusion levels, and higher local temperature linked to wound healing and pain reduction [28].

The antimicrobial activity of the broadband Vis + wIRA in combination with PSs has already been studied in conjunction with toluidine blue or chlorine e6 to eradicate in situ oral biofilms with outstanding results [26,29]. As previously described, a distinctive feature of this light source is its positive effect on the healing process. This property is important for the treatment of periodontal diseases and peri-implantitis [26,30]. As a result, the antimicrobial activity of the Vis + wIRA in combination with chlorine e6 has been tested against planktonic periodontal pathogens and subgingival biofilms with positive results [31].

To date, the combination of the good properties of ICG with those of broadband Vis + wIRA has only been tested against supragingival biofilms [30] and not yet against many representative periodontal bacteria or periodontal subgingival biofilms. Regarding the use of this drug in clinical practice, it is important to consider that a perfect aPDT must have a good antimicrobial activity without harmful side effects [7]. The cell toxicity of ICG in combination with Vis + wIRA has not been evaluated thus far.

Hence, this study aimed to evaluate the antimicrobial activity of ICG in combination with Vis + wIRA against planktonic periodontal pathogens and in situ subgingival biofilms from patients with chronic periodontitis. In addition, the cytotoxicity of this therapy was investigated for the first time in the present study.

2. Materials and Methods

2.1. Light Source

The light source used in this study was a combination of visible-light (Vis) wavelengths and water-filtered infrared-A (wIRA) wavelengths produced by a radiator (Hydrosun®750 FS, Hydrosun Medizintechnik, Müllheim, Germany) [26,29–31] The wIRA results after the filtration of the light produced by a halogen bulb with the help of a water cuvette (7 mm), which reduces the parts of the infrared radiation (most of the infra-red B, C and portions of the A filtrated by the water) that could cause a thermal load on the skin surface [32]. The additional orange filter BTE 31 was adapted instead to the traditional BTE 595, because it was reported that this filter allowed more effective integral radiation regarding the absorption spectrum of protoporphyrin IX [26]. That could induce damage in bacterial cells and improve the regeneration process and wound healing [33]. Compared to infrared unfiltered lamps, wIRA results in a smaller increase in the skin temperature after 30 min of irradiation [34].

The continuous water-filtered spectrum had a wavelength range from 570 nm to 1400 nm, with local minima at 970 nm, 1200 nm, and 1430 due to the water filter [34]. The applied irradiance of Vis + wIRA was measured directly using a thermopile radiometer (HBM1, Hydrosun, Müllheim, Germany) and it was approximately 48 mW cm^{-2} in the visible range and 152 mW cm^{-2} in the wIRA range for a total irradiance of 200 mW cm^{-2}, which was applied on the bacterial strains and oral biofilm for 5 min [30], and on the cells for 5, 10, and 20 min.

The photosensitizer used in this study was Indocyanine Green (Verdye®—Diagnostic Green, Aschheim-Dornach, Freiburg, Germany). ICGs' maximal light absorption is approximately 800 nm [35]. It was dissolved in water for injection (Aqua—B. Braun, Melsungen, Germany) according to the manufacturer's instructions to reach an initial concentration of 5 mg/mL. Subsequent dilutions were made in GC-HP-Bouillon medium (GC) (University Hospital, Freiburg, Germany) until final concentrations of 50 µg/mL, 150 µg/mL, 300 µg/mL, and 500 µg/mL were reached. The GC-HP-Bouillon is a culture medium that has been used for anaerobic bacteria prior to the determination of fatty acid composition of the cell envelope using a gas chromatograph (Hewlett Packard, Agilent Technologies, Poway, CA, USA) (Table S1). The ICG solutions were prepared immediately before the test to avoid light-induced photochemical attenuation. The ICG used in this study had an absorbance spectrum in GC medium of approximately 640–940 nm (i-control™, microplate reader software 2017, Tecan, Austria GmbH.), which is properly covered for the broad-band Vis + wIRA used in this study (Figure 1).

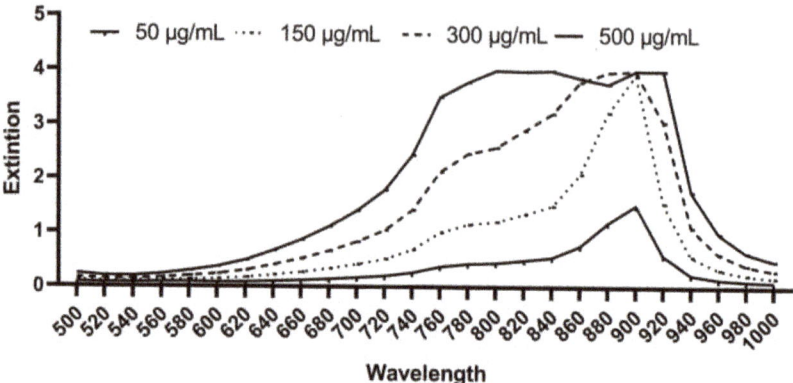

Figure 1. Absorption spectrum of ICG in GC medium at a concentration of 50 µg/mL, 150 µg/mL, 300 µg/mL, and 500 µg/mL (Tecan Infinite® 200 Reader).

2.2. Bacterial Strains

The first stage of the research focused on the following planktonic periodontal-related bacteria: *Parvimonas micra* (anaerobic), *Atopobium riame* (anaerobic), *Slackia exigua* (anaerobic), and *Actinomyces naeslundii* (aerobic) as Gram-positive; and *Porphyromonas gingivalis* (anaerobic), *Fusobacterium nucleatum* (anaerobic), *Aggregatibacter actinomycetemcomitans* (aerobic), and *Prevotella nigrescens* (anaerobic) as Gram-negative species.

The bacterial strains listed above were maintained in long-term storage at −80 °C as was established previously [36]. The aerobic bacteria were subcultured on Columbia agar with sheep blood plus (Oxoid™, Wesel, Germany) plates at 37 °C with 5% CO_2 under aerobic conditions, the anaerobic bacteria were subcultured on yeast extract cysteine blood agar (HCB) (University Hospital Freiburg, Germany) plates at 37 °C under anaerobic conditions (anaerobic jars, Anaerocult®, Merck, Darmstadt, Germany). The overnight cultures were prepared in Brain-Heart-Infusion (BHI) medium (Oxoid™) and GC-HP medium for aerobic and anaerobic bacteria, respectively [30,31].

2.3. Selection of the Patients

The following protocol was reviewed and approved by the Ethics Committee of the University of Freiburg (no. 502/13, Albert-Ludwigs-University of Freiburg, Germany). Subgingival plaque sampling was undertaken from five patients diagnosed with chronic periodontitis (CP) based on the periodontal disease classification system proposed by the International Workshop for a classification of Periodontal Diseases and Conditions in 1999 [37,38]. A periodontologist took the samples from teeth diagnosed with a CP with a periodontal pocket depth of ≥5 mm. The exclusion criteria for this research were a severe systemic disease, pregnancy or lactation, pus secretions from periodontal pockets, and the use of antibiotics or other antimicrobial agents within the last 6 months. The samples were stored in reduced transport fluid (RTF) (University Hospital Freiburg, Germany) at −80 °C until use [39].

2.4. aPDT of the Bacterial Strains and Subgingival Biofilm Samples

The cell concentration for the single bacteria and plaque samples was determined with the help of a serial dilution and a bacterial suspension with cell concentration of approximately 1×10^6 cells/mL in GC-HP medium was prepared, and the bacterial suspension was made at approximately 1×10^6 cells/mL according to the serial dilution of a "CFU" in CG-HP medium. Afterwards, the ICG was added at different concentrations (50 µg/mL, 150 µg/mL, 300 µg/mL, 500 µg/mL). A bacterial suspension without ICG served as a negative control. The positive control was the bacterial suspension with chlorhexidine 0.2% (CHX) (Pharmacy of the University Hospital Freiburg, Germany). All the groups were replicated in two equal multi-well plates (24-well plate, Grainer bio-one), and incubated for 2 min in the dark prior to irradiation. One of the multi-well plates was treated under irradiation for 5 min at 37 °C with Vis + wIRA.

In order to determine the colony forming units (CFU) number for each group, serial dilutions were made in basis medium (University Hospital Freiburg) a peptone-yeast medium (Table S2), and plated onto HCB (University Hospital Freiburg) for the planktonic aerobic bacteria and onto Columbia agar plates (OXOID) for the aerobic biofilm, prior to incubation at 37 °C and 5% CO_2.

The anaerobic planktonic bacteria and the anaerobic CFU of the oral biofilm were cultured on HCB at 37 °C in anaerobic jars (Anaerocult ®, Merck, Darmstadt, Germany). All the experiments were carried out twice in duplicate [31].

2.5. Cell Toxicity of aPDT with ICG and Vis + wIRA

The cell toxicity was tested using the AlamarBlue™ assay (BioRad, Hercules, CA, USA) according to the manufacturer's instructions.

Immortalized human gingival keratinocytes were seeded at a density of 2×10^5 cells/well in a 24-well cell culture plate and were cultivated in keratinocyte growth medium (Keratinocyte Growth Medium 2), containing supplements (KGM2, Promo Cell, Heidelberg, Germany) and antibiotics (kanamycin, 50 µg/mL; Sigma-Aldrich, Munich, Germany). This parental oral gingival keratinocyte cell line (GK) was established by immortalization with the E6 and E7 genes of the human papillomavirus 16 (HPV-16) [40].

On the day after seeding, the cells were treated with ICG and Vis + wIRA. For this purpose, 1:10 ICG stock solutions were prepared with Aqua dest. In each cell culture well, the medium was replaced with 450 µL KGM. Afterwards, 50 µL ICG in Aqua dest with appropriate concentrations (50, 150, 300, and 500 µg/mL) was added directly before irradiation with Vis + wIRA. For growth control without ICG, 50 µL Aqua dest was added analogously to the samples. Irradiation was performed either at room temperature or the cell culture plates were fixed in a water bath at 37 °C.

The cell culture plates were irradiated with Vis + wIRA for 5, 10, or 20 min without a lid on the cell culture plate. Immediately after irradiation, the temperature in the cell culture medium was measured (temperature module t3000 FC from Fluke, Washington, DC, USA). The ICG medium was subsequently aspirated, and the cells were washed three times with PBS buffer.

For the AlamarBlue assay, cells were incubated with KGM and 10% AlamarBlue in an incubator at saturated humidity, 37 °C, and 5% CO_2. Two hours later, the cell culture supernatant was removed, and the fluorescence intensity was measured in a Tecan Infinite 200 plate reader (excitation at 450 nm, measurement at 590 nm). The data were analyzed according to the AlamarBlue manufacturer's instructions in relation to growth control. As a positive control, all cells were killed with 60% isopropanol for 5 min. Unirradiated cells with ICG were placed in an incubator in the dark. All fluids were pre-warmed to 37 °C before being added to the cells. Three independent experiments were performed.

Light microscope images were taken after treatment and a washing step and before the addition of the AlamarBlue solution at 400× magnification.

2.6. Statistical Analysis

The means, standard deviations, and relative frequencies were computed for a descriptive evaluation of the data. An analysis of variance (ANOVA) was conducted to analyze the differences between the vitality results for the different groups. The p-values of pairwise comparisons were adjusted using the Student–Newman–Keuls method. In situations where no normal distribution could be assumed, the two-sample Wilcoxon rank-sum test was used. The significance level was set to $p = 0.05$. All the calculations were performed with the statistical software STATA 17.0 (StataCorp LLC, Texas, TX, USA).

3. Results

3.1. ICG in Combination with Vis + wIRA Reduces the Viability of Periodontal Planktonic Bacteria

3.1.1. Gram-Positive Bacteria

After the treatment of *P. micra* with ICG and Vis + wIRA, bactericidal activity was observed for all the tested ICG concentrations. The killing rate was $\geq$99.99% (4.6 $\log_{10}$ CFU) for 50 µg/mL (Figure 2a), $\geq$99.9% (3.2 $\log_{10}$ CFU) for 150 µg/mL (Figure 2b), $\geq$99.9% (3.8 $\log_{10}$ CFU) for 300 µg/mL (Figure 2c), and $\geq$99.9% (3.5 $\log_{10}$ CFU) for 500 µg/mL (Figure 2d). Against *A. rimae*, bactericidal activity was also observed for all the ICG concentrations, with a killing rate of $\geq$99.999% (5.5 $\log_{10}$ CFU) for 50 µg/mL (Figure 3a) and a reduction of $\geq$99.9% for 150 µg/mL, 300 µg/mL, and 500 µg/mL (3.5, 3.1, and 3.4 $\log_{10}$ CFU respectively) (Figure 3b–d). The treatment of *S. exigua* exhibited a bactericidal activity with concentrations of 50 µg/mL and 150 µg/mL; the killing rate was $\geq$99.99% (4.5 and $\log_{10}$ CFU) and $\geq$99.9% (3.8 $\log_{10}$ CFU), respectively (Figure 2a,b). The other concentrations (300 and 500 µg/mL) displayed a good effectivity with a killing rate $\geq$99% (2.5 and 2.4 $\log_{10}$ CFU, respectively) (Figure 2c,d). After the treatment of *A. naeslundii* with ICG and Vis + wIRA, the effectivity rate was lower than 1 $\log_{10}$ CFU with all the ICG concentrations (Figure 2a–d).

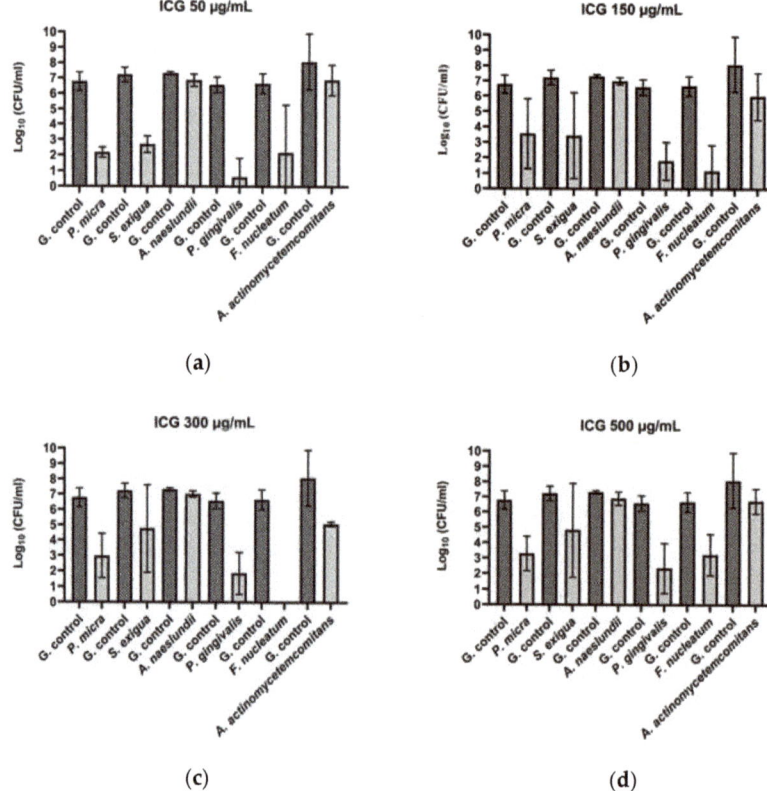

Figure 2. Photodynamic efficacy of ICG in combination with Vis + wIRA against periodontal bacteria. ICG was tested at concentrations of (**a**) 50 µg/mL, (**b**) 150 µg/mL, (**c**) 300 µg/mL, and (**d**) 500 µg/mL. The CFU numbers are given on a $\log_{10}$ scale per milliliter ($\log_{10}$ CFU/mL).

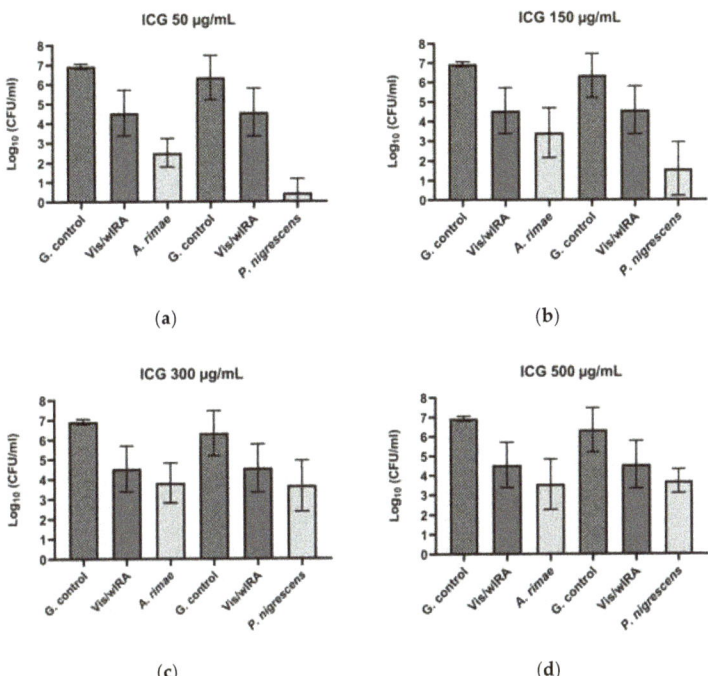

Figure 3. Photodynamic efficacy of ICG in combination with Vis + wIRA against *A. rimae* and *P. nigrensces*. ICG was tested at concentrations of (**a**) 50 µg/mL, (**b**) 150 µg/mL, (**c**) 300 µg/mL, and (**d**) 500 µg/mL. The CFU numbers are given on a log$_{10}$ scale per milliliter (log$_{10}$ CFU/mL).

3.1.2. Gram-Negative Bacteria

After the treatment with ICG in combination with Vis + wIRA, bactericidal activity against *P. gingivalis* was observed with a killing rate of ≥99.9999% with 50 µg/mL (6 log$_{10}$ CFU) (Figure 2a). The 150 µg/mL, 300 µg/mL, and 500 µg/mL ICG concentrations also exhibited bactericidal activity with a reduction of ≥99.99% (4 log$_{10}$ CFU) (Figure 2b–d). The same behavior was observed against *F. nucleatum*, with a bactericidal activity under all the tested ICG concentrations, expressed in a killing rate between ≥99.9999% (6.7 log$_{10}$ CFU) at 300 µg/mL (Figure 2c) concentration and ≥99.9% (3.4 log$_{10}$ CFU) at 500 µg/mL (Figure 2a–d). The experiment performed with *A. actinomycetemcomitans* showed a bactericidal activity of ICG at 300 µg/mL, where the killing rate was ≥99.9% (3 log$_{10}$ CFU) (Figure 2c), while for the last concentrations a reduction effect of ≥99% with 150 µg/mL (2.1 log$_{10}$ CFU) (Figure 2b) and 90% with 50 and 500 µg/mL (1 log$_{10}$ CFU) (Figure 2a,d) was observed. Against *P. nigrescens*, the bactericidal activity of ICG was achieved with a killing rate of ≥99,999% (5.9 log$_{10}$ CFU) and ≥99.99% (4.7 log$_{10}$ CFU) with 50 µg/mL and 150 µg/mL concentrations (Figure 3a,b), respectively, and a killing rate of ≥99% (2.6 log$_{10}$ CFU) for the two remaining concentrations (Figure 3c,d).

All calculations were performed in comparison with the untreated control. The positive controls (group treated with CHX 0.2%) exhibited a high bacterial killing rate (100%) for all Gram-negative and Gram-positive microorganisms.

After the comparison between the growth control groups in tested Gram-positive and Gram-negative bacteria and the growth control plus ICG without the effect of the irradiation with Vis + wIRA, no killing rate over 90% was observed.

The treatment with Vis + wIRA without ICG only exhibited a bacterial reduction over 90% for two bacteria, *A. rimae* (2.4 log$_{10}$ CFU) and *P. nigrescens* (1.8 log$_{10}$ CFU), in comparison to the untreated control (Figure 3).

3.2. ICG in Combination with Vis + wIRA Reduces the Viability of Subgingival Periodontal Biofilm

Figure 4 shows the behavior of ICG in four concentrations (50 µg/mL, 150 µg/mL, 300 µg/mL, and 500 µg/mL) in combination with Vis + wIRA against subgingival biofilm from five periodontal patients. After the comparison between the untreated group and the group treated with ICG 50 µg/mL plus Vis + wIRA, a highly significant difference (p-value 0.0079) was observed with a killing log rate of $\geq$90% (1 $\log_{10}$ CFU/mL) (Figure 4a). The comparison between the untreated group and the group treated with ICG 150 µg/mL plus Vis + wIRA showed a highly significant difference (p-value 0.007) and a killing rate lower than 90% (Figure 4b). The combination of Vis + wIRA and 500 µg/mL ICG revealed a significant difference with a p-value of 0.01 in comparison to the untreated control, although the killing rate was also lower than 90% (Figure 4d). For the group treated with ICG 300 µg/mL plus Vis + wIRA, no statistical differences were observed after the comparison to the untreated control group (Figure 4c). In the group treated with 0.2% CHX (positive control), no cultivable bacteria were determined (Figure 4a–d).

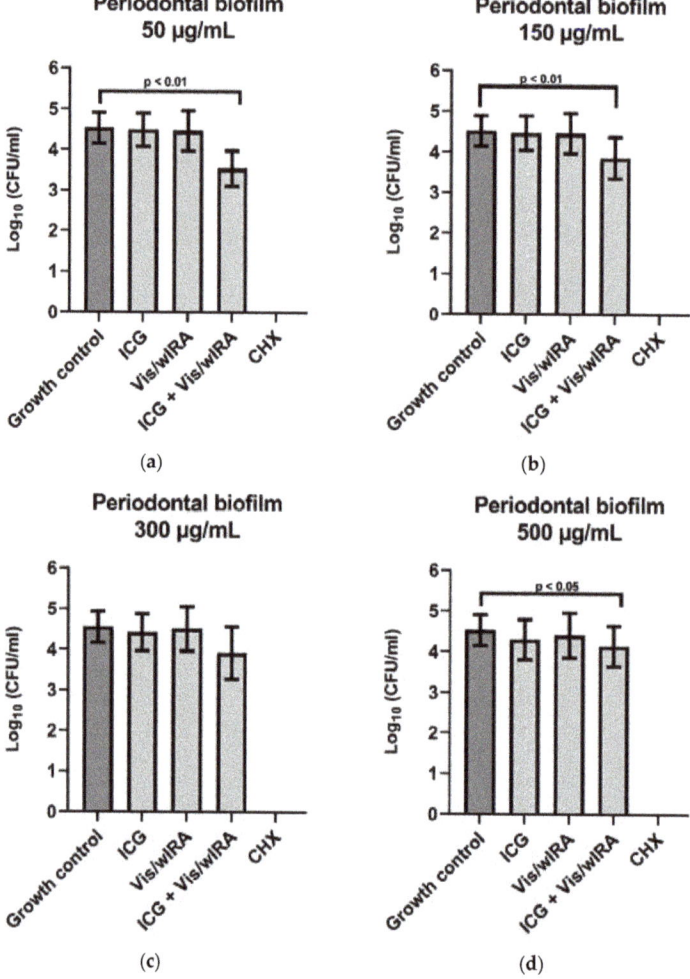

Figure 4. Photodynamic efficacy of ICG in combination with Vis + wIRA on periodontal biofilm. ICG was tested in concentrations of (**a**) 50 µg/mL, (**b**) 150 µg/mL, (**c**) 300 µg/mL, and (**d**) 500 µg/mL. The CFU numbers are given on a $\log_{10}$ scale per milliliter ($\log_{10}$ CFU/mL).

3.3. Vis + wIRA in Combination with ICG Affects the Cell Viability of Human Gingival Keratinocytes In Vitro

Vis + wIRA alone does not affect cell viability at room temperature (RT) or at 37 °C after 5 min, 10 min, or 20 min. Only after 10 min Vis + wIRA at 37 °C is a significant increase of metabolic activity (by 11%) measurable.

Figure 5a–d shows that 50 µg/mL ICG significantly reduces keratinocyte metabolic activity by 16% after 5 min, by 12% after 10 min, and not significantly by 6% after 20 min incubation compared to the growth control (Figure 5a). ICG alone at concentrations of 150 µg/mL, 300 µg/mL, and 500 µg/mL showed similar trends in cell viability, namely a significant decrease of cell survival between 14% and 34% (Figure 5b–d), while the highest applied concentration of 500 µg/mL for 10 min led to a reduction of 39% in metabolic activity. The combination of ICG with Vis + wIRA strongly increases cell toxicity. After 5 min of irradiation at RT and with 50 µg/mL only 25%, and with 150 µg/mL only 4% of the cells were viable (Figure 5a,b).

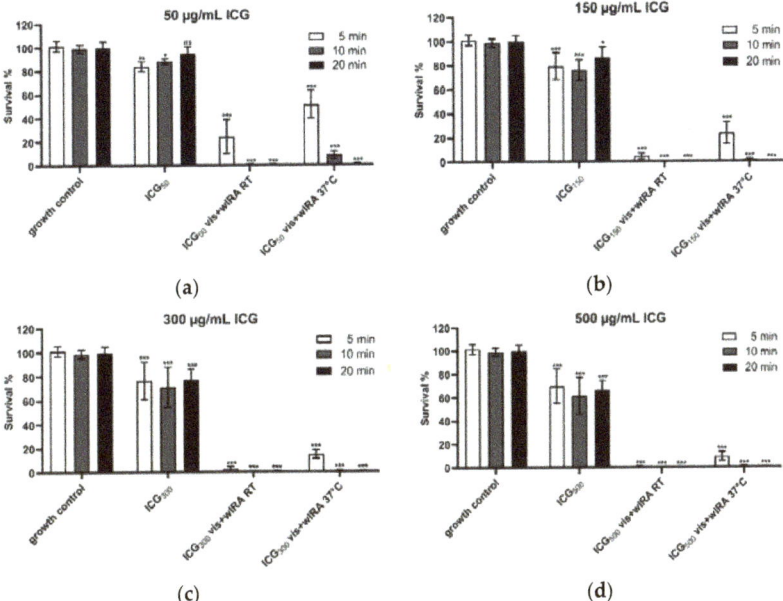

Figure 5. Cell viability after treatment with (**a**) 50, (**b**) 150, (**c**) 300, and (**d**) 500 µg/mL ICG and Vis + wIRA. Human gingival keratinocytes were incubated with different concentrations of ICG at RT or 37 °C with or without Vis + wIRA radiation for 5 min, 10 min, or 20 min. Cell viability was analyzed with the AlamarBlue assay. The associated p-values compared to the growth control are specified. ns: $p > 0.05$; * $p < 0.05$; ** $p < 0.01$; *** $p < 0.001$.

After 10 min and 20 min Vis + wIRA irradiation and ICG in all concentrations at RT, all cells were killed (Figure 5a–d). The treatment of the cells with Vis + wIRA and at 37 °C (water bath) for 5 min led to a cell survival rate of 51% with 50 µg/mL ICG (Figure 5a), 23.4% with 150 µg/mL ICG (Figure 5b), 14.5% with 300 µg/mL ICG (Figure 5c), and 9.2% with 500 µg/mL ICG (Figure 5d). After 10 min Vis + wIRA, only in the lowest ICG concentration (50 µg/mL) 8% of the cells survived compared to the growth control. All higher ICG concentrations led to complete cell death after 10 and 20 min (Figure 5a–d).

The light microscopic images after 5 min and simultaneous irradiation with Vis + wIRA confirmed the results of the AlamarBlue assay for all ICG concentrations. The images showed clear morphological changes after the combination of ICG with Vis + wIRA. The cellular damage was more clearly visible after irradiation at RT than after irradiation at 37 °C in a water bath. The keratinocytes of the growth control, ICG alone, and irradiation without ICG showed no morphological damage (Figure 6).

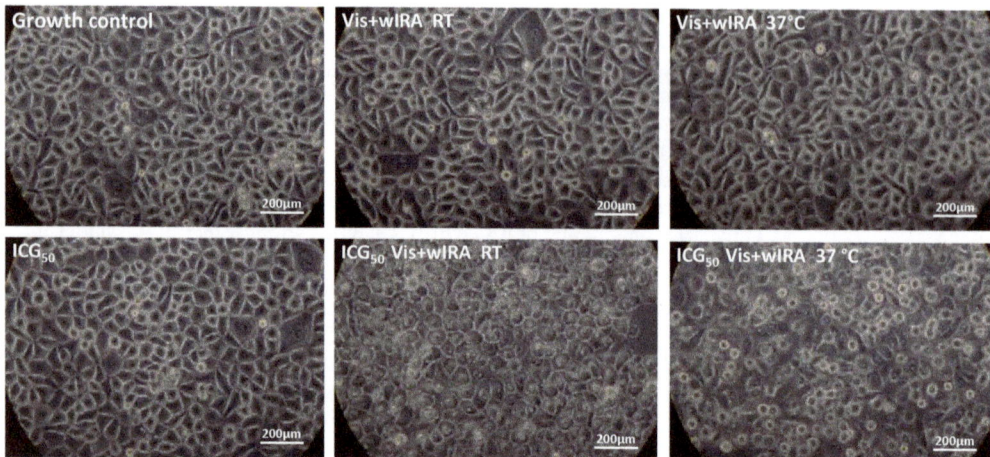

Figure 6. After only 5 min of treatment, 50 g/mL ICG and Vis + wIRA lead to morphological damage in cells. Human gingival keratinocytes were incubated with 50 µg/mL ICG and irradiated with Vis + wIRA at RT or at 37 °C in a water bath. All experimental approaches were washed twice after treatment with PBS buffer and microscopically examined at a magnification of 400×. The scale bar is shown on the bottom right. Additional light microscope images of the other ICG concentrations and time points are attached in the supplement.

4. Discussion

In order to provide an alternative to the traditional therapy for periodontal diseases and without forgetting the current antibiotics resistance crisis, the present study focused on the antimicrobial behavior and cytotoxicity of aPDT with ICG in combination with Vis + wIRA.

The effectiveness of a PS is correlated with its chemical structure and the composition of the bacterial cell membrane [9,41]. For this reason, it is important to evaluate the antimicrobial activity of a new therapy against Gram-positive and Gram-negative bacteria, and in previous studies, the efficacy of aPDT against both types of bacteria was already described [42]. Considering these findings, a group of representative Gram-positive and Gram-negative periodontal pathogens was evaluated in the present study.

Various PSs, such as methylene blue (MB), toluidine blue O (TBO), curcumin, and, recently, ICG, have been used in dentistry. ICG seems to be one of the best options due to its better penetration compared to other PSs and the fact that there is no evidence in dentistry of allergic or anaphylactic reactions related to its iodide component [43].

It was previously reported that ICG alone had no bactericidal effect against *Streptococcus salivarius* [44] and different planktonic oral bacteria [30]. These results are consistent with our observations, which dismissed the antimicrobial activity of ICG without irradiation against the tested planktonic periodontal bacteria.

The type of light used by the present research was a specific broad-band Vis + wIRA. One of the first attempts to use this specific broad-band Vis + wIRA light in aPDT was made by Al-Ahmad et al. [45], who showed prominent results against planktonic bacterial cultures and initial bacterial colonization. Further experiments of this novel aPDT revealed excellent results in eradicating initial and mature oral biofilm. Based on this work, the 5-min irradiation was selected for this study, as it can be considered safe and practical in dentistry and was shown to be effective in previous studies [29,30].

Excellent results were also observed with aPDT using Vis + wIRA against planktonic periodontal pathogens and subgingival biofilm from periodontal patients, this time in combination with chlorine e6. The authors emphasized the good results of this novel aPDT in addition to the indirect wound healing enhancement and innate immune response reported in other studies [31], which opens the possibility to use this light source in aPDT for the treatment of periodontal diseases.

In this context, in the present study, the antimicrobial behavior of both the PS ICG and the Vis + wIRA against periodontal pathogens was evaluated. This combination previously showed good antimicrobial results against other oral bacterial strains and total human salivary bacteria [30].

The aPDT with ICG plus Vis + wIRA in the present study showed good antimicrobial activity against seven of eight planktonic periodontal pathogens (Figures 2 and 3).

Studies with other PSs, such as curcumin-based irrigants and LED light [46], and methylene blue with a diode laser against *A. naeslundii* biofilm isolated from patients with osteonecrosis [47], yielded good antimicrobial activity [46,47]. These results are not consistent with our results, where the aPDT with ICG and Vis + wIRA did not display a good antimicrobial effect against this bacterium. The differences could be related to the relationship between antimicrobial effectivity of a specific PS and the physicochemical characteristics of the microorganism-PS interaction, which varies between species and strains [48]. In the present study, a strong reduction of *F. nucleatum* after the treatment with ICG plus Vis + wIRA was observed, and a complete reduction of all viable bacteria was detected at 300 µg/mL ICG (Figure 2), whereby these results are consistent with those of Burchard 2019 [30]. An earlier study investigated the effect of adding a water-soluble vitamin E analog Trolox^{TM} to ICG with a near-IR-laser light [49]. The authors detected no viable bacteria after the treatment with ICG 500 µg/mL and irradiation (100 J/cm^2), while a complete bacterial eradication was obtained at a much lower concentration with ICG (50 µg/mL) after the addition of Trolox and under the same irradiation conditions (100 J/cm^2) [49]. In the present study, the percentage of reduction at this concentration was ≥99.99%, which represents a good bactericidal activity.

As mentioned above, Kranz et al. ([49]) also evaluated the effect of the addition of a vitamin E analog Trolox^{TM} to ICG and a near-IR-laser light against *P. gingivalis* and *A. actinomycetemcomitans* with the total eradication of bacteria. In the present study, *P. gingivalis* was highly eradicated (99.9999% killing rate) after treatment with 50 µg/mL ICG plus Vis + wIRA (Figure 2). Regarding *A. actinomycetemcomitans*, previous authors reported no bacterial reduction with ICG (250 µg/mL) without the addition of the vitamin E analog, and a total reduction of viable bacteria with 250 µg/mL ICG with the vitamin E analog Trolox^{TM} [49]. The present results revealed a bactericidal activity of ICG (300 µg/mL) plus Vis + wIRA (99.9%) towards *A. actinomycetemcomitans* (Figure 2). Interestingly, a lower antimicrobial activity against *A. actinomycetemcomitans* was observed in both the present results and those of Kranz et al. and this behavior could be related to the high negative charge on its surface, its ability to avoid oxidative attack, and a small increase in the tolerance to thermal heat [49].

To the best of our knowledge, there are no previous reports on the effect of aPDT with ICG against planktonic *P. nigrescens*, *P. micra*, *A. rimae*, and *S. exigua*. However, in a randomized clinical trial, a reduction in the levels of *P. nigrescens* and *P. intermedia* after aPDT was found (MB plus diode laser) [50]. These results are similar to ours, where a bactericidal activity (99.9999%) was displayed against *P. nigrescens* (50 µg/mL) (Figure 3).

The same type of light used in the present research (Vis + wIRA) was previously tested, this time in combination with chlorine e6 against planktonic periodontal pathogens (*A. odontolyticus*, *F. nucleatum*, *A. actinomycetemcomitans*, *P. gingivalis*, *E. corrodens*, *P. micra*, *A. rimae*, and *S. exigua*) [31]. Interestingly, almost the same percentage of reduction (≥99.9%) was observed with both PSs chlorine e6 and 300 µg/mL of ICG plus Vis + wIRA against *A. actinomycetemcomitans* and against *F. nucleatum* with chlorine e6 [31] and ICG Vis + IRA (300 µg/mL). A slightly better performance was observed for the chlorine e6 dye against

P. micra and *A. rimae* [31] compared to our results, in this case, with the smaller concentration (Figures 2 and 3). In the present study, the bactericidal activity of aPDT with ICG against *S. exigua* (Figure 2) and *P. gingivalis* (Figure 2) was shown. A 100% killing rate with chlorine e6 was previously obtained by Al-Ahmad et al. [31], and, as was explained earlier, these differences in the activity of both PSs may be due to the different chemical structures that affect the microbial susceptibility of each bacterium in different ways [41].

Biofilms are the main cause of many chronic infections in different fields of medicine [51] and the main etiological factor of periodontitis [52]. In view of this, and in an effort to get closer to the clinical situation, the combination of ICG and Vis + wIRA against ex vivo periodontal subgingival biofilms was tested for the first time.

In a previous research, the effect of ICG plus Vis + wIRA on initial and mature oral biofilm was investigated. The authors reported a significant reduction of mature oral biofilm and complete eradication of initial biofilm at a concentration of 450 µg/mL [30]. These results are compatible with our results concerning the subgingival periodontal biofilm, where a significant difference was obtained compared to the untreated control. Unlike the results presented by Burchard et al. [30], in the present study, complete eradication of the subgingival periodontal biofilm was not observed for any ICG concentrations.

According to the present study, the effectiveness of aPDT using ICG and Vis + wIRA displays a different antimicrobial behavior against planktonic bacteria and biofilm. A similar trend was previously observed, where even at the same concentration ICG plus Vis + wIRA was less effective against mature biofilm than against bacteria in initial adhesion [30]. The behavior of aPDT on periodontal biofilm samples from patients has, so far, not been extensively investigated. Interestingly, a group of researchers obtained similar results on periodontal biofilms treated with methylene blue and diode laser, probably due to the fact that oral biofilms are more resistant against aPDT than planktonic bacteria [53].

On the other hand, the higher antimicrobial effectivity observed by Buchard et al. [30] compared to the results of the present study could probably be related to the different structures present in the subgingival periodontal biofilm, with predominantly Gram-negative anaerobic bacteria [54]. Previously, it was suggested that these kinds of bacteria are less susceptible to aPDT with ICG plus Vis + wIRA [55].

Furthermore, it is important to consider that in clinical practice subgingival periodontal biofilm is located in areas with a lower oxygen supply, which makes the ability of ICG to produce free radicals and singlet oxygen without oxygen supply important [18]. This situation was not tested in this research, and it could improve the behavior of ICG plus Vis + wIRA as an adjuvant to scaling and root planning (SRP) in the treatment of patients with chronic periodontitis. Although our positive control (CHX) displayed perfect antimicrobial activity, it is important to remember the side effects of this medicine, such as changes in the taste of patients, tooth pigmentations [56], and oral mucosa disturbances, among others [57]. Additionally, bacterial resistance has been reported, especially from Gram-negative bacteria [58].

In line with the concept that the perfect aPDT should integrate a good antimicrobial activity without harmful side effects and with easy handling [7], the cell toxicity of ICG in combination with Vis + wIRA at different temperatures (RT and 37 °C) was tested for the first time.

Our results showed that the cell viability was not affected by the irradiation with Vis + wIRA without ICG even after 20 min. These data sets are in the line with what was previously reported about the lack of cytotoxicity in eukaryotic cells under longer time exposition (20 min and beyond) and a higher dosage (3700 W/m^2) of Vis + wIRA [59].

A direct relationship between ICG concentration and cytotoxicity was observed by the present study and in human retinal pigment epithelial (ARPE-19) cells [60]. However, many authors have highlighted ICG without light activation has no significant cell toxicity [61,62], even at higher concentrations [63]. The present results on the effect of ICG in combination with Vis + wIRA showed a direct relationship between cell toxicity, time, the concentration of ICG, and temperature. The higher the concentration, temperature, and the longer the time of irradiation, the greater the cell toxicity (Figure 5). In previous research on human osteoblasts, cell viability and proliferation were not impaired at low ICG concentration (5 µM) and low irradiation time (less than 40 s) with a diode laser [62]. On immortalized human colon carcinoma HT-29 cells with diode laser and ICG, the cell viability decreased inversely proportionally to the ICG concentration (10–500 µM) [61]. Studies on retinal pigment epithelial cells (ARPE-19) with intense fiberoptic illumination and ICG (0.5–5.0 mg/mL) showed the same relationship between concentration and toxicity [64]. Meanwhile, Pourhajibagher et al. [63] observed that ICG (500–2000 µg/mL) plus diode laser leads to a significant increase in toxicity in human fibroblast cells (HuGu) with a decrease in ICG concentration and an increase in irradiation time.

The discrepancies between the results of the different studies could be related to the diversity of cell types, PS concentrations, duration of the PS-cells interaction, and light sources studied [63]. However, the potent cytotoxicity of this therapy remains latent.

It is still controversial whether the effect of ICG is photo-oxidative or only photothermal [30], and for this reason, the cell toxicity of aPDT with ICG plus Vis + wIRA was tested at RT and at 37 °C (water bath) (Figure 5).

In the present study, a direct relationship between ICG concentration and temperature increase by Vis + wIRA was observed. Irradiation in a 37 °C water bath resulted in a more constant temperature However, irradiation above 10 min and 50 µg/mL of ICG induced complete cell death under both conditions (RT or 37 °C) (Figure 5). The pronounced temperature increase was only achieved in the cell culture wells when ICG and Vis + wIRA were combined. In the absence of light or irradiation without ICG, there were no significant changes in the medium temperature (data not shown).

Wang et al. [65] studied extracellular vesicles loaded with ICG and paclitaxel (cytostatic) at different concentrations (6.25, 12.5, 25, and 50 µg/mL). A steady increase in temperature was observed during 5 min irradiation, with the temperature increasing in direct proportion to the concentrations of drug and laser power [65]. A steady temperature increase was also observed by Ruhi et al. [66] using ICG and a diode laser over 400 s of irradiation [66]. In contrast to our results, in a previous study, no correlation between temperature and aPDT was observed with ICG (500–2000 µg/mL) plus diode laser after 30 s, 60 s, and 2 × 30 s with a 1 min interval [63]. These contrasting results are probably explained by the shorter periods of irradiation time used by the authors.

It was previously established that a temperature increase to ≥ 42.5 °C produces a cytotoxic effect dependent on the principle dose-effect [67]. In the present study, after 5 min treatment at 37 °C, an ICG concentration of 50 µg/mL seems to be the most appropriate concentration because the temperature was below this range (data not shown) and within the safe temperature range to avoid pulp damage [68]. In addition, the 50 µg/mL ICG concentration with Vis + wIRA expressed the best antimicrobial behavior against the subgingival periodontal biofilm (Figure 4), which is possibly related to the decrease in the light absorption properties of ICG at higher concentrations because of aggregated ICG molecules [66]. Additionally, it was previously reported that ICG has a low singlet oxygen quantum yield [41], which decreases at high concentrations [66]. ICG aggregates in the presence of aqueous solutions, and this property is lower in plasma and blood [69]. For this reason, it would be interesting to evaluate this situation in a future study, given that it could affect the behavior of this therapy.

Whether the mechanism of action of ICG in aPDT is photochemical rather than photothermal on bacterial cells compared to eukaryotic cells is still unknown and requires further research. The studies by Ricci et al. [70] argued for a photochemical effect, as they showed that the addition of an oxygen singlet quencher could prevent apoptosis of retinal epithelial cells by ICG and laser irradiation [70]. A further investigation found that, in addition to photothermic effects, ICG was shown to have a photodynamic effect by generating ROS [71]. Since pathogens indicate various susceptibility for singlet oxygen and radical species, it is important for future studies to measure the ROS under the selected experimental conditions. This would lead to understanding the photoreaction mechanisms (I vs. II) and, consequently, mechanism of the applied aPDT.

The effectivity of aPDT with ICG and diode laser as an adjunct on periodontal therapy was already studied in clinical trials with prominent results and no adverse events reported; however, it is still necessary to evaluate variables such as light sources, ICG concentrations [72], irradiation time, and their relationship with cell toxicity in order to avoid possible negative side effects.

5. Conclusions

Within the limitations of this study, although the aPDT using ICG in combination with Vis + wIRA showed high antimicrobial activity against periodontal pathogens and subgingival oral biofilm, its use for the treatment of periodontal patients could lead to toxic effects towards gingival cells. For this reason, further investigation is necessary to evaluate the toxicity of this specific aPDT with different variables such as ICG concentrations and irradiation time. It would be also interesting to test this specific therapy with ICG under chemical or physical modifications, which could improve this behavior.

Supplementary Materials: The following supporting information can be downloaded at: https://www.mdpi.com/article/10.3390/biomedicines10050956/s1, Table S1: GC-HP-Bouillon is a culture medium that has been used for anaerobic bacteria prior to the determination of fatty acid 17 composition of the cell envelope using a gas chromatograph (Hewlett Packard, Agilent Technologies, Poway, CA,USA); Table S2: Basis medium is a peptone-yeast medium.

Author Contributions: D.L.G.S. and S.J.R. drafted and critically revised the manuscript, methodology, data analysis, and interpretation; E.H. critically revised the manuscript; K.V. performed the statistical analysis of the data; A.A.-A. conceived and designed the study, supervised, and critically revised the manuscript. All authors have read and agreed to the published version of the manuscript.

Funding: This study was supported by the Swiss Dr. Braun Science Foundation (ICG) and in part by the German Research Foundation (DFG; Grant AL 1179/4-1).

Institutional Review Board Statement: The study was conducted according to the guidelines of the Declaration of Helsinki, and approved by the local Ethics Committee of the University of Freiburg (no. 502/13, approved on 5 December 2013).

Informed Consent Statement: Informed consent was obtained from all subjects involved in the study.

Data Availability Statement: Data are available on request due to restrictions, e.g., privacy or ethical. The data presented in this study are available on request from the corresponding author.

Acknowledgments: Bettina Spitzmüller is acknowledged for skillful technical laboratory assistance.

Conflicts of Interest: The authors declare no conflict of interest. The funders had no role in the design of the study; in the collection, analyses, or interpretation of data; in the writing of the manuscript; or in the decision to publish the results.

References

1. WHO. Global Health Estimates: Life Expectancy and Leading Causes of Death and Disability. 2019. Available online: https://www.who.int/data/gho/data/themes/mortality-and-global-health-estimates (accessed on 3 December 2021).
2. WHO. Antimicrobial Resistance. 2021. Available online: https://www.who.int/news-room/fact-sheets/detail/antimicrobial-resistance (accessed on 17 November 2021).
3. FDI. Antibiotic Resistance in Dentistry. 2021. Available online: https://www.fdiworlddental.org/antibiotic-resistance-dentistry (accessed on 29 November 2021).
4. Wainwright, M.; Maisch, T.; Nonell, S.; Plaetzer, K.; Almeida, A.; Tegos, G.P.; Hamblin, M.R. Photoantimicrobials-are we afraid of the light? *Lancet Infect Dis.* **2017**, *17*, e49–e55. [CrossRef]
5. Raab, O. Über die Wirkung fluoreszcierender Stoffe aus Infusorien. *Z Biol.* **1900**, *39*, 524.
6. Jesionek, A.; von Tappeiner, H. Zur Behandlung der Hautcarcinome mit fluoreszierenden Stoffen. *Dtsch. Arch. Klin. Med.* **1905**, *85*, 223–239.
7. Cieplik, F.; Deng, D.; Crielaard, W.; Buchalla, W.; Hellwig, E.; Al-Ahmad, A.; Maisch, T. Antimicrobial photodynamic therapy–what we know and what we don't. *Crit. Rev. Microbiol.* **2018**, *44*, 571–589. [CrossRef] [PubMed]

8. Abrahamse, H.; Hamblin, M.R. New photosensitizers for photodynamic therapy. *Biochem. J.* **2016**, *473*, 347–364. [CrossRef] [PubMed]
9. Hu, X.; Huang, Y.Y.; Wang, Y.; Wang, X.; Hamblin, M.R. Antimicrobial Photodynamic Therapy to Control Clinically Relevant Biofilm Infections. *Front. Microbiol.* **2018**, *9*, 1299. [CrossRef] [PubMed]
10. Wainwright, M.; Crossley, K.B. Photosensitising agents—circumventing resistance and breaking down biofilms: A review. *Int. Biodeterior. Biodegrad.* **2004**, *53*, 119–126. [CrossRef]
11. Omar, G.S.; Wilson, M.; Nair, S.P. Lethal photosensitization of wound-associated microbes using indocyanine green and near-infrared light. *BMC Microbiol.* **2008**, *8*, 111. [CrossRef]
12. Reinhart, M.B.; Huntington, C.R.; Blair, L.J.; Heniford, B.T.; Augenstein, V.A. Indocyanine Green: Historical Context, Current Applications, and Future Considerations. *Surg. Innov.* **2016**, *23*, 166–175. [CrossRef]
13. Ptaszek, M. Rational design of fluorophores for in vivo applications. *Prog. Mol. Biol. Transl. Sci.* **2013**, *113*, 59–108. [CrossRef]
14. Saxena, V.; Sadoqi, M.; Shao, J. Indocyanine green-loaded biodegradable nanoparticles: Preparation, physicochemical characterization and in vitro release. *Int. J. Pharm.* **2004**, *278*, 293–301. [CrossRef] [PubMed]
15. Hoop, M. Die ICG-gestützte Photothermische Therapie (PTT). *ZMK* **2013**, *29*, 528–541.
16. Shirata, C.; Kaneko, J.; Inagaki, Y.; Kokudo, T.; Sato, M.; Kiritani, S.; Akamatsu, N.; Arita, J.; Sakamoto, Y.; Hasegawa, K.; et al. Near-infrared photothermal/photodynamic therapy with indocyanine green induces apoptosis of hepatocellular carcinoma cells through oxidative stress. *Sci. Rep.* **2017**, *7*, 13958. [CrossRef] [PubMed]
17. Cherrick, G.R.; Stein, S.W.; Leevy, C.M.; Davidson, C.S. Indocyanine green: Observations on its physical properties, plasma decay, and hepatic extraction. *J. Clin. Investig.* **1960**, *39*, 592–600. [CrossRef]
18. Raut, C.P.; Sethi, K.S.; Kohale, B.R.; Mamajiwala, A.; Warang, A. Indocyanine green-mediated photothermal therapy in treatment of chronic periodontitis: A clinico-microbiological study. *J. Indian Soc. Periodontol.* **2018**, *22*, 221–227. [CrossRef]
19. Baumgartner, J.C. Microbiologic and pathologic aspects of endodontics. *Curr. Opin. Dent.* **1991**, *1*, 737–743.
20. Beltes, C.; Sakkas, H.; Economides, N.; Papadopoulou, C. Antimicrobial photodynamic therapy using Indocyanine green and near-infrared diode laser in reducing Entrerococcus faecalis. *Photodiagnosis Photodyn. Ther.* **2017**, *17*, 5–8. [CrossRef]
21. Nagahara, A.; Mitani, A.; Fukuda, M.; Yamamoto, H.; Tahara, K.; Morita, I.; Ting, C.C.; Watanabe, T.; Fujimura, T.; Osawa, K.; et al. Antimicrobial photodynamic therapy using a diode laser with a potential new photosensitizer, indocyanine green-loaded nanospheres, may be effective for the clearance of Porphyromonas gingivalis. *J. Periodontal Res.* **2013**, *48*, 591–599. [CrossRef]
22. Pourhajibagher, M.; Chiniforush, N.; Ghorbanzadeh, R.; Bahador, A. Photo-activated disinfection based on indocyanine green against cell viability and biofilm formation of Porphyromonas gingivalis. *Photodiagnosis Photodyn. Ther.* **2017**, *17*, 61–64. [CrossRef]
23. Beytollahi, L.; Pourhajibagher, M.; Chiniforush, N.; Ghorbanzadeh, R.; Raoofian, R.; Pourakbari, B.; Bahador, A. The efficacy of photodynamic and photothermal therapy on biofilm formation of Streptococcus mutans: An in vitro study. *Photodiagnosis Photodyn. Ther.* **2017**, *17*, 56–60. [CrossRef]
24. Hill, G.; Dehn, C.; Hinze, A.V.; Frentzen, M.; Meister, J. Indocyanine green-based adjunctive antimicrobial photodynamic therapy for treating chronic periodontitis: A randomized clinical trial. *Photodiagnosis Photodyn. Ther.* **2019**, *26*, 29–35. [CrossRef] [PubMed]
25. Nikinmaa, S.; Moilanen, N.; Sorsa, T.; Rantala, J.; Alapulli, H.; Kotiranta, A.; Auvinen, P.; Kankuri, E.; Meurman, J.H.; Pätilä, T. Indocyanine Green-Assisted and LED-Light-Activated Antibacterial Photodynamic Therapy Reduces Dental Plaque. *Dent. J.* **2021**, *9*, 52. [CrossRef] [PubMed]
26. Karygianni, L.; Ruf, S.; Follo, M.; Hellwig, E.; Bucher, M.; Anderson, A.C.; Vach, K.; Al-Ahmad, A. Novel Broad-Spectrum Antimicrobial Photoinactivation of In Situ Oral Biofilms by Visible Light plus Water-Filtered Infrared A. *Appl. Environ. Microbiol.* **2014**, *80*, 7324–7336. [CrossRef] [PubMed]
27. Daeschlein, G.; Alborova, J.; Patzelt, A.; Kramer, A.; Lademann, J. Kinetics of physiological skin flora in a suction blister wound model on healthy subjects after treatment with water-filtered infrared-A radiation. *Skin Pharmacol. Physiol.* **2012**, *25*, 73–77. [CrossRef]
28. Hartel, M.; Hoffmann, G.; Wente, M.N.; Martignoni, M.E.; Büchler, M.W.; Friess, H. Randomized clinical trial of the influence of local water-filtered infrared A irradiation on wound healing after abdominal surgery. *Br. J. Surg.* **2006**, *93*, 952–960. [CrossRef] [PubMed]
29. Al-Ahmad, A.; Bucher, M.; Anderson, A.C.; Tennert, C.; Hellwig, E.; Wittmer, A.; Vach, K.; Karygianni, L. Antimicrobial Photoinactivation Using Visible Light Plus Water-Filtered Infrared-A (VIS + wIRA) Alters In Situ Oral Biofilms. *PLoS ONE* **2015**, *10*, e0132107. [CrossRef] [PubMed]
30. Burchard, T.; Karygianni, L.; Hellwig, E.; Follo, M.; Wrbas, T.; Wittmer, A.; Vach, K.; Al-Ahmad, A. Inactivation of oral biofilms using visible light and water-filtered infrared A radiation and indocyanine green. *Future Med. Chem.* **2019**, *11*, 1721–1739. [CrossRef] [PubMed]
31. Al-Ahmad, A.; Walankiewicz, A.; Hellwig, E.; Follo, M.; Tennert, C.; Wittmer, A.; Karygianni, L. Photoinactivation Using Visible Light Plus Water-Filtered Infrared-A (vis+wIRA) and Chlorine e6 (Ce6) Eradicates Planktonic Periodontal Pathogens and Subgingival Biofilms. *Front. Microbiol.* **2016**, *7*, 1900. [CrossRef]
32. Hoffmann, G. Principles and working mechanisms of water-filtered infrared-A (wIRA) in relation to wound healing. *GMS Krankenhhyg. Interdiszip.* **2007**, *2*, Doc54.
33. von Felbert, V.; Schumann, H.; Mercer, J.B.; Strasser, W.; Daeschlein, G.; Hoffmann, G. Therapy of chronic wounds with water-filtered infrared-A (wIRA). *GMS Krankenhhyg. Interdiszip.* **2008**, *2*, Doc52.

34. Piazena, H.; Kelleher, D.K. Effects of infrared-A irradiation on skin: Discrepancies in published data highlight the need for an exact consideration of physical and photobiological laws and appropriate experimental settings. *Photochem. Photobiol.* **2010**, *86*, 687–705. [CrossRef] [PubMed]
35. Engel, E.; Schraml, R.; Maisch, T.; Kobuch, K.; König, B.; Szeimies, R.M.; Hillenkamp, J.; Bäumler, W.; Vasold, R. Light-induced decomposition of indocyanine green. *Investig. Ophthalmol. Vis. Sci.* **2008**, *49*, 1777–1783. [CrossRef] [PubMed]
36. Jones, D. Maintance of bacteria on glass beads at −60 °C and to −70 °C. In *Maintenance of Microorganisms: A Manual of Laboratory Methods*; Kirsop, B.E., Snell, J.J.S., Eds.; Academic Press: London, UK, 1984; pp. 35–40.
37. Wiebe, C.B.; Putnins, E.E. The periodontal disease classification system of the American Academy of Periodontology—An update. *J. Can. Dent. Assoc.* **2000**, *66*, 594–597.
38. American Academy of Periodontology Task Force Report on the Update to the 1999 Classification of Periodontal Diseases and Conditions. *J. Periodontol.* **2015**, *86*, 835–838. [CrossRef] [PubMed]
39. Gajardo, M.; Silva, N.; Gómez, L.; León, R.; Parra, B.; Contreras, A.; Gamonal, J. Prevalence of periodontopathic bacteria in aggressive periodontitis patients in a Chilean population. *J. Periodontol.* **2005**, *76*, 289–294. [CrossRef] [PubMed]
40. Roesch-Ely, M.; Steinberg, T.; Bosch, F.X.; Müssig, E.; Whitaker, N.; Wiest, T.; Kohl, A.; Komposch, G.; Tomakidi, P. Organotypic co-cultures allow for immortalized human gingival keratinocytes to reconstitute a gingival epithelial phenotype in vitro. *Differentiation* **2006**, *74*, 622–637. [CrossRef] [PubMed]
41. George, S.; Hamblin, M.R.; Kishen, A. Uptake pathways of anionic and cationic photosensitizers into bacteria. *Photochem. Photobiol. Sci.* **2009**, *8*, 788–795. [CrossRef]
42. Raghavendra, M.; Koregol, A.; Bhola, S. Photodynamic therapy: A targeted therapy in periodontics. *Aust. Dent. J.* **2009**, *54* (Suppl. 1), S102–S109. [CrossRef]
43. Chiniforush, N.; Pourhajibagher, M.; Shahabi, S.; Bahador, A. Clinical Approach of High Technology Techniques for Control and Elimination of Endodontic Microbiota. *J. Lasers Med. Sci.* **2015**, *6*, 139–150. [CrossRef]
44. Meister, J.; Hopp, M.; Schäfers, J.; Verbeek, J.; Kraus, D.; Frentzen, M. *Indocyanine Green (ICG) as a New Adjuvant for the Antimicrobial Photo-Dynamic Therapy (aPDT) in Dentistry*; SPIE: Bellingham, WA, USA, 2014; Volume 8929.
45. Al-Ahmad, A.; Tennert, C.; Karygianni, L.; Wrbas, K.T.; Hellwig, E.; Altenburger, M.J. Antimicrobial photodynamic therapy using visible light plus water-filtered infrared-A (wIRA). *J. Med. Microbiol.* **2013**, *62*, 467–473. [CrossRef]
46. Sotomil, J.M.; Münchow, E.A.; Pankajakshan, D.; Spolnik, K.J.; Ferreira, J.A.; Gregory, R.L.; Bottino, M.C. Curcumin-A Natural Medicament for Root Canal Disinfection: Effects of Irrigation, Drug Release, and Photoactivation. *J. Endod.* **2019**, *45*, 1371–1377. [CrossRef] [PubMed]
47. Hafner, S.; Ehrenfeld, M.; Storz, E.; Wieser, A. Photodynamic Inactivation of Actinomyces naeslundii in Comparison With Chlorhexidine and Polyhexanide—A New Approach for Antiseptic Treatment of Medication-Related Osteonecrosis of the Jaw? *J. Oral Maxillofac. Surg.* **2016**, *74*, 516–522. [CrossRef] [PubMed]
48. Carrera, E.T.; Dias, H.B.; Corbi, S.C.T.; Marcantonio, R.A.C.; Bernardi, A.C.A.; Bagnato, V.S.; Hamblin, M.R.; Rastelli, A.N.S. The application of antimicrobial photodynamic therapy (aPDT) in dentistry: A critical review. *Laser Phys.* **2016**, *26*, 123001. [CrossRef] [PubMed]
49. Kranz, S.; Huebsch, M.; Guellmar, A.; Voelpel, A.; Tonndorf-Martini, S.; Sigusch, B.W. Antibacterial photodynamic treatment of periodontopathogenic bacteria with indocyanine green and near-infrared laser light enhanced by Trolox(TM). *Lasers Surg. Med.* **2015**, *47*, 350–360. [CrossRef] [PubMed]
50. Theodoro, L.H.; Assem, N.Z.; Longo, M.; Alves, M.L.F.; Duque, C.; Stipp, R.N.; Vizoto, N.L.; Garcia, V.G. Treatment of periodontitis in smokers with multiple sessions of antimicrobial photodynamic therapy or systemic antibiotics: A randomized clinical trial. *Photodiagnosis Photodyn. Ther.* **2018**, *22*, 217–222. [CrossRef] [PubMed]
51. Bjarnsholt, T. The role of bacterial biofilms in chronic infections. *APMIS Suppl.* **2013**, *136*, 1–51. [CrossRef] [PubMed]
52. Lamont, R.J.; Koo, H.; Hajishengallis, G. The oral microbiota: Dynamic communities and host interactions. *Nat. Rev. Microbiol.* **2018**, *16*, 745–759. [CrossRef]
53. Fontana, C.R.; Abernethy, A.D.; Som, S.; Ruggiero, K.; Doucette, S.; Marcantonio, R.C.; Boussios, C.I.; Kent, R.; Goodson, J.M.; Tanner, A.C.; et al. The antibacterial effect of photodynamic therapy in dental plaque-derived biofilms. *J. Periodontal. Res.* **2009**, *44*, 751–759. [CrossRef]
54. Maddi, A.; Scannapieco, F.A. Oral biofilms, oral and periodontal infections, and systemic disease. *Am. J. Dent.* **2013**, *26*, 249–254.
55. Burchard, T.; Karygianni, L.; Hellwig, E.; Wittmer, A.; Al-Ahmad, A. Microbial Composition of Oral Biofilms after Visible Light and Water-Filtered Infrared a Radiation (VIS+wIRA) in Combination with Indocyanine Green (ICG) as Photosensitizer. *Antibiotics* **2020**, *9*, 532. [CrossRef]
56. McCoy, L.C.; Wehler, C.J.; Rich, S.E.; Garcia, R.I.; Miller, D.R.; Jones, J.A. Adverse events associated with chlorhexidine use: Results from the Department of Veterans Affairs Dental Diabetes Study. *J. Am. Dent. Assoc.* **2008**, *139*, 178–183. [CrossRef] [PubMed]
57. James, P.; Worthington, H.V.; Parnell, C.; Harding, M.; Lamont, T.; Cheung, A.; Whelton, H.; Riley, P. Chlorhexidine mouthrinse as an adjunctive treatment for gingival health. *Cochrane Database Syst. Rev.* **2017**, *3*, Cd008676. [CrossRef] [PubMed]
58. Russell, A.D. Chlorhexidine: Antibacterial action and bacterial resistance. *Infection* **1986**, *14*, 212–215. [CrossRef] [PubMed]
59. Marti, H.; Koschwanez, M.; Pesch, T.; Blenn, C.; Borel, N. Water-filtered infrared a irradiation in combination with visible light inhibits acute chlamydial infection. *PLoS ONE* **2014**, *9*, e102239. [CrossRef] [PubMed]

60. Ho, J.D.; Tsai, R.J.; Chen, S.N.; Chen, H.C. Cytotoxicity of indocyanine green on retinal pigment epithelium: Implications for macular hole surgery. *Arch. Ophthalmol.* **2003**, *121*, 1423–1429. [CrossRef] [PubMed]
61. Bäumler, W.; Abels, C.; Karrer, S.; Weiss, T.; Messmann, H.; Landthaler, M.; Szeimies, R.M. Photo-oxidative killing of human colonic cancer cells using indocyanine green and infrared light. *Br. J. Cancer* **1999**, *80*, 360–363. [CrossRef] [PubMed]
62. Ateş, G.B.; Ak, A.; Garipcan, B.; Gülsoy, M. Indocyanine green-mediated photobiomodulation on human osteoblast cells. *Lasers Med. Sci.* **2018**, *33*, 1591–1599. [CrossRef]
63. Pourhajibagher, M.; Chiniforush, N.; Parker, S.; Shahabi, S.; Ghorbanzadeh, R.; Kharazifard, M.J.; Bahador, A. Evaluation of antimicrobial photodynamic therapy with indocyanine green and curcumin on human gingival fibroblast cells: An In Vitro photocytotoxicity investigation. *Photodiagnosis Photodyn. Ther.* **2016**, *15*, 13–18. [CrossRef]
64. Gale, J.S.; Proulx, A.A.; Gonder, J.R.; Mao, A.J.; Hutnik, C.M. Comparison of the in vitro toxicity of indocyanine green to that of trypan blue in human retinal pigment epithelium cell cultures. *Am. J. Ophthalmol.* **2004**, *138*, 64–69. [CrossRef]
65. Wang, M.; Lv, C.Y.; Li, S.A.; Wang, J.K.; Luo, W.Z.; Zhao, P.C.; Liu, X.Y.; Wang, Z.M.; Jiao, Y.; Sun, H.W.; et al. Near infrared light fluorescence imaging-guided biomimetic nanoparticles of extracellular vesicles deliver indocyanine green and paclitaxel for hyperthermia combined with chemotherapy against glioma. *J. Nanobiotechnol.* **2021**, *19*, 210. [CrossRef]
66. Ruhi, M.K.; Ak, A.; Gülsoy, M. Dose-dependent photochemical/photothermal toxicity of indocyanine green-based therapy on three different cancer cell lines. *Photodiagnosis Photodyn. Ther.* **2018**, *21*, 334–343. [CrossRef] [PubMed]
67. Schlemmer, M.; Lindner, L.H.; Abdel-Rahman, S.; Issels, R.D. Principles, technology and indication of hyperthermia and part body hyperthermia. *Radiologe* **2004**, *44*, 301–309. [CrossRef] [PubMed]
68. Zach, L.; Cohen, G. Pulp response to externally applied heat. *Oral Surg. Oral Med. Oral Pathol.* **1965**, *19*, 515–530. [CrossRef]
69. Mordon, S.; Devoisselle, J.M.; Soulie-Begu, S.; Desmettre, T. Indocyanine green: Physicochemical factors affecting its fluorescence in vivo. *Microvasc Res.* **1998**, *55*, 146–152. [CrossRef] [PubMed]
70. Ricci, F.; Pucci, S.; Sesti, F.; Missiroli, F.; Cerulli, L.; Spagnoli, L.G. Modulation of Ku70/80, clusterin/ApoJ isoforms and Bax expression in indocyanine-green-mediated photo-oxidative cell damage. *Ophthalmic Res.* **2007**, *39*, 164–173. [CrossRef]
71. You, Q.; Sun, Q.; Wang, J.; Tan, X.; Pang, X.; Liu, L.; Yu, M.; Tan, F.; Li, N. A single-light triggered and dual-imaging guided multifunctional platform for combined photothermal and photodynamic therapy based on TD-controlled and ICG-loaded CuS@mSiO$_2$. *Nanoscale* **2017**, *9*, 3784–3796. [CrossRef]
72. Bashir, N.Z.; Singh, H.A.; Virdee, S.S. Indocyanine green-mediated antimicrobial photodynamic therapy as an adjunct to periodontal therapy: A systematic review and meta-analysis. *Clin. Oral Investig.* **2021**, *25*, 5699–5710. [CrossRef]

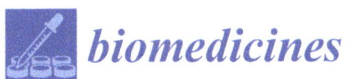

Article

Photodynamic Therapy (PDT) in Prosthodontics: Disinfection of Human Teeth Exposed to *Streptococcus mutans* and the Effect on the Adhesion of Full Ceramic Veneers, Crowns, and Inlays: An In Vitro Study

Corina Elena Tisler [1], Radu Chifor [2,*], Mindra Eugenia Badea [2], Marioara Moldovan [3], Doina Prodan [3], Rahela Carpa [4], Stanca Cuc [3,*], Ioana Chifor [2] and Alexandru Florin Badea [5]

[1] Department of Prosthetic Dentistry and Dental Materials, Iuliu Hatieganu University of Medicine and Pharmacy, 32 Clinicilor Street, 400006 Cluj-Napoca, Romania; tisler.corina@umfcluj.ro
[2] Department of Preventive Dental Medicine, Iuliu Hatieganu University of Medicine and Pharmacy, Avram Iancu 31, 400083 Cluj-Napoca, Romania; mebadea@umfcluj.ro (M.E.B.); ioana.chifor@umfcluj.ro (I.C.)
[3] Department of Polymer Composites, Institute of Chemistry "Raluca Ripan", University Babes-Bolyai, 400294 Cluj-Napoca, Romania; marioara.moldovan@ubbcluj.ro (M.M.); doina.prodan@ubbcluj.ro (D.P.)
[4] Department of Molecular Biology and Biotechnology, Faculty of Biology and Geology, Babeș Bolyai University, 1 M. Kogălniceanu Street, 400084 Cluj-Napoca, Romania; rahela.carpa@ubbcluj.ro
[5] Department of Morphological Sciences, Discipline of Anatomy and Embryology, Faculty of General Medicine, Iuliu Hatieganu University of Medicine and Pharmacy, 3–5 Clinicilor Street, 400006 Cluj-Napoca, Romania; alexandru.badea@umfcluj.ro
* Correspondence: chifor.radu@umfcluj.ro (R.C.); stanca.boboia@ubbcluj.ro (S.C.); Tel.: +40-742-195-229 (R.C.); +40-757-939-232 (S.C.)

Abstract: The use of PDT in prosthodontics as a disinfection protocol can eradicate bacteria from tooth surfaces by causing the death of the microorganisms to which the photosensitizer binds, absorbing the energy of laser light during irradiation. The aim of the study was to investigate the capacity of PDT to increase the bond strength of full ceramic restorations. In this study, 45 extracted human teeth were prepared for veneers, crowns, and inlays and contaminated with *Streptococcus mutans*. Tooth surfaces decontamination was performed using a diode laser and methylene blue as a photosensitizer. The disinfection effect and the impact on tensile bond strength were evaluated by scanning electron microscopy (SEM) and pull-out tests of the cemented ceramic prosthesis. Results show that the number of bacteria was reduced from colonized prepared tooth surfaces, and the bond strength was increased when PDT was used. In conclusion, the present study indicates that using PDT as a protocol before the final adhesive cementation of ceramic restorations could be a promising approach, with outstanding advantages over conventional methods.

Keywords: photodynamic therapy; biofilm; ceramic; adhesion; pull-out test; SEM

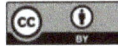

1. Introduction

In recent years, dentistry has experienced a wide development, and patient demands are aligned with the present restorative possibilities. All-ceramic restorations can regain lost functions, combining the strength of materials with a clearly superior and stable aesthetic over time, while adhesive cements ensure adequate bonding. Furthermore, these materials require minimum invasive preparations, as they are able to preserve and prolong teeth integrity.

Cementation in fixed prosthodontics as a final clinical step can be very challenging. The longevity of the restorations depends on the accuracy of the two main procedures that are performed in the last visit to the clinic—disinfection of the prepared tooth and cementation.

Photodynamic therapy is a non-invasive approach that involves a photosensitizer, a visible light of an appropriate wavelength, and the production of reactive oxygen species (mainly singlet oxygen), which immediately causes phototoxicity and leads to serious bacterial damage and death [1–5]. Its efficacy over *Streptococcus mutans* (a Gram-positive bacteria and the main responsible for dental caries) has been demonstrated, both in the stage of free microorganism and while organized in biofilms [4–7]. PDT is able to strongly reduce the number of bacteria from colonized dental surfaces.

The positive effect of photodynamic therapy can also extend to adhesion when used as a decontamination protocol before cementation. We did not find any studies able to reveal the impact of PDT on prosthodontic cementation, while in endodontics and orthodontics, it had a negative impact or was effectless on the bond strength and mechanical properties of dentin from the intracanal prosthetic space [8–11] and bond strength of orthodontic brackets [12].

Over the past several years, dental ceramics used in prosthodontics have been upgraded, achieving a great improvement of their mechanical properties due to the actual processing techniques and enhanced microstructures [13]. Lithium disilicate—the most representative material of glass ceramics—is a biocompatible and esthetic material with remarkable mechanical properties and a wide applicability, used for inlays, veneers, and crowns (anterior and posterior) fabrication [14]. These prostheses represent single-tooth restorations generally made of ceramic. Their major advantage is they require minimal preparations and allow dental tissues conservation. The highlighted advantages of inlays, veneers, and crowns are completed by adhesive cementation.

The adhesion of all-ceramic restorations has multiple advantages, such as higher retention and improved marginal adaptation. Resin-based adhesive cements are widely used for inlays, crowns, and veneers cementation, especially the dual-cured type, which gives a better polymerization control and an increased working time [15].

The substrate to which ceramic is bonded has great importance, as adhesion to the enamel is superior to the one that can be achieved onto dentin. In consequence, dental preparations limited to enamel have a higher bond strength than the ones at a depth that implies both enamel and dentin. For this reason, the bonding of ceramic veneers only to dentin should be avoided or performed with great caution [16].

Nevertheless, the examination of the tensile strength of luting cements can be performed by using a pull-out test to achieve axial oriented forces that lead to dislodgement of restorations cemented to extracted human teeth [17].

The novelty of the present research lies in the adhesion testing of three types of lithium disilicate prostheses before and after PDT, along with the antibacterial effect when an atypical protocol was used.

The aim of this study is to evaluate the efficiency of photodynamic therapy in the field of prosthodontics by simulating a clinical cementation protocol of all-ceramic restorations (inlays, veneers, and crowns) and to underline the double advantage that a single operation can have—simultaneous disinfection and bond strength enhancement. Our main purpose is to analyze the capacity of PDT of interfering with the adhesion of lithium disilicate ceramic prostheses by mechanically testing the bonded final restorations. The null hypothesis was that PDT had no effect on disinfecting prepared teeth or increasing the adhesion to all-ceramic restorations.

2. Materials and Methods

2.1. Prosthodontic Preparation

The samples were represented by 45 extracted human teeth (incisors, premolars, and molars) that were divided into 3 groups as follows: 15 teeth were prepared for veneers (with an extension of the preparation on the oral surface; noted from 1F to 15F), 15 for class I inlays (noted from 1I to 15I), and 15 for crowns (noted from 1C to 15C). All preparations were made using diamond burs fixed into a high-speed, high-torque handpiece (electric motor) at depths that afford the placement of ceramic restorations, using an identical preparation and finishing protocol. Due to the difficulties encountered during the collection, handling, and storage of real human saliva, artificial saliva was preferred as a storage material for teeth before and after prosthodontic preparation. Artificial saliva formulations were developed at the Department of Polymer Composites, Institute of Chemistry "Raluca Ripan" and contain Na_2HPO_4, $NaHCO_3$, $CaCl_2$, H_2O, and HCl.

2.2. Bacterial Contamination

The strain used was *Streptococcus mutans* ATCC 25,175 from the collection of the Laboratory of Microbiology, Faculty of Biology and Geology, UBB, Cluj.

To obtain the bacterial suspension, the BHI-T culture medium was inoculated with the *Streptococcus mutans* strain which was then incubated for 24 h at 37 °C. After the growing period, the bacterial suspension was used as the inoculum for the 45 tubes with BHI-T culture medium. A volume of 500 µL of 0.5 MacFarland bacterial suspension was inoculated into tubes with a BHI-T medium. Then, aseptically, one tooth was placed in each tube.

The tubes with teeth placed in the BHI-T culture medium and inoculated with the bacterium under study were incubated for 8 days at a temperature of 37 °C. Immediately after the incubation period, teeth were removed from the immersion environments and placed on aluminum stubs with the prepared surface facing upwards. The specimens were then examined using SEM at a low vacuum, at a pressure of 80 Pa, and with an acceleration voltage of 30 kV. Scanning electron microscopy (SEM-Inspect S, FEI) examination was performed to identify the presence of bacterial biofilm on prepared tooth surfaces at a magnification of $\times 5000$.

2.3. Photodynamic Therapy Protocol

PDT was performed using the SiroLaser Blue (Dentsply Sirona, New York, NY, USA) from the Department of Preventive Dental Medicine, Iuliu Hatieganu University of Medicine and Pharmacy, Cluj. Methylene blue (MB) was used as a photosensitizer and washed using a gradated syringe with Kaqun water (oxygen-rich, alkaline water).

For every group of teeth from 1 to 10 MB gel 1% was applied on the prepared surfaces for 3 min and then washed under an easy jet of 3 mL Kaqun water for 20 s. The MultiTip of 8 mm was chosen as the irradiation laser tip. The diode SiroLaser Blue with 660 nm wavelength was set at 100 mW power in the continuous mode and applied for 180 s. This protocol was repeated identically for every tooth from 1 to 10, while teeth from 11 to 15 from every group were washed only with 3 mL of Kaqun water for 20 s, without PS or laser irradiation. SEM examination was repeated to observe bacterial presence on teeth subjected to PDT.

2.4. Fabrication and Cementation of Prosthodontic Restorations (Veneers, Inlays, and Crowns)

Impressions of all teeth were taken with Variotime (Heraeus, Hanau, Germany) polyvinyl siloxane using the sandwich impression technique. Gypsum casts were poured, on which wax patterns were then modeled. After modeling, a prefabricated wax rod was placed on each wax model, parallel with the path of insertion. For the fabrication of the prosthesis, IPS e.max PRESS ceramic ingots were used. The selected color was A2 from the Vita Classical Shade Guide. Ceramic pressing was performed with Programat EP 3010 oven. Final restorations were not glazed, and the resulting ceramic rods were kept as a structure of the restorations.

After conducting the previously described PDT, cementation was performed for every tooth, according to the instructions of the manufacturer of Variolink Esthetic dual-cure (DC) luting composite. Restorations were placed on teeth using Variolink Esthetic try-in paste, and the adaptation was checked. Monobond Etch & Prime (self-etching glass-ceramic primer) was applied with a micro brush on the internal surfaces of restorations for 60 s and then spread with a strong stream of air. Prepared surfaces were etched using orthophosphoric acid gel 37%, for 15–30 s on enamel, and 10–15 s on dentin. The etching agent was rinsed thoroughly with a stream of water. Teeth surfaces were dried until the etched enamel appeared chalky white. Starting with the enamel, tooth surfaces were coated with Adhese Universal for 20 s and then dispersed with oil- and moisture-free compressed air. Light curing was performed for 10 s using Demi Plus Kerr Dental Curing Light. Variolink Esthetic DC was applied with an application tip directly to the internal surface of the restoration (for veneers and crowns) and in the cavity (for inlays). The ceramic prosthesis was then seated and held in place during excess removal. Excess material was light cured with a polymerization light for 2 s at 10–15 mm by running the light probe along the entire cement line and removed immediately with a scaler. Restoration margins were covered with liquid strips immediately after excess removal to prevent oxygen inhibition and light cured for 10 s. Margins and cement lines were polished with Kenda polishers. SEM examination was performed to explore the bond interface at the tooth–prosthesis junction.

2.5. Pull-Out Test

Each tooth was incorporated in self-curing acrylate at both ends—the ceramic rod and the root—leaving the crown free of acrylate. After the material setting, the whole assembly was kept in artificial saliva for 24 h.

Pull out-test was performed (Figure 1) by using a Lloyd LR5k Plus dual-column mechanical testing machine (Ametek/Lloyd Instruments, Germany, provided with a cell with a maximum recording force of 5KN), at a crosshead speed of 1 mm/min (ASTM D638 standard), and the data were processed using NexygenPlus software. For each investigated group, 15 evaluations (10 teeth with PDT and 5 teeth without PDT) were performed. Measurements that had a difference of ±15% of the measured average value were eliminated. The results were subjected to ANOVA one-way statistical analysis (α-0.05) and Tukey's ad hoc test using the Origin 2019b Graphing and Analysis (Origin Lab) software (Northampton, MA, USA). Fracture areas were evaluated by SEM and optical microscope (Zeiss Stemi 2000-C Stereo Microscope 6.5x–50x, Germany).

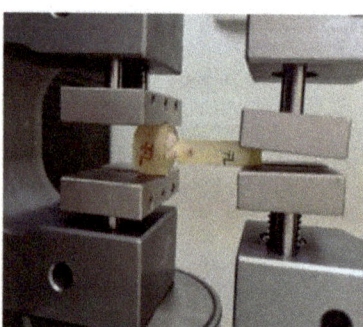

Figure 1. Pull-out mechanical test using LLOYD LR5k Plus.

3. Results

3.1. Effectiveness of Disinfection through Photodynamic Therapy

This study assessed the effectiveness of using PDT as a method of disinfection of prepared coronary surfaces of extracted teeth. SEM analysis of contaminated prepared dental surfaces showed the appearance of *Streptococcus mutans* biofilm consisting of an agglomeration of cocci that completely covered the dental structures (Figure 2a,c,e). The 8-day-old biofilm revealed cells with a particular arrangement—such as solitary cells positioned next to each other—which had lost their specific chain conformation.

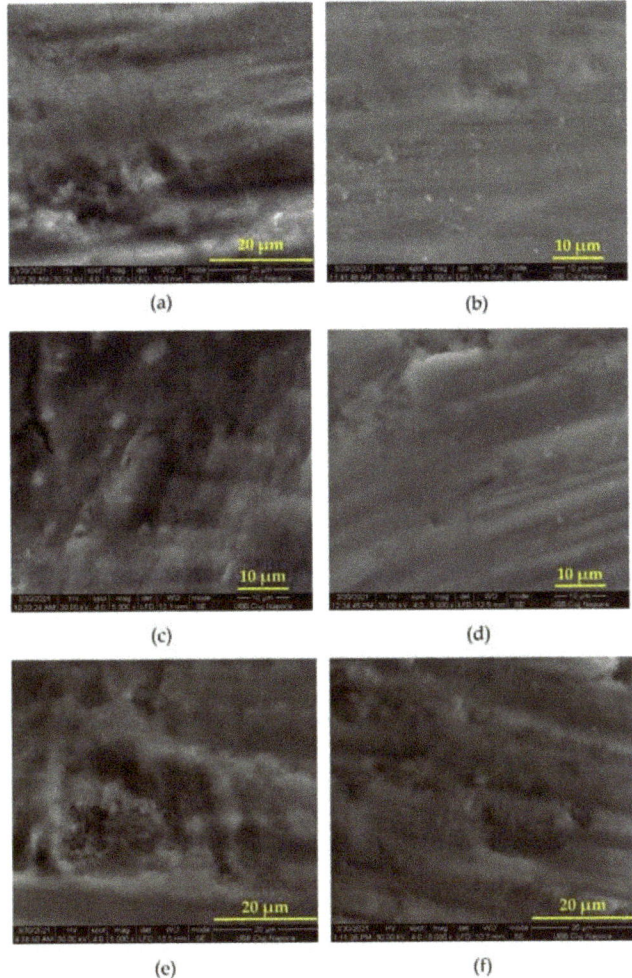

Figure 2. SEM images of contaminated teeth surface before and after PDT: (**a**) expansive colonization by *S. mutans*, biofilm covering entire veneer preparation; (**b**) SEM view after PDT on veneer preparation surface; (**c**) *S. mutans* biofilm on crown preparation; (**d**) crown preparation surface after PDT; (**e**) SEM image of *S. mutans* biofilm on inlay preparation; (**f**) inlay preparation surface after PDT.

The antibacterial effect on photodynamic therapy was highlighted by post-irradiation images that showed the disappearance of the bacterial biofilm and the presence of few solitary remaining bacteria (Figure 2b,d,f). PDT managed to reduce the number of colonizing streptococci on the surface of dental preparations.

3.2. Appearance of Tooth–Prosthesis Interface after Adhesive Cementation

SEM images of the adhesion between IPS e.max PRESS ceramic veneers, inlays, and crowns highlight qualitative cementation with an appropriate marginal adaptation to tooth structures (Figure 3).

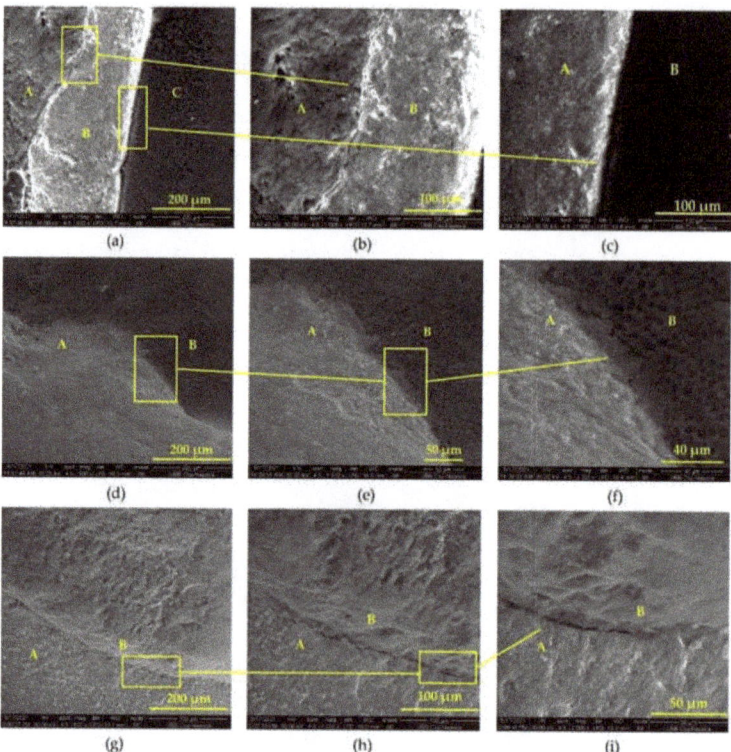

Figure 3. SEM representation of adhesion: (**a**) SEM image of the IPS e.max PRESS veneer interface area (A), adhesive cement (B), enamel area (C); (**b**) SEM image of the IPS e.max PRESS veneer (A), cement (B) interface; (**c**) SEM image of the interface adhesive cement (B), tooth enamel (C); (**d**) SEM view of ceramic inlay (A), tooth dentin (B), interface ×500; (**e**) SEM view of ceramic inlay (A), tooth dentin (B), interface ×1000; (**f**) SEM view of ceramic inlay (A), tooth dentin (B), interface ×2000; (**g**) SEM view of tooth enamel (A), ceramic crown (B), interface ×500; (**h**) SEM view of tooth enamel (A), ceramic crown (B), interface ×1000; (**i**) SEM view of tooth enamel (A), ceramic crown (B), interface ×2000.

3.3. Adhesion Pull-Out Test

The results of the pull-out test for the examined groups (crown, veneer, and inlay) are summarized in Table 1. The highest values of tensile strength of specimens treated with PDT (Figure 4) and comparison of load at upper yield between groups (Figure 5) are graphically represented. Based on the comparison of Anova one-way test results between the groups of teeth with and without photodynamic therapy, there were no different statistical semificatives between them for any of the groups of materials ($p \geq 0.05$). Based on the comparison of the values between all three groups (with and without photodynamic therapy) of restorations, there were different values of p, which did not show large statistically significant differences. In Tukey's test, groups with the same letter are without statistically significant differences (tensile strength), and those with different notations reflect significant differences between them (crown and veneer with inlay for load at maximum load and load at upper yield).

Table 1. Adhesion pull-out test.

Type of Prosthesis		Load at Maximum Load (N)	Tensile Strength (MPa)	Load at Upper Yield (N)
Crown	With PDT	265.82 ± 34.6781 [a]	84.6 ± 8.52369 [c]	209 ± 42.7055 [d]
	Without PDT	257.22 ± 51.8807 [a]	64.7 ± 12.7614 [c]	188 ± 55.1160 [d]
Veneer	With PDT	248.43 ± 20.9848 [a]	79.079 ± 7.64638 [c]	248.43 ± 35.0042 [d]
	Without PDT	239.55 ± 35.7009 [a]	80.571 ± 10.3334 [c]	228.88 ± 24.2239 [d]
Inlay	With PDT	305.98 ± 41.05021 [b]	97.396 ± 11.03891 [c]	290.83 ± 28.9973 [e]
	Without PDT	302.11 ± 84.5941 [b]	90.557 ± 15.2840 [c]	290.05 ± 20.9471 [e]
p value		0.00316	0.2135	0.02715

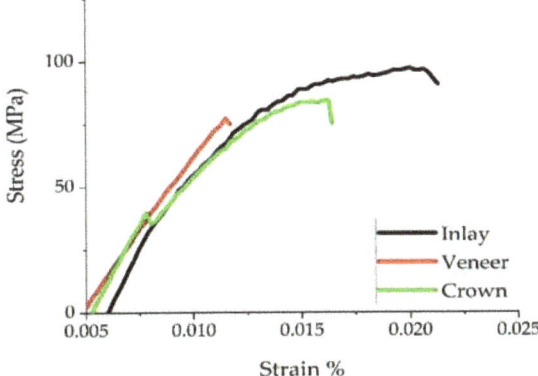

Figure 4. Comparison of the tensile strength highest values from each examined group when PDT was used.

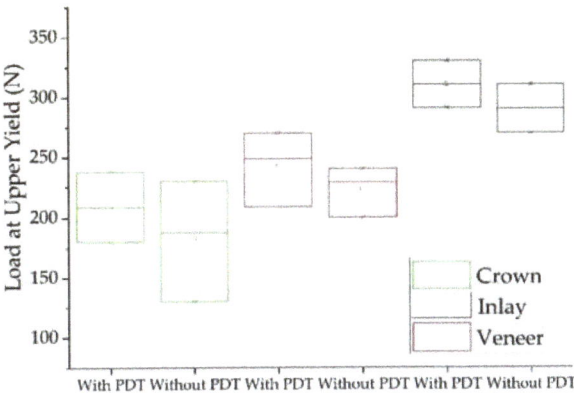

Figure 5. Comparison of load at upper yield between examined groups with and without PDT.

Fracture areas were highlighted by scanning electron microscopy (Figure 6) for veneer and crown groups, and prepared dentin was analyzed for debonded inlay group. SEM views revealed cracked subjacent dentin for veneers and crowns, fractured pieces of IPS e.max PRESS, and remaining Variolink Esthetic DC onto the dental surface alternating with areas where it was missing. For the inlay group, the specific detail was the presence of adhesive cement on the tooth, suggesting that fractures occurred at the cement–ceramic inlay interface. Optical microscopy images revealed veneers and crown specimens failure by fracture and inlay specimens failure by debonding (Figure 7).

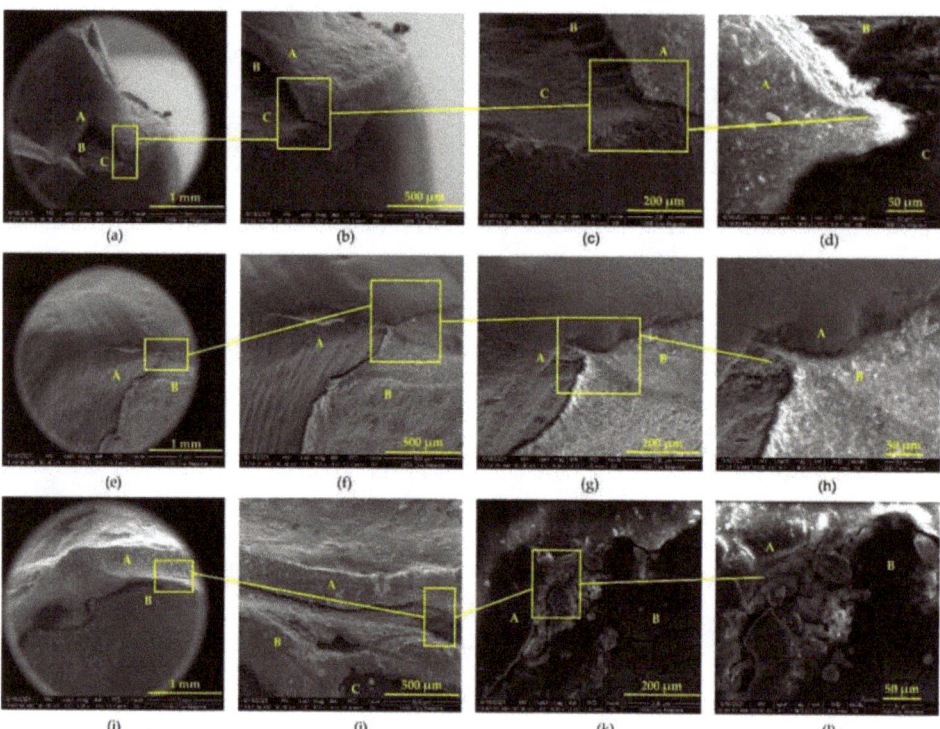

Figure 6. SEM examination of fracture areas after mechanical pull-out test: (**a**) SEM image of the veneer fracture zone: ceramic material (A), residual cement (B), tooth dentin (C) ×100; (**b**) SEM image of the veneer fracture zone: ceramic material (A), residual cement (B), tooth dentin (C) ×200; (**c**) SEM image of the veneer fracture zone: ceramic material (A), residual adhesive cement (B), tooth dentin (C) ×500; (**d**) SEM image of the veneer fracture zone: ceramic material (A), residual adhesive cement (B), tooth dentin (C) ×1000; (**e**) SEM view of the inlay cavity after debonding: prepared marginal dentin (A), residual adhesive cement (B) ×100; (**f**) SEM view of the inlay cavity after debonding: prepared marginal dentin (A), residual adhesive cement (B) ×200; (**g**) SEM view of the inlay cavity after debonding: prepared marginal dentin (A), residual adhesive cement (B) ×500; (**h**) SEM view of the inlay cavity after debonding: prepared marginal dentin (A), residual adhesive cement (B) ×1000; (**i**) SEM view of the fractured ceramic crown (A), tooth dentin (B) ×100; (**j**) SEM view of the fractured ceramic crown (A), residual adhesive cement (B), tooth dentin (C) ×200; (**k**) SEM view of the fractured ceramic crown (A), tooth dentin (B) ×500; (**l**) SEM view of the fractured ceramic crown (A), tooth dentin (B) ×1000.

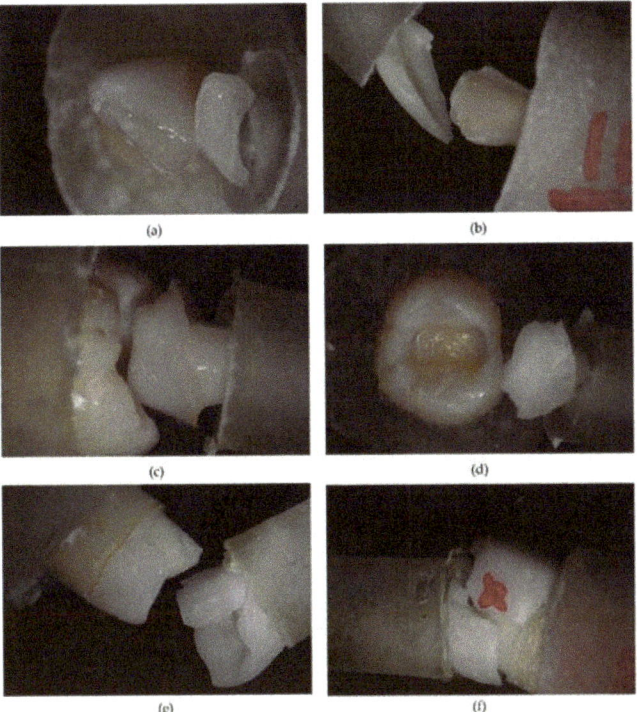

Figure 7. Optical microscope evaluation after mechanical pull-out test: (**a**) veneer fractured specimen; (**b**) fractured ceramic veneer after decementation; (**c**) inlay debonded specimen; (**d**) inlay restoration and preparation after debonding; (**e**) fractured crown restoration; (**f**) aspect of ceramic crown after decementation.

4. Discussion

Given the increased applicability of photodynamic therapy in dentistry, our goal was to explore a less addressed branch. We studied the use of this therapy in fixed prosthetics as an alternative to conventional procedures for disinfecting previously prepared dental abutments and explored possible effects on the immediate adhesive cementation of ceramic prostheses frequently performed by dentists in their current practice. Due to changes in the evaluated properties when PDT was applied, the null hypothesis was rejected.

For bacterial inoculation, we selected the *Streptococcus mutans* strain, given that it is mainly responsible for the appearance of caries processes. An essential feature of this bacterium is that it has receptors that enable it to adhere to the hard dental tissues [18]. The carious potential of this bacterium is accentuated by the ability to secrete glucan (which promotes bacterial adhesion and biofilm formation) and lactic acid, also by its acid tolerance mechanism [19]. Previous studies evaluated PDT's efficacy on *S. mutans* biofilms incubated for 5 days [4,7], 3 days [20], 48 h [21], respectively, while others [22] used a 7-day old biofilm. Our streptococcal biofilm also visibly developed on prepared teeth after 8 days. We chose this specific period considering that usually, a prosthetic restoration is finalized in about a week, during which the tooth is directly exposed to the oral bacterial flora if no provisional restorations are used or if they fracture.

Scanning electron microscopy is a common method of examining surface details by generating a three-dimensional image. This technique allows a direct examination performed at a high resolution [7,23]. In the present study, we verified the biofilm formation on the prepared areas of teeth. SEM images highlighted the presence of agglomerated cocci and poorly represented extracellular matrix structures, in accordance with other *S.mutans* biofilm exposures [7,22].

Although it was reported that the use of photodynamic therapy in fixed prosthodontics for dentinal decontamination before final cementation of crowns requires high-level laser therapy [24], this study investigated the antibacterial effect of this therapy at a minimum power of the used diode laser. In the present study, we used a SiroBlue diode laser at a wavelength of 660 nm. This chosen wavelength is specific to the photobiomodulation (PBM) protocol of this laser. Its applicability in tissue regeneration does not imply the use of a photosensitizer. The biomodulatory effect of diode lasers with different wavelengths was demonstrated [25,26]. A single laser-irradiation was performed, similarly to the process reported by another research [25].

Using tissue regeneration laser settings, as well as the addition of methylene blue as a photosensitizer and its washing with Kaqun water, represents an atypical protocol of PDT. Other studies have shown the effectiveness of various standard PDT protocols on both aerobic and anaerobic bacterial species [27–30]. The selection of the photosensitizer (MB) and laser power (100 mW) was based on previous works that demonstrated their efficacy [4,21,30]. MB had also a higher sterilizing effect [20] when compared with hematoporphyrin monomethyl ether (HMME). Post-PDT SEM images revealed a significant bacterial reduction; our results are in consensus with the antibacterial effect reported by other studies [4,6,20,21,31,32].

Moreover, this study evaluated the impact that photodynamic therapy had on the immediate adhesion of all-ceramic restorations. To our knowledge, no previous studies have evaluated the influence of PDT on veneers, inlays, and crowns adhesion to prepared coronary enamel and dentin, separately or together with the antimicrobial effect. Furthermore, e.max restorations are made from lithium disilicate ceramic, which provides excellent aesthetics and superior quality and strength. IPS e.max Press ceramic material contains a glass matrix, and 70% incorporated lithium disilicate crystals. IPS e.max PRESS is available as ingots with different shades and translucencies [33]. This material is used for veneers, inlays, and single crowns, as it is able to ensure translucency and resistance, with indications in both anterior and posterior teeth. The fracture resistance of lithium disilicate prosthesis is higher than that of zirconia or metal–ceramic prosthesis [34].

The longevity of indirect prosthetic restorations depends largely on the quality of the adhesion between the restorative material and the dental substrate. The veneer–cement-adhesive–tooth (enamel) interface revealed a homogeneous and uniformly thick layer of Variolink Esthetic DC adhesive cement. At the boundary between the veneer and the adhesive cement, there were areas with microcracks due to the contraction of the cement during light curing (Figure 3b), but the contact was intimate, without gaps, without areas of separation of the two materials, emphasizing a tight adhesion of cement to ceramics [35]. The evaluation of the junction between the adhesive cement and the tooth (enamel) showed very good adhesion, an adhesive system of uniform thickness, and a weakly represented but present hybrid layer (Figure 3c). No cracks, gaps, or discontinuities were identified at this level, indicating a good quality of adhesion between the adhesive cement and the tooth enamel. Our findings are similar to those reported by other studies that evaluated the adhesion of lithium disilicate ceramic bonded with the same cement that we used [36]. SEM images of tooth dentin–ceramic inlay (Figure 3d,e,f) and tooth dentin–ceramic crown (Figure 3g,h,i) highlighted a close adaptation of the prosthesis to tooth structures at different magnification levels. It is also worth mentioning that for heat-pressed lithium disilicate crowns and inlays, a marginal gap no higher than 100 µm is clinically acceptable [37,38].

In this study, we used ceramic prosthesis realized together with an occlusal or incisal bar parallel with their path of insertion, which served for assembling the universal testing machine and performing a mechanical pull-out test [39]. For every investigated group (crowns, veneers, and inlays) with and without PDT, testing was performed. Our results demonstrated that the antimicrobial protocol performed before adhesion did not statistically influence the examined parameters (load at maximum load, tensile strength, and load at upper yield). Noticeably, the obtained values were higher for every group when PDT was used (Table 1)—except for the tensile strength of veneers, which was approximatively the same with and without PDT. To our knowledge, no previous study has compared the tensile strength of cemented e.max ceramic prosthetic restorations before and after PDT using a pull-out retention test. All specimens from crown and veneer groups failed by fracture, while the inlay group failed by decementation. This is probably due to the difference in thickness between restorations—the inlays are thicker, in accordance with the cavity preparation. In our findings, load at maximum load for all the studied groups was similar when compared to the failure load reported by one study that used an unspecified luting composite for cementation [34]. Another study [40] reported higher values of the Load at maximum load than our results. This difference may appear due to the different protocol—the cementation was performed using adhesive cement different from ours, the occlusal surface was prepared flat, the wax patterns were designed digitally and milled, and because the internal surfaces of the restorations were etched with 9.5% hydrofluoric acid. A study with similar results [41] of the load at maximum load evaluated the retention of lithium disilicate crowns using bioactive cements. We did not find studies that evaluated tensile strength and load at upper yield for the types of restorations that we evaluated by pull-out test.

After assessing the results for every group of specimens, the authors evaluated the differences and similarities between them. Based on the results, we did not find any difference between veneer and crown groups when analyzing tensile strength, load at maximum load, and load at upper yield. A statistically significant difference was detected between them and the inlay group regarding load at maximum load ($p = 0.003$) and load at upper yield ($p = 0.027$). This difference may be due to the increased thickness of the inlay, compared with the other two preparations.

All specimens were submitted to SEM examination to investigate fracture areas on both tooth and ceramic surfaces. The microscopy images reveal dentin areas partially covered with the residual adhesive cement at the fracture zone of the ceramic prosthesis. The appearance of the fracture lines revealed small fragments of ceramic material above the cracked dental tissue. The adhesive cement covered the dental areas where the fracture occurred at the ceramic–cement interface and was absent where the bond had failed at the cement–tooth interface, similar to what other studies have reported [42,43].

The limitations of the present study are represented by the dehydration of samples during SEM examination. Additionally, observation of small sections may not fully reflect the characteristics of the whole sample under investigation. Concerning mechanical testing, the practitioner's skills in performing all cementation steps can influence mechanical results. Moreover, using a single bacterial species led to a complete lack of results of the evaluation under the conditions of a biofilm.

In our future research, we intend to use complex, multispecies biofilms. In this way, by collecting oral dental plaque for contamination, in vivo conditions and the structure of a biofilm can be simulated [44,45].

Within the limitations of the in vitro conditions, the present study demonstrates the effectiveness of photodynamic therapy when it is used as a part of the cementation protocol. Additionally, it opens the way for future research to increase the applicability and use of PDT in fixed prosthodontics from an antibacterial and adhesion point of view.

5. Conclusions

S. mutans adhesion on prepared teeth and development of the bacterial biofilm was highlighted by pre-irradiation microscopic examinations.

SEM images after PDT showed a bacterial reduction, demonstrating that 100 mW laser power was sufficient to decontaminate the prepared surfaces. PDT can be considered an appropriate disinfection protocol for coronary dental tissues before the restorative phase.

Evaluation of the adhesive cementation of lithium disilicate ceramic veneers, crowns, and inlays showed a good marginal adaptation. A mechanical pull-out test revealed improved adhesion for all examined groups when PDT was applied before cementation., However, the inlay group had better bond strength when compared with the veneer and crown groups.

More studies are needed to evaluate the effectiveness of different photosensitizers and lasers on disinfection and adhesion, to extend the use of lasers in dental prosthetics.

Author Contributions: Conceptualization, C.E.T.; methodology, C.E.T., R.C. (Radu Chifor), and S.C.; validation, M.M.; formal analysis, M.E.B. and A.F.B.; investigation, C.E.T., D.P., and R.C. (Radu Chifor); data curation, I.C.; writing—original draft preparation, C.E.T., S.C., and R.C. (Rahela Carpa); writing—review and editing, M.M.; supervision, M.E.B. All authors have read and agreed to the published version of the manuscript.

Funding: This research received no external funding.

Institutional Review Board Statement: Not applicable.

Informed Consent Statement: Not applicable.

Data Availability Statement: The data reported in the present study are available on request from the corresponding author.

Conflicts of Interest: The authors declare no conflict of interest.

References

1. Stájer, A.; Kajári, S.; Gajdács, M.; Musah-Eroje, A.; Baráth, Z. Utility of photodynamic therapy in dentistry: Current concepts. *Dent. J.* **2020**, *8*, 43. [CrossRef] [PubMed]
2. Merigo, E.; Conti, S.; Ciociola, T.; Manfredi, M.; Vescovi, P.; Fornaini, C. Antimicrobial Photodynamic Therapy Protocols on *Streptococcus mutans* with Different Combinations of Wavelengths and Photosensitizing Dyes. *Bioengineering* **2019**, *6*, 42. [CrossRef] [PubMed]
3. Ishiyama, K.; Nakamura, K.; Ikai, H.; Kanno, T.; Kohno, M.; Sasaki, K.; Niwano, Y. Bactericidal action of photogenerated singlet oxygen from photosensitizers used in plaque disclosing agents. *PLoS ONE* **2012**, *7*, e37871. [CrossRef]
4. Nemezio, M.A.; de Souza Farias, S.S.; Borsatto, M.C.; Aires, C.P.; Corona, S.A.M. Effect of methylene blue-induced photodynamic therapy on a *Streptococcus mutans* biofilm model. *Photodiagnosis Photodyn. Ther.* **2017**, *20*, 234–237. [CrossRef]
5. Misba, L.; Zaidi, S.; Khan, A.U. Efficacy of photodynamic therapy against *Streptococcus mutans* biofilm: Role of singlet oxygen. *J. Photochem. Photobiol. B* **2018**, *183*, 16–21. [CrossRef]
6. Garcia, M.T.; Pereira, A.H.C.; Figueiredo-Godoi, L.M.A.; Jorge, A.O.C.; Strixino, J.F.; Junqueira, J.C. Photodynamic therapy mediated by chlorin-type photosensitizers against *Streptococcus mutans* biofilms. *Photodiagnosis Photodyn. Ther.* **2018**, *24*, 256–261. [CrossRef]
7. Weber, K.; Delben, J.; Bromage, T.G.; Duarte, S. Comparison of SEM and VPSEM imaging techniques with respect to *Streptococcus mutans* biofilm topography. *FEMS Microbiol. Lett.* **2014**, *350*, 175–179. [CrossRef]
8. Shuwaish, M.S.B. Impact of photodynamic therapy on the push out bond strength of fiber post to root dentin: A systematic review. *Photodiagnosis Photodyn. Ther.* **2020**, *32*, 102010. [CrossRef]
9. Ramos, A.T.P.R.; Belizário, L.G.; Venção, A.C.; Jordão-Basso, K.C.F.; de Souza Rastelli, A.N.; de Andrade, M.F.; Kuga, M.C. Effects of photodynamic therapy on the adhesive interface of fiber posts cementation protocols. *JOE* **2018**, *44*, 173–178. [CrossRef]
10. Ramos, A.T.P.R.; Belizário, L.G.; Jordão-Basso, K.C.F.; Shinohara, A.L.; Kuga, M.C. Effects of photodynamic therapy on the adhesive interface using two fiber posts cementation systems. *Photodiagnosis Photodyn. Ther.* **2018**, *24*, 136–141. [CrossRef] [PubMed]
11. Sahyon, H.B.S.; da Silva, P.P.; de Oliveira, M.S.; Cintra, L.T.A.; Gomes-Filho, J.E.; dos Santos, P.H.; Sivieri-Araujo, G. Effect of photodynamic therapy on the mechanical properties and bond strength of glass-fiber posts to endodontically treated intraradicular dentin. *J. Prosthet. Dent.* **2018**, *120*, 317.E1–317.E7. [CrossRef]
12. Mirhashemi, A.; Hormozi, S.; Noroozian, M.; Chiniforush, N. The effect of antimicrobial photodynamic therapy on shear bond strength of orthodontic bracket: An in vitro study. *Photodiagnosis Photodyn. Ther.* **2021**, *34*, 102244. [CrossRef] [PubMed]
13. Silva, L.H.D.; Lima, E.D.; Miranda, R.B.D.P.; Favero, S.S.; Lohbauer, U.; Cesar, P.F. Dental ceramics: A review of new materials and processing methods. *Braz. Oral Res.* **2017**, *31* (Suppl. S1), 133–146. [CrossRef]
14. Warreth, A.; Elkareimi, Y. All-ceramic restorations: A review of the literature. *Saudi. Dent. J.* **2020**, *32*, 365–372. [CrossRef]
15. Kara, O.; Ozturk, A.N. The effect of surface treatments on the bonding strength of ceramic inlays to dentin. *J. Adhes. Sci. Tech.* **2017**, *31*, 2490–2502. [CrossRef]
16. Nada, H.E.; Ahmed, S.E.; Fayza, H.A. Shear bond strength of ceramic laminate veneers to enamel and enamel–dentine complex bonded with different adhesive luting systems. *ADJ* **2016**, *41*, 131–137. [CrossRef]

17. Stawarczyk, B.; Basler, T.; Ender, A.; Roos, M.; Özcan, M.; Hämmerle, C. Effect of surface conditioning with airborne-particle abrasion on the tensile strength of polymeric CAD/CAM crowns luted with self-adhesive and conventional resin cements. *J. Prosthet. Dent.* **2012**, *107*, 94–101. [CrossRef]
18. Carrera, E.T.; Dias, H.B.; Corbi, S.C.T.; Marcantonio, R.A.C.; Bernardi, A.C.A.; Bagnato, V.S.; Rastelli, A. The application of antimicrobial photodynamic therapy (aPDT) in dentistry: A critical review. *Laser Phys.* **2016**, *26*, 123001. [CrossRef] [PubMed]
19. Matsui, R.; Cvitkovitch, D. Acid tolerance mechanisms utilized by *Streptococcus mutans*. *Future Microbiol.* **2010**, *5*, 403–417. [CrossRef] [PubMed]
20. Liang, X.; Zou, Z.; Zou, Z.; Li, C.; Dong, X.; Yin, H.; Yan, G. Effect of antibacterial photodynamic therapy on *Streptococcus mutans* plaque biofilm in vitro. *J. Innov. Opt. Health Sci.* **2020**, *13*, 2050022. [CrossRef]
21. Azizi, A.; Shohrati, P.; Goudarzi, M.; Lawaf, S.; Rahimi, A. Comparison of the effect of photodynamic therapy with curcumin and methylene Blue on *streptococcus mutans* bacterial colonies. *Photodiagnosis Photodyn. Ther.* **2019**, *27*, 203–209. [CrossRef]
22. Asahi, Y.; Miura, J.; Tsuda, T.; Kuwabata, S.; Tsunashima, K.; Noiri, Y.; Hayashi, M. Simple observation of *Streptococcus mutans* biofilm by scanning electron microscopy using ionic liquids. *AMB Express* **2015**, *5*, 6. [CrossRef] [PubMed]
23. Borges, C.C.; Palma-Dibb, R.G.; Rodrigues, F.C.C.; Plotegher, F.; Rossi-Fedele, G.; de Sousa-Neto, M.D.; Souza-Gabriel, A.E. The effect of diode and Er, Cr: YSGG lasers on the bond strength of fiber posts. *Photobiomodul. Photomed. Laser Surg.* **2020**, *38*, 66–74. [CrossRef]
24. Gounder, R.; Gounder, S. Laser science and its applications in prosthetic rehabilitation. *J. Lasers Med. Sci.* **2016**, *7*, 209–213. [CrossRef]
25. Ladiz, M.A.R.; Mirzaei, A.; Hendi, S.S.; Najafi-Vosough, R.; Hooshyarfard, A.; Gholami, L. Effect of photobiomodulation with 810 and 940 nm diode lasers on human gingival fibroblasts. *Dent. Med. Probl.* **2020**, *57*, 369–376. [CrossRef] [PubMed]
26. Sterczała, B.; Grzech-Leśniak, K.; Michel, O.; Trzeciakowski, W.; Dominiak, M.; Jurczyszyn, K. Assessment of human gingival fibroblast proliferation after laser stimulation in vitro using different laser types and wavelengths (**1064**, *980*, 635, 450, and 405 nm)—preliminary report. *J. Pers. Med.* **2021**, *11*, 98. [CrossRef] [PubMed]
27. Kubasiewicz-Ross, P.; Hadzik, J.; Gedrange, T.; Dominiak, M.; Jurczyszyn, K.; Pitułaj, A.; Fleischer, M. Antimicrobial Efficacy of Different Decontamination Methods as Tested on Dental Implants with Various Types of Surfaces. *Med. Sci. Monit.* **2020**, *26*, e920513. [CrossRef]
28. Kubasiewicz-Ross, P.; Fleischer, M.; Pitułaj, A.; Hadzik, J.; Nawrot-Hadzik, I.; Bortkiewicz, O.; Jurczyszyn, K. Evaluation of the three methods of bacterial decontamination on implants with three different surfaces. *Adv. Clin. Exp. Med.* **2020**, *29*, 177–182. [CrossRef]
29. Dhaliwal, J.S.; Abd Rahman, N.A.; Ming, L.C.; Dhaliwal, S.K.S.; Knights, J.; Albuquerque Junior, R.F. Microbial Biofilm Decontamination on Dental Implant Surfaces: A Mini Review. *Front. Cell. Infect. Microbiol.* **2021**, *11*, 736186. [CrossRef]
30. Schneider, M.; Kirfel, G.; Berthold, M.; Frentzen, M.; Krause, F.; Braun, A. The impact of antimicrobial photodynamic therapy in an artificial biofilm model. *Lasers Med. Sci.* **2012**, *27*, 615–620. [CrossRef]
31. Rolim, J.P.; De-Melo, M.A.; Guedes, S.F.; Albuquerque-Filho, F.B.; De Souza, J.R.; Nogueira, N.A.; Rodrigues, L.K. The antimicrobial activity of photodynamic therapy against *Streptococcus mutans* using different photosensitizers. *J. Photochem. Photobiol. B.* **2012**, *106*, 40–46. [CrossRef]
32. Dascalu, L.M.; Moldovan, M.; Prodan, D.; Ciotlaus, I.; Popescu, V.; Baldea, I.; Carpa, R.; Sava, S.; Chifor, R.; Badea, M.E. Assessment and Characterization of Some New Photosensitizers for Antimicrobial Photodynamic Therapy (aPDT). *Materials* **2020**, *13*, 3012. [CrossRef] [PubMed]
33. Salem, S.K.; Shalaby, M.M. Fracture strength and marginal gap of re-pressed IPS E.max PRESS crowns with different concentrations. *E. D. J.* **2019**, *65*, 1939–1948. [CrossRef]
34. Mobilio, N.; Fasiol, A.; Mollica, F.; Catapano, S. Effect of different luting agents on the retention of lithium disilicate ceramic crowns. *Materials* **2015**, *8*, 1604. [CrossRef] [PubMed]
35. Mester, A.; Moldovan, M.; Cuc, S.; Tomuleasa, C.; Pasca, S.; Filip, M.; Piciu, A.; Onisor, F. Characteristics of Dental Resin-Based Composites in Leukemia Saliva: An In Vitro Analysis. *Biomedicines* **2021**, *9*, 1618. [CrossRef]
36. Chirca, O.; Biclesanu, C.; Florescu, A.; Burcea, A.; Motelica, L.; Holban, A. Comparative study on adhesion to the dental structure of the total ceramic crown with different adhesive cements. *Rom. J. Mater.* **2021**, *51*, 309–318.
37. Bastos, N.A.; Bitencourt, S.B.; Carneiro, R.F.; Ferrairo, B.M.; Strelhow, S.S.F.; Dos Santos, D.M.; Bombonatti, J.F.S. Marginal and internal adaptation of lithium disilicate partial restorations: A systematic review and meta-analysis. *J. Indian Prosthodont. Soc.* **2020**, *20*, 338. [CrossRef] [PubMed]
38. Riccitiello, F.; Amato, M.; Leone, R.; Spagnuolo, G.; Sorrentino, R. In vitro evaluation of the marginal fit and internal adaptation of zirconia and lithium disilicate single crowns: Micro-CT comparison between different manufacturing procedures. *Open Dent. J.* **2018**, *12*, 160. [CrossRef] [PubMed]
39. Heintze, S.D. Crown pull-off test (crown retention test) to evaluate the bonding effectiveness of luting agents. *Dent. Mater.* **2010**, *26*, 193–206. [CrossRef]
40. Johnson, G.H.; Lepe, X.; Patterson, A.; Schäfer, O. Simplified cementation of lithium disilicate crowns: Retention with various adhesive resin cement combinations. *J. Prosthet. Dent.* **2018**, *119*, 826–832. [CrossRef] [PubMed]
41. Streiff, K.R.; Lepe, X.; Johnson, G.H. Long-term retention of lithium disilicate crowns with a current bioactive cement. *J. Esthet. Restor. Dent.* **2021**, *33*, 621–627. [CrossRef] [PubMed]

42. Upadhyaya, V.; Arora, A.; Singhal, J.; Kapur, S.; Sehgal, M. Comparative analysis of shear bond strength of lithium disilicate samples cemented using different resin cement systems: An in vitro study. *J. Indian Prosthodont. Soc.* **2019**, *19*, 240. [CrossRef] [PubMed]
43. Levartovsky, S.; Bohbot, H.; Shem-Tov, K.; Brosh, T.; Pilo, R. Effect of Different Surface Treatments of Lithium Disilicate on the Adhesive Properties of Resin Cements. *Materials* **2021**, *14*, 3302. [CrossRef] [PubMed]
44. Alsaif, A.; Tahmassebi, J.F.; Wood, S.R. Treatment of dental plaque biofilms using photodynamic therapy: A randomised controlled study. *Eur. Arch. Paediatr. Dent.* **2021**, *22*, 791–800. [CrossRef] [PubMed]
45. Tahmassebi, J.; Drogkari, E.; Wood, S.R. A study of the control of oral plaque biofilms via antibacterial photodynamic therapy. *Eur. Arch. Paediatr. Dent.* **2015**, *16*, 433–440. [CrossRef]

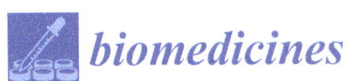

Article

Photodynamic Therapy in Combination with Doxorubicin Is Superior to Monotherapy for the Treatment of Lung Cancer

Joseph C. Cacaccio [1], Farukh A. Durrani [1], Joseph R. Missert [2] and Ravindra K. Pandey [1,*]

[1] Photodynamic Therapy Center, Cell Stress Biology, Roswell Park Comprehensive Cancer Center, Buffalo, NY 14263, USA; joseph.cacaccio@roswellpark.org (J.C.C.); farukh.durrani@roswellpark.org (F.A.D.)
[2] Photolitec, LLC, 73 High Street, Buffalo, NY 14223, USA; jmissert@photolitec.com
* Correspondence: ravindra.pandey@roswellpark.org

Abstract: We have previously shown that a radioactive (^{123}I)-analog of methyl 3-(1′-(iodohexyloxy) ethyl-3-devinylpyropheophorbide-a (PET-ONCO), derived from chlorophyll-a can be used for positron emission tomography (PET) imaging of a variety of tumors, including those where ^{18}F-FDG shows limitations. In this study, the photodynamic therapy (PDT) efficacy of the corresponding non-radioactive photosensitizer (PS) was investigated in a variety of tumor types (NSCLC, SCC, adenocarcinoma) derived from lung cancer patients in mice tumor models. The in vitro and in vivo efficacy was also investigated in combination with doxorubicin, and a significantly enhanced long-term tumor response was observed. The toxicity and toxicokinetic profile of the iodinated PS was also evaluated in male and female Sprague-Dawley rats and Beagle dog at variable doses (single intravenous injections) to assess reversibility or latency of any effects over a 28-day dose free period. The no-observed-adverse-effect (NOAEL) of the PS was considered to be 6.5 mg/kg for male and female rats, and for dogs, 3.45 mg/kg, the highest dose levels evaluated, respectively. The corresponding plasma C_{max} and AYC_{last} for male and female rats were 214,000 and 229,000 ng/mL and 3,680,000 and 3,810,000 h * ng/mL, respectively. For male and female dogs, the corresponding plasma C_{max} and AYC_{last} were 76,000 and 92,400 ng/mL and 976,000 and 1,200,000 h * ng/mL, respectively.

Keywords: photosensitizers; photodynamic therapy; toxicokinetics; chemotherapy; combination therapy

Citation: Cacaccio, J.C.; Durrani, F.A.; Missert, J.R.; Pandey, R.K. Photodynamic Therapy in Combination with Doxorubicin Is Superior to Monotherapy for the Treatment of Lung Cancer. *Biomedicines* **2022**, *10*, 857. https://doi.org/10.3390/biomedicines10040857

Academic Editors: Stefano Bacci and Kyungsu Kang

Received: 16 February 2022
Accepted: 1 April 2022
Published: 6 April 2022

Publisher's Note: MDPI stays neutral with regard to jurisdictional claims in published maps and institutional affiliations.

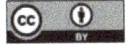

Copyright: © 2022 by the authors. Licensee MDPI, Basel, Switzerland. This article is an open access article distributed under the terms and conditions of the Creative Commons Attribution (CC BY) license (https://creativecommons.org/licenses/by/4.0/).

1. Introduction

Among a variety of cancer types, lung cancer is considered to be the leading cause of death related and the most commonly diagnosed form of such disease [1,2]. Lung cancer is divided into two broad histologic classes, which grow and spread differently: small-cell lung carcinomas (SCLCs) and non-small cell lung carcinomas (NSCLCs) [3]. Treatment options for lung cancer include surgery, chemotherapy and radiation therapy [4–7]. However, in many cases, cancer cells develop drug resistance and become nonresponsive to chemotherapy [8], thus necessitating the exploration of alternative and/or complementary treatment modalities. Photodynamic Therapy (PDT) has emerged as an effective treatment modality for various malignant neoplasia and tumors [9,10]. In PDT, the photochemical interaction of light, photosensitizer (PS) and molecular oxygen produces reactive oxygen species (ROS), mainly singlet oxygen ($^1O_2$), which is responsible for the destruction of tumor [11–15].

A large number of porphyrin-based photosensitizers (PS) has been investigated in-clinic for the treatment of lung cancer by PDT [16–22], and the initial response has been encouraging. However, some of the first-generation PSs showed limited tumor specificity and prolonged skin phototoxicity. Moreover, PDT being a localized treatment was not curative for those patients with metastasis. In most of the second-generation agents, especially with HPPH [3-(1′-hexyloxy) ethyl-3-devinylpyropheophorbide-a] [23], derived from chlorophyll-a, the long-term skin phototoxicity problem has been resolved [24], but it is potentially curative only for localized cancers. Therefore, efforts are currently underway to investigate the utility of PDT in combination with other treatment modalities, e.g., chemotherapy, immunotherapy, etc. [25,26]. The initial clinical results are promising but the treatment parameters need to be optimized in a large patient population.

For the past several years, one of the objectives of our laboratory has been to develop multi-functional agents for cancer-imaging (PET, MRI or fluorescence or of these combination) [27] and treatment of cancer by PDT, using a "See and Treat" approach. In one of our attempts, we have been able to develop an iodinated PS (methyl-3(1'-m-iodobenzyloxy) ethyl-3-devinyl pyropheophorbide-a), which in its radioactive form (^{124}I-) can be used to image a variety of tumors by PET imaging [28], and as a non-radioactive analog for NIR fluorescence-imaging and treatment of cancer by PDT. Thus, a single agent (in combination of radioactive + corresponding non-radioactive forms) can be used for imaging (PET, fluorescence) and therapy of cancer [28]. This product provides a unique opportunity to determine the stage of cancer (localized or metastasized) by PET imaging of the cancer patient with ^{124}I-labeled agent and select the treatment plan accordingly: either PDT alone (if cancer is localized) or PDT + chemotherapy (if the cancer is metastasized). Therefore, we initially investigated the PET imaging ability of the ^{124}I-labeled agent of this compound (PET-ONCO) in a variety of tumor types, including lung tumors, and excellent results were obtained [28]. This report presents (a) the utility of a corresponding non-labeled iodinated PS **1** for treating lung cancer with and without chemotherapy (doxorubicin) in a variety of lung tumors xenografts derived from lung cancer patients and (b) the toxicity and toxicokinetic profiles of the PS formulated in Pluronic F-127 at variable doses in male and female rats and dogs. We and others have previously shown the improved PDT efficacy of certain tetrapyrrolic photosensitizers in a Pluronic-based formulation either by encapsulation or by conjugating the PS with Pluronic F-127 with and without the combination of co-delivery of doxorubicin for overcoming drug resistance in cancer [29–31].

2. Results and Discussion

Chemistry: The PS **1** [(methyl-3-(1'-*meta*-iodo-benzyloxy) ethyl-3-devinylpyropheophorbide-a] was synthesized from Chlorophyll-a by following the methodology established in our laboratory [28]. See Figure 1.

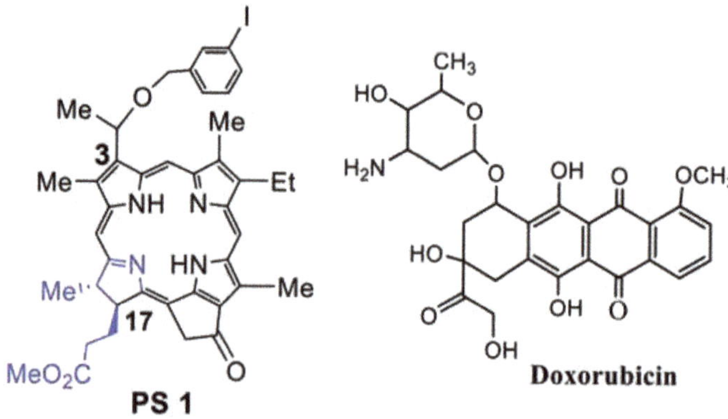

Figure 1. Doxorubicin, a chemotherapy agent [32] routinely used for the treatment of lung cancer patients, was purchased from Sigma Aldrich, USA.

In vitro Studies:

(a) *In vitro cell uptake and PDT efficacy of PS1 in Tween80 vs Pluronic F 127 formulations:* For *in vitro* studies, PDX 14541 cell line (a squamous cell carcinoma, SCC), derived from a lung cancer patient tumor was initially used to investigate the PDT efficacy of iodinated photosensitizer (PS) **1**. The PS was formulated in two different formulations (1% Tween 80/5% dextrose and 2% Pluronic F-127 in PBS) to determine the impact of delivery vehicle in PDT efficacy at various light and drug doses. Among the parameters used, PS **1** formulated in 2% Pluronic F-127 showed significantly higher efficacy when compared to the 1% Tween 80 formulation (Figure 2). At the light dose of 1 J/cm^2 (665 nm), the IC$_{50}$ values of PS **1** in Pluronic and Tween80 formulations were 662.5 nM and 5196 nM, respectively. Finally, neither formulation showed any dark toxicity with drug alone and no light treatment.

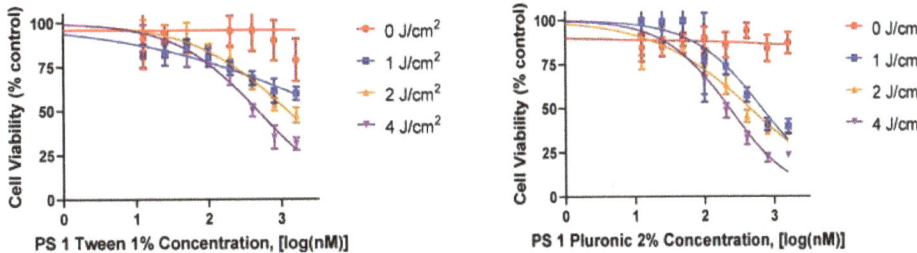

Figure 2. A comparative in vitro PDT efficacy of PS **1** formulated either in 1% Tween®-80 (left graph) or 2% Pluronic® F-127 (right graph) in lung cancer cell line 14541 derived from a lung cancer patient. The cells were incubated with PS **1** for 24 h, and then exposed to light (665 nm, 1–4 J/cm^2) 24 h. The PDT efficacy was determined by MTT assay, and the results were analyzed using GraphPad Prism 7 software.

(b) *Impact of PS **1** formulated in Tween and Pluronic in PDX 14541 cells and fibroblast co-culture*: Photosensitizers which specifically accumulate in tumor cells over normal cells is vital in minimizing adverse effects. To demonstrate PS **1** tumor specificity over normal lung cells, a co-culture system was prepared using PDX 14541 cells and normal lung fibroblast. Additionally, the normal lung fibroblast cells were transfected with GFP to distinguish the two cell types visually. In this system, PS **1** in both formulations (Tween®-80 and Pluronic® F-127) showed higher uptake in tumor cells over the normal cells. However, the Pluronic formulation had a better distribution across the tumor cells mass. In the Tween formulation, the PS concentration along the periphery of the tumor cell mass was higher compared to the center of the mass determined by its fluorescence intensity (Figure 3).

(c) *Comparative independent in vitro efficacy of PS 1-PDT and doxorubicin therapy:* PDT is an efficient modality in destroying localized tumors but has limitations in treating metastasis, where the delivery of the light could be problematic. To demonstrate the advantages of PDT in combination with doxorubicin, and its synergetic impact to treat lung cancer, the Bliss independence model of synergy was investigated in A549 lung cancer cells. The tumor cells were incubated with PS **1** at variable concentration for 24 h, washed with fresh media and exposed to variable light doses (1–4 J/cm^2), and the PDT efficacy was determined by MTT assay [33]. For determining the efficacy of doxorubicin, the A549 cells were treated with doxorubicin at variable concentration, incubated for 24, 48 or 72 h. The effective dose was determined via the MTT assay (Figure 4). The IC$_{50}$ values of the PS (conc. 300 nM), light dose (665 nm, 1 J/Cm^2) at 24 h post-incubation of the PS) and doxorubicin (625 nm, cells incubated for 48 h) were used to select the concentration of the PS and doxorubicin for determining the best treatment parameters.

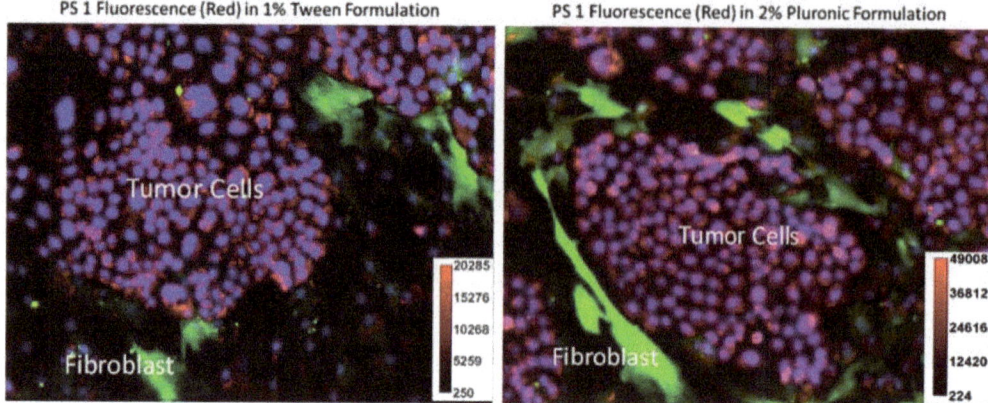

Figure 3. A co-culture system containing PDX 14541 tumor cells and normal lung-fibroblast cells transfected with GFP. PS **1** uptake (red) was observed in both Tween®-80 and Pluronic® F-127 formulations within the tumor cells. GFP-transfected fibroblast cells are shown in green. While both tumor cells and fibroblast demonstrated PS fluorescence, the PS concentration amount (fluorescence intensity) observed in normal fibroblast cells was significantly lower than in tumor cells. Compared to Tween 80 formulation, the PS **1** in Pluronic F-127 formulation showed more evenly PS distribution. Hoechst 33342 was used to stain the nucleus of the cells (blue). The PS **1** did not show any localization in cell nucleus. The fluorescence intensity of the PS **1** in Tween and Pluronic formulations was measured by ImageJ software (see scale bars).

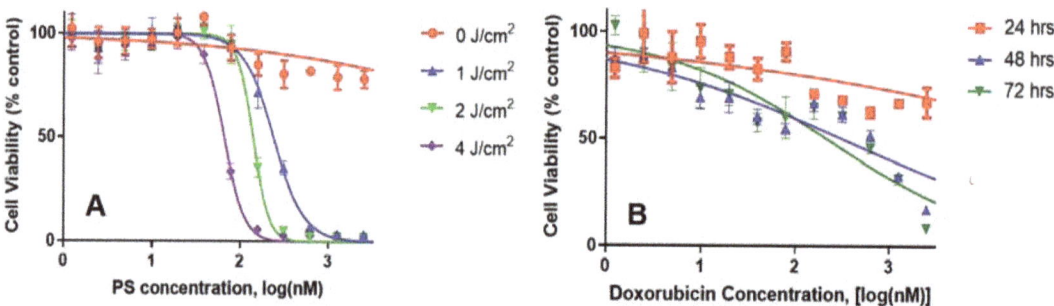

Figure 4. The in vitro cytotoxic effect of PS **1**-PDT at variable concentrations/light doses and doxorubicin efficacy at variable concentrations after incubating for 48 h were independently determined in A549 cell lines. For the PDT experiment, the cells were exposed to light at 24 h. Cells were then rested for 48 h and tested for cytotoxic effects via MTT assay. The cells were incubated with doxorubicin for 48 h and then tested for cytotoxicity by MTT assay.

(d) *PS **1**-PDT in combination with doxorubicin therapy shows a synergetic effect.* The impact of PS **1**-PDT in combination with doxorubicin was studied and analyzed by following the Bliss method. [34]. The Bliss independence model was generated by comparing the cell viability data from individual treatment, with those obtained by combining both the modalities in various PS and doxorubicin doses. A topological map was generated by graphing 36 different peaks of antagonism followed by valleys of synergy, indicated in red (Figure 5). A combination index that is less than 1 indicates synergy, while if the value is greater than 1, the combination was antagonistic. The in vitro model suggests that for best efficacy, doxorubicin and PS should be used in a molar ratio of 2:1. In a combination therapy experiment, the cell viability was reduced to 50% at 20 nM conc. of PS **1** and 10 nM conc. of doxorubicin, whereas PS **1** alone at 20 nM yielded 90% viability and doxorubicin alone at 10 nM showed 80% cell viability.

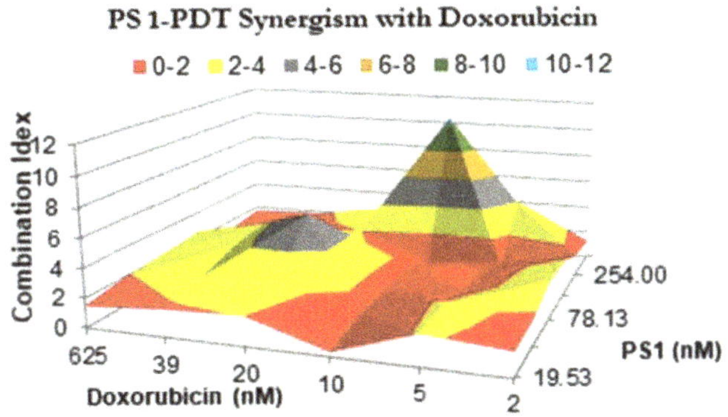

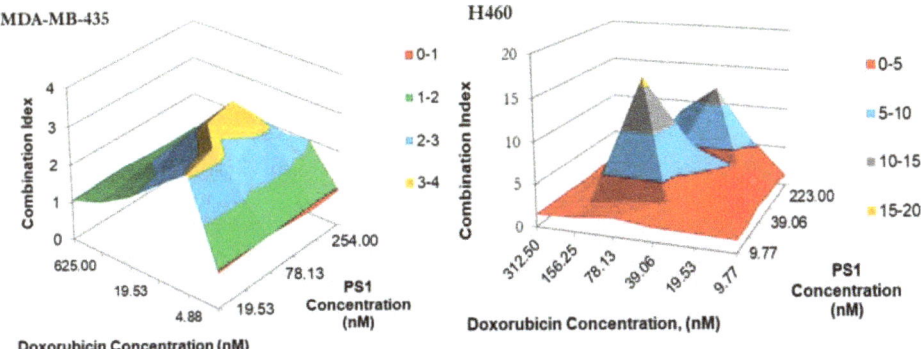

Figure 5. The synergism of PS **1** and doxorubicin were tested at varying drug doses. A549 cells were incubated with PS **1**. Cells were exposed to light (fluence: 1.0 J/cm^2, fluence rate: 75 mW/cm^2) applied at 24 h post-incubation. Doxorubicin was then added at various concentrations, and cells were incubated for 48 h, then assessed for cytotoxic effects. The combination indices were calculated for each point using the formula CI = [E$_{PS1}$ + E$_{dox}$ − E$_{PS1}$E$_{dox}$]/E$_{PS1*dox}$. Therefore, the combination index plotted above represents the ratio between the hypothetical efficacy and the observed efficacy of the combination. Peaks indicate antagonism, values near 1.0 indicate an additive effect, and valleys indicate synergism.

(e) <u>Synergetic Impact of PS **1**-PDT and doxorubicin in various cell lines:</u> Before initiating in vivo studies, additional in vitro experiments were preformed to investigate if synergetic trends remained consistent in two additional cell lines: H460 (non-small cell lung cancer) and MDA-MB-43 (breast cancer). H460 reacted similarly to A549, except the regions of antagonism were expanded. This includes the 2:1 combination yielding the highest degree of synergy. Meanwhile, MDA-MB-435 demonstrated almost no areas of synergy. Instead, most of the combinations yielded additive or antagonistic effects (Figures 6 and 7).

Figure 6. The synergism of PS **1** and doxorubicin tested MDA-MB-435 in H460 and at varying drug doses. Cells were plated and PS **1** was added. Cells were exposed to light (fluence: 1.0 J/cm^2, fluence rate: 75 mW/cm^2) at 24 h post-incubation. Doxorubicin at various doses was then added, and cells were incubated for 48 h, then assessed for cytotoxic effects. The combination indices were calculated for each point using the formula CI = [E$_{PS1}$ + E$_{Dox}$ − E$_{PS1}$E$_{Dox}$]/E$_{PS1+Dox}$. Peaks indicate antagonism, values near 1.0 indicate an additive effect, and valleys < 1.0 indicate synergism. Areas indicated in red denote synergetic concentrations and valleys < 1.0 indicate synergism. Areas indicated in blue and red denote synergetic concentrations.

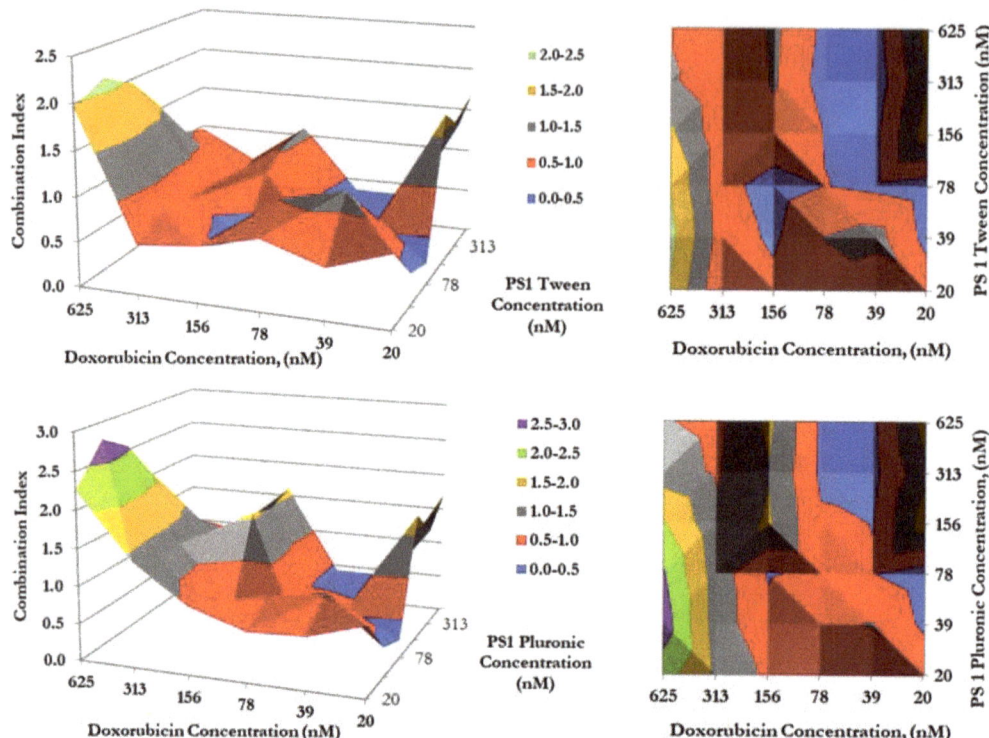

Figure 7. The synergism of doxorubicin in combination with PS **1** in either Tween or Pluronic formulation. Cells were plated and PS **1** was added. Cells were exposed to light (Fluence: 1.0 J/cm^2, Fluence rate: 75 mW/cm^2) at 24 h post-incubation. Doxorubicin was then added at variable concentrations, and cells were incubated for 48 h, then assessed for cytotoxic effects. The combination indices (C.I.) were calculated for each point using the formula C.I. = [E_{PS1} + E_{Dox} − $E_{PS1}E_{Dox}$]/$E_{PS1 \cdot Dox}$. Peaks indicate antagonism, values near 1.0 indicate an additive effect, and valleys <1.0 indicate synergism. Areas indicated in red and blue denote synergetic concentrations, while grey indicates an additive effect.

(f) *Impact of formulation (Tween vs. Pluronic formulation of PS) in combination with doxorubicin in combination therapy:* To determine if the photosensitizer delivery vehicle(s) had any influence in the mode of action of PDT in combination with doxorubicin therapy, a synergetic study was conducted by using both the formulations of PS **1**. The PS **1** dissolved in Tween80/5% Dextrose/ D5W yielded similar synergy with doxorubicin, as shown previously in Pluronic formulation (Figure 5), where the highest synergetic effect was observed when PS **1** and doxorubicin concentrations were in a ratio of 2:1.

In vitro Studies:

(a) *PS 1 shows high tumor-specificity and stability in Pluronic (2%) formulation* Similar to most of the porphyrin-based compounds the iodinated PS **1** also showed limited solubility in water. Therefore, it was formulated in two FDA approved formulations: (i) Tween 80/dextrose in water and (ii) Pluronic F-127/PBS at various concentrations, and the stability/concentration of PS in formulation solution was determined at 4 °C and −20 °C. In both formulations (1%Tween 80/5% Dextrose and 2% Pluronic/PBS), the photosensitizer could be dissolved in a high concentration, and was stable, with no loss of PS concentration at least for 24 months at −20 °C. PS **1** can also be formulated at lower concentrations of Pluronic (0.5%, 1.0%), but the long-term stability was low with a significant release of the PS. The concentration/stability/purity of PS **1** in both formulations was confirmed by spin filtration of the formulation, and then analyzing the filtrate(s) and retentate for the concentration of the PS by spectrophotometric and HPLC analyses.

To establish the treatment parameters of PDT (especially the optimal time for light irradiation to tumors), whole body fluorescence imaging of the desired PS over variable timepoints was performed in four PDX models (NSCLC 148070, NSCLC 0229042, SCC 14541 and lung Adenocarcinoma 15021). The mice (SCID, 3 mice/group) were injected with the PS **1** (0.47 mmol/kg) formulated in 2% Pluronic F-127/PBS and the whole-body fluorescence imaging was performed via epi-illumination on an IVIS-in vivo system. Image analysis was carried out with Living Image Acquisition and Analysis Software. The fluorescence was measured using an excitation wavelength at 640 nm and emission at 680 nm as the instrument was most sensitive to detect fluorescence of PS using this filter set. Images were analyzed for average radiant efficiency over three regions of interest (ROI) covering the tumor, liver and skin, and results were expressed as the mean average radiant efficiency +/− standard deviation. The highest fluorescence was observed at 24 h post-injection in all tumor models. Interestingly, the greatest difference in PS uptake in tumor vs. liver and skin determined by fluorescence imaging was also seen at the same time point (Figure 8).

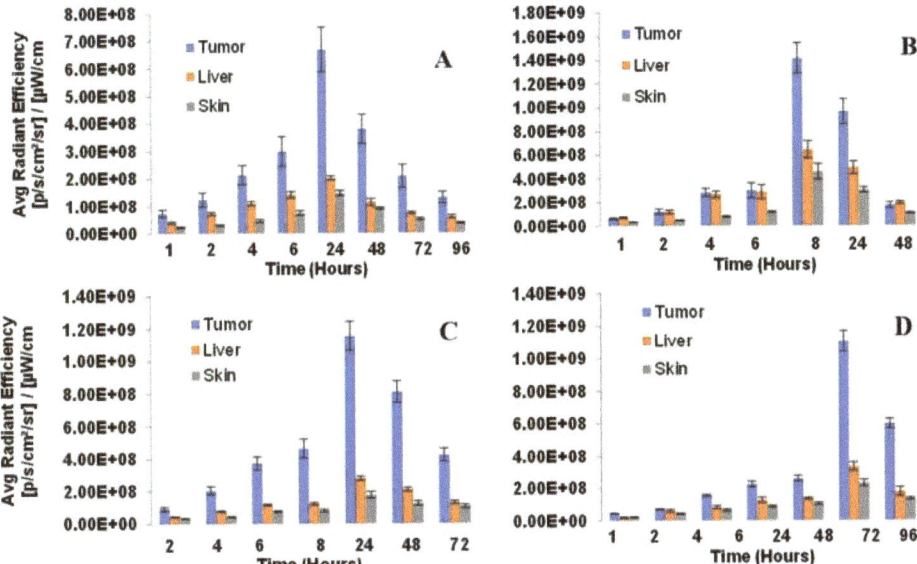

Figure 8. Biodistribution of PS in lung PDX models: (**A**) NSCLC148070, (**B**) NSCLC 0229047, (**C**) SCC 14541 and (**D**) Lung Adenocarcinoma 15021. SCID mice (3 mice/group) were implanted with lung xenografts on the right flank. Tumors were grown until reaching approximately 5 mm diameter. PS **1** (formulated in 2% Pluronic F-127, at a dose of 0.47 µmol/kg was administered retro-orbitally (alternate for tail vein injection). Tumor, liver and skin uptake was measured by an IVIS Spectrum using Living Image acquisition and analysis software at 2, 4, 6, 8, 24, 48 and 72 h. Excitation and emission filters were 640–660 nm and >720 nm respectively. In all tumor types, the maximum uptake was observed at 24 h post-injection of the PS.

(b) *Determination of PDT Efficacy of PS **1** in PDX Models* We have previously investigated the in vivo PDT efficacy of **PS 1** in mice bearing FaDu, Colon26, UMUC3 and U87 tumors, and the most effective drug dose was determined to be 1.0 mmol/kg, and light dose: 135 J/cm^2, 75 mW/cm^2. Therefore, we used the same treatment parameters for evaluating its efficacy in a variety of lung PDX models (NSCLC148070, NSCLC 15021, SCLC14541, SCLC 0229047).

(c) *Imaging of PDX tumors Small Cell Lung Carcinoma (SCLC) and Non-Small Cell Lung Carcinoma (NSCLC): SCLC (A) 14541 (B) 0229047 and NSCLC (C) 15021 (D) 148070 using PS1 at 0.47 μmol PS **1** in 2% Pluronic® F-127*: Similar to most of the pyropheophorbides, PS **1** is also a highly fluorescent molecule with long wavelength absorption at 665 nm and emission at 670 nm/720 nm.

The success of PDT depends on the PS uptake and retention in tumor(s), availability of oxygen and exposure with an appropriate wavelength of light. For the present study, the female SCID mice were implanted with xenografts on the right flank. The tumors were grown until reaching approximately 5 mm diameter. The PS was then injected intravenously at a dose of 1 μmol/kg and whole-body fluorescence imaging via epi-illumination was performed by an IVIS Spectrum system. Image analysis was carried out with Living Image acquisition and analysis software. The image obtained using Ex: 640–660 nm, Em: >680 nm was used as the instrument was most sensitive to detect fluorescence of PS 1 using this filter set. Images were analyzed for average radiant efficiency over three regions of interest (ROIs) covering the tumor, liver and skin (shaved), and results were expressed as the mean average radiant efficiency ± standard deviation. The time for highest uptake of the PS was determined by fluorescence at variable time points after injecting PS **1**.

(d) *PDT efficacy of PS **1** in treating SCLC PDX tumors: 14541 and 0229047*: PDT treatment was performed and replicated using 1 μmol/kg PS **1** in 2% Pluronic® F-127 in female SCID mice bearing SCLC tumors irradiated with light at 665 nm at a dose of 135 J/cm^2 and fluence rate of 75 mW/cm^2 (Figure 9). Mice were followed for 60 days post-PDT treatment, and palpable tumors were monitored via caliper measurement. Tumor volume was calculated as length x width x $\frac{1}{2}$ width. The cure rates (CR) in both SCLC tumors at 60 days were 15/23 = 65% and 19/20 = 95%, respectively, with a significant *p* value of 0.0001 in both PDX types.

(e) *PDT efficacy of PS **1** in treating of NSCLC PDX tumors: 15,021 and 48,070*: PS **1**-PDT was also evaluated in SCID mice bearing SCLC tumors (PDX 15,021 and 48,070) at a dose of 1.0 μmol/kg in 2% Pluronic® F-127. At 24 h post-injection of the PS, the tumors were irradiated with light at 665 nm at a light dose of 135 J/cm^2 and fluence rate of 75 mW/cm^2. The tumor regrowth in each mouse was followed for 60 days post-PDT treatment, and palpable tumors were monitored via caliper measurement. Tumor volume was calculated as length × width × $\frac{1}{2}$ width. The cure rates (CR) in both NSCLC tumors at day 60 were 10/13 = 77% and 7/14 = 50%, respectively, with a significant *p* value of 0.0001 in both PDX types (Figure 9).

(f) *PS **1**-PDT in combination with doxorubicin enhances long-term tumor cure*: To investigate the impact of PDT in combination with chemotherapy, PDT treatment was performed first using female SCID mice bearing SCLC 14541 tumors (PDX). In brief, PS **1** at a dose of 1 μmol/kg was injected. At 24 h post-injection, the tumors were exposed to light (665 nm, light dose: 135 J/cm^2, 75 mW/cm^2) and then the PDT treated mice were injected (*i.v.*) only one time with doxorubicin at a dose of 2.5 mg/kg. Mice were monitored for 60 days post-PDT treatment, and palpable tumors were measured via caliper measurement. Tumor volume was calculated as length × width × $\frac{1}{2}$ width. The cure rates (CR) in SCLC tumors at 60 days were 15/23 = 65% and in combination with doxorubicin were 4/5 = 80%, respectively, with a significant P value calculated by Mantel-Cox software in both treatment types. The tumor response depicted in Figure 10 shows a significant improvement in long-term cure by PDT in combination with doxorubicin therapy.

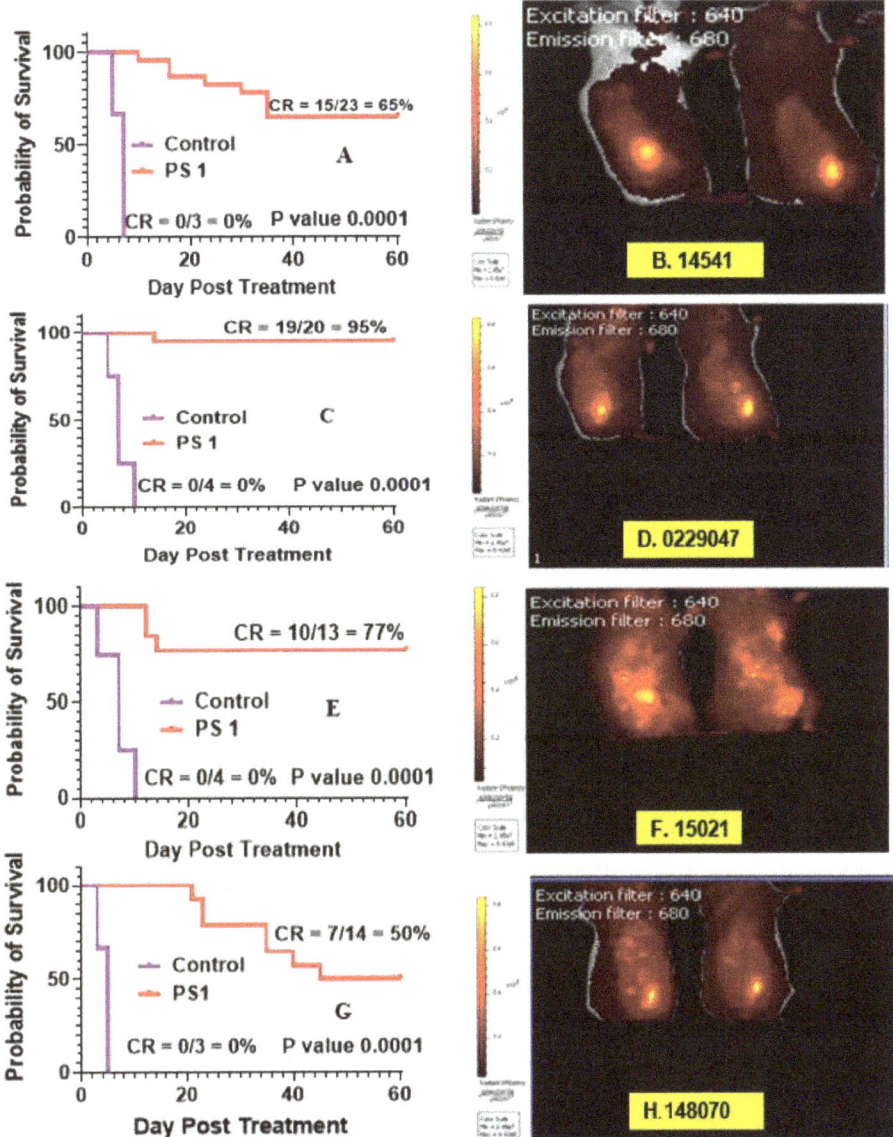

Figure 9. Fluorescence imaging and PDT efficacy of SCID mice bearing PDX lung tumors: (**A**) PDT efficacy of mice bearing SCLC 14541 tumors and (**B**) tumor images; (**C**) PDT efficacy of mice bearing SCLC 2229047 tumors and (**D**) tumor images; (**E**) PDT efficacy of mice bearing NSCLC 15021 tumors and (**F**) tumor images; (**G**) PDT efficacy of mice bearing NSCLC 148070 tumor and (**H**) tumor images. For determining long-term efficacy, mice were injected (i.v.) with PS **1** (1 mmol/kg), and at 24 h post-injection, the tumors were exposed with light (665 nm, 135 J/cm^2, 75 mW/cm^2), and tumor growth was monitored daily for 60 days.

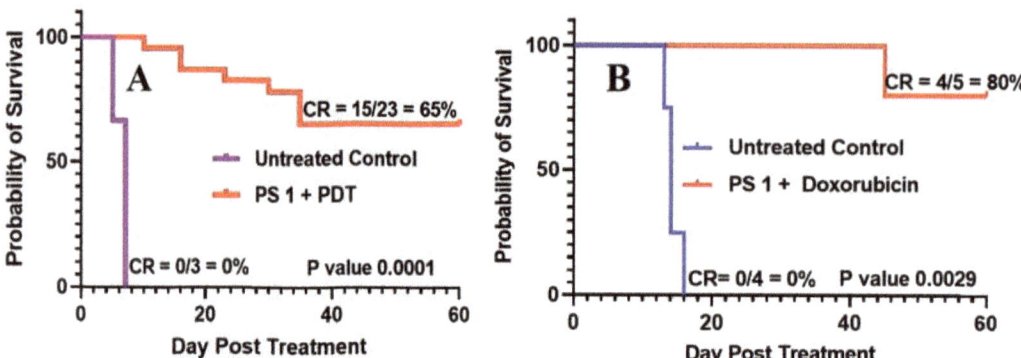

Figure 10. (**A**) SCID mice were injected intravenously with PS **1** at a dose of 1.0 µmol/kg; the tumors were irradiated with light (665 nm, light dose: 135 J/cm^2, 75 mW/cm^2) at 24 h post-injection. (**B**) In a second set of experiments, five SCID mice bearing SCLC 14541 tumors after PDT treatment as discussed above were injected (i.v.) with doxorubicin (2.5 mg/kg × 1 dose), and tumor regrowth of mice in both sets of experiments was monitored daily for 60 days. If there is any tumor regrowth, the mice were euthanized on that day. On day 60, mice with no tumor regrowth (cure) were also euthanized following an approved protocol procedure.

(g) *STAT3 dimerization as a bio-marker to PDT response:* We have previously shown that the STAT3 dimerization is an efficient biomarker for predicting the outcome of PDT treatment both in vitro and in vivo [35]. Various in vivo experiments conducted in animals, and the clinical PDT using HPPH as a PS have shown that a significant amount of the HPPH was not bleached (destroyed) after the light treatment (PDT), and those patients who showed limited STAT3 dimerization on further light treatment gave improved long-term tumor cure. Thus, STAT3 dimerization could be a valuable biomarker in evaluating the PDT response in cancer patients. Therefore, in this particular study, the percentage of STAT3 dimerization after light treatment was measured in mice bearing various lung cancer tumors, and the preliminary results shown in Figure 11 indicate that all the tumors showed a certain percentage of STAT3 dimerization, but this was not directly proportional to the tumor response (Figure 9). These results are certainly interesting; however, further in vivo studies are needed to confirm a direct correlation between the percentage of STAT3 dimerization and long-term PDT efficacy using a larger group of mice bearing a variety of tumor types with variable vascularity.

(h) *Impact of Pluronic F-127 formulation in photophysical properties of PS 1:* Similar to most of the tetrapyrrole-based PS, e.g., HPPH^{30}, the PS **1** derived from chlorophyll-a, on formulating in Pluronic F-127/PBS solution forms aggregation, which significantly reduces its absorption and fluorescence intensities. However, in the presence of HSA (human serum albumin) or BSA (bovine serum albumin), the PS self-aggregation disaggregates, and exhibit photophysical properties similar to the respective monomers observed in organic solvents (e.g., methanol or tetrahydrofuran).

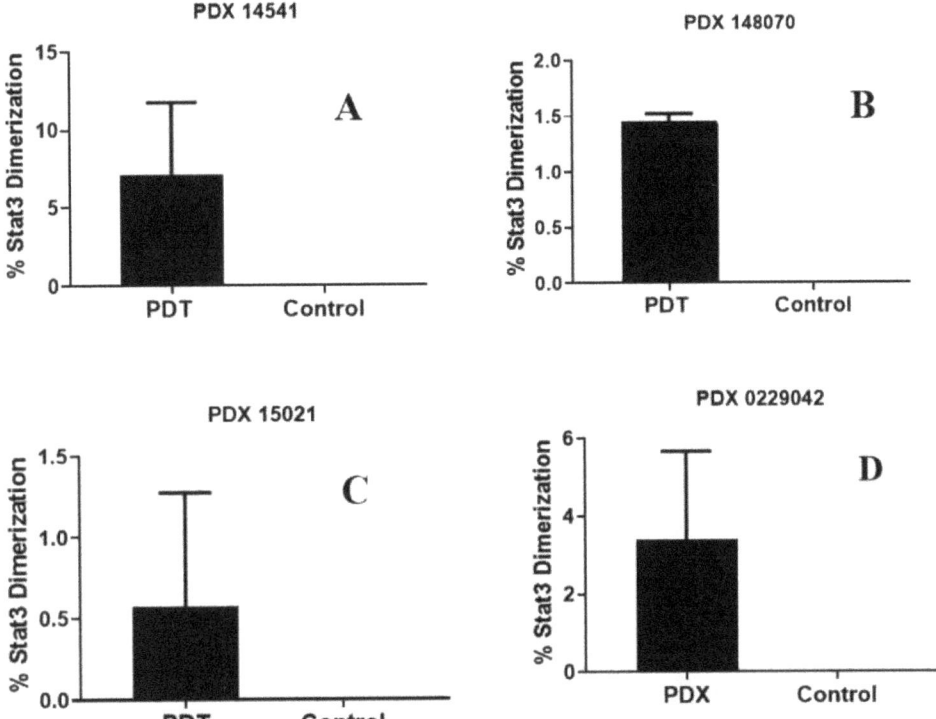

Figure 11. Percentage of STAT3 dimerization measured after in vivo PDT in SCID mice (3 mice/group) bearing tumors on the flank with patient-derived lung cell carcinoma SCC 14541 (**A**), USCLC 148070 (**B**), adenocarcinoma NSCLC 15021 (**C**), and squamous cell carcinoma, SCC 0229047 (**D**). Tumors were grown for approximately 2 weeks until they reached 6–10 mm diameter; the mice were then injected with 1.0 µmol/kg PS **1** in 2% Pluronic® F-127 formulation. In each set of experiments, PDT treatment was given to two mice at 24 h with light at 665 nm at a dose of 135 J/cm² and fluence rate of 75 mW/cm². One mouse in each experiment also received PS **1**, but no light treatment and used as a control.

3. PS 1 Toxicity at Variable Doses in Rats and Dogs

The objectives of this study were to evaluate the toxicity and toxicokinetic profiles following bolus intravenous (IV) administration of PS **1** (formulated in 2% Pluronic F-127/PBS) to male and female Sprague-Dawley rats and Beagle Dogs after a single dose to assess reversibility of latency of any effects over a 28-day free period. These studies were performed under the guidelines set by the United States Food and Drug Administration, in a GMP Facility (Frontage Laboratories, Cleveland, OH, USA).

(a) Rats' toxicity results: The iodinated PS **1** was administered to male and female rats, by a single iv injection, at target dose levels of 0, 1, 4 or 8 mg/kg (Table 1). The control and high-dose animals were administered 0 or 8 mg/kg of the test article in 2% Pluronic F-127 (*w/v*) in DPBS. The low dose animals were administered 1 mg/kg of the test article in 0.25% luronic F-127 and the mid-dose animals were administered 4 mg/kg of the test article in Pluronic F-127 (2% *w/v* in PBS). The Group 1–4 animals were terminated the day after dose administration (Day 2, ten rats/sex/group) or after a 28-day recovery period (Day 29, ten rats/sex/group). Separate groups 3 rats/sex/group of animals were used for toxicokinetic evaluation (3 rats/sex/group in vehicle control group and 9 rats/sex/group in the drug treatment group).

Table 1. Group assignments and dose levels (rat study).

Dose Group	Number of Animals (M/F)	Test Article	Target		Actual [a]		Dose Volume (mL/Kg)	Number of Animals For Necropsy (M/F)	
			Dose Level (mg/kg)	Dose Conc. (mg/mL)	Dose Level (mg/kg)	Dose Conc. (mg/kg)		Main (Day 2)	Recovery (Day 29)
					Toxicity Groups				
1	20/20	PS 1	0	0	0	0	10	10/10	10/10
2	20/20	PS 1	1	0.1	1.11	0.111	10	10/10	10/10
3	20/20	PS 1	4	0.4	3.32	0.332	10	10/10	10/10
4	20/20	PS 1	8	0.8	6.55	0.655	10	10/10	10/10
					Toxicokinetic Groups				
5	3/3	PS 1	0	0	0	0	10	NA [b]	NA
6	9/9	PS 1	1	0.1	1.11	0.111	10	NA	NA
7	9/9	PS 1	4	0.4	3.32	0.332	10	NA	NA
8	9/9	PS 1	8	0.8	6.55	0.655	10	NA	NA

[a] Based on the analysis of initial samples only. [b] NA = Not Applicable

Analysis of samples collected from the 0.1, 0.4 and 0.8 mg/mL dose formulations demonstrated that these formulations were homogeneous (CV</− 1.4%). The mean concentrations of the 0.1, 0.4 and 0.8 mg/mL homogeneity samples were 111, 83.0 and 81.9% of the target, respectively, which were outside of the accuracy criteria (+/− 10%) of the target concentration. Analysis of backup samples confirmed the initial results. The actual dose levels were 1.11, 3.32 and 6.55 mg/kg, respectively.

There was no mortality or moribundity and no PS related effects on: clinical observations, body weight, food consumption (recovery animals only), ophthalmology clinical pathology (hematology, coagulation, clinical chemistry and urinalysis), gross pathology, organ weights and histopathology or microscopic findings.

On day 2, the most notable changes were several-fold elevations in serum cholesterol and triglycerides concentrations for both males and females of Group 1 (vehicle) and Group 4 (high dose). On day 29, both cholesterol and triglycerides values returned to the normal range. These changes were potentially Pluronic F-127 related (a vehicle component). In addition, statistically significant changes were observed in multiple serum chemistry on Day 2. These changes were not considered adverse due to their scattered small magnitude nature. The T_{max} ranged from 0.083 to 1000 h. The elimination half-life ranged from 7.03 to 9.90 h. Increases in C_{max} were approximately dose proportional and increases in $ACCl_{ast}$ were greater than dose proportional. These values were similar in males and females. Single intravenous injections of PS **1** to male and female rats at dose levels of 0, 1.11, 3.32 and 6.55 mg/kg was well tolerated with no adverse test article-related effects. The no-observed-adverse-effect level (NOAEL) for the PS was considered to be 6.55 mg/kg for male and female rats, the highest dose level evaluated (Table 2).

Table 2. Toxicokinetic parameters of PS **1** in rats.

Group	Pyroanalog 531 Dose (mg/kg)	Sex	T_{max} (h)	$T_{1/2}$	Cmax (ng/mL)	AUC_{last} (h ng/mL)	$AUC_{0-\infty}$ (h * ng/mL)
6	1.11	M	0.500	7.94	33,700	367,000	417,000
		F	0.500	7.45	37,000	378,000	435,000
7	3.32	M	0.083	7.03	111,000	1,180,000	1,290,000
		F	0.083	9.13	128,000	1,340,000	1,600,000
8	6.55	M	1.000	9.45	214,000	3,120,000	3,381,000
		F	0.500	9.90	229,000	3,180,000	3,810,000

(b) **Dogs' toxicity results:** Photosensitizer **1** was administered to male and female Beagle dogs, by a single intravenous injection, at dose levels of: 0, 0.5, 2 or 4 mg/kg.

The low-dose animals were administered 0.5 mg/kg or the test article of 0. 25 Pluronic F-127 (*w/v*) in DPBS and the mid-dose animals were administered 2 mg/kg of the test article in 1% Pluronic F-127 (*w/v*) in Dulbecco's Phosphate Buffered Saline (DPBS). There were 6 dogs/sex in each dose group with 3 dogs/sex terminated the day after the final dose and 3 dogs/sex terminated after a 28-day recovery period. The study design is shown in Table 3.

Table 3. Group assignments and dose levels (dog study).

	Number of Animals (M/F)	Test Article	Target		Actual [a]		Dose Volume (mL/Kg)	Number of Animals for Necropsy (M/F)	
			Dose Level (mg/kg)	Dose Conc. (mg/mL)	Dose Level (mg/kg)	Dose Conc. (mg/kg)		Main (Day 2)	Recovery (Day 29)
					Toxicity Groups				
1	6/6	PS 1	0	0	0	0	5	3/3	3/3
2	6/6	PS 1	0.5	0.1	0.42	0.0847	5	3/3	3/3
3	6/6	PS 1	2	0.4	1.52	0.304	5	3/3	3/3
4	6/6	PS 1	4	0.8	3.45	0.690	5	3/3	3/3
					Toxicokinetic Groups				
5	6/6	PS 1	0	0	0	0	5	NA	NA
6	6/6	PS 1	0.5	0.1	0.42	0.0847	5	NA	NA
7	6/6	PS 1	2	0.4	1.52	0.304	5	NA	NA
8	6/6	PS 1	4	0.8	3.45	0.690	5	NA	NA

[a] Based on the analysis of initial samples, only dose animals were administered 0 or 4 mg/kg of the test article in 2% Pluronic.

Analysis of samples collected from 0.1, 0.4 and 0.8 mg/mL formulations demonstrated that these formulations were homogenous (RSD </−). The mean concentrations of the samples were 84.7, 76.0 and 86.3% of the target, respectively, which were outside of the accuracy criteria. The actual dose levels were 0.42, 1.52 and 3.45 mg/kg, respectively.

Similar to the study discussed above on rats, there was no mortality and there were no adverse evaluations in triglycerides levels or moribundity and no PS-related effects on: clinical observations, body weight, food consumption (recovery animals only), ophthalmology clinical pathology (hematology, coagulation, clinical chemistry and urinalysis), gross pathology, organ weights and histopathology or microscopic findings. The triglyceride values returned to within the normal range by Day 29.

The T_{max} ranged from 0.083 to 0.458 h. The elimination half-life was 13.7 h. Increase in C_{max} and AUC_{last} were 76,000 and 92,000 ng/mL and 976,000 and 1,2000,000 hr * ng/mL for males and females, respectively. The no-observed-adverse-effect level (NOAEL) for PS **1** was observed to be 3.45 mg/kg for male and female dogs, the highest dose level evaluated (Table 4).

Table 4. Mean toxicokinetic parameters of PS **1** in dogs.

Group	Pyro Analog 531 Dose (mg/kg)	Sex	T_{max} (hr)	$T_{1/2}$	Cmax (ng/ML)	AUC_{last} (hr*ng/mL
2	0.42	M	0.458	NR	5330	83,100
		F	0.153	13.7	7000	110,000
3	1.52	M	0.389	NR	28,500	365,000
		F	0.083	NR	31,100	392,000
4	3.45	M	1.153	NR	76,000	976,000
		F	0.3.75	NR	92,400	1,200,000

4. Conclusions

The results presented in this article show that the iodinated PS **1** derived from chlorophyll-a is an efficient photosensitizer for the treatment of a variety of l PDX lung cancer tumors. Interestingly, PS1-PDT in combination with doxorubicin at a single dose enhanced the long-term cure in SCID mice bearing SCLC 14541 tumors. These results are exciting, and in a future study, the optimization of treatment parameters at variable doses of PS and chemotherapy agents (either doxorubicin or cisplatin) may further improve long-term cure with reduced toxicity. This approach will certainly help to select the best treatment parameter for treating lung cancer patients. The advantages of the iodinated compound are due to its unique ability to image the cancer in radioactive form (^{124}I-), and as a non-radioactive analog it can be used for fluorescence guided photodynamic therapy of cancer. A "true" tri-functional (MR, fluorescence imaging and image-guided therapy).

The toxicity and toxicokinetic profiles of PS **1** in 2% Pluronic F-127 formulation was investigated at variable doses in rats and dogs in a GMP facility, following the United States FDA guidelines. Under the doses tested, even at higher than the therapeutic dose, no significant toxicity was observed.

5. Experimental Methods

<u>Chemistry</u>: The iodinated PS **1** was derived from chlorophyll-a in a multistep synthesis following our own methodology. [33]. The GMP material for toxicity and toxicokinetic studies in rats and dogs was synthesized in a GMP facility following the guidelines of the United States FDA.

<u>Cell Culture and establishing patient-derived xenograft cell line</u>: Lung cancer cell lines (A549 and H460) and breast cancer cell line (MDAMB435) were acquired from ATCC. Cells were grown in 75 cm cm^2 flask with 10% Fetal bovine serum and 5% Penicillin Streptomycin-supplemented media were used to grow the cells under normoxic conditions of 5% CO_2 at 37 °C.

Patient-derived mouse-carried xenografts (PDX) were isolated and grown as epithelial cell lines. Briefly, to establish a cell line from tumor chunks, the tumors were digested in trypsin and DNase I. The epithelial cells were mechanically separated from the tumor and allowed to grow on collagen coated plates. These PDX cell lines were used to investigate tumor specificity of PET-ONCO compared to normal fibroblast cells as well as investigate PDT efficacy in vitro.

<u>Co-culture system of PDX 14541 cells and normal lung fibroblast</u>: PDX 14541 tumor cells were plated in a 6-well plate at around 1000 cells per well. After 24 h, normal lung fibroblast cells that had been pre-transfected with GFP (provided by Dr. Heinz Baumann, Molecular & Cellular Biology, Roswell Park Comprehensive Cancer Center) were plated next at about 5000 cells per well. The cells were allowed to grow to confluency and then were dosed with 1 µM PS**1**. Next, 24 h after dosing, the cells were stained with Hoechst 2422 and imaged using a Zeiss fluorescent microscope.

Determination of in vivo Imaging/PDT efficacy:

Fluorescence Imaging: The SCID mice with PDX Lung tumors of 200–250 mm^3 were injected intravenously (i.v) with photosensitizer PS **1** at dose of 1 µmol/kg in Pluronic formulations. The PS uptake in tumors was determined by fluorescence imaging using a PerkinElmer IVIS Spectrum at variable time points, and maximum uptake was observed at 24 h post-injection.

PDT Efficacy/Tumor Response: At this timepoint, the tumors were irradiated with light (fluence: 135 J/cm^2; fluence rate: 75 mW/cm^2) for 30 min at 665 nm using a Lightwave™ laser diode. Mice were restrained without anesthesia in plexiglass holders designed to expose only the tumor and a 2–4 mm annular margin of skin to light. Two axes (mm) of tumor (L, longest axis; W, shortest axis) were measured with the aid of a Vernier caliper. The tumor assessment and measurements were taken daily, then three times a week for 4 weeks, and twice a week thereafter for a total of 60 days post treatment. Tumor volume (mm^2) was estimated using a formula: tumor volume = $\frac{1}{2}$ (L × W^2). The complete tumor regression (CR) was defined as the inability to detect tumor by palpation at the initial site of tumor appearance for more than two-month post-therapy. Partial tumor regression (PR) was defined as ≥50% reduction in initial tumor size. The edema, erythema and scar formation in the treatment field was observed and recorded. Tumor response for each treatment was evaluated for the tumor response. For statistical analysis, the log-rank Mantel-Cox test, a standard analysis method, was used.

Author Contributions: J.C.C. and F.A.D. conducted the *in vitro and in vivo* experiments, respectively, and analyzed the data, J.R.M. prepared the photosensitizer and formulated it in various formulations. R.K.P. proposed the project, provided the financial assistance and discussed the project with all the members of the research team on regular basis. All authors have read and agreed to the published version of the manuscript.

Funding: This research was funded by the NIH (SBIR Contract: HHSN26120120024C), Photolitec LLC, Buffalo, NY, USA, and a partial funding from NIH grant P30 CA016066.

Institutional Review Board Statement: The animal studies were conducted in accordance with the protocol (537 M) approved by Roswell Park Institutional ethics committee (IACUC).

Informed Consent Statement: The patients' tumor sample were obtained from the institute's tumor bank.

Data Availability Statement: The data presented in this manuscript are available on request to Pandey.

Acknowledgments: The authors are highly thankful to NIH (SBIR Contract: HHSN261201700024C)) and Photolitec, LLC, as well as to the partial support from the shared resources of the Roswell Park Comprehensive Cancer Support Grant (P30 CA016056). The help rendered by Frontage Laboratory, Ohio, USA for toxicity and toxicokinetic studies of PS **1** at variable drug doses is highly appreciated.

Conflicts of Interest: The authors declare no conflict of interest.

References

1. Sung, H.; Farley, J.; Rebecca, L.; Siegel, M.P.H.; Laversanne, M.; Soerjomataram, I.; Jemal, A.; Bray, F. Global Cancer Statistics 2020: GLOBOCAN estimates of incidence and mortality worldwide for 36 cancers in 185 countries. *CA Cancer J. Clin.* **2021**, *71*, 209–249. [CrossRef] [PubMed]
2. Torre, L.A.; Siegel, R.I.; Jernal, A. Lung cancer statistics. *Adv. Exp. Med. Biol.* **2016**, *893*, 1–19. [CrossRef] [PubMed]
3. Ferone, G.; Lee, M.C.; Sage, J.; Berns, A. Cells of origin of lung cancers: Lessons from mouse studies. *Genes Dev.* **2022**, *34*, 1017–1032. [CrossRef] [PubMed]
4. Gattamachi, A.; Johnson, J. What are the treatment options for lung cancer. *Med. News* **2021**.
5. Raman, V.; Yang, C.F.J.; Deng, J.Z.; Amico, T.A. Surgical treatment for early stage non-small cell lung cancer (NSCLC). *J. Thorasic. Dis.* **2018**, *10*, S898–S904. [CrossRef]
6. Lee, S.H. Chemotherapy for lung cancer in the era of personalized medicine. *Tuberic. Respir. Dis.* **2019**, *82*, 178–189. [CrossRef]
7. Vinod, S.K.; Hau, E. Radiotherapy treatment for lung cancer: Current status and future directions. *Respirology* **2020**, *25*, 61–71. [CrossRef]
8. Wang, X.; Zhang, H.; Chen, X. Drug resistance and combating drug resistance in cancer. *Cancer Drug Resist.* **2019**, *2*, 141–160. [CrossRef]
9. His, R.A.; Rosenthal, D.I.; Glatstein, E. Photodynamic therapy in the treatment of cancer: Current state of the art. *Drugs* **1999**, *57*, 725–734.
10. Hu, T.; Wang, Z.; Shen, W.; Liang, R.; Yan, D.; Wei, M. Recent advances in innovative strategies for enhanced cancer photodynamic therapy. *Theranostics* **2021**, *11*, 3278–3300. [CrossRef]
11. Kessel, D.; Oleinick, N.L. Cell death pathways associated with photodynamic therapy: An update. *Photochem. Photobiol.* **2018**, *94*, 213–218. [CrossRef] [PubMed]
12. Calli, J.P.; Spring, B.Q.; Rizvi, I.; Evans, C.L.; Samkos, K.S.; Varma, S.; Pague, B.; Hassan, T. Imaging and photodynamic therapy: Mechanism, Monitoring and Optimization. *Chem. Rev.* **2010**, *110*, 2795–2838.
13. Luby, B.M.; Waosh, C.D.; Zheng, G. Advanced photosensitizer activation strategies for smarter photodynamic therapy beacons. *Angew. Chem.* **2019**, *58*, 2558–2569. [CrossRef] [PubMed]
14. Lee, H.; Han, J.; Shin, H.; Han, H.; Na, K.; Kim, H. Combination of chemotherapy and photodynamic therapy for cancer treatment with sonoporation effects. *J. Control. Release* **2018**, *10*, 190–199. [CrossRef]
15. Che, Y.; Zhang, L.; Li, F.; Sheng, J.; Xu, C.; Li, D.; Yu, H.; Liu, W. Combination of chemotherapy and photodynamic therapy with oxygen self-supply in the form of mutual assistance for cancer therapy. *Int. J. Nanomed.* **2021**, *16*, 3779–3794.
16. Okunaka, T.; Kato, H.; Konaka, C.; Furukawa, K.; Harada, M.; Yamamoto, Y. Photodynamic therapy of lung cancer with bronchial artery infusion of Photofrin. *Diagn. Ther. Endosc.* **1996**, *2*, 202–206. [CrossRef]
17. Senapathy, G.J.; George, E.P.; Abrahamse, H. Enhancement of phthalocyanine mediated photodynamic therapy of lung cancer cells. *Molecules* **2020**, *25*, 4874. [CrossRef]
18. Dong, W.; Li, K.; Qiu, L.; Liu, Q.; Xie, M.; Lim, J. Targeted photodynamic therapy of lung cancer with biotinylated silicon (IV) phthalocyanine. *Curr. Pharm. Biotechnol.* **2021**, *22*, 414–422. [CrossRef]
19. Kato, H. Photodynamic therapy of lung cancer–A revirw of 19 years' experience. *J. Photochem. Photobiol. B Biol.* **1998**, *42*, 96–99. [CrossRef]

20. Allison, R.; Moghissi, K.; Downie, G.; Dixon, K. Photodynamic therapy (PDT) of lung cancer. *Photodiagn. Photodyn. Ther.* **2011**, *8*, 231–239. [CrossRef]
21. Nwogu, C.; Pera, P.; Bshara, W.; Attwood, K.; Pandey, R.K. Photodynamic therapy of human lung cancer xenografts in mice. *J. Surg. Res.* **2016**, *200*, 8–12. [CrossRef] [PubMed]
22. Karwicka, M.; Pucelik, B.; Gonet, M.; Elas, M.; Dabrowski. Effects of photodynamic therapy with Radaporfin on tumor oxygenation and blood flow in a lung cancer mouse model. *Sci. Rep.* **2019**, *9*, 12655. [CrossRef] [PubMed]
23. Dhillon, S.S.; Demmy, T.L.; Yendamuri, S.; Loewen, G.; Nwogu, C.; Cooper, M.; Henderson, B.W. A Phase I Study of Light Dose for Photodynamic Therapy (PDT) Using 2-[1-hexyloxyethyl]-2 devinyl Pyropheophorbide-a (HPPH) for Treatment of Non-small Cell Carcinoma in situ or Non-small Cell Microinvasive Bronchogenic Carcinoma. A Dose Ranging Study. *J. Thorac. Oncol.* **2016**, *11*, 234–241. [CrossRef] [PubMed]
24. Bellnier, D.A.; Greco, W.R.; Loewen, G.M.; Nava, H.; Oseroff, A.R.; Pandey, R.K.; Tsuchida, T.; Dougherty, T.J. Population pharmacokinetics of the photodynamic therapy agent 2.(1-hexyloxyethyl]-2-devinyl pyropheophorbide0a in cancer patients. *Cancer Res.* **2003**, *63*, 1806–1813.
25. Yuan, Z.; Fan, G.; Wu, H.; Liu, C.; Zhan, Y.; Qiu, Y.; Shou, C.; Gao, F.; Zhang, J.; Yin, P.; et al. Photodynamic therapy synergies with PD-L1 checkpoint blockade for immunotherapy of CRC by multifunctional nanoparticles. *Mol. Ther.* **2021**, *29*, 2931–2948. [CrossRef]
26. Siddiqui, M.R.; Railkr, R.; Sanford, T.; Crooks, D.R.; Eckhaus, M.A.; Haines, D.; Choyke, P.L.; Kobayashi, H.; Agarwal, P.K. Targeting Epidermal Growth Factor Receptor (EGFR) and Human Epidermal Growth Factor Receptor 2 (HER2) Expressing Bladder Cancer Using Combination Photoimmunotherapy (PIT). *Nat. Sci. Rep.* **2019**, *8*, 2084. [CrossRef]
27. Zhang, S.; Cheruku, R.R.; Dukh, M.; Tabaczynski, W.; Patel, N.J.; White, W.H.; Missert, J.R.; Spernyak, J.A.; Pandey, R.K. The structures of Gd(III) chelates conjugated at the periphery of HPPH have a significant impact on the imaging and therapy of cancer. *Chem. Med. Chem.* **2020**, *15*, 2058–2070. [CrossRef]
28. Srivatsan, A.; Pera, P.; Joshi, P.; Marko, A.J.; Durrani, F.; Missert, J.R.; Curtin, L.; Sexton, S.; Yao, R.; Sajjad, M. Highlights on the imaging (nuclear/fluorescence) and phototherapeutic potential of a tri-functional chlorophyll-a analog with no significant toxicity in mice and rats. *J. Photochem. Photobiol. B Biol.* **2020**, *211*, 111988. [CrossRef]
29. Pucelik, B.; Arnaut, L.G.; Stochel, G.; Dabrowski, J.M. Design of Pluronic-based formulation for enhanced redaporfin-photodynamic therapy against pigmented melanoma. *ACS Appl. Mater. Interfaces* **2016**, *8*, 22039–22055. [CrossRef]
30. Cacaccio, J.; Durrani, F.; Cheruku, R.R.; Borah, B.; Ethirajan, M.; Tabaczynski, W.; Pera, P.; Missert, J.R.; Pandey, R.K. Pluronic F-127: An Efficient Delivery Vehicle for 3-(1'-hexyloxy)ethyl-3-devinylpyropheophorbide-a (HPPH or Photochlor). *Photochem. Photobiol.* **2020**, *96*, 625–635. [CrossRef]
31. Park, H.; Park, W.; Na, K. Doxorubicin loaded singlet-oxygen producible polymeric micelle based on chlorine e6 conjugated Pluronic F127 for overcoming drug resistance in cancer. *Biomaterials* **2014**, *35*, 7963–7969. [CrossRef] [PubMed]
32. Otterson, G.A.; Vallalona-Calero, M.A.; Hicks, W.; Pan, X.; Ellerton, J.A.; Gettinger, S.N.; Murren, J.R. Phase I/II study of inhaled doxorubicin combined with platinum-based therapy for advanced non-small cell lung cancer. *Clin. Cancer Res.* **2010**, *16*, 2466–2473. [CrossRef] [PubMed]
33. Meerlo, J.V.; Kaspers, G.J.L.; Cloos, J. Cell sensitivity assays: The MTT assay. *Methods Mol. Biol.* **2011**, *731*, 237–245.
34. Liu, O.; Yin, X.; Languino, L.; Altieri, D. Evaluation of drug combination effect using a Bliss independence dose response surface model. *Stat. Biopharm. Res.* **2018**, *10*, 112–122. [CrossRef] [PubMed]
35. Liu, W.; Oseroff, A.R.; Baumann, H. Photodynamic therapy causes cross-linking of signal transducer and activator of transcription proteins and attenuation of interleukin-6 cytokine responsiveness in epithelial cells. *Cancer Res.* **2004**, *64*, 6579–6587. [CrossRef] [PubMed]

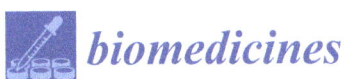

Article

Antitumor Effect and Induced Immune Response Following Exposure of Hexaminolevulinate and Blue Light in Combination with Checkpoint Inhibitor in an Orthotopic Model of Rat Bladder Cancer

Laureline Lamy [1,2], Jacques Thomas [3], Agnès Leroux [3], Jean-François Bisson [4], Kari Myren [5,†], Aslak Godal [5,‡], Gry Stensrud [5,§] and Lina Bezdetnaya [1,2,*]

1. Centre de Recherche en Automatique de Nancy, Centre National de la Recherche Scientifique, UMR 7039, Université de Lorraine, Campus Sciences, Boulevard des Aiguillette, 54506 Vandoeuvre-lès-Nancy, France; la.lamy@nancy.unicancer.fr
2. Research Department, Institut de Cancérologie de Lorraine, 6 Avenue de Bourgogne, 54519 Vandoeuvre-lès-Nancy, France
3. Service de Biopathologie, Institut de Cancérologie de Lorraine, 54506 Vandoeuvre-Lès-Nancy, France; j.thomas@nancy.unicancer.fr (J.T.); a.leroux@nancy.unicancer.fr (A.L.)
4. ETAP-Lab., 13 Rue du Bois de la Champelle, 54500 Vandoeuvre-les-Nancy, France; jfbisson@etap-lab.com
5. Photocure ASA, Hoffsveien 4, 0275 Oslo, Norway; myren@oncoinvent.com (K.M.); asgodal@online.no (A.G.); gry.stensrud@lytixbiopharma.com (G.S.)
* Correspondence: l.bolotine@nancy.unicancer.fr
† Current employment: Oncoinvent AS, Gullhaugveien 7, 0484 Oslo, Norway.
‡ Deceased in September 2021.
§ Current employment: Lytix Biopharma, Sandakerveien 138, 0484 Oslo, Norway.

Abstract: Previous studies have found that use of hexaminolevulinate (HAL) and blue light cystoscopy (BLC) during treatment of bladder cancer had a positive impact on overall survival after later cystectomy, indicating a potential treatment effect beyond improved diagnostic accuracy. The aim of our study was to determine whether HAL and BL mimicking clinically relevant doses in an orthotopic rat model could have therapeutic effect by inducing modulation of a tumor-specific immune response. We also assessed whether administration with a checkpoint inhibitor could potentiate any effects observed. Rats were subjected to HAL BL alone and in combination with anti-PD-L1 and assessed for anti-tumor effects and effects on immune markers. Positive anti-tumor effect was observed in 63% and 31% of rats after, respectively, 12 and 30 days after the procedure, together with a localization effect of CD3+ and CD8+ cells after 30 days. Anti-tumor effect at 30 days increases from 31% up to 38% when combined with intravesical anti-PD-L1. In conclusion, our study demonstrated treatment effects with indications of systemic immune activation at diagnostic doses of HAL and blue light. The observed treatment effect seemed to be enhanced when used in combination with intravesically administrated immune checkpoint inhibitor.

Keywords: bladder cancer; Hexvix®; photodiagnosis; PDT; immune checkpoints

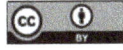

1. Introduction

Urothelial carcinoma is the fifth most prevalent cancer worldwide, where non-muscle-invasive bladder cancer (NMIBC) constitutes 75% of primary diagnosis [1]. NMIBC is characterized by frequent recurrences and progression to muscle-invasive bladder cancer within 24 months after treatment with transurethral resection of bladder tumor (TURBT) followed by intravesical bacillus Calmette–Guérin (BCG) instillation [2].

Use of the photosensitizer hexaminolevulinate (HAL, Hexvix®) and blue light cystoscopy (BLC®) has been introduced to increase detection of tumors during diagnosis and surgical treatment of bladder cancer [3]. HAL induces preferential accumulation of intracellular protoporphyrin IX (PpIX) in neoplastic tissue. Illumination with blue light (BL; 380–440 nm) produces a clearly demarcated red fluorescence from malignant tissue. Increased detection leads to more complete tumor resection, resulting in improved short and sustained long-term recurrence rates [4,5]. BLC with HAL is recognized and recommended across international and national guidelines [6,7].

Whereas photodynamic diagnosis (PDD) is a diagnostic modality, photodynamic therapy (PDT) is a promising technology in the treatment of various cancer types. PDT combines the administration of a photosensitizer with the illumination of light of specific wavelength to generate cytotoxic singlet oxygen. PDT destroys tumor cells via direct cell destruction and indirectly via vascular shutdown and induction of acute local inflammatory response resulting in immune system activation [8–12]. HAL-mediated PDT with WL was earlier tested with curative purpose in patients with urothelial carcinoma after TUR and demonstrated efficacy of the treatment without major side effects [13]. Intriguingly, two studies have demonstrated positive impact on patient outcomes after cystectomy in patients who had undergone BLC prior to their cystectomy compared to WL-TURB, indicating an additional effect of BLC beyond pure detection [14,15]. Both overall survival and cancer-specific survival were significantly higher in the BLC group, and prior BLC with HAL was found to be an independent predictor of survival after radical cystectomy [15].

A promising new age of immunotherapy has arrived in the form of checkpoint inhibition [16]. Tumor cells can escape immune surveillance by upregulating PD-L1/PD-1 expression in cells of tumor microenvironment. The anti-PD-1 and anti-PD-L1 antibodies bind, respectively, to PD-1 on T cells and PD-L1 on cancer cells preventing the interaction of PD-1 and PD-L1, thus reactivating the anti-tumor immune response of cytotoxic T cells [17]. For bladder cancer treatment, five such drugs have been approved by the FDA for use in different settings, including pembrolizumab for BCG-unresponsive high-risk NMIBC [18,19]. Immune checkpoint inhibitors have demonstrated a higher benefit in heavy CD8+ infiltrated tumors and in tumors with high tumor mutational burden [19]. The role of checkpoint inhibition in NMIBC has been summarized by Hahn and coworkers [20].

Several studies on the combined effect of PDT with photosensitizers and immune checkpoint inhibition in preclinical models aiming to improve the therapeutic efficiency have been reported [21]. Enhanced anti-tumor efficacy was demonstrated in murine tumor models including breast, subcutaneous, melanoma, renal cell carcinoma, and colon through a combined action of checkpoint inhibitors and PDT. The local treatment of tumor together with the systemic administration of checkpoint inhibitors primed an immune response resulting in increased infiltration of activated CD8+ T cells in the primary tumor, but also in secondary tumors/metastases indicating an abscopal effect. Moreover, an immunological memory effect was developed as PDT-treated tumor-free mice were protected against developing new tumors when re-challenged [21–25].

We hypothesized that the positive impact on patient outcomes in patients who had undergone BLC prior to cystectomy could be caused by a direct anti-tumor effect and/or activation of the immune system as seen with PDT. Therefore, as a proof-of principle study for future translation study, we investigated whether intravesical administration of HAL followed by a diagnostic blue light illumination regime (PDD) could have an anti-tumor and immune modulating effects, as well as increasing susceptibility to PD-1/PD-L1 pathway inhibition in a preclinical model. Rats were therefore treated with HAL and BL in an orthotopic model of bladder cancer and subjected to histopathological analysis and assessment of immune markers. Co-administration of HAL BL with a checkpoint inhibitor was further tested in this model aiming to assess for potentiation of anti-tumor effects.

2. Materials and Methods

2.1. Tumor Cells Culture

The rat bladder TCC cell line AY-27 has been established as a primary bladder tumor in Fischer 344 rats by feeding the rats with N-(4-[5-nitro-2-furyl]-2-thiazolyl) formamide. The bladder tumor cells were cultured in vitro as a monolayer at 37 °C in a humidified 5% CO_2

and 95% air atmosphere in RPMI 1640 culture media (Sigma, Saint-Quentin Fallavier, France) complemented with 9% FCS, 1% L-glutamine and 1% antibiotic/antimycotic solution. Cells were passaged when nearly confluent. The cell culture medium and other culture ingredients and PBS were obtained from Sigma (France).

2.2. Orthotopic Tumor Model

Nine-week-old female Fischer rats (Charles River Laboratories, Chatillon-sur-Chalronne France) weighing 140–165 g were housed in groups of 4 rats per cage in a room with 12-h inverted light/dark cycle and controlled temperature (22 ± 2 °C). Animal care protocols were used in accordance with the guidelines of the European Communities Council Directive on the approximation of laws, regulations, and administrative provisions of the Member States regarding the protection of animals used for scientific purposes, the National Institutes of Health Guide for the care and use of laboratory animals, and the ASAB Ethical Committee. The studies received approval from the French Ministry of Higher Education and Research (agreements no. APAFIS#14510 on 9 July 2018, and no. APAFIS#23597 on 3 March 2020). Animal supervision was performed daily. All efforts were made to prevent animal suffering.

Tumors were induced as initially described by Xiao et al. [26]. Briefly, animals were anaesthetized with an intraperitoneal injection (i.p.) of ketamine/xylazine mixture (54/6 mg·kg^{-1}) to maintain ~1.5 h of anesthesia and fixed on animal boards kept at 37 °C. The anesthesia was completed by i.p. injection of 0.01 mg/kg opioid-based buprenorphine. After urethral catheterization of the bladder with a 16-gauge plastic intravenous cannula, the bladder urothelium was first conditioned with 0.5 mL HCl (0.1 N) for 15 s, neutralized with 0.5 mL (0.1 N) NaOH for 15 s, and immediately washed several times with sterile physiological serum. Then, a suspension of AY-27 cells (106 cells) in 0.5 mL of medium was instilled into the bladder via the catheter for 1 h.

2.3. Hexylaminolevulinate Preparation and Administration

Hexylaminolevulinate (HAL HCl (Mw 251)) was kindly provided by Photocure ASA, Oslo, Norway. HAL was dissolved in RPMI medium (without serum) immediately before instillation and 0.5 mL 8 mM were instilled intravesically and kept for 1 h. After bladder evacuation, bladders were washed three times with the PBS solution followed by illumination.

2.4. Illumination of Rat Bladders

Whole bladder illumination with blue light (BL) was performed at day 5 after tumor cell implantation using a 200 mW Modulight laser model ML 6500 with excitation wavelength at 405 nm, coupled to fiber with a cylindrical diffuser (1 × 5 mm, Medlight) placed in a central position in the bladder filled with 0.5 mL PBS. During illumination the irradiance was fixed at 7 mW/cm^2 and a total light dose was 7.5 J/cm^2. The illumination parameters were selected to mimic the irradiance and light doses used during a clinical blue light cystoscopy. The selected parameters were in the same range as reported by Karl Storz for their D-Light C Photodynamic Diagnosis (PDD) system [27].

2.5. Combination Therapy

Mouse PD-L1 monoclonal antibody (clone 10F.9G2; Bio-XCell) was delivered by manufacturer as a liquid stock solution (7.50 mg/mL) and stored at 4 °C. Immunotherapy was conducted using two administration routes of anti-PD-L1: intravesical (ives) and intraperitoneal (i.p.). Treatment scheme was selected based on prior studies in rodents of combined action of immune checkpoints inhibitors with either radiotherapy or PDT [22,28]. Treatment scheme is presented in Figure 1.

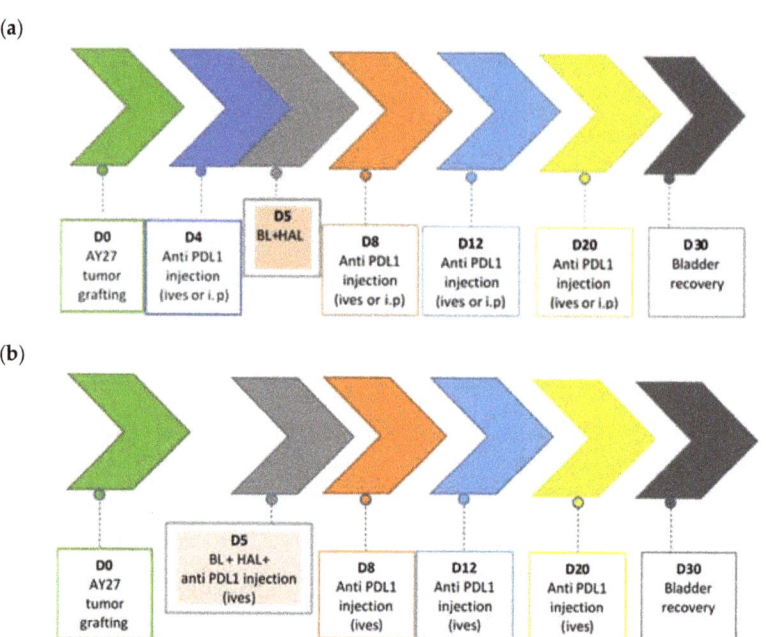

Figure 1. Experimental scheme of HAL BL treatment alone and in combination with anti PD-L1 injections. (**a**) Intraperitoneal (i.p.) and intravesical (ives) administrations; (**b**) anti PD-L1 co-administration with HAL (same syringe).

2.5.1. Intraperitoneal Injections (i.p.)

For i.p. injections, no additional anesthesia was required. Stock PD-L1 solution was diluted in endotoxin-free PBS immediately before use. At each of four PD-L1 injections, rats received 100 µL/rat of anti-mouse PD-L1 antibody at the concentration of 2 mg/mL. A treatment dose of 0.2 mg/rat/injection was selected based on prior published experience [28]. Injections were performed at days 4, 8, 12, and 20 after tumor implantation (Figure 1).

2.5.2. Intravesical Instillations (ives)

Instillation was done during 1 h under ketamine/xylazine anesthesia. At each of four PD-L1 ives instillations, rats received 500 µL/rat of antibody at the concentration 7.5 mg/mL. The dose of 3.75 mg/rat/injection was selected to represent the dose used in clinical settings [29], recalculated for equivalent doses in rats. Two schedules of anti-PD-L1 ives instillations were used: on days 4, 8, 12, and 20 or on days 5, 8, 12, and 20 after tumor cells implantation. In the second schedule, the first anti-PDL1 instillation (on day 5) was co-administered together with HAL (in one syringe) (Figure 1).

2.6. Pathological and Immunological Analysis

The rats were sacrificed by intracardiac overdose of pentobarbital at 7, 12, and 30 days after tumor cell inoculation for pathological and immunological analysis.

2.6.1. Hematoxylin-Eosin-Safran (HES) Analysis

Cystectomy specimens were fixed with 4% formaldehyde before paraffin embedding for about 4 h. Afterwards, the bladders were cut in four parts and placed in cassette. After approximately 48 h in dehydratation bath, the bladders were paraffined. Two sections (5 µm) obtained serially at 0.2 mm intervals were stained with hematoxylin-Eosin-Safran (automatic methods).

Therapeutic efficacy in rat bladders was graded into 4 groups (Table 1), based on modified Dworak TGR (tumor regression rate) system [30]. These four groups stand for No Response (NR), Moderate Response (MR), Near Complete Response (near CR) and Complete Response (CR). Typical images corresponding to each of four grades are depicted in Figure 2. Positive anti-tumor effect was considered as a sum of near CR and CR.

Table 1. Tumor response grades (adapted with modification from [30]).

No Response (NR)	Moderate Response (MR)	Near Complete Response (Near CR)	Complete Response (CR)
Rat with strong muscle-infiltrative tumor	Rats with few tumor cells or islets of tumor cells in several areas	Rats with singular islet of tumor cells or very few tumor cells	Absence of tumor cells

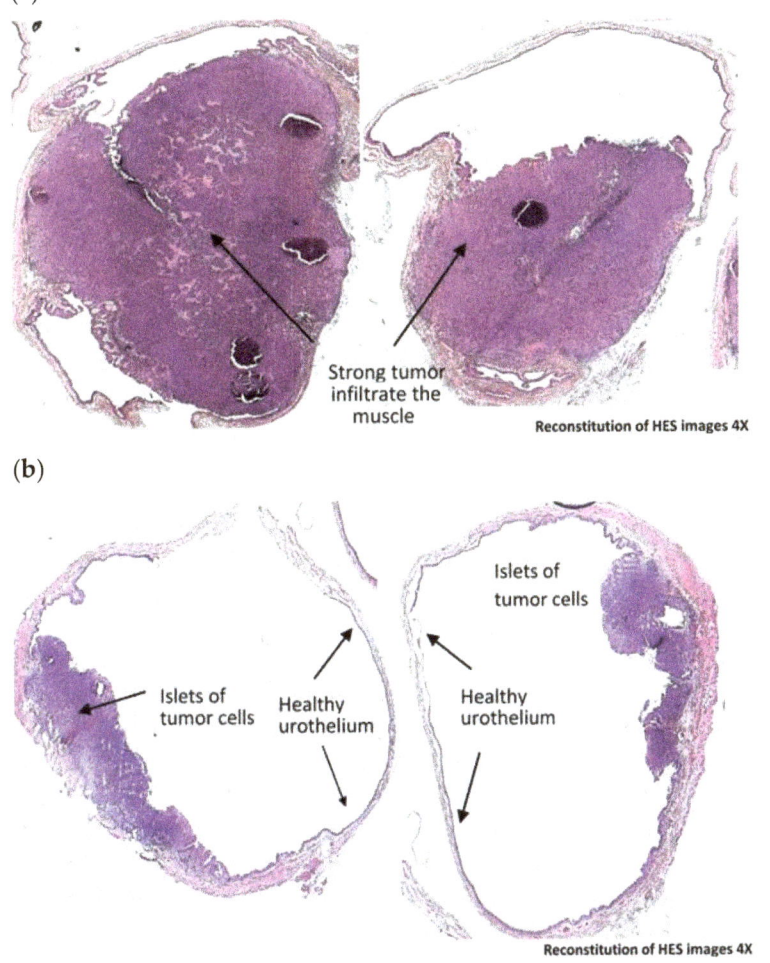

Figure 2. *Cont.*

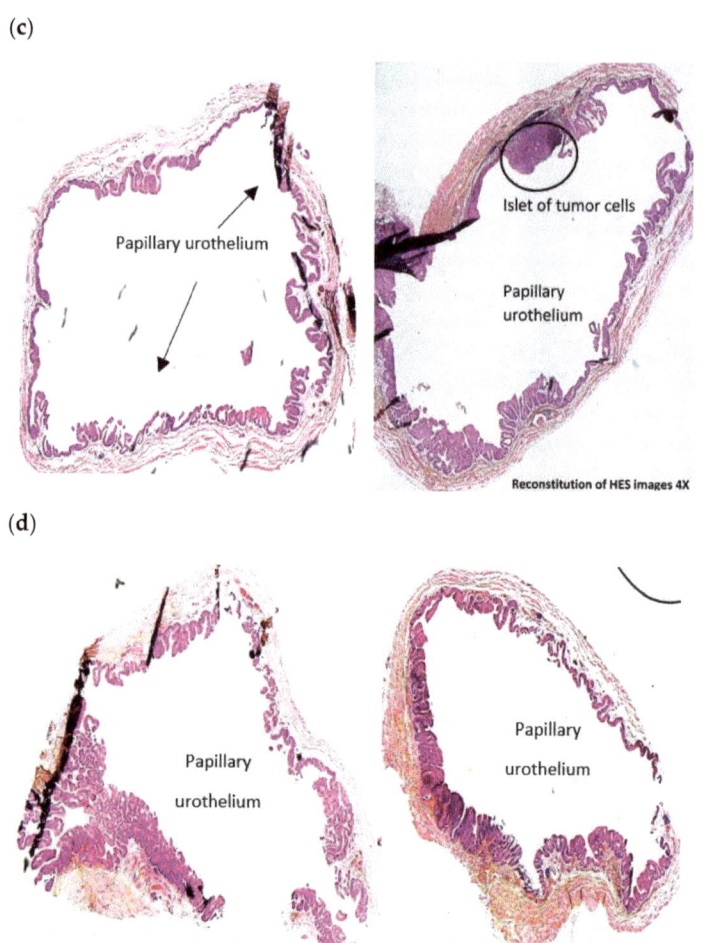

Figure 2. Tumor response grades (adapted with modification from [30]) and bladder tumor typical images corresponding to different response rates. (**a**) No response (NR): bladders with strong muscle-infiltrative tumor; (**b**) Moderate response (MR): bladders with few tumor cells or islets of tumor cells in several areas; (**c**) Near Complete Response (Near CR); (**d**) Complete Response (CR).

2.6.2. Assessment of Immune Cells in Tissues

Inflammatory cells were evaluated by CD3+, CD8+, and CD4+ lymphocytes labeling. CD8+ and CD4+ antibodies staining protocol was adapted from a protocol published by Bressenot [31] with slight modifications. CD4+ lymphocytes labeling was performed according to manufacturer recommendations. CD8+ and CD4+ immunohistochemistry (IHC) was carried out on 4 μm thick deparaffinized sections in a manual mode. Before staining, the sections were subjected to heat-induced epitope retrieval by incubation in 0.01 M Tris/EDTA solution (pH 8) at 95 °C for 40 min, followed by 10 min of cooling. Slices were briefly rinsed with water. The sample on the slide was spotted with dakopen. PBS Tween (0.1 M phosphate buffer, pH 7.4, 0.1% (v/v) Tween 20) was added to each spotted sample for 30 min. Endogenous peroxydase activity at each spot was blocked by 5 min incubation in a 3% hydrogen peroxide solution in distilled water. Primary antibody was diluted in 1% (m/v) BSA. With this aim, purified mouse anti-RatCD8a (1: 100 diluted, BD Pharmingen) was incubated at room temperature for 1 h and mouse anti-rat CD4 W3/25

(1: 200 diluted, Bio-Rad, Marnes-La- Coquette, France) was incubated at 4 °C overnight. After that, the slices were washed twice with PBST, each for 10 min and incubated with secondary antibody, biotinylated goat anti-mouse Ig (multiple adsorption), diluted 1:100 for CD8, and biotinylated donkey anti-mouse IgG, diluted 1:50 for CD4. Secondary antibody remained on the slides for 1 h at room temperature.

Afterwards, the slices were washed twice with PBST, each for 10 min, followed by incubation with streptavidin-peroxidase (BD Pharmingen) for 30 min at room temperature. The slices were washed twice with PBST (each for 5 min). The Novared TR system (Abcys, Paris, France) was used to detect bound peroxidase (12 min). Nuclear counterstaining was performed with twice diluted Harris hematoxylin (1 min). At the end of the procedure, the slices were dehydrated in three baths of alcohol (95/100/xylen) and covered by lamellas. IHC CD3 was carried out on 4μm thick deparaffinized sections and further staining was performed with automated immunostainer (BenchMark ULTRA instrument) with flex rabbit polyclonal anti-CD3+ human antibody (Agilent) as primary antibody.

Inflammation was assessed by the expression of CD8+, CD4+ and CD3+ lymphocytes. The ratio of all cell nuclei (Olympus, X40) at several images (4 or 5) achieving totally about 1000 cells to CD8+, CD4+, and CD3+ lymphocytes was calculated.

2.6.3. PD-L1 Expression in Tumor Cells

PD-L1 expression was assessed according to manufacturer recommendations. PD-L1 protein detection in paraffin-embedded bladders was determined with mouse monoclonal anti-PD-L1 antibody, Clone 22C3 against PD-L1 (Agilent). Staining was performed by using an automated immunostainer (BenchMark ULTRA instrument). The OptiView DAB IHC Detection Kit (OptiView) is an indirect, biotin-free system for detecting rabbit primary antibody. After this labeling, the slides were visualized by white light microscopy. In the first lieu, assessment at low magnification was performed to identify homogeneity of staining. Afterwards, at high magnification, the areas of interest were analyzed to separate immune PD-L1 positives cells from tumor cells. Finally, PD-L1 positive tumor cells were quantified.

PD-L1 expression was evaluated according to Percentage Staining (PS) of tumor cells used in conventional clinical practice. PS was graded into strong (50 < PD-L1 < 100%); moderate (1 < PD-L1 < 49%) and weak expression (PD-L1 < 1%). Typical images corresponding to different levels of PD-L1 expression are indicated in Figure 3.

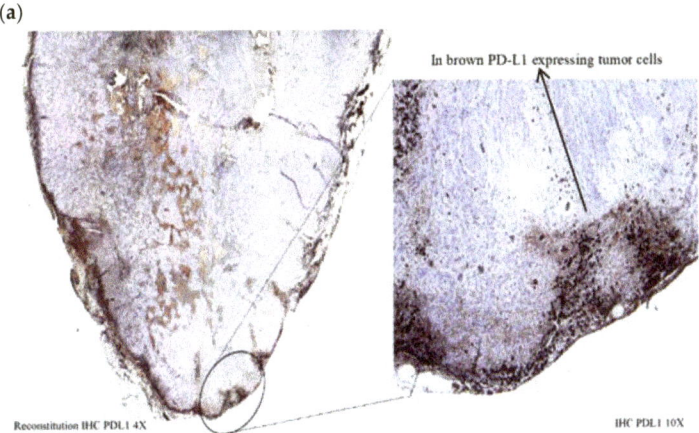

Figure 3. Cont.

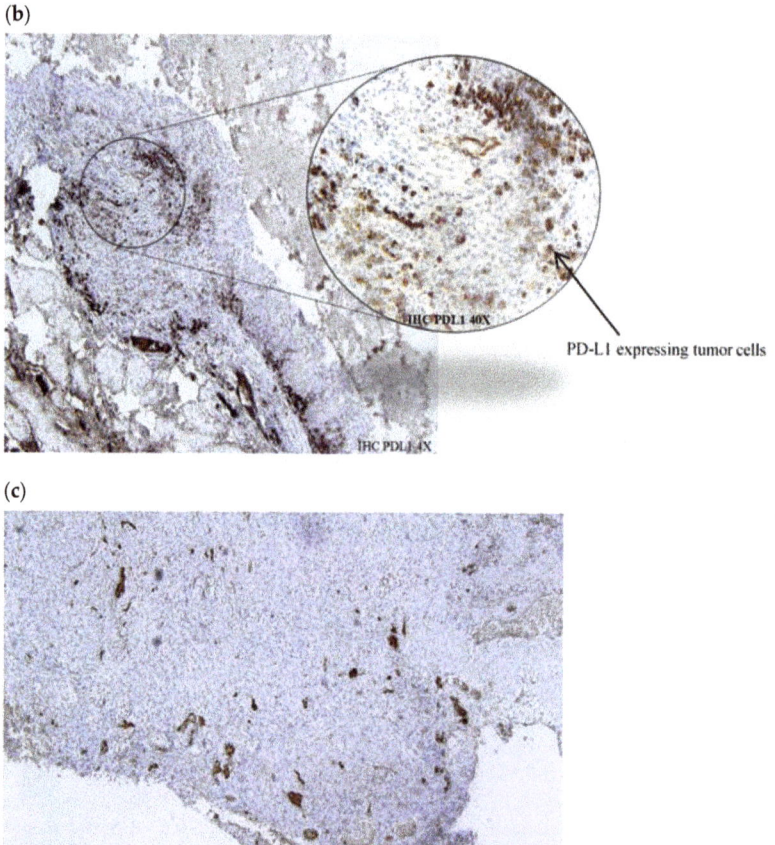

Figure 3. Representative images of PD-L1 staining. (**a**) Typical image of strong membranous PD-L1 expression (>50%). Example of bladder sample treated with HAL BL. Membranous PD-L1 expression in tumor cells (10×). Photo captured at 12 days post-grafting; (**b**) typical image of moderate membranous PD-L1 expression (1 < PD-L1 < 49%). Example of bladder sample treated with BL. Membranous PD-L1 expression in tumor cells (×4). Photo captured at 30 days post-grafting; (**c**) typical image of weak membranous PD-L1 expression (<1%). Example of bladder sample treated with HAL BL (×4). Photo captured at 30 days post-grafting.

2.7. Statistical Analysis

The overall number of animals used in this study was 85. The number of rats differed in each group. For the HES-assessed anti-tumor effect, the numbers of rats in each group were between 6 and 13. For the IHC-assessed PD-L1 expression, the numbers of rats in each group were from 4 to 12.

Expression of T lymphocytes is presented as mean ± SEM; comparison between groups was performed using non-parametric Mann–Whitney U test. p values < 0.05 were considered statistically significant.

The correlation between variables and responses was determined by partial least squares regression. The significant main, interaction, and squared terms were found by the backward selection procedure removing one-by-one of the most insignificant terms until only significant terms remained ($p < 0.05$). The statistical calculations were performed by the statistical software Modde Pro version 12.0.1, Sartorius Stedim data analytics AB.

3. Results

3.1. HAL-PDD-Mediated Therapeutic Effect in AY27 Orthotopic Bladder Tumors

We studied the therapeutic effect of HAL and BL illumination at different time points after tumor cell inoculation. Intravesical instillation of HAL and BL illumination was performed five days after tumor grafting. A significant positive therapeutic outcome (63%; $p < 0.05$) was demonstrated when the rats subjected to HAL BL were assessed 12 days after tumor grafting (n = 8) (Table 2). Five rats were either tumor-free (CR) or with few tumor cells (Near CR), while two rats responded moderately (MR). In the last case, we observed a tumor confined to bladder wall but without entire wall invasion. In one rat the treatment was ineffective (NR) (Table 2).

Table 2. HES assessed therapeutic efficacy in rat bladders at 7, 12, and 30 days after tumor inoculation in control and experimental groups.

Time after Grafting (d)	Treatments	Tumor Response Grades					
		NR	MR	Near CR	CR	Near CR + CR	
12	HAL BL (n = 8)	1/8	2/8	3/8	2/8	5/8	63%
30	CTR ND NL (n = 12)	12/12	0/12	0/12	0/12	0/12	0%
	CTR BL (n = 6)	6/6	0/6	0/6	0/6	0/6	0%
	HAL BL (n = 13)	8/13	1/13	0/13	4/13	4/13	31%

HAL BL: HAL and blue light, CTR ND NL: control no drug no light, CTR BL: control blue light only, NR: no response, MR; moderate response, CR; complete response.

The positive therapeutic outcome was not sustained in rats sacrificed 30 days post-grafting where the beneficial effect was significantly reduced to 31% (n = 13; $p < 0.05$). After 30 days, four out of 13 rats were tumor-free (CR), one rat responded moderately (MR), but 8 out of 13 bladders demonstrated strong muscle-infiltrative tumors (NR) (Table 2). Two control groups were also assessed 30 days after tumor grafting. In the untreated control tumor group (CTR ND NL; n = 12) HES demonstrated muscle invasive tumors in the chorion in all rats (Table 2). In control rats subjected to BL illumination only (CTR BL; n = 6), the bladders of all six rats were heavily invaded with tumor (Table 2). All rats in all treatment group survived without any visible sign of suffering.

3.2. Assessment of Immunological Markers

In all treated groups we observed a strong inflammation, and therefore in the next step we assessed the recruitment of lymphocytes. The CD3+ inflammatory marker and two subsets of T cells, namely, CD4+ T helper cells and CD8+ cytotoxic T lymphocytes were quantified and their localization was assessed in extracted tumors at different times after tumor grafting.

Expression of CD3+ in untreated control tumors (CTR ND NL) at 12 days post grafting was 17% (data not shown) and increased significantly to 29% at 30 days post tumor grafting ($p < 0.01$) (Figure 4). This increase in CD3+ expression in untreated tumors confirms a chronic inflammatory status inherent to tumor presence. CD3+ expression in rat bladders subjected to HAL BL was significantly lower (19%; $p < 0.05$) than that in non-treated group (CTR ND NL) but not different from the control BL group (23%) (Figure 4).

CD8+ expression was not significantly different between tested groups 30 days after tumor grafting and varied between 18% and 21% (data not shown). The expression of CD4+ was overall lower than that of CD8+ and varied between 7% and 11% but was not significantly different between tested groups ($p > 0.1$) (data not shown).

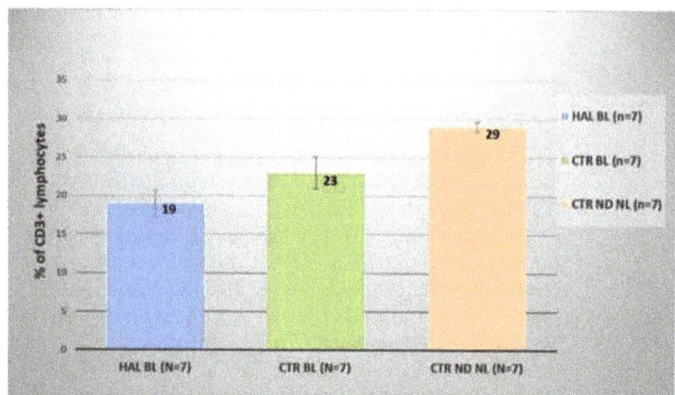

Figure 4. Expression of CD3+ lymphocytes in rat bladder tumors 30 days after tumor grafting in control and experimental groups.

Albeit no quantitative difference was observed in the expression of CD3+ after HAL BL compared to BL only, close examination of the slides revealed a different localization of the CD3+ lymphocytes. A strong CD3+ localization around tumor cells was observed in the HAL BL group, whereas in the CTR BL group, CD3+ lymphocytes were mostly localized on the periphery of tumor sample (Figure 5a,b). The same distribution pattern was observed for CD8+ lymphocytes (Figure 5c,d), but unlike CD3+ cells, partial localization was also seen in the control BL group. CD4+ cells were distributed on the periphery in both experimental groups (data not shown). Periphery localization of CD3+, CD4+ and CD8+ was also observed for untreated control tumors (data not shown). The localization of CD3+ and CD8+ lymphocytes around tumor cells in HAL BL-treated rat bladders could indicate a stimulation of the immune system explaining the anti-tumor effect (Table 2). Therefore, in the next step we studied whether the anti-tumor effect could be improved by combining exposure of HAL and BL with anti-PD-L1 immunotherapy.

(a)

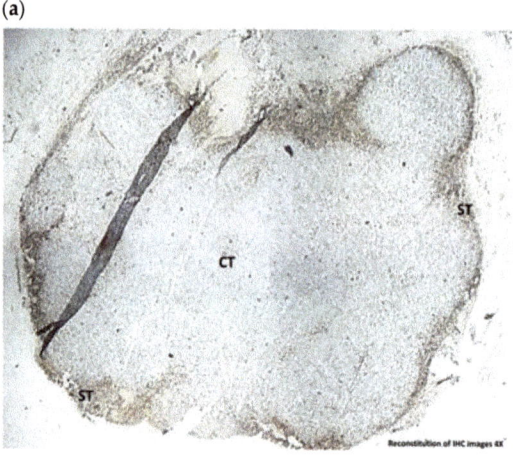

Figure 5. *Cont.*

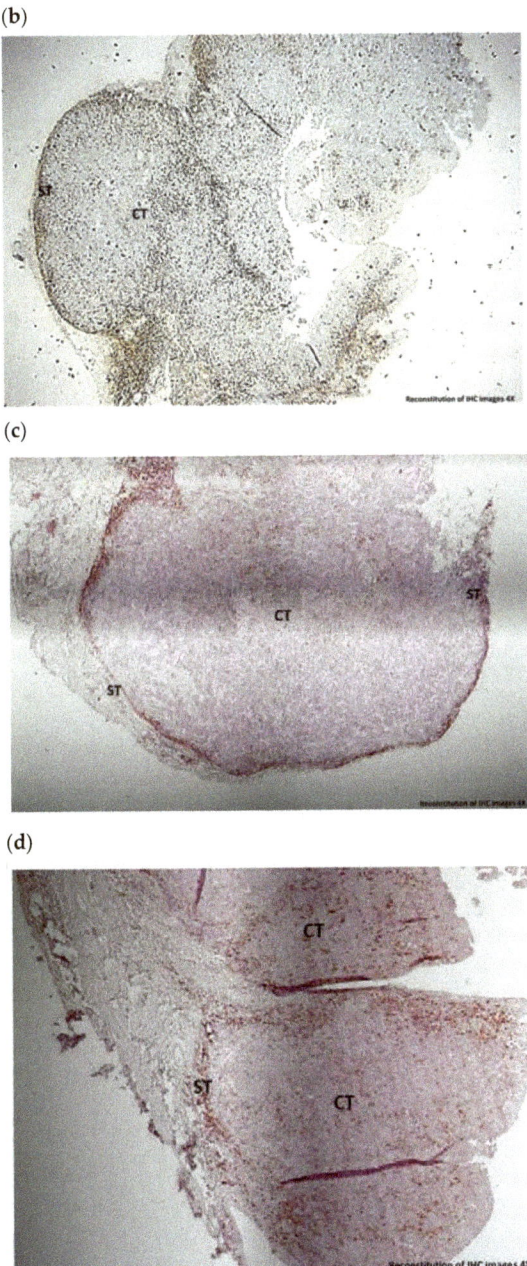

Figure 5. Typical images of CD3+ lymphocytes (**a,b**) and CD8+ lymphocytes (**c,d**) in bladder tumors 30 days post-grafting. (**a**) CD3+ lymphocytes in CTR BL sample displaying peripheral localization in stroma regions (ST) (×4); (**b**) CD3+ lymphocytes in HAL BL sample displaying localization around tumor cells in the center of tumor (CT) (×4); (**c**) CD8+ lymphocytes in CTR BL sample displaying peripheral localization in stroma regions (ST) (×10); (**d**) CD8+ lymphocytes in HAL BL sample displaying localization around tumor cells in the center of tumor (CT) (×10).

3.3. IHC-Assessed PD-L1 Expression in Bladder Tumor Cells

PD-L1 expression was assessed in tumor cells collected from rats exposed to HAL BL, BL only and untreated control tumor at 7 days, 12 days, and 30 days after tumor grafting (Table 3). Only weak/moderate expression of PD-L1 was seen in the HAL BL and CTR BL groups at 7 days after tumor grafting (Table 3). Twelve days after tumor grafting, a transient increase to strong PD-L1 expression was observed in all experimental groups (Table 3; Figure 3a) but did not sustain. Indeed, 30 days after tumor grafting the PD-L1 expression returned back to weak/moderate levels (Table 3; Figure 3b,c).

Table 3. IHC-assessed PD-L1 expression at 7, 12, and 30 days after tumor inoculation in control (CTR ND NL, CTR BL) and HAL BL-treated bladder tumors.

Time after Grafting (Days)	Treatments	50 < PD-L1 < 100% Strong	1 < PD-L1 < 49% Moderate	PD-L1 < 1% Weak
7	HAL BL (n = 4)	0/4	1/4	3/4
12	CTR ND NL (n = 4)	3/4	1/4	0/4
	CTR BL (n = 4)	3/4	1/4	0/4
	HAL BL (n = 6)	4/6	0/6	2/6
30	CTR ND NL (n = 11)	2/11	1/11	8/11
	CTR BL (n = 5)	2/5	2/5	1/5
	HAL BL (n = 12)	0/12	1/12	11/12

3.4. Therapeutic Effect of Immune Checkpoint Therapy in AY27 Orthotopic Bladder Tumors

The increased PD-L1 expression 12 days after tumor grafting justified further experiments with anti-PD-L1 immunotherapy. Two different administration routes of anti-PD-L1 were performed: intravesical (ives) and intraperitoneal (i.p.) and two different dosing regimens (Figure 1). No anti-tumor effect was observed in the controls treated with anti-PD-L1 ives or i.p. alone 30 days after tumor grafting (Table 4). However, all groups exposed to HAL showed a positive anti-tumor effect. This effect was significant for rats exposed to HAL BL alone and in combination with anti-PDL-1 immunotherapy compared with control groups ($p < 0.05$). A treatment regime with intravesical co-administration of HAL BL and anti-PD-L1 seemed to be more advantageous (38%) compared to the other groups, although the difference was not statistically significant ($p > 0.05$) (Table 4). It is important to note that no signs of suffering were noted with the combination with checkpoints inhibitors.

Table 4. HES-assessed anti-tumor effect in rat bladders 30 days after tumor inoculation. Tumor bearing rats were subjected to ives (intravesical) or i.p. (intraperitoneal) anti- PD-L1 immunotherapy.

Treatments	Tumor Response Grades					
	NR	MR	Near CR	CR	Near CR + CR	
CTR PDL1 ives (n = 9)	9/9	0/9	0/9	0/9	0/9	0%
CTR PDL1 i.p (n = 10)	10/10	0/10	0/10	0/10	0/10	0%
HAL BL PDL1 i.p (n = 9)	7/9	0/9	1/9	1/9	2/9	22%
HAL BL PDL1 ives (n = 10)	6/10	1/10	0/10	3/10	3/10	30%
HAL BL PD-L1 ives co-administered (n = 8)	3/8	2/8	2/8	1/8	3/8	38%
HAL BL * (n = 13)	8/13	1/13	0/13	4/13	4/13	31%

HAL BL: HAL and blue light, CTR: control no drug no light, NR: no response, MR; moderate response, CR; complete response. * Taken from Table 2.

4. Discussion

In our study, we used blue light illumination after intravesical instillation of hexylaminolevulinate alone and in combination with checkpoint inhibitor in rat bladders with orthotopic tumors. This tumor model mimics bladder cancer in humans standing mostly for NMIBC, with a progression to MIBC (stages II-III) [26,32,33]. Studies of photodynamic therapy (PDT) with HAL and red light has been performed in this orthotopic bladder cancer model, demonstrating a positive short-term (48 h–168 h) therapeutic effect [34,35]. Therefore, this model should be suitable for our experiments.

In terms of dosimetry, the idea was to mimic the light doses used during a clinical blue light cystoscopy (PhotoDynamic Diagnosis, PDD). Based on measurements of blue light intensity from the tip of the cystoscope, the average range of light intensities was calculated at the distance between the scope and tumor during a PDD bladder investigation assuming a working distance between 3 and 5 cm. Furthermore, the age of the lamp was considered since its intensity varies with lamp age between 100–60% (lower limit) of full intensity. Based on the above, a range of irradiances of 1.8–12.3 mW/cm^2 (mean 7.0 mW/cm^2) was obtained. In our case, the delivered light doses were calculated by multiplying the above range with the range of typical blue light exposure times during tumor-resection (2–20 min) yielding a range of light doses of 0.2–14.8 J/cm^2 (mean 7.5 J/cm^2). Precise light dosing in in vivo studies, especially in hollow organs, is difficult to conduct due to variations in multiply parameters e.g., light diffusion, light scattering, and exact tumor localization. Therefore, certain caution is needed while interpreting the results. Based on these calculations, we used a fixed irradiance at 7 mW/cm^2 and a total light dose of 7.5 J/cm^2. This is in the same range as documented by Karl Storz for their D-Light C Photodynamic Diagnosis (PDD) system [27]. They report irradiance of blue light (mW/cm^2) of 1.3, 3.5, and 32 for distances from tissue of 5, 3, and 1 cm, respectively.

In this study, we found a significant anti-tumor effect at observation end point, which was fixed at 30 days after tumor grafting with complete response (CR) in 31% (4/13 rats) of animals exposed to HAL and BL (Table 2). At the same time, we observed a strong tumor infiltration with CD3+ and CD8+ T cells in this experimental group indicating a T cell-mediated immune response. Enhancement of T cell activation has also been reported in studies of HAL red light PDT in a similar orthotopic bladder cancer model in rats [32]. The T cells infiltration is a result of an alteration in the tumor microenvironment, stimulating the release of different mediators and recruiting lymphocytes from the circulating blood to the tumor [36,37]. It appears that exposure of HAL BL as used during a diagnostic PDD procedure may result in a similar immune stimulation with activating of the innate and adaptive pathways [9,11,12]. It is likely that this immune system activation is the reason for the anti-tumor effect in the rats exposed to HAL and BL. A higher proportion of rats showed an anti-tumor effect 12 days after being exposed to HAL BL. At this time point, 63% of the rats showed CR (2/8 rats) or near CR (3/8) (Table 2). During the time period between 12 and 30 days, T cell dysfunction, exhaustion, and tolerance may happen due to the ligation of PD-1 with PD-L1 ligand, thus contributing to diminishing of HAL BL long-term effect. PD-1 or PD-L1 blockade can lead to an enhancement of anti-tumor activity [20]. It is also possible that the immune stimulation following single exposure to HAL and BL is not strong enough to control the tumor growth in this model. With the aim of achieving a sustained anti-tumor effect and to assess whether there could be an additional treatment effect we applied a combination of HAL and BL with targeted anti-PD-1 immunotherapy. PD-L1 is strongly expressed in MIBC but also in advanced stages of NMIBC [28]. Two administration routes of anti-PD-1 were tested in this model, intravesical and intraperitoneal. Irrespective of intravesical or intraperitoneal administration, targeted immunotherapy administered alone was ineffective as none of the tested rats responded positively (Table 4). Contrary, all groups exposed to HAL showed a positive anti-tumor effect although this effect was statistically significant only for rats exposed to HAL BL and where HAL BL was combined with intravesical administered anti-PDL-1 immunonotherapy. A treatment regime where HAL BL and anti-PD-L1 were co-administered intravesically at the same day provided the best antitumor effect where 38% of the rats showed near CR and CR. The somewhat lower anti-tumor effect when anti-PD-1 was administered i.p. (22%) compared to ives (30%) might also be explained by the lower concentration of anti-PD-1 used for this administration route.

The rather modest incremental effect seen when combining HAL BL with anti-PD-1 might be explained by the weak PD-L1 expression on the tumor cells. In our study, IHC-assessed PD-L1 expression in bladder cancer samples clearly showed that a strong expression of PD-L1 was evident 12 days after tumor implantation but it did not sustain (Table 3). Although expression of PD-L1 in tumors is correlated with higher response to therapy, this is not definite, and it is argued that an absence of PD-L1 expression in biopsies does not preclude response to anti-PD-1/PD-L1 immunotherapy [22]. It has earlier been reported that radiotherapy upregulates the PD-L1 expression on tumors cells, justifying the combination with anti-PD1/anti-PD-L1 inhibitors [28]. Moreover, CD8+ T cells are shown to be vital for the local and systemic therapeutic effects seen after combining radiation with checkpoint inhibitors [28]. As tumor infiltration with CD8+ T cells was not observed in our study until 30 days after tumor grafting, a potential upregulation of the PD-L1 expression as a consequence of T cell tumor infiltration amplifying the effect of the anti-PD-1 checkpoint inhibitor was not possible to rule out at observation end point for our study.

A recent study of Kirschner et al. compared efficacy of intravesical versus systemic (intraperitoneal) administration of an anti-PD-1 inhibitor in the treatment of localized bladder cancer in an orthotopic mouse model [38]. Intravesical anti-PD-1 administration had trend to improved survival thus providing effective anti-tumor treatment for bladder tumors. Further, increased CD8+ T cells infiltration in tumors was observed, especially after intravesical administration. Our study also demonstrated that intravesical administration of anti-PD-L1 combined with HAL BL has an improved survival over systemic i.p. administration, probably due to a higher local drug concentration after ives administration. Local immunotherapy administration into the bladder could represent a substantial clinical benefit, reducing systemic exposure and side effects. Our study in rats and the study reported by Kirschner et al. [38] in mice are encouraging in this respect. However, additional clinical trials are warranted before intravesical instillation of anti-PD-L1 could be widely used in humans alone or in combination with HAL and BL.

This is to the best of our knowledge the first proof-of principle study demonstrating an anti-tumor effect and indication of immune activation following HAL and BL exposure in vivo. Our hypothesis of immune activation could be strengthened by performing T cell depletion using anti-CD3. Moreover, IHC assessments could be supplemented by flow cytometry to give more conclusive results. Future studies can benefit from analysis of other immune markers including cytokine panels, antigen-specific CD8+, and granzyme B production.

5. Conclusions

We have demonstrated an anti-tumor effect of HAL and blue light when trying to mimic the dosing regimen of a photodynamic diagnostic procedure in an orthotropic bladder cancer model in rats. The anti-tumor effect is most probably pertaining to stimulation of the immune system as evident by tumor infiltration of CD3+ and CD8 + T cells. These results support our hypothesis that the positive impact on patient outcomes observed in patients who had undergone BLC prior to cystectomy could be explained by systemic immune activation induced by HAL and blue light. Combination of HAL and blue light with intravesical anti-PD-L1 resulted in increased anti-tumor effects. Further studies are warranted to explore the long-term effects of HAL and blue light alone or in combination with checkpoint inhibitors which should extend to investigate any systemic (abscopal) effects. The idea that local treatment with HAL and blue light can prime an immune response with potential additional effect of checkpoint inhibitors is also intriguing.

Author Contributions: Investigation, methodology, L.L.; formal analysis, validation, J.T.; formal analysis, investigation, A.L.; methodology, supervision, J.-F.B.; Writing—review and editing, K.M.; Conceptualization, project administration, writing—original draft, A.G.; funding acquisition, Methodology, writing—original draft, writing—review and editing, G.S.; project administration, supervision, writing—original draft, writing—review and editing, L.B. All authors have read and agreed to the published version of the manuscript.

Funding: This work was supported by Photocure ASA (Oslo, Norway) which also supplied Hexvix®. Aslak Godal, Gry Stensrud and Kari Myren were employed by Photocure ASA during the course of this study.

Institutional Review Board Statement: The study was conducted according to the guidelines of the European Communities Council Directive on the approximation of laws, regulations, and administrative provisions of the Member States regarding the protection of animals used for scientific purposes, the National Institutes of Health Guide for the care and use of laboratory animals and the ASAB Ethical Committee. The studies received approval from the French Ministry of Higher Education and Research (agreements no. APAFIS#14510 on 9 July 2018, and no. APAFIS#23597 on 3 March 2020).

Data Availability Statement: The dataset generated and analyzed in this study is not publicly available but may be obtained from the corresponding author upon reasonable request.

Acknowledgments: The authors thank Knut Dyrstad, KD Metrix, for his expertise and assistance with the statistical analysis used in this manuscript.

Conflicts of Interest: The authors declare no conflict of interest.

References

1. Miranda-Filho, A.; Bray, F.; Charvat, H.; Rajaraman, S.; Soerjomataram, I. The world cancer patient population (WCPP): An updated standard for international comparisons of population-based survival. *Cancer Epidemiol.* **2020**, *69*, 101802. [CrossRef] [PubMed]
2. Matulewicz, R.S.; Steinberg, G.D. Non-muscle-invasive bladder cancer: Overview and contemporary treatment landscape of neoadjuvant chemoablative therapies. *Rev. Urol.* **2020**, *22*, 43–51. [PubMed]
3. Di Stasi, S.M.; De Carlo, F.; Pagliarulo, V.; Masedu, F.; Verri, C.; Celestino, F.; Riedl, C. Hexaminolevulinate hydrochloride in the detection of nonmuscle invasive cancer of the bladder. *Ther. Adv. Urol.* **2015**, *7*, 339–350. [CrossRef] [PubMed]
4. Stenzl, A.; Burger, M.; Fradet, Y.; Mynderse, L.A.; Soloway, M.S.; Witjes, J.A.; Kriegmair, M.; Karl, A.; Shen, Y.; Grossman, H.B. Hexaminolevulinate guided fluorescence cystoscopy reduces recurrence in patients with nonmuscle invasive bladder cancer. *J. Urol.* **2010**, *184*, 1907–1914. [CrossRef] [PubMed]
5. Grossman, H.B.; Stenzl, A.; Fradet, Y.; Mynderse, L.A.; Kriegmair, M.; Witjes, J.A.; Soloway, M.S.; Karl, A.; Burger, M. Long-term decrease in bladder cancer recurrence with hexaminolevulinate enabled fluorescence cystoscopy. *J. Urol.* **2012**, *188*, 58–62. [CrossRef]
6. Chang, S.S.; Boorjian, S.A.; Chou, R.; Clark, P.E.; Daneshmand, S.; Konety, B.R.; Pruthi, R.; Quale, D.Z.; Ritch, C.R.; Seigne, J.D.; et al. Diagnosis and treatment of non-muscle invasive bladder cancer: AUA/SUO guideline. *J. Urol.* **2016**, *196*, 1021–1029. [CrossRef]
7. EAU Guidelines: Non-Muscle-Invasive Bladder Cancer. Available online: https://uroweb.org/guideline/non-muscle-invasive-bladder-cancer/ (accessed on 5 January 2022).
8. Garg, A.D.; Nowis, D.; Golab, J.; Agostinis, P. Photodynamic therapy: Illuminating the road from cell death towards anti-tumour immunity. *Apoptosis* **2010**, *15*, 1050–1071. [CrossRef]
9. Mroz, P.; Hashmi, J.T.; Huang, Y.; Lange, N.; Hamblin, M.R. Stimulation of anti-tumor immunity by photodynamic therapy. *Expert Rev. Clin. Immunol.* **2011**, *7*, 75–91. [CrossRef]
10. Reginato, E.; Wolf, P.; Hamblin, M.R. Immune response after photodynamic therapy increases anti-cancer and anti-bacterial effects. *World J. Immunol.* **2014**, *4*, 1–11. [CrossRef]
11. Anzengruber, F.; Avci, P.; de Freitas, L.F.; Hamblin, M.R. T-cell mediated anti-tumor immunity after photodynamic therapy: Why does it not always work and how can we improve it? *Photochem. Photobiol. Sci.* **2015**, *14*, 1492–1509. [CrossRef]
12. Hwang, H.S.; Shin, H.; Han, J.; Na, K. Combination of photodynamic therapy (PDT) and anti-tumor immunity in cancer therapy. *J. Pharm. Investig.* **2018**, *48*, 143–151. [CrossRef] [PubMed]
13. Bader, M.J.; Stepp, H.; Beyer, W.; Pongratz, T.; Sroka, R.; Kriegmair, M.; Dirk, Z.; Mona, W.; Derya, T.; Christian, G.S.; et al. Photodynamic therapy of bladder cancer—A phase I study using hexaminolevulinate (HAL). *Urol. Oncol. Semin. Orig. Investig.* **2013**, *31*, 1178–1183. [CrossRef] [PubMed]
14. Gakis, G.; Ngamsri, T.; Rausch, S.; Mischinger, J.; Todenhöfer, T.; Schwentner, C.; Schmid, M.A.; Hassan, F.A.-S.; Renninger, M.; Stenzl, A. Fluorescence-guided bladder tumour resection: Impact on survival after radical cystectomy. *World J. Urol.* **2015**, *33*, 1429–1437. [CrossRef] [PubMed]

15. Renninger, M.; Fahmy, O.; Schubert, T.; Schmid, M.A.; Hassan, F.; Stenzl, A.; Gakis, G. The prognostic impact of hexaminolevulinate-based bladder tumor resection in patients with primary non-muscle invasive bladder cancer treated with radical cystectomy. *World J. Urol.* **2019**, *38*, 397–406. [CrossRef] [PubMed]
16. Pardoll, D.M. The blockade of immune checkpoints in cancer immunotherapy. *Nat. Rev. Cancer* **2012**, *12*, 252–264. [CrossRef]
17. Song, D.; Powles, T.; Shi, L.; Zhang, L.; Ingersoll, M.A.; Lu, Y. Bladder cancer, a unique model to understand cancer immunity and develop immunotherapy approaches. *J. Pathol.* **2019**, *249*, 151–165. [CrossRef]
18. Kim, H.S.; Seo, H.K. Emerging treatments for bacillus Calmette–Guérin-unresponsive non-muscle-invasive bladder cancer. *Investig. Clin. Urol.* **2021**, *62*, 361–377. [CrossRef]
19. Lopez-Beltran, A.; Cimadamore, A.; Blanca, A.; Massari, F.; Vau, N.; Scarpelli, M.; Cheng, L.; Montironi, R. Immune checkpoint inhibitors for the treatment of bladder cancer. *Cancers* **2021**, *13*, 131. [CrossRef]
20. Hahn, N.M.; Necchi, A.; Loriot, Y.; Powles, T.; Plimack, E.R.; Sonpavde, G.; Roupret, M.; Kamat, A.M. Role of checkpoint inhibition in localized bladder cancer. *Eur. Urol. Oncol.* **2018**, *1*, 190–198. [CrossRef]
21. Anand, S.; Chan, T.; Hasan, T.; Maytin, E. Current prospects for treatment of solid tumors via photodynamic, photothermal, or ionizing radiation therapies combined with immune checkpoint inhibition (a review). *Pharmaceuticals* **2021**, *14*, 447. [CrossRef]
22. O'Shaughnessy, M.J.; Murray, K.S.; La Rosa, S.P.; Budhu, S.; Merghoub, T.; Somma, A.; Monette, S.; Kim, K.; Corradi, R.B.; Scherz, A.; et al. Systemic antitumor immunity by PD-1/PD-L1 inhibition is potentiated by vascular-targeted photodynamic therapy of primary tumors. *Clin. Cancer Res.* **2017**, *24*, 592–599. [CrossRef] [PubMed]
23. Gao, L.; Zhang, C.; Gao, D.; Liu, H.; Yu, X.; Lai, J.; Wang, F.; Lin, J.; Liu, Z. Enhanced anti-tumor efficacy through a combination of integrin αvβ6-targeted photodynamic therapy and immune checkpoint inhibition. *Theranostics* **2016**, *6*, 627–637. [CrossRef] [PubMed]
24. Kleinovink, J.W.; Fransen, M.F.; Löwik, C.W.; Ossendorp, F. Photodynamic-Immune checkpoint therapy eradicates local and distant tumors by CD8+ T cells. *Cancer Immunol. Res.* **2017**, *5*, 832–838. [CrossRef]
25. Liu, Q.; Tian, J.; Tian, Y.; Sun, Q.; Sun, D.; Wang, F.; Xu, H.; Ying, G.; Wang, J.; Yetisen, A.K.; et al. Near-infrared-ii nanoparticles for cancer imaging of immune checkpoint programmed death-ligand 1 and photodynamic/immune therapy. *ACS Nano* **2021**, *15*, 515–525. [CrossRef] [PubMed]
26. Xiao, Z.; McCallum, T.J.; Brown, K.M.; Miller, G.G.; Halls, S.B.; Parney, I.; Moore, R. Characterization of a novel transplantable orthotopic rat bladder transitional cell tumour model. *Br. J. Cancer* **1999**, *81*, 638–646. [CrossRef] [PubMed]
27. Summary of Safety and Effectiveness (SSED). Karl Storz D-Light C Photodynamic Diagnosis (PDD) System. PMA Number P050027. Available online: https://fda.report/PMA/P050027/5/P050027B.pdf (accessed on 9 February 2022).
28. Wu, C.-T.; Chen, W.-C.; Chang, Y.-H.; Lin, W.-Y.; Chen, M.-F. The role of PD-L1 in the radiation response and clinical outcome for bladder cancer. *Sci. Rep.* **2016**, *6*, 19740. [CrossRef] [PubMed]
29. Efficacy of Durvalumab in Non-Muscle-Invasive Bladder Cancer. Available online: https://www.clinicaltrials.gov/ct2/show/NCT03759496?term=PD-L1&cond=NMIBC&rank=1 (accessed on 7 February 2022).
30. Kim, S.H.; Chan, P.S.; Kim, D.Y.; Park, J.W.; Baek, J.Y.; Kim, S.Y.; Park, S.C.; Oh, J.H.; Byung-Ho, N.; Nam, B.-H. What is the ideal tumor regression grading system in rectal cancer patients after preoperative chemoradiotherapy? *Cancer Res. Treat.* **2016**, *48*, 998–1009. [CrossRef]
31. Bressenot, A.; Marchal, S.; Bezdetnaya, L.; Garrier, J.; Guillemin, F.; Plénat, F. Assessment of apoptosis by immunohistochemistry to active caspase-3, active caspase-7, or cleaved PARP in monolayer cells and spheroid and subcutaneous xenografts of human carcinoma. *J. Histochem. Cytochem.* **2009**, *57*, 289–300. [CrossRef]
32. Arum, C.-J.; Gederaas, O.A.; Larsen, E.L.P.; Randeberg, L.L.; Hjelde, A.; Krokan, H.E.; Svaasand, L.O.; Chen, D.; Zhao, C.-M. Tissue responses to hexyl 5-aminolevulinate-induced photodynamic treatment in syngeneic orthotopic rat bladder cancer model: Possible pathways of action. *J. Biomed. Opt.* **2011**, *16*, 028001. [CrossRef]
33. Lilge, L.; Roufaiel, M.; Lazic, S.; Kaspler, P.; Munegowda, M.A.; Nitz, M.; Bassan, J.; Mandel, A. Evaluation of a Ruthenium coordination complex as photosensitizer for PDT of bladder cancer: Cellular response, tissue selectivity and in vivo response. *Transl. Biophotonics* **2020**, *2*, 2. [CrossRef]
34. Larsen, E.L.P.; Randeberg, L.L.; Gederaas, O.A.; Arum, C.-J.; Hjelde, A.; Zhao, C.-M.; Chen, D.; Krokan, H.E.; Svaasand, L.O. Monitoring of hexyl 5-aminolevulinate-induced photodynamic therapy in rat bladder cancer by optical spectroscopy. *J. Biomed. Opt.* **2008**, *13*, 044031. [CrossRef] [PubMed]
35. François, A.; Salvadori, A.; Bressenot, A.; Bezdetnaya, L.; Guillemin, F.; D'Hallewin, M.A. How to avoid local side effects of bladder photodynamic therapy: Impact of the fluence rate. *J. Urol.* **2013**, *190*, 731–736. [CrossRef] [PubMed]
36. Rocha, L.B.; Gomes-Da-Silva, L.C.; Dąbrowski, J.M.; Arnaut, L.G. Elimination of primary tumours and control of metastasis with rationally designed bacteriochlorin photodynamic therapy regimens. *Eur. J. Cancer* **2015**, *51*, 1822–1830. [CrossRef] [PubMed]
37. Preise, D.; Oren, R.; Glinert, I.; Kalchenko, V.; Jung, S.; Scherz, A.; Salomon, Y. Systemic antitumor protection by vascular-targeted photodynamic therapy involves cellular and humoral immunity. *Cancer Immunol. Immunother.* **2009**, *58*, 71–84. [CrossRef]
38. Kirschner, A.N.; Wang, J.; Rajkumar-Calkins, A.; Neuzil, K.E.; Chang, S.S. Intravesical anti-pd-1 immune checkpoint inhibition treats urothelial bladder cancer in a mouse model. *J. Urol.* **2020**, *205*, 1336–1343. [CrossRef]

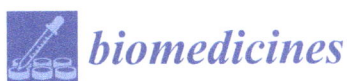

Article

Chlorin Endogenous to the North Pacific Brittle Star *Ophiura sarsii* for Photodynamic Therapy Applications in Breast Cancer and Glioblastoma Models

Antonina Klimenko [1,†], Elvira E. Rodina [1,†], Denis Silachev [2,†], Maria Begun [1], Valentina A. Babenko [2], Anton S. Benditkis [3], Anton S. Kozlov [3], Alexander A. Krasnovsky [3], Yuri S. Khotimchenko [1] and Vladimir L. Katanaev [1,4,*]

[1] Institute of Life Sciences and Biomedicine, Far Eastern Federal University, 690922 Vladivostok, Russia; klimenko.am@dvfu.ru (A.K.); rodina.ee@dvfu.ru (E.E.R.); begun.ma@dvfu.ru (M.B.); khotimchenko.ys@dvfu.ru (Y.S.K.)

[2] A.N. Belozersky Research Institute of Physico-Chemical Biology, Moscow State University, 119899 Moscow, Russia; proteins@mail.ru (D.S.); babenkova@belozersky.msu.ru (V.A.B.)

[3] Federal Research Center of Biotechnology of the Russian Academy of Sciences, 119071 Moscow, Russia; anton93benditkis@yandex.ru (A.S.B.); anton4ikk_06@mail.ru (A.S.K.); phoal@mail.ru (A.A.K.)

[4] Translational Research Center in Oncohaematology, Department of Cell Physiology and Metabolism, Faculty of Medicine, University of Geneva, 1211 Geneva, Switzerland

* Correspondence: vladimir.katanaev@unige.ch

† These authors contributed equally to this work.

Abstract: Photodynamic therapy (PDT) represents a powerful avenue for anticancer treatment. PDT relies on the use of photosensitizers—compounds accumulating in the tumor and converted from benign to cytotoxic upon targeted photoactivation. We here describe (3S,4S)-14-Ethyl-9-(hydroxymethyl)-4,8,13,18-tetramethyl-20-oxo-3-phorbinepropanoic acid (ETPA) as a major metabolite of the North Pacific brittle stars *Ophiura sarsii*. As a chlorin, ETPA efficiently produces singlet oxygen upon red-light photoactivation and exerts powerful sub-micromolar phototoxicity against a panel of cancer cell lines in vitro. In a mouse model of glioblastoma, intravenous ETPA injection combined with targeted red laser irradiation induced strong necrotic ablation of the brain tumor. Along with the straightforward ETPA purification protocol and abundance of *O. sarsii*, these studies pave the way for the development of ETPA as a novel natural product-based photodynamic therapeutic.

Keywords: porphyrin; chlorin; singlet oxygen; photodynamic therapy; ophiura; cancer; breast cancer; glioblastoma; mouse models

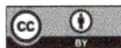

1. Introduction

Photodynamic therapy (PDT) relies on the use of photosensitizers—compounds that are relatively benign until excited by light of a particular wavelength that converts them into an activated state resulting in the generation of reactive oxygen species [1–3]. PDT finds multiple applications in medicine, particularly in anticancer therapy, where it has been approved to treat cancers in the skin (basal cell carcinoma), lungs, or esophagus [2,3]. Other forms of cancer, such as in the breast or brain (e.g., glioblastoma) have so far evaded approved PDT applications [2,3].

A number of photosensitizers have been marketed for PDT in different countries, and the search for novel compounds never ceases [3,4]. Photosensitizers activatable in the red part of the spectrum are particularly sought, as the red light can penetrate deeper in biological tissues [1,3]. Derived from chemical synthesis, these complex compounds weigh upon the costs of PDT; stability in body fluids is another issue with synthetic photosensitizers [3,4].

Natural products have always been one of the major sources of new drugs, including oncology therapeutics [5–7]. Porphyrin-type compounds such as chlorins can act as efficient photosensitizers and have been found in diverse living groups [4,8]. In a search for novel anticancer compounds from ophiuras [9], we have recently discovered the chlorin (3S,4S)-14-Ethyl-9-(hydroxymethyl)-4,8,13,18-tetramethyl-20-oxo-3-phorbinepropanoic acid (ETPA) from a North Pacific brittle star *Ophiura sarsii*—the first-ever porphyrin identified in Ophiuroidea (phylum Echinodermata) [10]. This discovery was unexpected, as Ophiuroidea were believed to lack porphyrin/chlorin synthesis [11] and raised the hypothesis that the *Ophiura sarsii* chlorin was the result of dietary (and perhaps seasonal) consumption by these marine invertebrates [10].

In the current work, we provide evidence that ETPA production is endogenous to *Ophiura sarsii* and is independent of their food consumption. As a major metabolite in this abundant brittle star species and amenable to simple purification, the 663 nm light-absorbing chlorin shows sub-micromolar phototoxicity against a panel of cancer cells in vitro and serves as an efficient PDT against glioblastoma in a mouse model. Our findings pave the way for the development of ETPA as a natural photosensitizer in a broad spectrum of PDT applications.

2. Materials and Methods

2.1. Species Collection and Food Deprivation

Brittle stars *Ophiura sarsii* were collected at the depths of 15–18 m near the Vyatlin Cape (Russky Island) in the Peter the Great Gulf, Sea of Japan, in December 2020. Sample collection was performed by the standards approved by the Ministry of Science and Higher Education (Russia); all efforts were made to minimize animal suffering. Brittle stars (wet weight—25 g) were separated into two groups. The first group, after thorough 2× running water rinsing, was frozen and stored at −80 °C. The second was placed into a clean spacious aquarium regularly refilled with fresh sterilized and filtered seawater without any source of food. Gradual emptying of the animals' digestive tracks could be visually seen in the first days of such fasting. After 12 days, the food-deprived animals were rinsed and stored as the first group.

2.2. Homogenization and Extraction

O. sarsii were mechanically homogenized and then sequentially placed in solvents with increasing polarity: hexane, chloroform, ethanol, and water (125 mL each) at room temperature for 8–12 h, with constant stirring on a PSU-10i shaker (Biosan, Riga, Latvia). The ratio of solvents to the homogenized mass was 5:1 (volume). The resulting extracts were cleared through paper filters and concentrated on a Hei-VAP Value Rotary Evaporator (Heidolph, Schwabach, Germany) at 37–40 °C under vacuum (chemical vacuum station PC 3002 VARIO (Vacuubrand, Wertheim, Germany)). The chlorin (3S,4S)-14-Ethyl-9-(hydroxymethyl)-4,8,13,18-tetramethyl-20-oxo-3-phorbinepropanoic acid (ETPA) localized to the ethanol fraction [10] that contained 721.5 mg (control brittle stars) and 579 mg (fasted brittle stars) dry weight. To remove salts from the ethanol extract, liquid-liquid extraction was performed. The ethanol extract was dissolved in 30 mL n-butanol and 50 mL water and transferred to a separatory funnel. The organic (butanol) phase was extracted 3× with 50 mL water. Then, n-butanol was removed from the fraction using the rotary evaporator, followed by dissolution of the precipitate in methanol for subsequent chromatography.

2.3. Analytical and Semi-Preparative HPLC

Analytical and Semi-Preparative HPLC was performed on a Shimadzu system (Shimadzu, Kyoto, Japan) equipped with LC-20AP modular pumps, an SPD-20A spectrophotometric detector, and an FRC-10A fraction collector. Analytical separation was performed on a Shim-pack SHIMADZU GIST C18 column (250 mm × 4.6 mm, particle size 5 µm). MeOH was used as the mobile phase solution A, and water acidified with 0.1% formic acid—as solution B. Chromatography was performed at a rate of 0.6 mL/min at 40 °C, with a maximum pressure of 10 MPa. Elution was achieved with a gradient: from 50 to 95% MeOH solution in 55 min, then 95% solution for 10 min, then returned to 50% MeOH in 5 min. Reanalysis was performed after complete conditioning of the column. Detection was carried out on a spectrophotometric detector at wavelengths of 210 nm and 366 nm.

Separation of extracts was carried out on a Shim-pack SHIMADZU GIST C18 column (250 mm × 10.00 mm, particle size 5 µm) with a mobile phase of methanol (solution A) and water acidified with 0.1% formic acid (solution B). Chromatography was performed at a rate of 2.6 mL/min at 23 °C. The gradient was from 80 to 97% solution in 50 min, 97% solution A in 8 min, then return to 80% MeOH in 7 min with UV detection at 210 nm and 366 nm.

2.4. High-Resolution Spectrophotometry

High-Resolution Spectrophotometry of the chromatographic fraction containing ETPA dissolved in methanol was performed by a UV-1800 spectrophotometer (Shimadzu, Kyoto, Japan) in the wavelength range from 200 to 800 nm.

2.5. Cells and Medium

Human breast cancer cells MCF-7, BT-20 and MDA-MB-231 (all from ATCC, atcc.org), rat C6 glioma cells and human embryonic kidney (HEK-293 cells, both from Collection of vertebrate cell cultures, Institute of Cytology, Russian Academy of Sciences (incras.ru/wp-content/uploads/2019/06/katalog_rccc_v_2018_rus.pdf, accessed on 21 December 2021) were cultured in DMEM + GlutaMAX medium (Gibco, Waltham, MA, USA) supplemented with 10% fetal bovine serum (Biosera, Nuaille, France) and 1% antibiotic–antimycotic (Gibco, USA). Cell cultures were grown in a CO_2 incubator with a Galaxy 48R cell vitality monitoring and vitality system (Eppendorf, Hamburg, Germany) at 37 °C and 5% CO_2.

2.6. Photoxicity Assays

ETPA was dissolved in DMSO. In 96-well microculture plates, human breast cancer and glioma cells were seeded at the density of 3000 cells/well and cultured overnight in a CO_2 incubator at 37 °C. After medium removal, 50 µL DPBS with serial dilutions of ETPA was added for 2 h (the resultant concentration of DMSO in the wells was <0.2%). Cells in pure DPBS served as a positive control; wells with DPBS without cells served as a negative control. Next, the cells were irradiated with red light in the wavelength range from 580 to 780 nm using a 2000–4000 lux LED lamp for 30 min. Removal of ETPA immediately before light exposure did not reduce/influence the resulting phototoxicity. Photosynthetic photon flux density (PPFD) was measured in 12 randomly chosen wells using the LI-190R Quantum Sensor (LI-COR Biosciences, Lincoln, NE, USA) and found to vary from 217–580 µmol/m^2/s. Fluence was measured (using a Newport Optical Power Meter 842-PE, MKS Instruments, Norwood, MA, USA) to be 16.04 J/cm^2. Next, a 200 µL culture medium was added to each well for additional incubation for 72 h in a CO_2 incubator at 37 °C.

To assess cell death, the culture medium was removed and 50 µL of MTT (triazolyl blue tetrazolium bromide) reagent (DIA-M, Moscow, Russia) dissolved in DPBS at 0.5 mg/mL was added for 3 h incubation at 37 °C. After aspiration of the liquid, 100 µL DMSO was added to each well for 5 min before measuring the optical density at wavelengths of 570 and 630 nm using a Cytation 5 multifunctional plate reader (BioTek, Winooski, VT, USA). MTT was separately performed for C6 and HEK-293 cells in the dark to obtain light-independent cytotoxicity. IC_{50} and standard error of the mean (SEM) were obtained by standard dose–response curve fitting using GraphPad Prism 8.

2.7. Determination of the Singlet Oxygen Quantum Yield of ETPA

Singlet oxygen was detected using two methods. One of them was based on the measurement of the rates of chemical trapping of singlet oxygen by 1,3-diphenylisobenzofuran (DPIBF) (Acros Organics, Geel, Belgium, >99%) as described [12,13]; see Supplementary

Figure S1. Having a strong absorption maximum at 414 nm, DPIBF is efficiently oxidized by singlet oxygen forming colorless products having no absorption maxima in the visible spectral region. The rate of DPIBF bleaching is directly proportional to the rate of $^1O_2$ production by irradiation of a photosensitizer. The absorption spectra of the trap solutions were recorded with the SF-56 spectrophotometer (LOMO Spektr, St. Petersburg, Russia). For irradiation, a xenon lamp and grating monochromator were employed.

Another method was based on detection of the infrared phosphorescence of singlet oxygen at 1270 nm, which arises due to the energy transfer from the triplet state of the photosensitizer molecules to oxygen, followed by the population of singlet oxygen (the reactive excited singlet ($^1\Delta_g$) state of oxygen molecules); see Supplementary Figure S2. Measurements were carried out using a laser/LED spectrometer assembled at the Federal Research Center of Biotechnology of the Russian Academy of Sciences [14]. The spectrometer allowed phosphorescence detection upon excitation by pulses of LED with the emission maxima at 399 nm (Polironik, Moscow, Russia). Phosphorescence was recorded at a 90° angle with respect to the excitation beam through the cut-off filter that transmitted IR light at $\lambda > 1000$ nm and one of three interchangeable interference filters with transmission maxima at 1230, 1270, and 1310 nm and half-width of 10 nm. The photodetector was an FEU-112 photomultiplier (Ekran Optical Systems, Novosibirsk, Russia) (PMT), with the S-1 spectral response cooled to -35 °C. PMT impulses were sent to a broadband (0–200 MHz) preamplifier and then to a USB computer board, which was launched by additional electric pulses synchronous with the pulses of the LED. The signal of the board was processed by a personal computer with the Parsec (Dubna, Russia) software. As a result, the time interval between pulses was divided into 256, 512, or 1024 channels, and the computer showed the number of PMT impulses accumulated in each channel during the irradiation time, thus forming the kinetic curves of singlet oxygen phosphorescence after LED pulses.

The phosphorescence method provides more information on singlet oxygen than the trapping method. However, the trapping method is much more sensitive. Acetone was employed as the solvent for the singlet oxygen measurements because ETPA is readily soluble in it. The absorption spectrum of ETPA in acetone is shown in Supplementary Figure S3.

2.8. Mouse Experimentation

Mouse Experimentation was conducted in accordance with the ethical standards and recommendations for accommodation and care of laboratory animals covered by the Council Directives of the European community 2010/63/EU on the use of animals for experimental studies. The animal protocols were approved by the institutional animal ethics committee of A.N. Belozersky Research Institute of Physico-Chemical Biology, Approval Code: Protocol 8/21, Approval Date: 7 September 2021.

2.9. Cell Culture and Intracranial Tumor Implantation

C6 glioma cells were harvested with trypsin/versene while in the logarithmic phase of growth before intracranial stereotaxic implantation as a single cell suspension (1×10^6 cells/mL) into young C57BL/6 female mice (18 ± 3 g). Under isoflurane anesthesia (2–2.5% in air) by the SomnoSuite® system (Kent Scientific Corporation, Torrington, CT, USA), the mouse was placed in a stereotactic frame, and the skull was exposed through a midline incision cleared of connective tissue and dried. Implantation was performed at the following coordinates: ML, -2.5; AP, -1.0; DV, -3.0, as previously described [15]. C6 glioma cells (5×10^5 per mouse) were implanted with Robot Stereotaxic (Neurostar, Tubingen, Germany) using a Hamilton microsyringe at the speed of 3 µL/min in 10 µL PBS.

2.10. Glioma Photodynamic Therapy (PDT)

PDT was performed 7 days after intracranial tumor implantation. Anatomical positioning of the tumor was obtained by brain magnetic resonance imaging (MRI) visualization. Tumor-bearing mice were sensitized via intravenous injection into the jugular vein of ETPA at 40 mg/kg of body weight 6 h pre-PDT; the drug dose regime was chosen following the study by [16]. Application of ETPA and PDT were conducted under isoflurane anesthesia. The brain skull in the illumination area was thinned with a milling cutter and illuminated for 30 min with a red laser light source (L04-1H, 650 nm, output power 100 mW) producing a 1.5 mm diameter light beam, positioned on the region corresponding to the stereotaxic coordinates of the prior tumor injection. The surface of the skull was constantly cooled with saline to avoid thermal damage to the brain. Rectal temperature was kept constant at 37.0 ± 0.2 °C using a heating pad. After PDT, the animals were returned to cages, provided with water and food ad libitum, and continually monitored for any signs of neurological deficit. The tumor-bearing group included 5 mice.

2.11. Magnetic Resonance Imaging and Histological Studies of the Tumor Injury

PDT-induced tumor injury was identified by analyzing brain MRI scans obtained 5 days after PDT on a 7-T magnet (Bruker BioSpec 70/30 USR; Bruker BioSpin, Ettlingen, Germany) using an 86 mm volume resonator for radiofrequency transmission and a phased array mice head surface coil for the reception. Before scanning, the animals were anesthetized with isoflurane 2–2.5% in a mixture of oxygen and air. Mice were placed in a prone position on a water-heated bed. The heads of the mice were immobilized using a nose mask and masking tape. The imaging protocol included a T2-weighted image sequence (time to repetition = 4500 ms, time to echo = 12 ms, slice thickness = 0.5 mm). After MRI, the animals were sacrificed, and the brains were removed, fixed, sectioned, and stained by hematoxylin–eosin.

3. Results

3.1. Chlorin Is Endogenous to O. sarsii

Since Ophiuroidea as the class of the Echinodermata phylum were considered porphyrin-free [11], we hypothesized that the chlorin (3S,4S)-14-Ethyl-9-(hydroxymethyl)-4,8,13,18-tetramethyl-20-oxo-3-phorbinepropanoic acid (ETPA) we previously discovered in the North Pacific *Ophiura sarsii* could result from the dietary consumption; the resulting seasonal variability in the ETPA content was also considered possible [10]. To address this issue, we performed a new *O. sarsii* collection in the same location but another season (December vs. May in [10]). Analytical HPLC (Figure 1A) of the butanol fraction of the ethanol extract of the freshly collected *O. sarsii* contained a major peak at a wavelength of 366 nm at the retention time of 52 min, which corresponds to ETPA as the major 366 nm absorbing compound from our previous study [10], arguing against a seasonal diversity in the new chlorin compound in the brittle stars.

In order to directly rule out that ETPA could be a dietary derivative of *O. sarsii*, we separated the fresh catch of the brittle stars into two portions, one subjected to direct freezing and processing and the other fasted for 12 days prior to processing for preparative isolation (see Methods). Briefly, 15 mg and 20 mg of the butanol fraction of the EtOH extracts from non-fasted and fasted brittle stars, respectively, were subjected to semi-preparative chromatography (Figure 1B). Identical chromatograms were obtained for fasted and non-fasted preparations, with the major 366 nm absorption peak (retention time 34–37 min), corresponding to ETPA from our prior work [10], collected for subsequent analyses.

To control the identity of the compound in the collected fractions, spectrophotometry was performed in the wavelength range of 200–800 nm. The resulting absorbance spectra were identical for the compound isolated from the fasted and non-fasted brittles stars and revealed the absorption typical for chlorins, with the absorbance peaks at 204, 293, 409, and 663 nm (Figure 2A), also fully coinciding with ETPA isolated by us from *O. sarsii* previously [10].

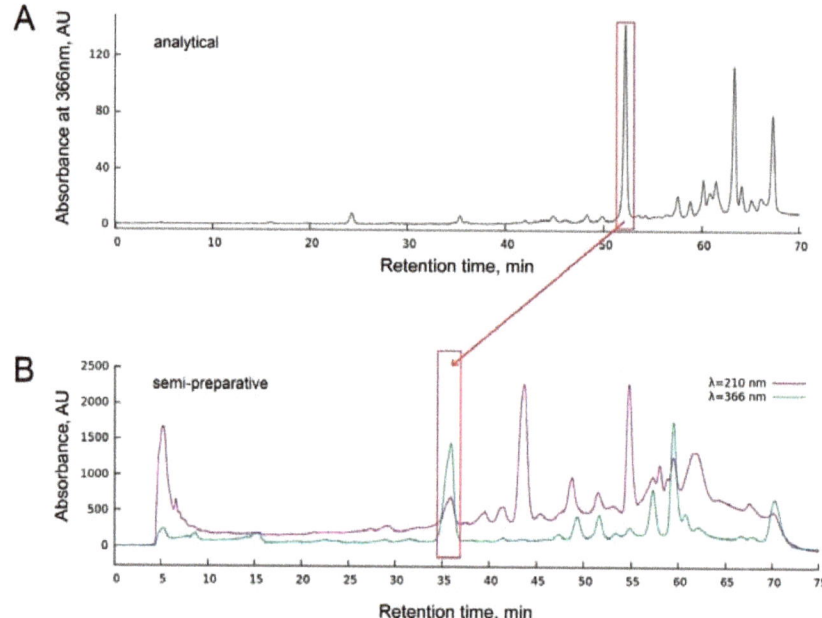

Figure 1. Analytical (**A**) and semi-preparative (**B**) chromatography of the butanol fraction of the EtOH extract of *O. sarsii*, absorption intensity at the wavelength of 366 nm (**A**) and 210 nm/366 nm (**B**). The major peak at the retention time of 52 min (**A**) and 35 min (**B**) corresponds to ETPA (chlorin) from our previous study [10]. Chromatograms from non-fasted ophiuras are shown in both panels; samples from the fasted ophiuras show identical chromatograms.

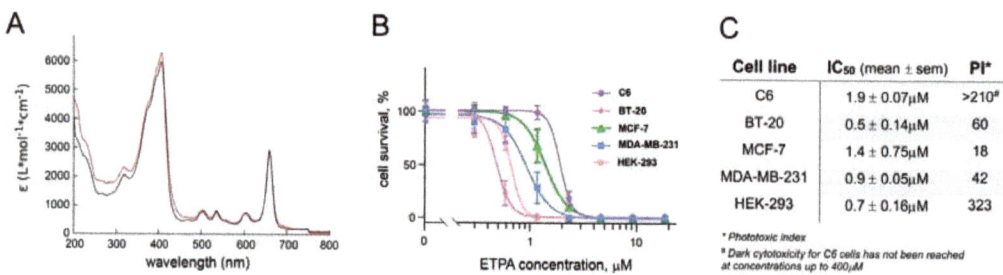

Figure 2. (**A**) Absorbance spectra of the chlorin compound isolated from the butanol fraction of the EtOH extract from control (red) and fasted (black) *O. sarsii* reveal absorbance peaks typical for chlorins, identical between the two preparations; (**B**) cell survival (MTT test) to evaluate the strong phototoxicity of ETPA after red-light irradiation. Data are given as mean ± SEM, n = 8 (3 for HEK-293 cells); (**C**) ETPA phototoxicity IC_{50} and the phototoxicity index (PI, calculated as IC_{50} in the dark/IC_{50} in the light [17]). Cell survival data in the dark are taken from [10] (breast cancer cell lines) or measured separately (C6 and HEK-293 cells, see Supplementary Figure S4).

The final yield of the chlorin compound was 0.56 mg from the non-fasted and 0.6 mg from the fasted ophiuras, or 3.7% and 3%, respectively. With these essentially identical yields, and with the lack of seasonal variability in the chlorin content, we concluded that ETPA is not part of the dietary preferences of the brittle stars but is endogenously synthesized by them.

3.2. Phototoxicity of ETPA against a Panel of Cancer Lines

The chlorin (ETPA) isolated from *O. sarsii* has shown dark cytotoxicity against a panel of breast cancer cell lines, with IC_{50}s in the range of 25–45 µM [10]. In order to assess whether the anticancer effect could be increased upon illumination of the compound to grant potential applicability for PDT, we next studied the phototoxic effect of ETPA.

Breast cancer cells lines BT-20, MCF-7, and MDA-MB-231, along with the glioma cell line C6 and non-cancerous HEK-293 cells, were preincubated for 2 h with increasing concentrations of ETPA before irradiation with a red-light LED lamp (580 to 780 nm) for 30 min (fluence = 16.04 J/cm^2). Cell growth in the subsequent 72 h was assessed with the MTT assay (see Methods). Resulting data (Figure 2B,C) show striking phototoxicity of ETPA, with the sub-micromolar to low-micromolar IC_{50}s and impressive phototoxic indices (PI, measured as IC_{50} in the dark/IC_{50} in the light [17], Figure 2C), arguing for the strong potential of this natural chlorin in PDT applications. Notably, dark phototoxicity for the glioma C6 cells was not achieved at the highest concentrations of ETPA tested (Figure 2C and Supplementary Figure S4).

3.3. Singlet Oxygen Production by ETPA

Two methods to measure singlet oxygen production by ETPA upon illumination were employed (see Methods). The first was based on the chemical trapping of singlet oxygen by 1,3-diphenylisobenzofuran (DPIBF) and bleaching of DPIBF at 414 nm upon ETPA irradiation. The ETPA excitation was produced by the monochromatic 660 nm red light corresponding to the ETPA absorption maximum, which is not absorbed by DPIBF (Figure 2A and Supplementary Figure S3). Figure 3A shows the time-dependent decay in DPIBF 414 nm absorbance upon red-light illumination in the presence of ETPA. When comparing the efficiency of ETPA with that of meso-tetraphenylporphyrin (TPP, Figure 3B) known to produce singlet oxygen with the quantum yield of 0.7 [12,13], the absolute quantum yield of singlet oxygen generation by ETPA was determined as 0.83. Taking into consideration the relative error for such measurements at ±10% of the average value, the singlet oxygen yield for ETPA can be estimated as 0.8 ± 0.1 from the trapping experiment.

The second method was based on detection of the infrared phosphorescence of singlet oxygen (see Methods), comparing the phosphorescence intensities (Figure 3C) in solutions of ETPA and phenalenone—one of the most efficient photosensitizers of singlet oxygen generation, with the quantum yield of this process close to one [14]. For calculations, so-called zero-time intensities (I_0) of phosphorescence were used, which were obtained by extrapolation of the semilogarithmic kinetic plots to the zero time. The obtained I_0 values were then normalized to the absorption coefficients ($1-10^{-A}$) of the pigments at the wavelength of excitation. The resulting data are summarized in Figure 3D.

Thus, both methods indicate that the quantum yield of singlet oxygen production by ETPA is close to 0.8, identifying ETPA as very a strong photosensitizer of singlet oxygen generation with promising for biomedical applications.

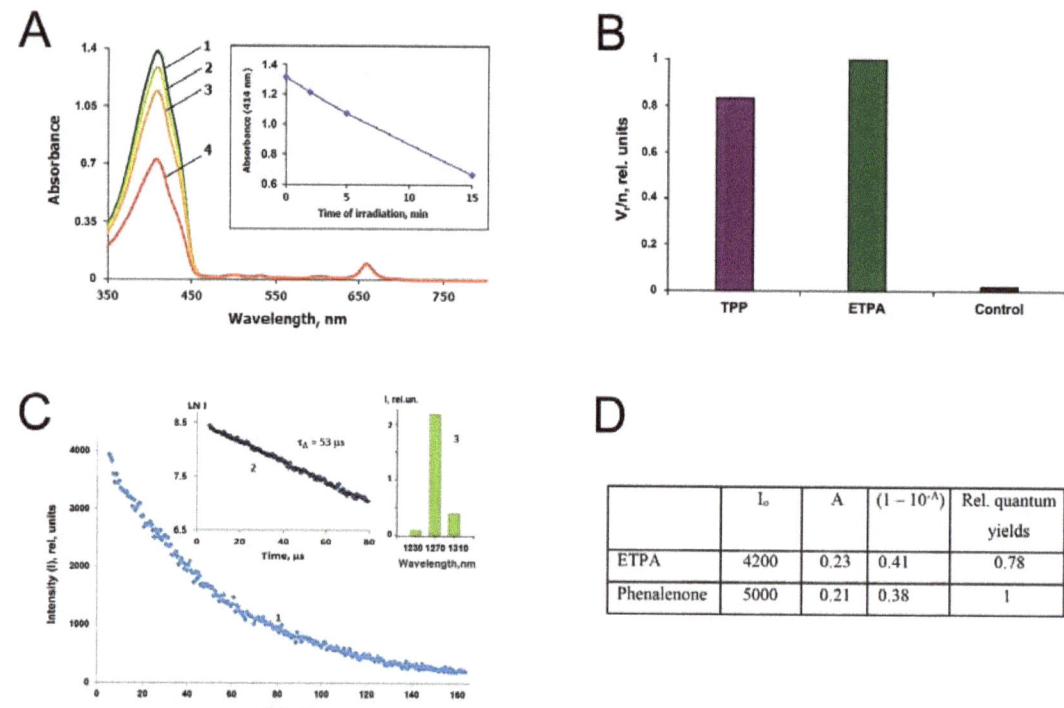

Figure 3. ETPA efficiently generates singlet oxygen: (**A**) changes in the absorption spectrum of DPIBF (curves 1–4) in the mixture of DPIBF with ETPA in acetone during irradiation by monochromatic red light (660 nm) absorbed by ETPA. Here, "2" corresponds to 2 min, "3" refers to 5 min, and "4" to 15 min irradiation. Power of exciting light was 83 μW. Inset shows the time course of 414 nm absorption fall of DPIBF. ETPA bleaching was not observed; (**B**) the relative quantum yields of DPIBF oxidation (V_r/n) upon irradiation of TPP and ETPA. The rate of spontaneous DPIBF bleaching in the dark without sensitizer and irradiation is defined as "Control". For TPP, irradiation time was 10 min, excitation wavelength was 512 nm, irradiation power was 105 μW, and absorbance of TPP at 512 nm was 0.024. For ETPA, irradiation time was 2 min, excitation wavelength was 660 nm, excitation power was 83 μW, and absorbance at 660 nm was 0.095; (**C**) kinetic trace of photosensitized phosphorescence of singlet oxygen upon excitation of ETPA by 5 μs pulses of violet LED (399 nm) in cartesian (1) and semilogarithmic (2) coordinates. Pulse repetition rate was 5 kHz, average LED power was 30 mW, and irradiation (averaging) time was 10 min. The PMT signal was accumulated using a time-resolved computer photon counting. The duration of one channel was 640 ns, and the number of channels was 256. Absorbance of the solution at 396 nm was 0.246 in a 1 cm quartz cell. Here, "3" indicates phosphorescence emission spectrum estimated using three interchangeable interference filters. I corresponds to the phosphorescence intensity just after the end (5 μs) of the LED pulse. The decay time (τ_Δ) of the phosphorescence exactly coincided with the known value of singlet oxygen lifetime in acetone; (**D**) calculation of the quantum yield of singlet oxygen by ETPA in comparison with phenalenone.

3.4. Photodynamic Therapy with ETPA in a Mouse Model of Brain Tumor

Inspired by the strong phototoxicity of ETPA against a panel of cancer cell lines in vitro, and by the especially high phototoxic index of our compound against glioma cells (Figure 2C), we next aimed at performing in vivo experiments of anticancer PDT with the brittle star-derived chlorin compound. Glioblastoma is the most common form of brain tumor, characterized by low responsiveness to treatment and poor prognosis (median survival < 2 years) [18]. Rat glioma C6 cells simulate human glioblastoma when injected into rats [19], and mouse brains [20,21] and have been a popular model in glioblastoma research [22]. We implanted C6 glioma cells in mouse brains (see Methods). After 7 days, IV administration of ETPA was performed, 6 h prior to brain MRI-guided targeted tumor illumination with a red laser (650 nm, see Methods and Figure 4A).

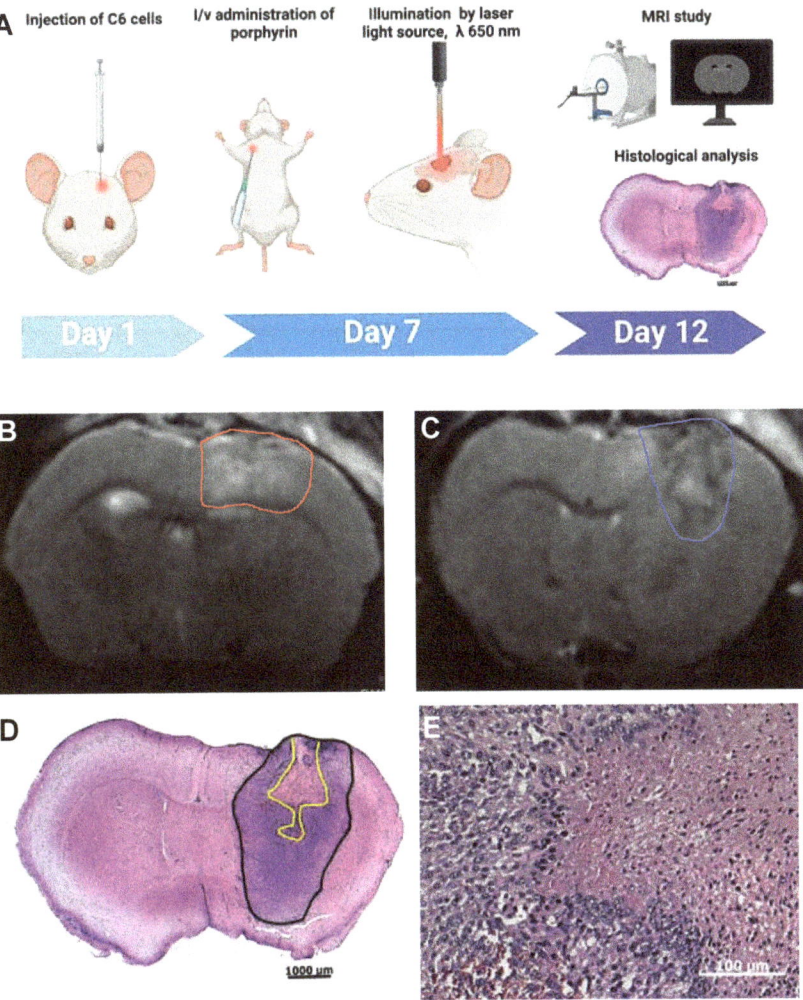

Figure 4. PDT using ETPA in a mouse model of glioblastoma: (**A**) scheme of the experiment; (**B**,**C**) representative T2-weighted MR images from coronal brain sections (0.5 mm thick) obtained 5 days after PDT. The area outlined with a red line refers to hyperintensities regions (edema, **B**). The area outlined with a blue line refers to PDT-induced glioma necrosis (**C**); (**D**) a representative histological section, stained with eosin–hematoxylin, demonstrates the tumor boundaries (outlined in black) and the presence of necrotic loci in the area of laser illumination (outlined in yellow); (**E**) enlarged area showing the boundaries of necrotic and intact tumor tissues. Images shown are representative of 3 animals.

Five days post PDT (Figure 4A), brain anatomical and histological analyses were performed. Through brain MRI, analysis of T2W-images revealed a strong signal change in the area exposed to laser irradiation. Figure 4B illustrates that in the tumor area exposed to laser irradiation, a hyperintense signal prevails indicating accumulation of water molecules in this area, i.e., tissue edema as the result of the photodynamic tissue damage. In the central part of the tumor (Figure 4C), the signal is mixed with zones of the hyperintense signal. Further histological analysis confirmed that this area corresponds to the area of necrosis (Figure 4D). Most of one hemisphere is occupied by a tumor consisting of poorly differentiated fusiform cells with large nuclei and narrow cytoplasm; many mitotic cells can also be seen. The stroma is poorly expressed. In the center of the tumor, there is an area of necrosis (a hypereosinophilic region devoid of nuclei), in the form of a pyramid with a broken apex. The area of necrosis occupies approximately 15% of the area of the tumor tissue in the section. At the border between dead and living tissue (Figure 4E), there are no reactive phenomena such as inflammation or connective tissue proliferation, and only blood vessels' dilatation can be noticed, along with numerous shapes (karyorrhexis, karyopycnosis, apoptotic bodies) of apoptotic cells. Notably, sham-operated and laser-irradiated mice reveal no noticeable brain damage ([23]; data not shown).

Our findings are consistent with prior studies demonstrating the high efficiency of PDT for C6 glioma in vivo, with glioma damage observed in deep brain regions [16]. A synthetic porphyrin compound, 2,4-(a43-dihydroxyethyl)deuteroporphyrin IX tetrakiscarborane carboxylate ester (BOPP), was used in this study [16,20]. Other porphyrin-based photo-sensitizers (e.g., Photofrin) have been applied for PDT of brain tumors in rats [24] and in clinical studies [25]. Similarly, chlorin-based photosensitizers (Photolon, Talaporfin) have also been tested [26,27]. However, none has yet reached clinical approval for brain malignancies [2,3,28].

A single dose (40 mg ETPA/kg mouse body weight) was used in our study. This drug dose regime in our mouse model was chosen following prior studies on PDT in rat models of brain tumors (keeping in mind the drug dose interspecies conversion rate [29]). The dose consisted of 2.5 mg/kg for Photolon [26], 25 mg/kg for BOPP [16], 40 mg/kg for hematoporphyrin derivative [30], or 100 mg/kg for 5-aminolevulinic acid [31]. The purpose of our work was not to find optimal concentrations/conditions for PDT but rather to provide a proof-of-concept demonstration of the potential of a natural chlorin—ETPA from *O. sarsii*—to provide photodynamic damage to the brain tumor. It is worth noting that we chose a low illumination regime (10 times less, as compared with [16]) to avoid thermal damage to the brain. Despite this sparing regime, we managed to achieve necrotic death within the irradiated area, indicating the high potential of ETPA for PDT.

4. Discussion

Porphyrin derivatives as unique molecules showing powerful phototherapeutic effects have found applications in anticancer PDT [4]. In our previous work, a new natural chlorin from the Pacific brittle star *Ophiura sarsii* was discovered [10]. In this current work, we uncovered multiple novel elements to the biology of this compound, (3S,4S)-14-Ethyl-9-(hydroxymethyl)-4,8,13,18-tetramethyl-20-oxo-3-phorbinepropanoic acid (ETPA) and its development toward PDT applications.

Although known in some marine invertebrates including some Echinodermata such as the sea urchin *Strongylocentrotus purpuratus* [8], porphyrins were considered absent in the class of Ophiuroidea [11]. Thus, following our discovery of ETPA in *Ophiura sarsii*, we hypothesized that this chlorin compound could be derived from a food source—perhaps a seasonal one—of these brittle stars [10]. However, our current data unequivocally demonstrate that ETPA is endogenous to this marine invertebrate. Subsequent research might be directed to the delineation of the biosynthetic routes of this first-ever Ophiuroidea porphyrin. Porphyrin biosynthesis has been well studied, with one of the conserved enzymes, aminolevulinic acid (ALA) synthase, producing the key intermediate 5-aminolevulinic acid from glycine and succinyl–CoA [8]. The *Strongylocentrotus purpuratus* genome encodes an

ALA synthase 62% identical to the mouse ortholog [8,32]. ALA synthase has been cloned from other marine invertebrates such as the bivalve *Patinopecten yessoensis*, and conserved gene sequences have been identified across taxonomic groups [33]. It is thus conceivable that despite the lack of the brittle star *O. sarsii* genomic data, its ALA synthase could be cloned in the future, along with the genes encoding other components of the porphyrin biosynthetic route. Further investigations could also be directed to the question of the role ETPA plays in the brittle star. As a major metabolite that can be isolated in large quantities, this chlorin compound is likely to play an important biological role in *O. sarsii*, such as participation in the electron transfer processes or protection from predators.

To investigate the medical utility of ETPA, we here performed proof-of-concept PDT studies in vitro and in vivo. The former assessed the phototoxic properties of ETPA against a panel of breast cancer and glioma cell lines, revealing sub-micromolar efficiency upon red-light irradiation. The latter relied on a popular animal model of glioblastoma demonstrating a remarkable PDT effect. Six hours post IV injection of ETPA, targeted red laser irradiation produced a dramatic photoablation in the brain tumor, leading to glioma necrosis. Notably, in the course of our experimentation, we did not observe any acute toxicity in the mice due to IV injection of ETPA, agreeing with studies with other photosensitizers on the good tolerability (and brain barrier permeability) of this group of compounds (e.g., [16,20]). More detailed pharmacokinetics and pharmacodynamics studies will be performed in the future, along with the broader assessment of the laser irradiation protocols, to further optimize the applicability of ETPA for the treatment of brain tumors (and other tumors) in animal models. A modification of the method can also be conceivable using fiber optic implantation into deeper brain regions to achieve maximal and maximally focused irradiation in the desired area [34]. Such future developments could be promising given the fact that none of the currently available photosensitizers has yet been approved for brain tumor PDT [2,3] despite several reaching clinical studies [25,27,28].

The abundance of ETPA in *O. sarsii* and the ease of its purification, along with its promising applications in PDT, make it attractive to consider upscaling of production of this natural product. Its abundance in its host is multiplied by the abundance of this brittle star species, wide-spread from Northern Atlantic, over the Arctic, and all the way to Northern Pacific, inhabiting waters from shallow to deep [35,36]. These features prompt considering mariculture of *O. sarsii* as has proven successful for other North Pacific invertebrates [37]. These possibilities, along with the preclinical developments of ETPA for PDT applications, may lead to the emergence of natural product-based novel photodynamic therapeutics.

Supplementary Materials: The following are available online at https://www.mdpi.com/article/10.3390/biomedicines10010134/s1, Supplementary Figure S1: Mechanism of photosensitized DPIBF oxygenation, Supplementary Figure S2: Mechanism of photosensitized IR phosphorescence of singlet oxygen, Supplementary Figure S3: Absorption spectrum of ETPA in acetone, Supplementary Figure S4: Dark cytotoxicity of ETPA against C6 and HEK-293 cells.

Author Contributions: Conceptualization, V.L.K. and Y.S.K.; methodology, M.B., V.A.B., A.S.B., A.S.K. and A.A.K.; validation, A.K., E.E.R. and D.S.; formal analysis, A.K., D.S. and A.A.K.; investigation, A.K., E.E.R. and D.S.; writing—original draft preparation, A.K., D.S., A.A.K. and V.L.K.; writing—review and editing, V.L.K.; supervision, A.A.K., Y.S.K. and V.L.K.; project administration, Y.S.K.; funding acquisition, V.L.K. and Y.S.K. All authors have read and agreed to the published version of the manuscript.

Funding: This research was funded by the Ministry of Science and Higher Education of Russian Federation, grant 13.1902.21.0012 "Fundamental problems of investigation and preservation of deep-sea ecosystems of potentially ore-bearing regions of the Northwestern Pacific" (Contract No. 075-15-2020-796). The researchers of the Federal Research Center (FRC) of Biotechnology were supported within the framework of the FRC State assignment.

Institutional Review Board Statement: The animal protocols were approved by the institutional animal ethics committee of A.N. Belozersky Research Institute of Physico-Chemical Biology, Approval Code: Protocol 8/21, Approval Date: 7 September 2021.

Informed Consent Statement: Not applicable.

Data Availability Statement: The data presented in this study are fully available in the main text and supplementary materials of this article.

Acknowledgments: Figure 4A was created with BioRender.com. Accessed on 29 December 2021. Agreement number: HR23DJH3U2. We thank A. Begun for assisting in the fluence measurement.

Conflicts of Interest: The authors declare no conflict of interest.

References

1. Dougherty, T.J. Introduction. In *Methods in Molecular Biology*; Springer Science + Business Media: Berlin/Heidelberg, Germany, 2010; Volume 635, pp. 1–6. [CrossRef]
2. Li, X.; Lovell, J.F.; Yoon, J.; Chen, X. Clinical development and potential of photothermal and photodynamic therapies for cancer. *Nat. Rev. Clin. Oncol.* **2020**, *17*, 657–674. [CrossRef]
3. Baskaran, R.; Lee, J.; Yang, S.G. Clinical development of photodynamic agents and therapeutic applications. *Biomater. Res.* **2018**, *22*, 25. [CrossRef] [PubMed]
4. Pandey, R.K.; Goswami, L.N.; Chen, Y.; Gryshuk, A.; Missert, J.R.; Oseroff, A.; Dougherty, T.J. Nature: A rich source for developing multifunctional agents. Tumor-imaging and photodynamic therapy. *Lasers Surg. Med.* **2006**, *38*, 445–467. [CrossRef]
5. Cragg, G.M.; Newman, D.J. Nature: A vital source of leads for anticancer drug development. *Phytochem. Rev.* **2009**, *8*, 313–331. [CrossRef]
6. Katanaev, V.L.; Blagodatski, A.; Xu, J.; Khotimchenko, Y.; Koval, A. Mining Natural Compounds to Target WNT Signaling: Land and Sea Tales. In *Handbook of Experimental Pharmacology*; Springer: Cham, Switzerland, 2021; Volume 269, pp. 215–248. [CrossRef]
7. Katanaev, V.L.; Di Falco, S.; Khotimchenko, Y. The Anticancer Drug Discovery Potential of Marine Invertebrates from Russian Pacific. *Mar. Drugs* **2019**, *17*, 474. [CrossRef]
8. Calestani, C.; Wessel, G.M. These Colors Don't Run: Regulation of Pigment—Biosynthesis in Echinoderms. In *Results and Problems in Cell Differentiation*; Springer: Cham, Switzerland, 2018; Volume 65, pp. 515–525. [CrossRef]
9. Blagodatski, A.; Cherepanov, V.; Koval, A.; Kharlamenko, V.I.; Khotimchenko, Y.S.; Katanaev, V.L. High-throughput targeted screening in triple-negative breast cancer cells identifies Wnt-inhibiting activities in Pacific brittle stars. *Sci. Rep.* **2017**, *7*, 11964. [CrossRef] [PubMed]
10. Klimenko, A.; Huber, R.; Marcourt, L.; Chardonnens, E.; Koval, A.; Khotimchenko, Y.S.; Ferreira Queiroz, E.; Wolfender, J.L.; Katanaev, V.L. A Cytotoxic Porphyrin from North Pacific Brittle Star Ophiura sarsii. *Mar. Drugs* **2021**, *19*, 11. [CrossRef]
11. Kennedy, G.Y. Porphyrins in invertebrates. *Ann. N. Y. Acad. Sci.* **1975**, *244*, 662–673. [CrossRef] [PubMed]
12. Krasnovsky, A.A., Jr.; Kozlov, A.S.; Roumbal, Y.V. Photochemical investigation of the IR absorption bands of molecular oxygen in organic and aqueous environment. *Photochem. Photobiol. Sci.* **2012**, *11*, 988–997. [CrossRef]
13. Krasnovsky, A.A.; Kozlov, A.S. Photonics of dissolved oxygen molecules. Comparison of the rates of direct and photosensitized excitation of oxygen and reevaluation of the oxygen absorption coefficients. *J. Photochem. Photobiol. A Chem.* **2016**, *329*, 167–174. [CrossRef]
14. Krasnovsky, A.A.; Benditkis, A.S.; Kozlov, A.S. Kinetic Measurements of Singlet Oxygen Phosphorescence in Hydrogen-Free Solvents by Time-Resolved Photon Counting. *Biochemistry* **2019**, *84*, 153–163. [CrossRef] [PubMed]
15. Irtenkauf, S.M.; Sobiechowski, S.; Hasselbach, L.A.; Nelson, K.K.; Transou, A.D.; Carlton, E.T.; Mikkelsen, T.; deCarvalho, A.C. Optimization of Glioblastoma Mouse Orthotopic Xenograft Models for Translational Research. *Comp. Med.* **2017**, *67*, 300–314.
16. Hill, J.S.; Kahl, S.B.; Stylli, S.S.; Nakamura, Y.; Koo, M.S.; Kaye, A.H. Selective tumor kill of cerebral glioma by photodynamic therapy using a boronated porphyrin photosensitizer. *Proc. Natl. Acad. Sci. USA* **1995**, *92*, 12126–12130. [CrossRef]
17. Padrutt, R.; Babu, V.; Klingler, S.; Kalt, M.; Schumer, F.; Anania, M.I.; Schneider, L.; Spingler, B. Highly Phototoxic Transplatin-Modified Distyryl-BODIPY Photosensitizers for Photodynamic Therapy. *ChemMedChem* **2021**, *16*, 694–701. [CrossRef]
18. Tan, A.C.; Ashley, D.M.; Lopez, G.Y.; Malinzak, M.; Friedman, H.S.; Khasraw, M. Management of glioblastoma: State of the art and future directions. *CA Cancer J. Clin.* **2020**, *70*, 299–312. [CrossRef] [PubMed]
19. Auer, R.N.; Del Maestro, R.F.; Anderson, R. A simple and reproducible experimental in vivo glioma model. *Can. J. Neurol. Sci.* **1981**, *8*, 325–331. [CrossRef]
20. Hill, J.S.; Kahl, S.B.; Kaye, A.H.; Stylli, S.S.; Koo, M.S.; Gonzales, M.F.; Vardaxis, N.J.; Johnson, C.I. Selective tumor uptake of a boronated porphyrin in an animal model of cerebral glioma. *Proc. Natl. Acad. Sci. USA* **1992**, *89*, 1785–1789. [CrossRef] [PubMed]
21. Fan, Y.; Cui, Y.; Hao, W.; Chen, M.; Liu, Q.; Wang, Y.; Yang, M.; Li, Z.; Gong, W.; Song, S.; et al. Carrier-free highly drug-loaded biomimetic nanosuspensions encapsulated by cancer cell membrane based on homology and active targeting for the treatment of glioma. *Bioact. Mater.* **2021**, *6*, 4402–4414. [CrossRef]
22. Grobben, B.; De Deyn, P.P.; Slegers, H. Rat C6 glioma as experimental model system for the study of glioblastoma growth and invasion. *Cell Tissue Res.* **2002**, *310*, 257–270. [CrossRef]
23. Romanova, G.A.; Silachev, D.N.; Shakova, F.M.; Kvashennikova, Y.N.; Viktorov, I.V.; Shram, S.I.; Myasoedov, N.F. Neuroprotective and antiamnesic effects of Semax during experimental ischemic infarction of the cerebral cortex. *Bull. Exp. Biol. Med.* **2006**, *142*, 663–666. [CrossRef]

24. Zhang, X.; Jiang, F.; Kalkanis, S.N.; Yang, H.; Zhang, Z.; Katakowski, M.; Hong, X.; Zheng, X.; Chopp, M. Combination of surgical resection and photodynamic therapy of 9L gliosarcoma in the nude rat. *Photochem. Photobiol.* **2006**, *82*, 1704–1711. [CrossRef]
25. Aziz, F.; Telara, S.; Moseley, H.; Goodman, C.; Manthri, P.; Eljamel, M.S. Photodynamic therapy adjuvant to surgery in metastatic carcinoma in brain. *Photodiagnosis Photodyn. Ther.* **2009**, *6*, 227–230. [CrossRef] [PubMed]
26. Tzerkovsky, D.A.; Osharin, V.V.; Istomin, Y.P.; Alexandrova, E.N.; Vozmitel, M.A. Fluorescent diagnosis and photodynamic therapy for C6 glioma in combination with antiangiogenic therapy in subcutaneous and intracranial tumor models. *Exp. Oncol.* **2014**, *36*, 85–89. [PubMed]
27. Akimoto, J.; Haraoka, J.; Aizawa, K. Preliminary clinical report on safety and efficacy of photodynamic therapy using talaporfin sodium for malignant gliomas. *Photodiagnosis Photodyn. Ther.* **2012**, *9*, 91–99. [CrossRef]
28. Quirk, B.J.; Brandal, G.; Donlon, S.; Vera, J.C.; Mang, T.S.; Foy, A.B.; Lew, S.M.; Girotti, A.W.; Jogal, S.; LaViolette, P.S.; et al. Photodynamic therapy (PDT) for malignant brain tumors—where do we stand? *Photodiagnosis Photodyn. Ther.* **2015**, *12*, 530–544. [CrossRef] [PubMed]
29. Nair, A.B.; Jacob, S. A simple practice guide for dose conversion between animals and human. *J. Basic Clin. Pharm.* **2016**, *7*, 27–31. [CrossRef] [PubMed]
30. Kaye, A.H.; Morstyn, G. Photoradiation therapy causing selective tumor kill in a rat glioma model. *Neurosurgery* **1987**, *20*, 408–415. [CrossRef]
31. Olzowy, B.; Hundt, C.S.; Stocker, S.; Bise, K.; Reulen, H.J.; Stummer, W. Photoirradiation therapy of experimental malignant glioma with 5-aminolevulinic acid. *J. Neurosurg.* **2002**, *97*, 970–976. [CrossRef]
32. Cameron, R.A.; Samanta, M.; Yuan, A.; He, D.; Davidson, E. SpBase: The sea urchin genome database and web site. *Nucleic Acids Res.* **2009**, *37*, D750–D754. [CrossRef]
33. Mao, J.; Zhang, Q.; Yuan, C.; Zhang, W.; Hu, L.; Wang, X.; Liu, M.; Han, B.; Ding, J.; Chang, Y. Genome-wide identification, characterisation and expression analysis of the ALAS gene in the Yesso scallop (*Patinopecten yessoensis*) with different shell colours. *Gene* **2020**, *757*, 144925. [CrossRef]
34. Cho, J.; Kwon, D.H.; Kim, R.G.; Song, H.; Rosa-Neto, P.; Lee, M.C.; Kim, H.I. Remodeling of Neuronal Circuits After Reach Training in Chronic Capsular Stroke. *Neurorehabilit. Neural Repair* **2016**, *30*, 941–950. [CrossRef] [PubMed]
35. Lütken, C.F. Contribution to knowledge about the brittle stars. II. Overview of the West Indian ophiuras (title in Danish). *Vidensk. Medd. Dan. Nat. Förening Kjøbenhavn* **1856**, *7*, 1–19.
36. Harris, J.L.; MacIsaac, K.; Gilkinson, K.D.; Kenchington, E.L. Feeding biology of Ophiura sarsii Lutken, 1855 on Banquereau bank and the effects of fishing. *Mar. Biol.* **2009**, *156*, 1891–1902. [CrossRef]
37. Gavrilova, G.S.; Kucheryavenko, A.V. Commercial rearing of the sea cucumber Apostichopus japonicus in Peter the great bay: Methodical peculiarities and results of the work of a mariculture farm in Sukhodol Bight. *Russ. J. Mar. Biol.* **2010**, *36*, 539–547. [CrossRef]

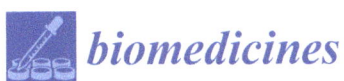

Article

Autophagy and Apoptosis Induced in U87 MG Glioblastoma Cells by Hypericin-Mediated Photodynamic Therapy Can Be Photobiomodulated with 808 nm Light

Viktoria Pevna [1], Georges Wagnières [2] and Veronika Huntosova [3],*

[1] Department of Biophysics, Institute of Physics, Faculty of Science, P.J. Safarik University in Kosice, Jesenna 5, 041 54 Kosice, Slovakia; viktoria.pevna@student.upjs.sk
[2] Laboratory for Functional and Metabolic Imaging, Institute of Physics, Swiss Federal Institute of Technology in Lausanne (EPFL), Station 6, Building CH, 1015 Lausanne, Switzerland; georges.wagnieres@epfl.ch
[3] Center for Interdisciplinary Biosciences, Technology and Innovation Park, P.J. Safarik University in Kosice, Jesenna 5, 041 54 Kosice, Slovakia
* Correspondence: veronika.huntosova@upjs.sk

Citation: Pevna, V.; Wagnières, G.; Huntosova, V. Autophagy and Apoptosis Induced in U87 MG Glioblastoma Cells by Hypericin-Mediated Photodynamic Therapy Can Be Photobiomodulated with 808 nm Light. *Biomedicines* **2021**, *9*, 1703. https://doi.org/10.3390/biomedicines9111703

Academic Editor: Kyungsu Kang

Received: 21 October 2021
Accepted: 15 November 2021
Published: 17 November 2021

Publisher's Note: MDPI stays neutral with regard to jurisdictional claims in published maps and institutional affiliations.

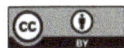

Copyright: © 2021 by the authors. Licensee MDPI, Basel, Switzerland. This article is an open access article distributed under the terms and conditions of the Creative Commons Attribution (CC BY) license (https://creativecommons.org/licenses/by/4.0/).

Abstract: Glioblastoma is one of the most aggressive types of tumors. Although few treatment options are currently available, new modalities are needed to improve prognosis. In this context, photodynamic therapy (PDT) is a promising adjuvant treatment modality. In the present work, hypericin-mediated PDT (hypericin-PDT, 2 J/cm^2) of U87 MG cells is combined with (2 min, 15 mW/cm^2 at 808 nm) photobiomodulation (PBM). We observed that PBM stimulates autophagy, which, in combination with PDT, increases the treatment efficacy and leads to apoptosis. Confocal fluorescence microscopy, cytotoxicity assays and Western blot were used to monitor apoptotic and autophagic processes in these cells. Destabilization of lysosomes, mitochondria and the Golgi apparatus led to an increase in lactate dehydrogenase activity, oxidative stress levels, LC3-II, and caspase-3, as well as a decrease of the PKCα and STAT3 protein levels in response to hypericin-PDT subcellular concentration in U87 MG cells. Our results indicate that therapeutic hypericin concentrations can be reduced when PDT is combined with PBM. This will likely allow to reduce the damage induced in surrounding healthy tissues when PBM-hypericin-PDT is used for in vivo tumor treatments.

Keywords: glioblastoma cells; autophagy; photodynamic therapy; photobiomodulation; apoptosis; microscopy; hypericin

1. Introduction

Glioblastomas are among the most aggressive primary tumors of the central nervous system. They are characterized by aggressive proliferation, invasiveness, diffuse infiltration and often high resistance to anticancer drugs [1,2]. For this reason, the prognosis for patient survival is poor. Researchers have made great efforts to develop therapeutic modalities that eliminate the ability of cells to resist treatments and induce cell death [3].

Photodynamic therapy (PDT) is a modern trend of adjuvant therapy in which a photosensitive molecule—a photosensitizer (PS), light at an appropriate wavelength absorbed by the PS, and oxygen are involved in the photoreactions that lead to photodestruction of the tumor [4]. In recent years, PDT has been used clinically to cure lung, head and neck, brain, prostate, colon, pancreatic, cervical, breast, and skin cancers [5]. The penetration depth of light is a major obstacle in PDT [6,7]. Light sources emitting in the red and near-infrared parts of the electromagnetic spectrum can be used to enable excitation of PSs relatively deep in tissues [6]. In addition, interstitial optical fiber-based cylindrical light distributors are also sometimes used to deliver light into bulky lesions. Therefore, surgical intervention in combination with PDT is a promising approach for the treatment of glioblastomas [8].

Hypericin is an interesting PS, which can be used for both PDT and photodiagnosis of cancer [9]. Hypericin is a naphthodianthrone characterized by a high hydrophobicity, the formation of non-fluorescent aggregates in aqueous solutions and a fluorescence emission of its monomers around 600 nm [10,11]. Hypericin dissolves well in the lipidic environment found in cell membranes [12]. Photodamages are induced in cells by singlet oxygen produced during the photoreaction taking place between hypericin molecules excited in their triplet and molecular oxygen [13–15].

The molecular mechanisms of PDT involve, in particular, the triggering of signaling pathways that lead to apoptosis of cancer cells. We have previously reported that the protein kinase C (PKC) signaling pathway is involved in the apoptotic response of glioblastoma cells to hypericin-mediated PDT [16–18]. We also observed the activation of PKCα and phosphorylation of Bcl2 in U87 MG glioblastoma cells after hypericin-mediated PDT [17,19]. The subcellular localizations of hypericin have been identified: the Golgi apparatus, lysosomes, plasma membrane and, in a few reports, in mitochondria [16,20–24]. The influence of hypericin on Bax and Bak, members of the Bcl2 protein family, suggests that hypericin plays an important role in the regulation of mitochondrial functions [25,26].

It has been reported that photobiomodulation (PBM) with light at 808 nm has beneficial effects on damaged mitochondria in cells [27–31]. In recent years, PBM has become an increasingly attractive modality to modulate reactive oxygen species in cells [32]. An approach to reduce inflammatory and oxidative stress markers by PBM at 810 nm has been demonstrated in hair cells [33]. The ease of application of light in different tissues gave rise to the idea of combining PBM and PDT. PBM at 660 nm was used to treat oral mucosa in combination with curcumin-mediated PDT at 468 nm [34]. For example, antimicrobial PDT with methylene blue and PBM has been used to improve and accelerate the healing process in the treatment of palatal ulcers [35]. The combination of PBM and PDT has even been proposed as an innovative approach for COVID-19 treatments [36].

While previous studies using curcumin and methylene blue-mediated PDT focused on antimicrobial treatment and PBM aimed at healing damaged tissues, the present work aims to demonstrate the efficacy of PBM at 808 nm and hypericin-mediated PDT in treating U87 MG glioblastoma cells. In our approach, hypericin forms non-fluorescent aggregates in the cytoplasm of cells that cannot be used for PDT. The use of PBM prior to hypericin application results in the formation of vesicles associated with the plasma membrane (of lipidic origin), which help to transport and dissolve hypericin intracellularly so that it is in a biologically active/fluorescent form for PDT. This further increases the production of lactate dehydrogenase and the efficacy of PDT. Various methods for detecting the metabolic activity of cancer cells and visualizing morphological changes by confocal fluorescence microscopy were used to detect the differences between cells treated with hypericin-PDT and PBM-hypericin-PDT. The interplay of autophagy and apoptosis, the two main modes of cell death, was studied by flow cytometry and Western blot of apoptotic and autophagic markers in U87 MG cells.

2. Materials and Methods

2.1. Cell Culture and Therapeutical Protocols

U87 MG human glioblastoma cells (cell culture was obtained from Cells Lines Services, Eppelheim, Germany) were grown in DMEM (Dulbecco's modified Eagle medium, high glucose, GlutaMAX™, with pyruvate, Gibco-Invitrogen, Life Technologies Ltd., Paisley, UK) supplemented with 10% FBS (fetal bovine serum, Gibco-Invitrogen, Life Technologies Ltd., Paisley, UK) and 1% (w/w) penicillin/streptomycin (Gibco-Invitrogen, Life Technologies Ltd., Paisley, UK) to 80% confluency, in the dark, under humidified atmosphere, 5% CO_2 and 37 °C.

Six therapeutical protocols were applied (see Figure 1). All protocols were stopped at the same time interval. PBM (808 nm diode laser (MDL-III-808/1~2500 mW, Changchun New Industries Optoelectronics Tech. Co. Ltd., Changchun, China), 2 min, 1.8 J/cm^2, 15 mW/cm^2) was applied shortly before hypericin administration into the cell culture medium. Hypericin at concentrations of 200 and 500 nM was administered for 3 h before PDT (590 nm light emitting diodes (homemade system), 2 min, 2 J/cm^2, 16.7 mW/cm^2).

Cell responses were examined 5 and 24 h after PDT. Mitochondrial stress and damages to the Golgi apparatus were induced with 100 nM and 10 µM rotenone (Sigma-Aldrich, Darmstadt, Germany) for 24 h. Phorbol 12-myristate 13-acetate (PMA, Sigma-Aldrich) at a concentration of 1 µM was applied to stimulate protein kinase C.

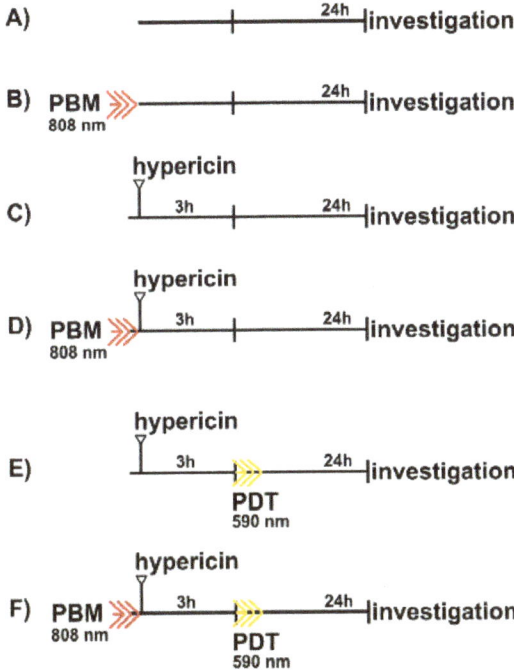

Figure 1. Schemes of therapeutical protocols: (A) control, (B) PBM, (C) hypericin in dark, (D) PBM-hypericin, (E) hypericin-PDT, and (F) PBM-hypericin-PDT.

2.2. Confocal Fluorescence Microscopy

U87 MG human glioblastoma cells were grown in confocal petri dishes embedded with cover slide (SPL, Gyeonggi-do, Korea). Mitochondria were labeled with 5 µM Rhodamine 123 (Rh123, Sigma-Aldrich, Darmstadt, Germany) for 15 min (excitation at 488 nm and emission in the spectral range 490–560 nm). Cell nuclei were labeled with 10 µg/mL Hoechst 33258 (ThermoFisher Scientific, Waltham, MA, USA) for 30 min (excitation at 405 nm and emission in the spectral range 450 ± 40 nm). Lysosomes were labeled with 400 nM LysoTracker Blue (ThermoFisher Scientific) (excitation at 405 nm and emission in the spectral range 450 ± 40 nm). NucView® 488 caspase-3 substrate (Biotium, Fremont, CA, USA) was used to detect caspase level in cells according to the supplier protocol (excitation at 488 nm and emission in the spectral range 490–560 nm). Plasma membranes were stained with Cell Mask Orange (ThermoFisher Scientific) according to the supplier protocol (excitation at 488 nm and emission in the spectral range >560 nm). Hypericin was detected in the spectral range >590 nm after excitation at 555 nm. The fluorescence intensity profile was analyzed using fluorescence images where the intensity was normalized to the hypericin fluorescence in the dark without PBM. Images with increased fluorescence intensity (HI) and normalized to the brightest signal (pixel) in the image were used to identify hypericin localization in cells.

Giantin and Protein Interacting with C Kinase—1 (PICK1) were visualized in cells with immunostaining. Cells were fixed with ice-cold (−20 °C) acetone (Centralchem, Bratislava, Slovakia) for 5 min at −20 °C and washed in ice-cold phosphate-buffered saline (PBS,

Sigma-Aldrich, Darmstadt, Germany). Cells were blocked in 5% bovine serum albumin (BSA, Sigma-Aldrich, Darmstadt, Germany) in PBS at room temperature (25 °C) for 1 h. The primary antibodies were dissolved in 5% BSA: anti-Giantin (1:300, ab80864, Abcam, Cambridge, UK) and PICK1 (1:300, Cell Signaling Technology, MA, USA) and incubated with the cells for 1 h at room temperature. After incubation, cells were washed with ice-cold PBS. The secondary antibody conjugated with AlexaFluor 488 (1:1000, ab150077, Abcam, Cambridge, UK) for Giantin and AlexaFluor 405 (1:1000, ab175652, Abcam, Cambridge, UK) for PICK1 were diluted in 1% BSA and applied to the cells for 1 h at room temperature. Fluorescence was detected in the following spectral domains: AlexaFluor 488 (excitation at 488 nm and emission in the spectral range 490–530 nm) and AlexaFluor 405 (excitation at 405 nm and emission in the spectral range 450 ± 40 nm).

Fluorescence images were acquired using a confocal fluorescence microscope system (LSM 700, Zeiss, Oberkochen, Germany), a 40× water immersion objective (NA 1.2, Zeiss), and a CCD camera (AxioCam HRm, Zeiss). Fluorescence images were analyzed using Zen 2011 software (Zeiss).

2.3. Cell Metabolism Assay and Lactate Dehydrogenase Assay

U87 MG human glioblastoma cells were seeded in 24-well plates. Cells were treated according to the protocols presented in Figure 1. After the treatments (24 h), 10 µL aliquots from the cell culture media were subjected to lactate dehydrogenase assay (LDH, Abcam) according to the supplier protocol. The absorbance of the LDH color assay was measured at 490 nm.

Detection of cellular metabolism was performed according to the supplier's protocol. In this assay, 3-(4,5-dimethylthiazol-2-yl)-2,5-diphenyltetrazolium bromide (MTT, Sigma-Aldrich, St. Louis, MO, USA) is converted to purple formazan, which is then dissolved in dimethyl sulfoxide (DMSO, Sigma-Aldrich) and detected using 96-well plate reader (GloMax TM-Multi1Detection system with Instinct Software, Madison, WI, USA) at 560 nm. The mean values from 8 measurements were plotted in histograms. The error bars represent the standard deviations. The levels of significant differences were calculated using one way ANOVA-test: a (dark), b (PBM), c (PDT), d (PBM + PDT) < 0.05, * $p < 0.05$, ** $p < 0.01$, *** $p < 0.001$.

2.4. Flow Cytometric Assay

Human U87 MG glioblastoma cells were treated according to the protocols in Figure 1. Five hours after PDT, cells were collected by trypsin/EDTA (ThermoFisher Scientific) and centrifuged at 600 rpm. Cell pellets were resuspended in Annexin V binding buffer (Mitenyi Biotec B.V. & Co. KG, Bergisch Gladbach, Germany), into which AnnexinV/FITC (Mitenyi Biotec B.V. & Co. KG, Bergisch Gladbach, Germany) or NucView® 488 caspase-3 substrate was added. Propidium iodide (PI, Mitenyi Biotec B.V. & Co. KG, Bergisch Gladbach, Germany) was added to the cell suspension just before detection by flow cytometer (MACSQuant® Analyzer, Miltenyi, Bergisch Gladbach, Germany) in channels B1 and B3. Hypericin fluorescence was detected in B2 channel.

2.5. Western Blot Assay

Cells at a density of 10^6 were lysed and homogenized in radioimmunoprecipitation buffer (RIPA) (150 mM sodium chloride, 1% Triton X-100, 0.5% sodium deoxycholate, 0.1% sodium dodecyl sulfate, 50 mM Tris, pH 8; all chemicals were purchased from Sigma-Aldrich, Darmstadt, Germany) with the inhibitor cocktail (2 × 1:100, Halt™ Protease and Phosphatase Inhibitor Cocktail, ThermoFisher Scientific, Waltham, MA, USA). Whole lysates (120 µg total protein amount) were diluted to 60 µg of final protein amount in 2× Laemmli buffer (Sigma-Aldrich, Darmstadt, Germany), loaded onto 7% or 15% polyacrylamide gels and subjected to electrophoresis. Proteins were transferred to a nitrocellulose membrane (0.22 µm; AppliChem, Darmstadt, Germany). Immunodetection was performed using the Western Breeze Chromogenic Kit (ThermoFisher Scientific, Waltham,

MA, USA). Proteins in the membrane were blocked with 5% BSA for 1 h at room temperature, washed, and then incubated overnight at 4 °C with primary antibodies: anti-LC3B (1:3000, ab221794, Abcam, Cambridge, UK), anti-PKCα (1:3000, ab4124, Abcam, Cambridge, UK), anti-STAT3 (1:1000, ab109085, Abcam, Cambridge, UK) and anti-GAPDH (1:1000, ab181602, Abcam, Cambridge, UK) were determined as housing protein. For protein visualization, secondary antibodies from the Western Breeze Chromogenic Kit were used to detect the primary rabbit antibodies. Analysis of the optical densities (O.D.) of the proteins in the membrane was performed using ImageJ software [37]. The normalized O.D. values presented in the histograms are the means of 3 measurements. The error bars represent the standard deviations.

3. Results

3.1. PBM Decreases Cell Metabolic Activity and Increases LDH Activity after Hypericin-PDT of U87 MG Cells

The metabolic activity of cells was detected in U87 MG glioblastoma cells after different treatment conditions. Two concentrations of rotenone were chosen to intoxicate the cells. It was found that the lower concentration of 100 nM rotenone inhibited complex I of the mitochondrial respiratory chain. At this concentration, the metabolic activity of the cells was not significantly affected compared to untreated controls (Figure 2A), although mitochondrial morphology was expected to undergo a fission. In contrast, 10 μM rotenone significantly decreased the metabolic activity of U87 MG cells (*** p). This concentration of rotenone leads not only to mitochondrial fission, but also to fragmentation of the Golgi apparatus, as later shown by confocal fluorescence microscopy. Neither PDT nor PBM affected the metabolic activity of the cells damaged by rotenone. Administration of 500 nM hypericin for 3 h in the dark and after PBM (see protocols in Figure 1) resulted in no significant differences compared with the untreated control. A significant decrease in the metabolic activity of U87 MG cells was only observed with the combined treatment of 10 μM rotenone for 24 h (Figure 2A). However, PDT of cells treated with hypericin (hypericin-PDT) resulted in quite dramatic changes. Indeed, the metabolic activity of treated cells decreased to below 50% compared to the activity of untreated control cells maintained in the dark. This effect was also observed with the combined treatment with both rotenone concentrations. In addition, PBM of U87 MG cells performed before hypericin administration (PBM-hypericin-PDT) increased the efficacy of PDT. The increased phototoxicity of PBM-hypericin-PDT was confirmed by the LDH assay, in which LDH production increased by up to 300% of untreated control cells (Figure 2B). A marked increase in LDH production was also observed in cells after hypericin-PDT. However, this effect was weaker (<250%) than that observed after PBM-hypericin-PDT. The presence of rotenone had no significant effect on hypericin-PDT and PBM-hypericin-PDT (Figure 2B).

3.2. PBM Decreases Hypericin Fluorescence in U87 MG Cells

The efficacy of PDT can be increased by increasing the concentration of hypericin. It can be assumed, in a first approximation, that the biological activity of hypericin is proportional to its fluorescent form in cells. Therefore, we studied the subcellular distribution of hypericin and its fluorescence in U87 MG cells. The hypericin concentration was reduced to 200 nM to decrease the phototoxic effect during the fluorescence measurements. The fluorescence intensity of 200 nM hypericin detected by flow cytometry in U87 MG cells 5 h after PDT is shown in Figure 3A. The fluorescence intensity of hypericin increased in cells after PDT (hypericin-PDT). In contrast, hypericin fluorescence decreased in cells treated with PBM-hypericin and PBM-hypericin-PDT. This observation was confirmed by confocal fluorescence microscopy (Figure 3B–D). The fluorescence of hypericin administered for 3 h in the dark (Figure 3B) was more intense than that of PBM-hypericin (Figure 3C). This difference is clearly seen in the hypericin fluorescence intensity profiles of selected cells (labeled 1 and 2 in Figure 3D). Hypericin fluorescence intensity correction (images labeled HI) and normalization to the brightest signal (pixel) in the image were used to identify the subcellular distribution of hypericin. In both treatments, a homogeneous localization of hypericin with bright intensity can be observed in the perinuclear region associated with the Golgi apparatus.

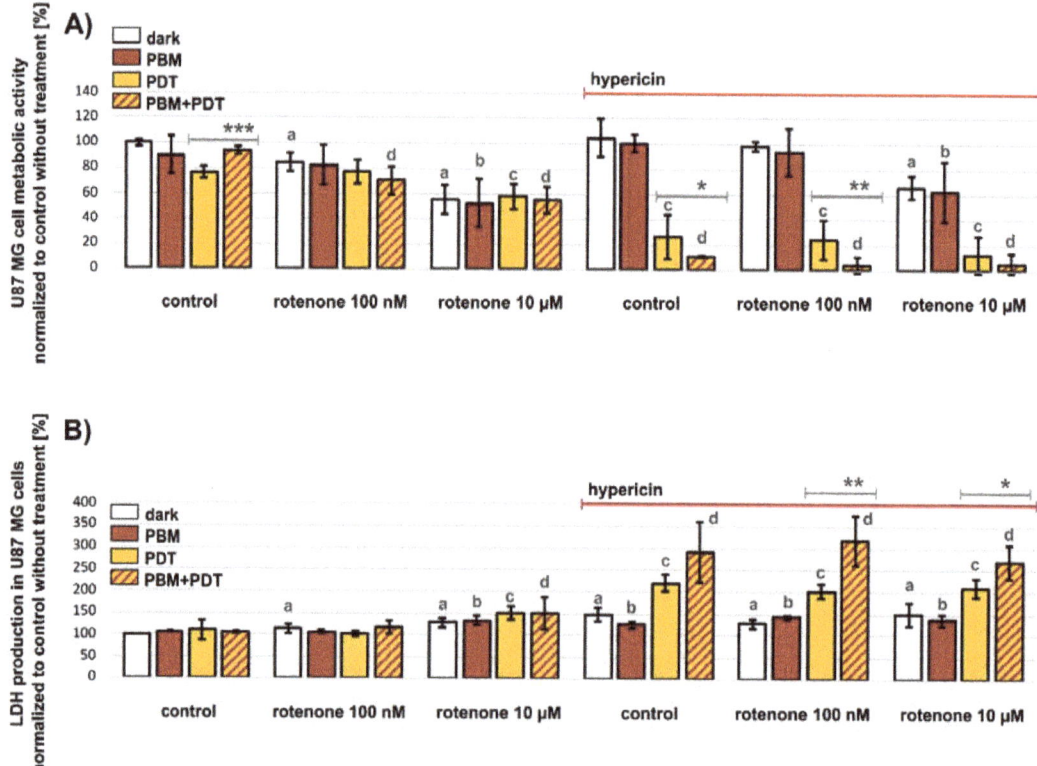

Figure 2. (**A**) Metabolic activity of U87 MG cells and (**B**) LDH activity in the dark (white columns), after PBM (red columns), hypericin-PDT (orange columns) and PBM-hypericin-PDT (orange columns with red patterns). Hypericin concentration was 500 nM (administered to cells for 3 h). Cell damage was also induced by 100 nM and 10 μM rotenone for 24 h. Significance level (against controls without hypericin treatment) was estimated using the one-way ANOVA-test: a (dark), b (PBM), c (PDT), d (PBM + PDT) < 0.05, * $p < 0.05$, ** $p < 0.01$, *** $p < 0.001$.

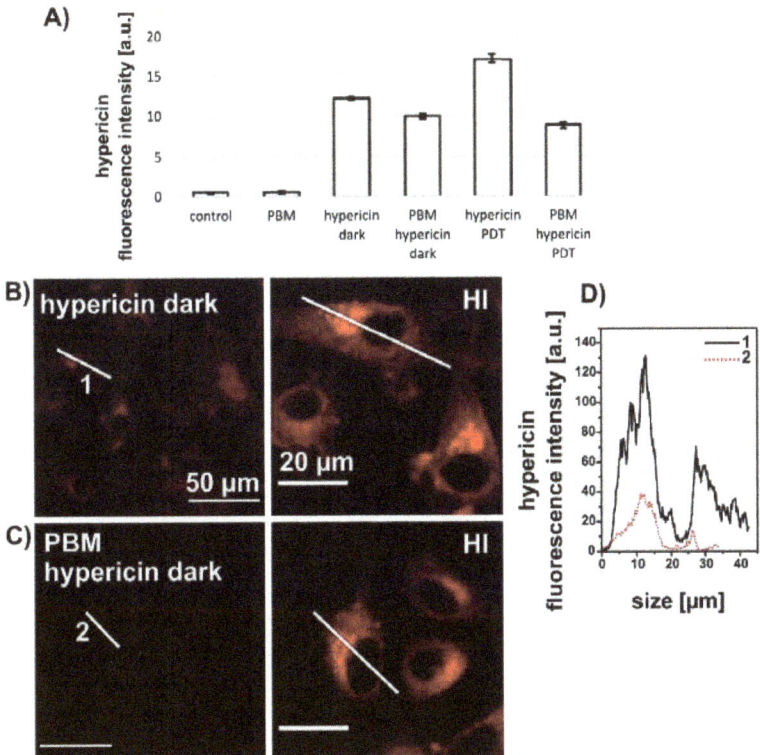

Figure 3. (**A**) Fluorescence intensity of 200 nM hypericin detected by flow cytometry in U87 MG cells under different conditions. Detection was performed 5 h after PDT. (**B**) Fluorescence distribution of 200 nM hypericin (3 h) in cells without and (**C**) with PBM. HI indicates high intensity correction to allow localization of hypericin. Scale bar—50 μm. White lines were drawn along selected cells to show the distribution of the hypericin fluorescence intensity in the cell along these lines. (**D**) Representative fluorescence distribution along lines 1 and 2 shown in (**B**,**C**), respectively.

3.3. Lysosomes Degradation, Mitochondria Destabilization and Fragmentation of Golgi Apparatus Are Induced by Hypericin-PDT and PBM-Hypericin-PDT

The organelles of main interest in the present study were mitochondria, lysosomes, Golgi apparatus and plasma membrane. These organelles were stained with specific fluorescent probes as shown in Figure 4.

Two treatments were chosen: 1 μM PMA and 10 μM rotenone administered over 5 h. Under these conditions, mitochondrial and lysosomal oriented oxidative stress can be induced, as can be seen by the morphology of mitochondria, which is different from the control (Figure 4A). Increased numbers of lysosomes were also observed (Figure 4B–C). While mitochondria and lysosomes were stressed and centralized around the nucleus after PMA treatment (see zoom in Figure 4B), rotenone stimulated a scattered distribution of lysosomes and mitochondria in the cytoplasm (see zoom in Figure 4C).

The morphology and localization of selected organelles observed in U87 MG cells after hypericin treatment in the dark resembled the untreated control (Figure 5A). To confirm the changes induced by massive nonphysiological oxidative stress, hydrogen peroxide was administered to these cells (Figure 5B). Destabilization and degradation of lysosomes resulted in translocation of LysoTracker Blue (lysosomal probe—blue color) into the nuclei of U87 MG cells. The mitochondrial membrane potential was dissipated by hydrogen peroxide and the mitochondrial probe (rhodamine 123—green color) diffused into the cytoplasm.

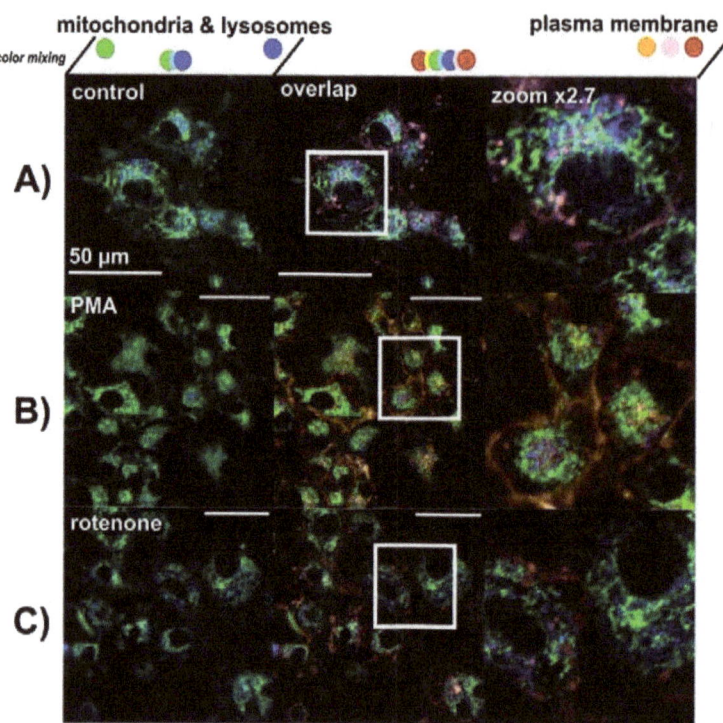

Figure 4. Confocal fluorescence images of rhodamine 123—mitochondria (green), LysoTracker Blue—lysosomes (blue), and Cell Mask Orange—plasma membrane (orange and red) in (**A**) U87 MG cells without treatment, (**B**) treated with 1 µM PMA, and (**C**) 10 µM rotenone for 5 h. The overlapping images were magnified to better see the organelles detected. Scale bar—50 µm.

Hypericin-PDT (Figure 5C) and PBM-hypericin-PDT (Figure 5D) triggered dramatic changes in the cells. Mitochondrial fission, an increase in the number of lysosomes, mitochondria membrane potential depletion, and lysosome destabilization were observed in the cells. When mitochondria and lysosomes could be observed, a perinuclear localization of these organelles was noted. If we subdivide the cells according to the stress induced by the previous treatments with PMA, rotenone and hydrogen peroxide, all three types of cell effects could be found after hypericin-PDT and PBM-hypericin-PDT. It should be noted that the red fluorescence consists of hypericin and Cell Mask Orange signals bleeding into the same detection channel.

The localization of hypericin was observed in the Golgi apparatus. For this reason, we immunostained Giantin localized in the Golgi apparatus of U87 MG cells. For better identification, a skeleton of U87 MG cells was detected with an antibody against PICK1. Beautiful cisternae of the Golgi apparatus localized in the perinuclear region can be detected in untreated control (Figure 6A), PMA (Figure 6B) and hypericin (Figure 6D) treated cells. Hypericin can be detected by its red fluorescence. Fragmentation of the Golgi apparatus and scattered localization of cisternae in the cytoplasm were observed in cells treated with rotenone (Figure 6C). Destabilization and fragmentation of the Golgi apparatus was also observed after hypericin-PDT and PBM-hypericin-PDT cells.

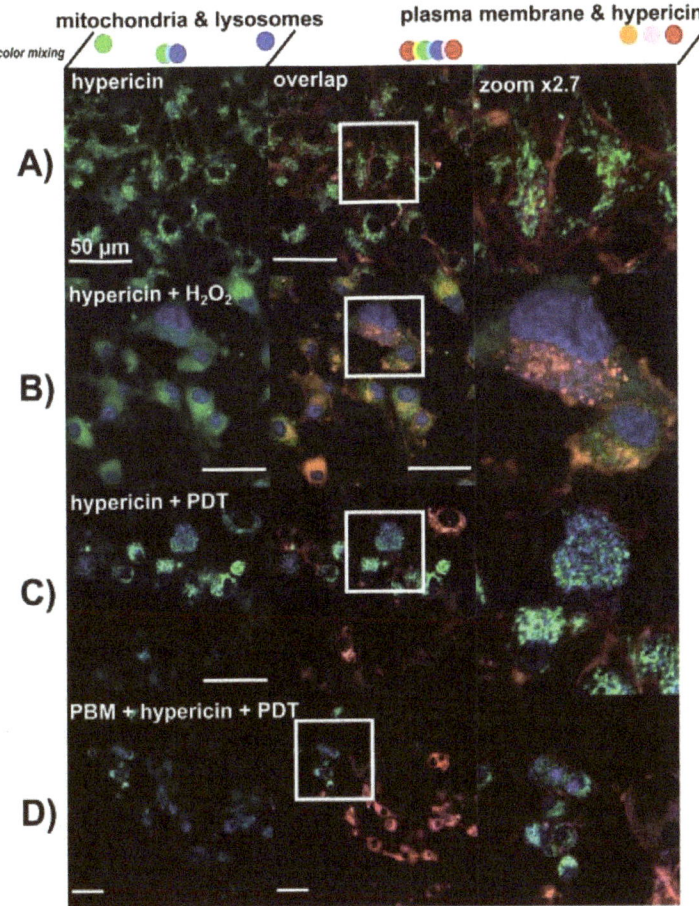

Figure 5. Confocal fluorescence images of rhodamine 123—mitochondria (green), LysoTracker Blue—lysosomes (blue), hypericin (orange and red) and Cell Mask Orange—plasma membrane (orange and red) in (**A**) U87 MG cells treated with 500 nM hypericin for 3 h, (**B**) hypericin in A + 1 mM H_2O_2 for 10 min, (**C**) hypericin-PDT and (**D**) PBM-hypericin-PDT detected 5 h after PDT. Overlapping images were magnified to better identify the organelles detected. Scale bar—50 µm.

3.4. PBM Increases Autophagy in U87 MG Cells after Hypericin-PDT

While the cells in the untreated control and hypericin treatment in the dark have the typical shape of U87 MG glioblastoma cells, those irradiated (PDT) have a round shape. Such a shape is typical of cells undergoing apoptosis and death. Subcellular localization of the NucView® 488 caspase-3 substrate was imaged in U87 MG cells treated as in the previous Section 3.3. These cells were stained with Cell Mask Orange and Hoechst to reveal the plasma membrane and nucleus. This combination led to the visualization of green fluorescence in the plasma membrane originating from Cell Mask Orange (see Figure 7A,B). On the other hand, cytosolic localization of green fluorescence belongs to the NucView® 488 caspase-3 substrate as observed in cells after rotenone treatment (Figure 7C). Typical apoptotic nuclei stained with Hoechst are indicated by white arrows in Figure 7C.

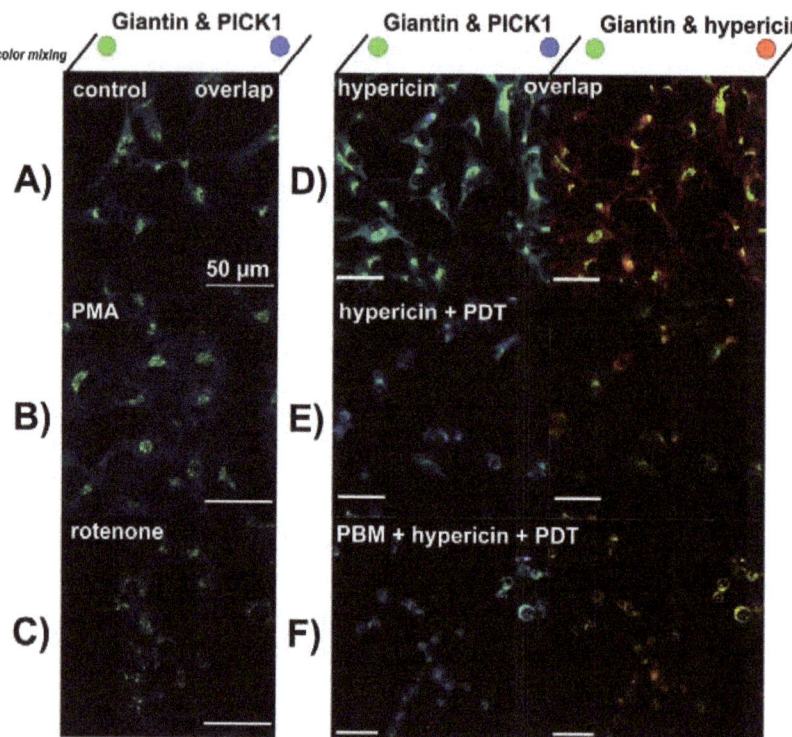

Figure 6. Confocal fluorescence images of Giantin (green), PICK1 (blue) and hypericin (red) in (**A**) U87 MG cells without treatment, (**B**) treated with 1 µM PMA and (**C**) 10 µM rotenone for 5 h. (**D**) cells treated with 500 nM hypericin for 3 h, (**E**) hypericin-PDT and (**F**) PBM-hypericin-PDT detected 5 h after PDT. Scale bar—50 µm.

Hypericin-PDT and PBM-hypericin-PDT resulted in cytosolic localization of the NucView® 488 caspase-3 substrate and condensation of chromatin visualized with Hoechst (Figure 7E,F). This was not observed in cells treated with hypericin in the dark (Figure 7D).

The increase of NucView® 488 caspase-3 substrate in U87 MG cells after hypericin-PDT and PBM-hypericin-PDT was confirmed by flow cytometry (green histograms in Figure 8A,C). Apoptotic cell populations with AnnexinV/FITC and PI staining were observed after these treatments (Figure 8B,D).

It should be noted that flow cytometry, in contrast to confocal fluorescence microscopy, was performed on cells treated with 200 nM hypericin to reduce the number of completely damaged/fragmented cells after PDT.

Since STAT3, LC3B and PKCα are involved in cancer cell migration, autophagy and apoptosis, Western blot analysis of their protein levels in cells was performed. The results are shown in Figure 9. The protein levels of STAT3 and PKCα decreased in the cells treated with 200 nM hypericin after PDT and PBM-hypericin-PDT. The bands decreased in the cells treated with 500 nM hypericin after PDT and PBM-hypericin-PDT.

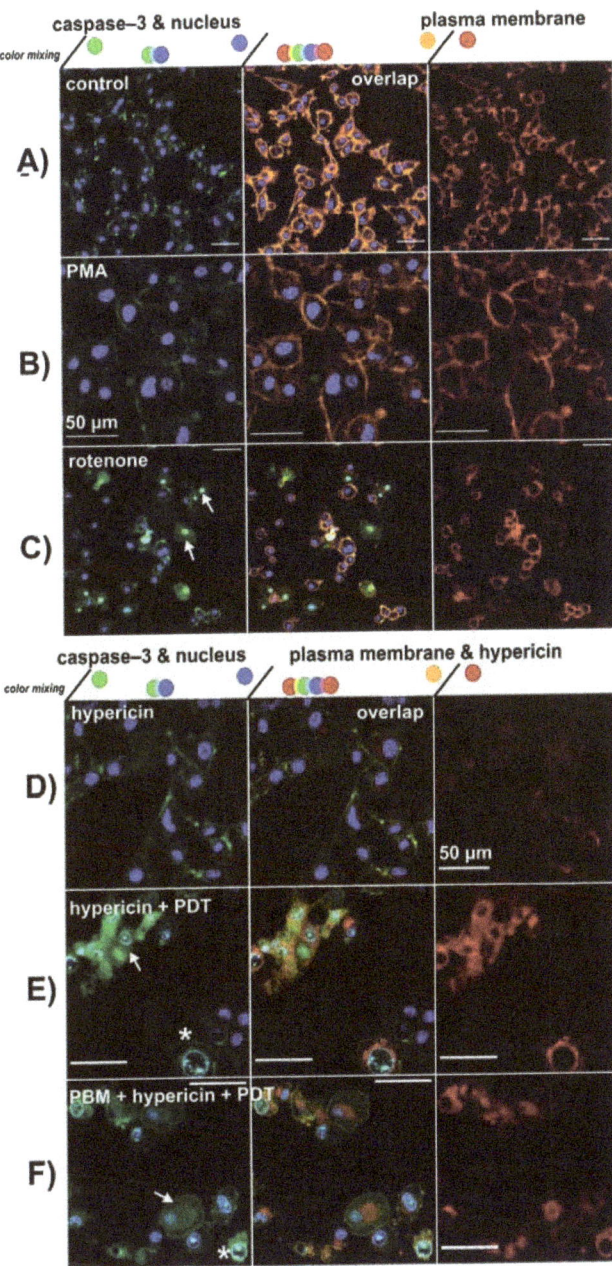

Figure 7. Confocal fluorescence images of NucView® 488 caspase-3 substrate (green), Hoechst—nucleus (blue), hypericin (red) and Cell Mask Orange—plasma membrane (orange and red) in (A) U87 MG cells without treatment, (B) treated with 1 µM PMA and (C) 10 µM rotenone for 5 h. (D) U87 MG cells treated with 500 nM hypericin for 3 h, (E) hypericin-PDT and (F) PBM-hypericin-PDT detected 5 h after PDT. Scale bar—50 µm. White asterisks indicate cells with typical apoptotic features stained with Hoechst. White arrows indicate localization of NucView® 488 caspase-3 substrate in the cytoplasm and nucleus.

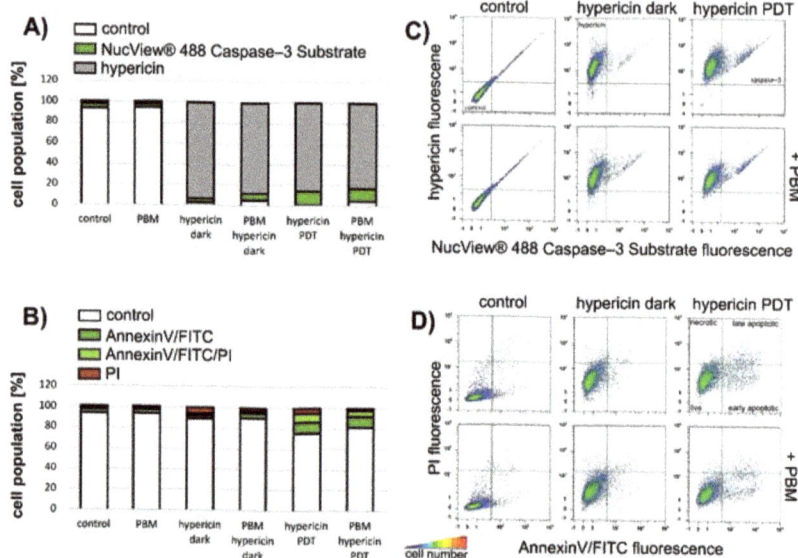

Figure 8. Flow cytometric analysis of (**A**) caspase-3 production (stained with NucView® 488 caspase-3 substrate (green histograms)) and (**B**) apoptosis/necrosis (stained with AnnexinV/FITC (green histograms) and PI (red histograms)) in U87 MG cells without treatment and treated with PBM, 200 nM hypericin in the dark, after PBM and PDT, as shown in the histograms. Detection was performed 5 h after PDT. White histograms show cells without staining and gray histograms show cells labeled with hypericin. (**C**) Correlation plots of the fluorescence intensities of hypericin and NucView® 488 caspase-3 substrate in the detected cells. (**D**) Correlation plots for the intensity of fluorescence of PI and AnnexinV/FITC in the detected cells. Cell number is color-coded (blue—minima, red—maxima).

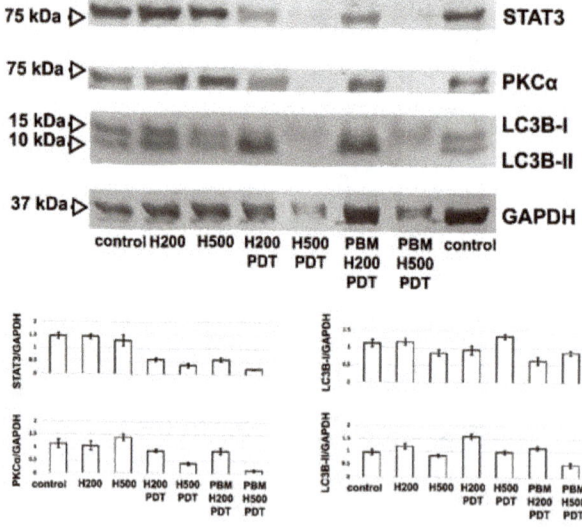

Figure 9. Western blot analysis of PKCα, STAT3 and LC3B protein levels in U87 MG cells without treatment and treated with PBM, 200 nM (H200) and 500 nM (H500) hypericin in the dark, after PBM and PDT, as shown in the images and histograms. GAPDH was used as the housing protein. The histograms show the optical densities of the detected bands.

LC3B is divided into two bands: LC3B-I and LC3B-II. Both LC3B bands were detected in the untreated control and hypericin-treated cells. However, LC3B-II was increased in the cells treated with 200 nM hypericin-PDT and PBM-hypericin-PDT (Figure 9). In contrast, LC3B-I was present in the cells treated with 500 nM hypericin-PDT and PBM-hypericin-PDT.

4. Discussion

The anti-glioblastoma activity of hypericin has been demonstrated without light application [38]. It has been suggested that hypericin may cause epigenetic changes, modulation of neuroglial tumor cell differentiation, modifications of the cytoarchitecture, and cell cycle alterations. Moreover, hypericin is known to inhibit the activity of PKC, which is involved in proliferation and cell death [39,40]. Therefore, the increase of its intracellular concentration by PBM could contribute to the enhancement of its biological activity in the dark and even improve its proapoptotic function in cancer cells after PDT.

Five proposed treatments were evaluated in this study. Only PBM was applied to improve glioblastoma cell status without administration of a photosensitizer (hypericin). The combination of PBM with hypericin without further illumination (no PDT) was compared with the biological activity of hypericin in the dark. No significant differences in the metabolic activities (detected with MTT) of these cells were observed, but some significant increase in LDH production was observed. This may be attributed to an increased oxygen consumption during PBM, which may temporarily switch the cell to anaerobic glycolysis. This effect was also observed in cells treated with hypericin-PDT, where LDH increased tremendously due to oxygen consumption. Consequently, PBM-hypericin-PDT resulted in the best treatment effect, i.e., proliferation was inhibited and LDH increased significantly. This effect was even better observed in the cells to which rotenone, an inhibitor of mitochondrial respiration, was applied. The destruction and alteration of subcellular organelles by hypericin-PDT and PBM-hypericin-PDT provided the impetus for autophagy and apoptosis signaling.

PDT has been shown to modulate the effect of hypericin on PKC isoform activity in glioblastoma cells [16,17]. This signaling molecule was also investigated in the present study. It was found that PKCα isoform, which is considered as an anti-apoptotic factor, was strongly affected by PDT. The protein level of PKCα decreased in glioblastoma cells after PDT depending on the concentration of hypericin. While PBM did not affect 200 nM hypericin-PDT, a higher concentration of 500 nM hypericin-PDT resulted in a greater reduction of PKCα in glioblastoma cells pretreated with PBM (PBM-hypericin-PDT). It should be noted that the drastic decrease in PKCα protein level is related to the translocation of PKCα from the cytosol to the plasma membrane, where it plays an important role in the apoptotic response of cancer cells. PBM was also shown to increase PKCα protein levels in untreated U87 MG cells and maintain PKCα localization in the perinuclear region.

The protein Signal Transducer and Activator of Transcription (STAT)-3, which is involved in the protection of cells from apoptosis, was also identified as a protein regulated by PKC [41,42]. In the present study, STAT3 protein level in U87 MG cells decreased similarly to PKCα after hypericin-PDT and PBM-hypericin-PDT. Downregulation and inhibition of STAT3 after PDT leading to apoptosis was observed in cancer cells treated with 5-aminolevulinic acid, 2-[1-hexyloxyethyl]-2devinyl pyropheophorbide-a and benzoporphyrin derivative [43–45]. This inhibition has been associated with inhibition of proliferation, infiltration of cancer cells, and induction of apoptosis in solid tumors.

Several studies have reported that hypericin-PDT induces apoptosis through the activation of caspase-3 and the release of cytochrome c with the recruitment of BH3-interacting domain death agonists (Bid, Bax, Bac, Bcl2) [25,46,47]. In our study, both hypericin-PDT and PBM-hypericin-PDT led to an increase in caspase-3 and apoptosis. However, our fluorescence microscopy results showed that not only mitochondria but also lysosomes and Golgi apparatus were strongly affected by hypericin-PDT.

The process of autophagy is often triggered in cancer, inflammation and neurodegeneration to maintain homeostasis in the cell, especially during the degradation of lysosomes [48,49]. In this process, LC3 plays an important role. In particular, lipidated LC3-II is associated with the formation of double-membrane autophagosomes [50]. We have shown here that 200 nM hypericin-PDT increased LC3B-II and 500 nM hypericin-PDT increased LC3B-I protein levels in U87 MG cells. Application of PBM prior to PDT reduced the effects observed in cells without PBM. Therefore, our results suggest that PBM-hypericin-PDT promotes apoptosis before autophagy. However, the balance between autophagy and apoptosis may be modulated by hypericin concentration in addition to PBM. The reduction in hypericin fluorescence intensity observed by flow cytometry and fluorescence microscopy after PBM may be explained by PBM-induced detoxification. We hypothesize that PBM-induced autophagy may be related to the detoxification processes in the cell.

As mentioned in the introduction, PBM has already been used in combination with PDT, but the aim of PBM application was to heal the treated area [34,35]. Enhancement of endogenous protoporphyrin IX production and homogenization in U87 MG cells by PBM has recently been addressed as a promising protocol for PDT and photodiagnostics [51]. To the best of our knowledge, this is the first time that PBM has been used in combination with PDT to eliminate cancer cells with photoactivated hypericin.

In our study, we showed that glioblastoma cells strive to reduce the photodamages induced by PBM-hypericin-PDT. However, metabolic activity and LDH levels in cells were significantly and much more severely affected by PBM-hypericin-PDT than by hypericin-PDT. Since LDH is important for both anaerobic metabolism and glycolysis, the effect of PBM may be attributed to oxygen consumption and glycolysis. The treatment efficacy was also higher in cells with damaged mitochondria and a Golgi apparatus stimulated with rotenone. This suggests that the elimination of cells by apoptosis may be enhanced by PBM-PDT in the case of mitochondrial and Golgi apparatus dysfunction, which is expected under less oxygen-rich conditions.

In conclusion, the application of PBM in our conditions was such that hypericin was not excited by the PBM light, but the biological activity of hypericin after PDT was affected by PBM. While PBM alone stimulates the detoxification of glioblastoma cells and decreases the hypericin intensity, consequently, probably due to its intracellular concentration, faster than its natural release, application of PDT to cells pretreated by PBM results in a more potent destructive effect than hypericin-PDT alone. Therefore, we hypothesize that this combination of light treatments led to an improvement in hypericin-PDT efficacy and to the identification of this PBM-hypericin-PDT combination as a promising treatment for glioblastomas. This treatment strategy is probably also of interest for solid tumors with heterogeneous metabolism and oxygenation.

Author Contributions: Conceptualization, V.P. and V.H.; methodology, V.P., V.H. and G.W.; validation, V.P. and V.H.; investigation, V.P. and V.H.; data curation, V.P. and V.H.; writing—original draft preparation, V.P., V.H. and G.W.; visualization, V.P., V.H. and G.W. All authors have read and agreed to the published version of the manuscript.

Funding: This research was funded by the Ministry of education, science, research, and sport of the Slovak Republic, grant number VEGA 1/0421/18, internal grant of Faculty of Science UPJS in Kosice vvgs-pf-2021-1788, the Swiss National Science Foundation (project 315230 185262/1) and European Union's Horizon 2020 research and innovation programme under grant agreement No. 952333, project CasProt (Fostering high scientific quality in protein science in Eastern Slovakia). This publication is the result of the project implementation: Open scientific community for modern interdisciplinary research in medicine (Acronym: OPENMED), ITMS2014+: 313011V455 supported by the Operational Program Integrated Infrastructure, funded by the ERDF.

Institutional Review Board Statement: Not applicable.

Informed Consent Statement: Not applicable.

Data Availability Statement: Data are presented in this work.

Conflicts of Interest: The authors declare no conflict of interest.

References

1. Kristensen, B.W.; Priesterbach-Ackley, L.P.; Petersen, J.K.; Wesseling, P. Molecular pathology of tumors of the central nervous system. *Ann. Oncol.* **2019**, *30*, 1265–1278. [CrossRef] [PubMed]
2. Hanif, F.; Muzaffar, K.; Perveen, K.; Malhi, S.M.; Simjee, S.U. Glioblastoma multiforme: A review of its epidemiology and pathogenesis through clinical presentation and treatment. *Asian Pac. J. Cancer Prev.* **2017**, *18*, 3–9.
3. Zhang, H.; Wang, R.; Yu, Y.; Liu, J.; Luo, T.; Fan, F. Glioblastoma treatment modalities besides surgery. *J. Cancer* **2019**, *10*, 4793–4806. [CrossRef] [PubMed]
4. Sorrin, A.J.; Kemal Ruhi, M.; Ferlic, N.A.; Karimnia, V.; Polacheck, W.J.; Celli, J.P.; Huang, H.C.; Rizvi, I. Photodynamic Therapy and the Biophysics of the Tumor Microenvironment. *Photochem. Photobiol.* **2020**, *96*, 232–259. [CrossRef]
5. Gunaydin, G.; Gedik, M.E.; Ayan, S. Photodynamic Therapy for the Treatment and Diagnosis of Cancer–A Review of the Current Clinical Status. *Front. Chem.* **2021**, *9*, 686303. [CrossRef] [PubMed]
6. Kim, M.M.; Darafsheh, A. Light Sources and Dosimetry Techniques for Photodynamic Therapy. *Photochem. Photobiol.* **2020**, *96*, 280–294. [CrossRef] [PubMed]
7. Mallidi, S.; Anbil, S.; Bulin, A.L.; Obaid, G.; Ichikawa, M.; Hasan, T. Beyond the barriers of light penetration: Strategies, perspectives and possibilities for photodynamic therapy. *Theranostics* **2016**, *6*, 2458–2487. [CrossRef] [PubMed]
8. Cramer, S.W.; Chen, C.C. Photodynamic Therapy for the Treatment of Glioblastoma. *Front. Surg.* **2020**, *6*, 81. [CrossRef]
9. Lenkavska, L.; Blascakova, L.; Jurasekova, Z.; Macajova, M.; Bilcik, B.; Cavarga, I.; Miskovsky, P.; Huntosova, V. Benefits of hypericin transport and delivery by low- and high-density lipoproteins to cancer cells: From in vitro to ex ovo. *Photodiagn. Photodyn. Ther.* **2019**, *25*, 214–224. [CrossRef]
10. Joniova, J.; Rebič, M.; Strejčková, A.; Huntosova, V.; Staničová, J.; Jancura, D.; Miskovsky, P.; Bánó, G. Formation of Large Hypericin Aggregates in Giant Unilamellar Vesicles—Experiments and Modeling. *Biophys. J.* **2017**, *112*, 966–975. [CrossRef]
11. Miskovsky, P. Hypericin—A New Antiviral and Antitumor Photosensitizer: Mechanism of Action and Interaction with Biological Macromolecules. *Curr. Drug Targets* **2005**, *3*, 55–84. [CrossRef]
12. Huntosova, V.; Alvarez, L.; Bryndzova, L.; Nadova, Z.; Jancura, D.; Buriankova, L.; Bonneau, S.; Brault, D.; Miskovsky, P.; Sureau, F. Interaction dynamics of hypericin with low-density lipoproteins and U87-MG cells. *Int. J. Pharm.* **2010**, *389*, 32–40. [CrossRef] [PubMed]
13. Darmanyan, A.; Burel, L.; Eloy, D.; Jardon, P. Singlet oxygen production by hypericin in various solvents. *J. Chim. Phys.* **1994**, *91*, 1774–1785. [CrossRef]
14. Varchola, J.; Želonková, K.; Chorvat, D.; Jancura, D.; Miskovsky, P.; Bánó, G. Singlet oxygen produced by quasi-continuous photo-excitation of hypericin in dimethyl-sulfoxide. *J. Lumin.* **2016**, *177*, 17–21. [CrossRef]
15. Ehrenberg, B.; Anderson, J.L.; Foote, C.S. Kinetics and Yield of Singlet Oxygen Photosensitized by Hypericin in Organic and Biological Media. *Photochem. Photobiol.* **1998**, *68*, 135–140. [CrossRef]
16. Misuth, M.; Joniova, J.; Horvath, D.; Dzurova, L.; Nichtova, Z.; Novotova, M.; Miskovsky, P.; Stroffekova, K.; Huntosova, V. The flashlights on a distinct role of protein kinase C δ: Phosphorylation of regulatory and catalytic domain upon oxidative stress in glioma cells. *Cell. Signal.* **2017**, *34*, 11–22. [CrossRef] [PubMed]
17. Dzurová, L.; Petrovajova, D.; Nadova, Z.; Huntosova, V.; Miskovsky, P.; Stroffekova, K. The role of anti-apoptotic protein kinase Cα in response to hypericin photodynamic therapy in U-87 MG cells. *Photodiagn. Photodyn. Ther.* **2014**, *11*, 213–226. [CrossRef] [PubMed]
18. Lenkavska, L.; Tomkova, S.; Horvath, D.; Huntosova, V. Searching for combination therapy by clustering methods: Stimulation of PKC in Golgi apparatus combined with hypericin induced PDT. *Photodiagn. Photodyn. Ther.* **2020**, *31*, 101813. [CrossRef] [PubMed]
19. Stroffekova, K.; Tomkova, S.; Huntosova, V.; Kozar, T. Importance of Hypericin-Bcl2 interactions for biological effects at subcellular levels. *Photodiagn. Photodyn. Ther.* **2019**, *28*, 38–52. [CrossRef]
20. Huntosova, V.; Nadova, Z.; Dzurova, L.; Jakusova, V.; Sureau, F.; Miskovsky, P. Cell death response of U87 glioma cells on hypericin photoactivation is mediated by dynamics of hypericin subcellular distribution and its aggregation in cellular organelles. *Photochem. Photobiol. Sci.* **2012**, *11*, 1428–1436. [CrossRef] [PubMed]
21. Theodossiou, T.A.; Hothersall, J.S.; De Witte, P.A.; Pantos, A.; Agostinis, P. The multifaceted photocytotoxic profile of hypericin. *Mol. Pharm.* **2009**, *6*, 1775–1789. [CrossRef]
22. Han, C.; Zhang, C.; Ma, T.; Zhang, C.; Luo, J.; Xu, X.; Zhao, H.; Chen, Y.; Kong, L. Hypericin-functionalized graphene oxide for enhanced mitochondria-targeting and synergistic anticancer effect. *Acta Biomater.* **2018**, *77*, 268–281. [CrossRef]
23. Thomas, C.; MacGill, R.S.; Miller, G.C.; Pardini, R.S. Photoactivation of hypericin generates singlet oxygen in mitochondria and inhibits succinoxidase. *Photochem. Photobiol.* **1992**, *55*, 47–53. [CrossRef]
24. Theodossiou, T.A.; Noronha-Dutra, A.; Hothersall, J.S. Mitochondria are a primary target of hypericin phototoxicity: Synergy of intracellular calcium mobilisation in cell killing. *Int. J. Biochem. Cell Biol.* **2006**, *38*, 1946–1956. [CrossRef] [PubMed]
25. Balogová, L.; Maslaňáková, M.; Dzurová, L.; Miškovský, P.; Štroffeková, K. Bcl-2 proapoptotic proteins distribution in U-87 MG glioma cells before and after hypericin photodynamic action. *Gen. Physiol. Biophys.* **2013**, *32*, 179–187. [CrossRef] [PubMed]

26. Huntosova, V.; Novotova, M.; Nichtova, Z.; Balogova, L.; Maslanakova, M.; Petrovajova, D.; Stroffekova, K. Assessing light-independent effects of hypericin on cell viability, ultrastructure and metabolism in human glioma and endothelial cells. *Toxicol. In Vitro* **2017**, *40*, 184–195. [CrossRef] [PubMed]
27. Silveira, P.C.L.; Ferreira, G.K.; Zaccaron, R.P.; Glaser, V.; Remor, A.P.; Mendes, C.; Pinho, R.A.; Latini, A. Effects of photobiomodulation on mitochondria of brain, muscle, and C6 astroglioma cells. *Med. Eng. Phys.* **2019**, *71*, 108–113. [CrossRef]
28. Chang, S.Y.; Lee, M.Y.; Chung, P.S.; Kim, S.; Choi, B.; Suh, M.W.; Rhee, C.K.; Jung, J.Y. Enhanced mitochondrial membrane potential and ATP synthesis by photobiomodulation increases viability of the auditory cell line after gentamicin-induced intrinsic apoptosis. *Sci. Rep.* **2019**, *9*, 19248. [CrossRef]
29. Yang, L.; Youngblood, H.; Wu, C.; Zhang, Q. Mitochondria as a target for neuroprotection: Role of methylene blue and photobiomodulation. *Transl. Neurodegener.* **2020**, *9*, 19. [CrossRef]
30. Foo, A.S.C.; Soong, T.W.; Yeo, T.T.; Lim, K.L. Mitochondrial Dysfunction and Parkinson's Disease—Near-Infrared Photobiomodulation as a Potential Therapeutic Strategy. *Front. Aging Neurosci.* **2020**, *12*, 89. [CrossRef]
31. Hamblin, M.R. Mechanisms and Mitochondrial Redox Signaling in Photobiomodulation. *Photochem. Photobiol.* **2018**, *94*, 199–212. [CrossRef]
32. Engel, K.W.; Khan, I.; Arany, P.R. Cell lineage responses to photobiomodulation therapy. *J. Biophotonics* **2016**, *9*, 1148–1156. [CrossRef]
33. Bartos, A.; Grondin, Y.; Bortoni, M.E.; Ghelfi, E.; Sepulveda, R.; Carroll, J.; Rogers, R.A. Pre-conditioning with near infrared photobiomodulation reduces inflammatory cytokines and markers of oxidative stress in cochlear hair cells. *J. Biophotonics* **2016**, *9*, 1125–1135. [CrossRef]
34. Pires Marques, E.C.; Piccolo Lopes, F.; Nascimento, I.C.; Morelli, J.; Pereira, M.V.; Machado Meiken, V.M.; Pinheiro, S.L. Photobiomodulation and photodynamic therapy for the treatment of oral mucositis in patients with cancer. *Photodiagn. Photodyn. Ther.* **2020**, *29*, 101621. [CrossRef] [PubMed]
35. Maya, R.; Costa Ladeira, L.L.; Maya, J.E.P.; Gonçalves, L.M.; Bussadori, S.K.; Paschoal, M.A.B. The combination of antimicrobial photodynamic therapy and photobiomodulation therapy for the treatment of palatal ulcers: A case report. *J. Lasers Med. Sci.* **2020**, *11*, 228–233. [CrossRef]
36. Fekrazad, R. Photobiomodulation and Antiviral Photodynamic Therapy as a Possible Novel Approach in COVID-19 Management. *Photobiomodul. Photomed. Laser Surg.* **2020**, *38*, 255–257. [CrossRef] [PubMed]
37. Schneider, C.A.; Rasband, W.S.; Eliceiri, K.W. NIH Image to ImageJ: 25 years of image analysis. *Nat. Methods* **2012**, *9*, 671–675. [CrossRef]
38. Dror, N.; Mandel, M.; Lavie, G. Unique Anti-Glioblastoma Activities of Hypericin Are at the Crossroad of Biochemical and Epigenetic Events and Culminate in Tumor Cell Differentiation. *PLoS ONE* **2013**, *8*, e73625. [CrossRef] [PubMed]
39. Utsumi, T.; Okuma, M.; Utsumi, T.; Kanno, T.; Yasuda, T.; Kobuchi, H.; Horton, A.A.; Utsumi, K. Light-dependent inhibition of protein kinase c and superoxide generation of neutrophils by hypericin, an antiretroviral agent. *Arch. Biochem. Biophys.* **1995**, *316*, 493–497. [CrossRef] [PubMed]
40. Zhang, W.; Law, R.E.; Hinton, D.R.; Couldwell, W.T. Inhibition of human malignant glioma cell motility and invasion in vitro by hypericin, a potent protein kinase C inhibitor. *Cancer Lett.* **1997**, *120*, 31–38. [CrossRef]
41. Kamran, M.Z.; Patil, P.; Gude, R.P. Role of STAT3 in cancer metastasis and translational advances. *Biomed Res. Int.* **2013**, *2013*, 421821. [CrossRef]
42. Jain, N.; Zhang, T.; Kee, W.H.; Li, W.; Cao, X. Protein kinase C δ associates with and phosphorylates Stat3 in an interleukin-6-dependent manner. *J. Biol. Chem.* **1999**, *274*, 24392–24400. [CrossRef]
43. Edmonds, C.; Hagan, S.; Gallagher-Colombo, S.M.; Busch, T.M.; Cengel, K.A. Photodynamic therapy activated signaling from epidermal growth factor receptor and STAT3: Targeting survival pathways to increase PDT efficacy in ovarian and lung cancer. *Cancer Biol. Ther.* **2012**, *13*, 1463–1470. [CrossRef]
44. Liu, W.; Oseroff, A.R.; Baumann, H. Photodynamic therapy causes cross-linking of signal transducer and activator of transcription proteins and attenuation of interleukin-6 cytokine responsiveness in epithelial cells. *Cancer Res.* **2004**, *64*, 6579–6587. [CrossRef]
45. Qiao, L.; Xu, C.; Li, Q.; Mei, Z.; Li, X.; Cai, H.; Liu, W. Photodynamic therapy activated STAT3 associated pathways: Targeting intrinsic apoptotic pathways to increase PDT efficacy in human squamous carcinoma cells. *Photodiagn. Photodyn. Ther.* **2016**, *14*, 119–127. [CrossRef] [PubMed]
46. Vantieghem, A.; Assefa, Z.; Vandenabeele, P.; Declercq, W.; Courtois, S.; Vandenheede, J.R.; Merlevede, W.; De Witte, P.; Agostinis, P. Hypericin-induced photosensitization of HeLa cells leads to apoptosis or necrosis: Involvement of cytochrome c and procaspase-3 activation in the mechanism of apoptosis. *FEBS Lett.* **1998**, *440*, 19–24. [CrossRef]
47. Barathan, M.; Mariappan, V.; Shankar, E.M.; Abdullah, B.J.; Goh, K.L.; Vadivelu, J. Hypericin-photodynamic therapy leads to interleukin-6 secretion by HepG2 cells and their apoptosis via recruitment of BH3 interacting-domain death agonist and caspases. *Cell Death Dis.* **2013**, *4*, e697. [CrossRef]
48. Bento, C.F.; Renna, M.; Ghislat, G.; Puri, C.; Ashkenazi, A.; Vicinanza, M.; Menzies, F.M.; Rubinsztein, D.C. Mammalian Autophagy: How Does It Work? *Annu. Rev. Biochem.* **2016**, *85*, 685–713. [CrossRef]
49. Rubinsztein, D.C. The roles of intracellular protein-degradation pathways in neurodegeneration. *Nature* **2006**, *443*, 780–786. [CrossRef] [PubMed]

50. Runwal, G.; Stamatakou, E.; Siddiqi, F.H.; Puri, C.; Zhu, Y.; Rubinsztein, D.C. LC3-positive structures are prominent in autophagy-deficient cells. *Sci. Rep.* **2019**, *9*, 10147. [CrossRef] [PubMed]
51. Joniová, J.; Kazemiraad, C.; Gerelli, E.; Wagnières, G. Stimulation and homogenization of the protoporphyrin IX endogenous production by photobiomodulation to increase the potency of photodynamic therapy. *J. Photochem. Photobiol. B Biol.* **2021**, *225*, 112347. [CrossRef] [PubMed]

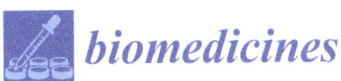

Article

Feasibility of Photodynamic Therapy for Glioblastoma with the Mitochondria-Targeted Photosensitizer Tetramethylrhodamine Methyl Ester (TMRM)

Alex Vasilev [1,2,†], Roba Sofi [2,3,†], Stuart J. Smith [4], Ruman Rahman [4], Anja G. Teschemacher [2] and Sergey Kasparov [1,2,*]

1. School of Life Sciences, Immanuel Kant Baltic Federal University, Universitetskaya Str., 2, 236041 Kaliningrad, Russia; otherlife@bk.ru
2. School of Physiology, Pharmacology and Neuroscience, University of Bristol, University Walk, Bristol BS8 1TD, UK; roba.sofi@bristol.ac.uk or rasafi@kau.edu.sa (R.S.); anja.teschemacher@bristol.ac.uk (A.G.T.)
3. Faculty of Medicine, King Abdul-Aziz University, Alehtifalat St., Jeddah 21589, Saudi Arabia
4. Children's Brain Tumour Research Centre, Nottingham Biodiscovery Institute, School of Medicine, University of Nottingham, Nottingham NG7 2RD, UK; stuart.smith@nottingham.ac.uk (S.J.S.); ruman.rahman@nottingham.ac.uk (R.R.)
* Correspondence: sergey.kasparov@bristol.ac.uk; Tel.: +44-117-331-2275
† Equal contributions.

Abstract: One of the most challenging problems in the treatment of glioblastoma (GBM) is the highly infiltrative nature of the disease. Infiltrating cells that are non-resectable are left behind after debulking surgeries and become a source of regrowth and recurrence. To prevent tumor recurrence and increase patient survival, it is necessary to cleanse the adjacent tissue from GBM infiltrates. This requires an innovative local approach. One such approach is that of photodynamic therapy (PDT) which uses specific light-sensitizing agents called photosensitizers. Here, we show that tetramethylrhodamine methyl ester (TMRM), which has been used to asses mitochondrial potential, can be used as a photosensitizer to target GBM cells. Primary patient-derived GBM cell lines were used, including those specifically isolated from the infiltrative edge. PDT with TMRM using low-intensity green light induced mitochondrial damage, an irreversible drop in mitochondrial membrane potential and led to GBM cell death. Moreover, delayed photoactivation after TMRM loading selectively killed GBM cells but not cultured rat astrocytes. The efficacy of TMRM-PDT in certain GBM cell lines may be potentiated by adenylate cyclase activator NKH477. Together, these findings identify TMRM as a prototypical mitochondrially targeted photosensitizer with beneficial features which may be suitable for preclinical and clinical translation.

Keywords: glioblastoma; photodynamic therapy; photosensitizer; mitochondria

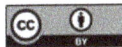

1. Introduction

Glioblastoma (GBM) is the deadliest adult brain cancer. Among possible cellular sources of GBM are neural stem cells (NSC), oligodendrocyte progenitor cells and astrocytes [1]. GBMs exhibit a highly heterogeneous molecular makeup and are characterized by genomic instability and high tendency for infiltration. GBM exists in a variety of molecular phenotypes, including isocitrate dehydrogenase wild type, mutant type and some others [2]. Molecular heterogeneity greatly reduces chances of finding a highly potent and universally useful drug against any one specific molecular target for this type of cancer.

The global standard of care, known as the Stupp protocol [3], consists of surgical resection followed by administration of the alkylating agent temozolomide (TMZ) in combination with radio-therapy. However, the Stupp protocol only extends median survival to ~14 months from diagnosis compared to 12 months when using radio-therapy alone [3].

This treatment protocol and the resultant survival prognosis have not significantly changed for the last 15 years.

Considering that GBM does not metastatically spread around the body and that primary tumors are often reasonably well localized, it is surprising that we are still making so little progress in improving treatment outcomes. The key reason for this is that, despite maximal surgical resection, the tumor inevitably reoccurs. Interestingly, most secondary tumors arise within <2 cm of the resection edge [4]. These recurrences originate from the infiltrating GBM cells which spread from the leading edge into non-neoplastic tissue parenchyma. Today, the macroscopic boundaries of the primary tumor are usually identified by neurosurgeons using specific staining with 5-aminolevulinic acid (5ALA, trade name Gliolan®) which was approved by the Food and Drug Administration in 2017 for the optical detection of GBM. 5ALA is fairly selectively converted into protoporphyrin IX in cancer cells [5]. Thus, by illuminating the tumor by near-UV blue light and monitoring resultant red fluorescence, surgeons are able to detect macroscopic boundaries of GBM. However, this does not allow visualization of the microscopic infiltrations. Moreover, in many cases, even though surgeons suspect infiltrations in certain areas, they are unable to remove residual disease due to the risk of severe neurological deficits.

Poor prognosis for patients with GBM necessitates research into alternative approaches for the treatment of this disease. One such approach is photodynamic therapy (PDT), as we have recently reviewed [6]. PDT is based on a photochemical reaction triggered by the absorption of photons of light by the molecules of a photosensitizer. Singlet oxygen and reactive oxygen species released by this reaction damage cellular macromolecules and eventually kill the cells. Even though quite a few molecules could theoretically be used as photosensitizers, only 5ALA has been extensively explored as a photosensitizer for GBM therapy, including in clinical trials [7]. The motivation for working with 5ALA is mainly the selective accumulation of fluorescent protoporphyrin IX in cancer cells which may intuitively suggest that PDT should only damage the malignant cells and not the healthy tissue. However, so far, experimental and clinical applications of 5ALA as a PDT agent have not been particularly successful [6] as 5ALA appears to be a poor photosensitizer, unable to generate sufficient amounts of free radicals to induce a powerful effect. High-power red light at approximately ~630 nm was used for its photoactivation in the published trials [8–10]. This contrasts with the peak absorption of protoporphyrin IX which is near 420 nm [8–12] This was largely motivated by the much better penetration of red light through brain tissue, but clearly, it cannot be efficient in terms of triggering the required photochemistry.

Over the past 10 years, the application of light to the brains of living animals has become a major tool in experimental neuroscience (a technology known as "optogenetics"), and a wealth of information is now available from these experiments. Hundreds of studies have used light to control cells, which are induced to express light-sensitive proteins. The wavelengths used for excitation are typically below 550 nM (blue-green-yellow). Despite the accepted notion that infra-red light (~700 nm and above) penetrates deeper into the tissue, which could be an advantage in the case of PDT, the vast experience accumulated with optogenetics unequivocally demonstrates that large quantities of light energy are damaging for a healthy brain. Moreover, light, especially the longer-wave red and infra-red light, easily releases heat which destroys brain cells (for further discussion, see [6]).

These considerations led us to investigate whether we might be more successful using another photosensitizer with a different principle of action and selectivity.

By serendipity, we discovered that one of the dyes routinely used to image mitochondrial membrane potential (MMP), tetramethylrhodamine (TMRM), acts as an efficient photosensitizer in patient-derived primary GBM cell lines and that it is possible to achieve at least partial selectivity over non-malignant primary rat astrocytes (RA). TMRM, which is a rhodamine derivative driven into the mitochondria by their negative membrane potential has been in routine laboratory use as a research reagent but never tested as a potential therapeutic. After brief (<1 min) illumination with a green light of moderate intensity,

TMRM causes the rapid and irreversible depolarization of GBM mitochondria, which ultimately leads to the apoptosis-mediated death of these cells. Here, we explored the effectiveness of TMRM as a photosensitizer for PDT (TMRM-PDT). We also attempted to increase the efficacy of TMRM-PDT using the cAMP-elevating compound NKH477 (a water-soluble analogue of forskolin) and a glycolysis inhibitor clotrimazole.

2. Materials and Methods

2.1. Primary Cultures of RA

Primary cultures of RA were prepared from the cerebral cortices, cerebellum and brainstem of Wistar rat pups (P2) as previously described [13]. Briefly, the brains of terminally anesthetized Wistar P2 pups were dissected out, crudely cross-chopped and incubated with agitation at 37 °C for 15 min in a solution containing HBSS, DNase I (0.04 mg/mL), trypsin from bovine pancreas (0.25 mg/mL) and BSA (3 mg/mL). Trypsinization was terminated by the addition of equal volumes of culture media comprised of DMEM, 10% heat-inactivated FBS, 100 U/mL penicillin, and 0.1 mg/mL streptomycin and the suspension was then centrifuged at 2000 rpm, at room temperature (RT) for 10 min. The supernatant was aspirated, and the remaining pellet was resuspended in 15 mL HBSS containing BSA (3 mg/mL) and DNase I (0.04 mg/mL) and gently triturated. After the cell debris settled, the cell suspension was filtered through a 40 μm cell strainer (BD Falcon, BD Biosciences, Franklin Lakes, NJ, USA) and cells were collected after centrifugation. Cells were seeded in a T75 flask containing the culture media (see above) and maintained at 37 °C with 5% CO_2. Once the cultures reached confluence and 1 week later, the flasks were mildly shaken overnight to remove microglia and oligodendrocytes.

2.2. GBM Cell Lines

UP007 and UP029 were kindly provided by Prof. J. Pilkington (University of Portsmouth) and maintained using standard laboratory protocols in media containing 10% serum and 1% penicillin/streptomycin (0.1 mg/mL penicillin, 100 units/mL streptomycin). In some experiments, we also used primary GBM cell lines specifically derived from the infiltrative edge of surgically removed tumors as described in Smith et al. [6]. These are designated as glioblastoma invasive margin (GIN) cell lines. Their culturing conditions and handling were the same as those for UP cell lines. All of the cell lines used were of the IDH-wildtype genetic background.

2.3. Measurement of Cell Viability

Cytotoxicity was assessed by lactate dehydrogenase (LDH), 3-(4,5-dimethylthiazol-2-yl)-2,5-diphenyltetrazolium bromide (MTT), and PrestoBlue™ (Invitrogen, Paisley, UK) assays.

2.3.1. LDH Assay

LDH is an intracellular enzyme that is released from cells upon the disruption of the cell membrane or cell lysis. Thermo Scientific™ Pierce™ LDH Cytotoxicity Assay (cat no. 88954) was used to determine the toxicity of TMRM in the absence of light illumination. This is a colorimetric assay where the amount of LDH in a sample is proportional to the amount of red formazan product produced by the consumption of NADH generated by the LDH-mediated conversion of L-lactate. After adding reaction buffers to the sample culture media, color intensity in wells was measured using an Infinite® 200 PRO microplate reader.

2.3.2. MTT Assay

The MTT assay was used to assess the potential detrimental effects of prolonged TMRM loading on cells. RA and GBM cell lines were seeded in a 96-well culture plate at 1×10^4 cells/mL in 10% FBS culture media at 37 °C in 5% CO_2 atmosphere and allowed to attach overnight. After 24 h, the culture media were replaced with fresh media containing different concentrations of TMRM (50 nM, 100 nM, 300 nM, 800 nM) and the plates were incubated for 48 h protected from light. Tests were done in triplicates. After incubation, the MTT reagent was added into the media at a final concentration of 0.5 mg/mL and incubated for 2 h 37 °C under low light conditions. Then, the MTT reagent was removed and 100 µL DMSO in each well was added and the cells were incubated at 37 °C for 30 min to dissolve the formazan crystal precipitates. Absorbance was measured at 570 nm. Cell viability was calculated by the following formula:

$$\left(\text{Absorbance}_{\text{experimental group}} / \text{Absorbance}_{\text{control group}} \right) \times 100\%$$

2.3.3. PrestoBlue™ Assay

To assess the viability of the cells after photoactivation with different illumination durations, we performed the PrestoBlue™ cell viability assay (Invitrogen) on UP007, UP029 and GIN8 cell lines. This assay does not require the fixation of cells and can be performed on the same set of cells several times. Cells were seeded in 96-well plates using the technique described above. Twenty-four hours later, cell lines were loaded with TMRM (300 nM × 40 min) and photoactivated for 45 s and 90 s (1.06 mW/mm^2). PrestoBlue assay was performed on day 2, 5 and 10 after the photoactivation of TMRM, following the manufacturer's instructions. Briefly, 10 µL of PrestoBlue reagent was added to each well and incubated for 20 min. Fluorescence was measured at 560 nM, thus reflecting the amount of the fluorescent product of the conversion of the reagent.

2.4. Assessment of Basal Mitochondrial Membrane Potential (MMP) Using Potential-Driven Dye TMRM

Cells were plated in 96-well plates and allowed to attach overnight. The following day, cells were loaded with 200 nM TMRM for 1 h. Images were taken using a ZOE (Bio-Rad, Watford, UK) fluorescent cell imager. Fluorescence intensity (as an estimate for MMP) was measured using the Fiji image processing tool and compared across cell types. Image acquisition parameters were fixed across all measurements.

2.5. Measurements of Mitochondrial Depolarization Dynamics Caused by TMRM

TMRM decay dynamics was tested using the following protocol. The cells were plated onto glass cover slips coated with type 1 rat tail collagen at a concentration of 0.25 mg/mL to enhance the attachment of the cells. Cover slips were placed inside small corning dishes at a density of 5×10^4 cells/mL. Dishes were incubated overnight in standard culture conditions. The next day, cells were loaded with 200 nM TMRM for 1 h. Before the photoactivation of TMRM, baseline images using a standard rhodamine filter block of Leica microscopes (excitation 515 nm–560 nm, emission-high pass filter 580 nm) were obtained as a sequence of six images, one every 10 s, for a total of one minute. This was followed by constant illumination with same green light for 30 s (photoactivation) followed by a series of 20 images every 10 s, for a total of 3 min. Imaging was conducted using a Leica DMIRB Inverted florescent microscope connected to a R6 Retiga digital camera and controlled by the Micromanager software. Imaging parameters such as exposure time and light intensity (1.4 mW/mm^2, 10× objective) were fixed throughout all imaging sessions. ImageJ software was used to process the images.

2.6. Assessment of MMP Recovery after TMRM-PDT

In this and all other series, we used ×5 objectives (unless specifically indicated) to illuminate large areas with numerous cells to achieve a uniform biological outcome across the whole pool of cells in an individual dish. Since two different makes of microscopes were used (Zeiss and Leica) the light power density was slightly different between some datasets (1.4 and 1.06 mW/mm^2 for Leica vs. 1.4 mW/mm^2 for Zeiss); however, this did not qualitatively affect the outcomes.

To ensure that all cells were evenly illuminated, we used a special plating technique which ensured that they were localized in the center of the well. This was important because in the preliminary experiments, we found that the cells located at the margins of the wells and their walls do not receive sufficient quantities of light and therefore do not react to PDT.

To this end, cells were plated as 3 µL drops, containing an average of ~300–350 cells/drop at the centers of the wells in a 96-well plate. After 45 min, when cells had attached to the bottom, wells were filled with 100 µL of fresh media and incubated overnight. This plating approach was used for all experiments involving TMRM-PDT. The next day, cells were incubated with 300 nM TMRM for 40 min, and TMRM was photoactivated for 40 s using a ×5 objective (1.06 mW/mm^2). Media in the wells were replaced and cells were returned into the incubator. Mitochondrial potential was measured 24 h later using TMRM.

2.7. TMRM-PDT

2.7.1. Evaluating the Efficacy of TMRM as a Photosensitizer: Effect of TMRM Photoactivation on Cell Viability

Cells were plated in the centers of the well as described above and loaded with 300 nM TMRM for 45 min. Photoactivation of TMRM was carried out for 40 s (1.06 mW/mm^2). Green light was used using standard filter blocks of Leica microscopes with a pass-band of ~520 nm–540 nm. Media were then replaced and the cells were incubated for 72 h. Fixation, nuclear staining, imaging and analysis were carried out as indicated above in this and further experiments in this section.

2.7.2. Concentration-Response Test for PDT with TMRM-PDT

On day 1, cells were plated following the previously described plating protocol, and were then allowed to grow in a cell culture incubator overnight. On day 2, media were removed, and cells were loaded with TMRM (100 nM, 300 nM, 800 nM) for 40 min. The center of each well was then illuminated by green light (~530 nm–580 nm) using a LSM780 ZEISS confocal microscope with a ×5 objective at 1.4 mW/mm^2 for 30 s. After the photoactivation, the media were exchanged and cells were incubated for 72 h. After 3 days incubation, the cells were fixed in 4% paraformaldehyde (PFA) for 15 min, washed in PBS three times and stained with 1 µg/mL DAPI for 10 min. Images were taken using a confocal microscope with objective power x5 to include all DAPI positive cells in one image for each well.

2.7.3. Exposure-Dependence of TMRM-PDT

Cells were seeded as described above and loaded with TMRM (100 nM) for 40 min. Photoactivation was carried out for 30 s, 60 s or 90 s at 1.4 mW/mm^2. Media were replaced and cells were then incubated for 72 h.

2.7.4. Retention of TMRM in Mitochondria of RA and GBM Cells

Cells were seeded as described above. Cells were loaded with different concentrations of TMRM for 40 min. After 40 min, TMRM was removed and fresh media was added. After 24 h, photoactivation was performed for 30 s at 1.4 mW/mm^2. Media were replaced with fresh media and the cells were incubated for 72 h.

2.7.5. Assessment of the Effect of Green Light Alone Using Presto Blue Viability Assay

UP007, UP029 and RA were plated in the centers of the wells in a 96-well plate as described above. The next day, the cells were irradiated with green light without TMRM staining for 60 s or 120 s (1.4 mW/mm^2). Note that the strength of this stimulus considerably exceeded all illumination regimes applied in other tests. After 3 days, cell viability was assessed with PrestoBlue assay following the manufacturer protocol.

2.7.6. Incubation with NKH477, Clotrimazole and Photoactivation

Cells were seeded in 96 well-plates using the technique described above. Milder TMRM-PDT conditions were used in these experiments in order to more easily reveal any additive or synergistic effects of the combined treatment. Specifically, 200 nM TMRM was used to load the cells instead of 300 nM. A Leica EC3 florescent microscope was used to illuminate the cells with a ×5 objective lens, light dose of 1.06 mW/mm^2 and the duration of illumination of 17 s only. To test whether NKH477 can enhance TMRM-PDT, GBM cells were pre-incubated with 10 μM NKH477 for 24 h before TMRM-PDT was conducted. The PDT outcome was tested on day 3 as previously described. We also tested whether we could potentiate the outcome of PDT with clotrimazole (a glycolysis inhibitor). Immediately after TMRM-PDT, 10 μM of the drug was also added to the wells. Cells were incubated with clotrimazole for three days before evaluating the outcome by the nuclear count as described above.

2.8. Assessment of Caspase Activation after PDT

To confirm that GBM cells affected by PDT undergo apoptosis, we used a genetic reporter of apoptosis CA-GFP (Caspase Activated Green fluorescent protein) as described in [14]. During apoptosis, caspase is activated via proteolytic cleavage. In CA-GFP, GFP fluorescence is completely quenched by a quenching peptide attached via the four amino acid caspase-7 cleavage motif Asp–Glu–Val–Asp. After the initiation of apoptosis, proteolytic removal of the quenching peptide by caspase-8 and caspase-9 results in restored GFP fluorescence. In order to stably express the reporter in dividing GBM cells, we generated a lentiviral vector where CA-GFP was expressed under control of the EF1α promoter, which is highly active and stable in GBM (own unpublished observation). GBM cells were loaded with TMRM (300 nM × 40 min) and photoactivated for 90 s (1.06 mW/mm^2). The plates were kept for 10 days and the surviving cells were then fixed, stained with DAPI and imaged using a ZOE imager.

2.9. Lentiviral Production

The full protocol was described in our previous study [15]. Briefly, for lentiviral production, Lenti-X™293 T Cell Line (Clontech, San Francisco, CA, USA) was transfected with plasmids pNHP (7.5 μg), pHEF-VSVG (3.1 μg), pCEP4-tat (0.7 μg) and pTYF-EF1α-CA-GFP (3.9 μg). Cells were then placed in an incubator under standard cell culture conditions. Culture media were collected after approximately 30 and 48 h after transfection and stored at 4 °C. Then, the media were filtrated and centrifuged in 20% sucrose at 74,000× g for 2 h. The supernatant was aspirated and 25 μL PBS was added. The following day, the lentiviral vector pellet was resuspended, aliquoted and frozen at −80 °C.

2.10. Statistical Analysis

The data were shown as mean ± SEM; the numbers of independent experiments are indicated on the figures and in the text. Statistical analysis was performed using one-way or two-way ANOVA using Prism software version 8.00. Differences were considered statistically significant at $p < 0.05$.

3. Results

3.1. Green Light Triggers Immediate Release of TMRM from the Mitochondria

Brief exposures of TMRM-loaded (200 nM) RA and GBM cells to green light (200–300 ms every 10 s), which are required for taking images, did not affect TMRM mitochondrial localization. TMRM intensity remained stable for 30 min or more in all cell lines (data not shown).

Nuclei, under resting conditions, usually contain little TMRM but once TMRM leaves the mitochondria, it spreads into other cellular compartments including the nucleus. Therefore, results are presented as a ratio of mitochondrial/nuclear TMRM florescence intensity (Figure 1a,b).

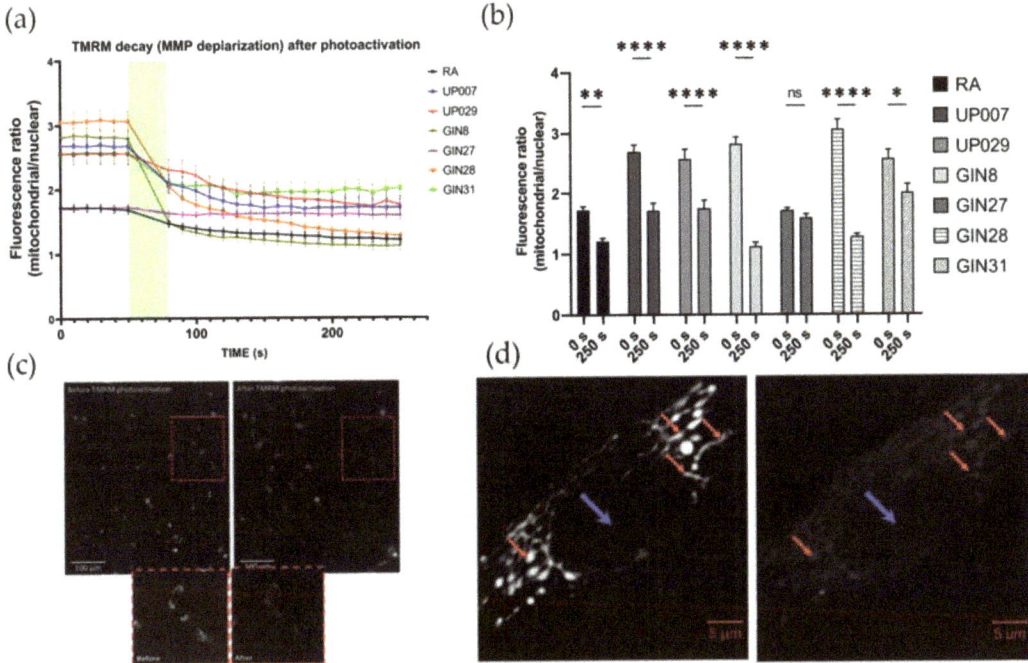

Figure 1. Light activation of TMRM triggers an immediate mitochondrial depolarization and results in dye re-distribution. (**a**) Mitochondria/nucleus fluorescence ratio dropped by 50% within 60 s and further decayed for the next 4–7 min. n: 24 cells from 4 independent exp. (**b**) Mitochondria/nucleus fluorescence ratios decreased after 250 s following light activation. (**c**) Representative images showing loss of TMRM from mitochondria over time and appearance of the dye in the nucleus. Red squares point to an enlarged area demonstrating a few cells at higher magnification (below). Note the redistribution of fluorescence from the bright clusters of mitochondria and its exit from the cells. The brightness of the images on the inset (lower images) is increased to facilitate viewing. For measurements, only raw images were used. (**d**) An example of a typical response to TMRM-PDT of a GBM GIN8 cell. Initially (left image), TMRM is localized exclusively to the mitochondria (red arrows) while the nucleus (blue arrow) is almost completely devoid of the staining. After photoactivation (right image), TMRM leaves the mitochondria and the contrast between mitochondria and nucleus is lost—hence the ratio mitochondria/nucleus drops). For clarification, images were taken at high magnification using LSM780 confocal microscope. (*) p value < 0.005, (**) p value < 0.001, (****) p value < 0.0001. ns—not significant.

Baseline MMP was stable before photoactivation (Figure 1a). Photoactivation of TMRM for 30 s resulted in the rapid exit of the dye from the mitochondria, most probably due to the loss of mitochondrial potential, decreasing the mitochondrial/nucleus fluorescence ratio (Figure 1a,b). Typical examples of TMRM distribution in GIN8 cell line before and after photoactivation are shown in Figure 1c,d. During this initial control period (1–30 s), it was evident that the GBM cell lines had significantly greater MMP (hyperpolarized mitochondria as reflected by the absolute intensity of TMRM staining) than normal RA, except the GIN27 cell line (Figure 2a, Supplementary Figure S3).

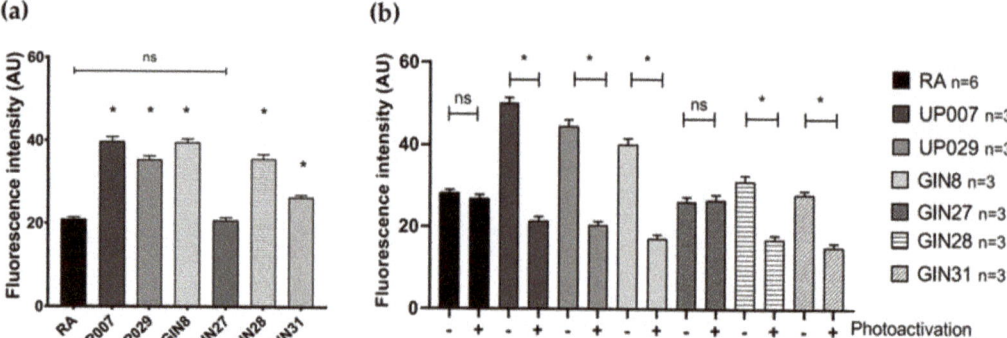

Figure 2. Mitochondrial membrane potential in RA and GBM cells, as reflected by TMRM florescence intensity. (**a**) Baseline MMP. GBM cells, except for GIN27, have greater basal MMP than normal RA. (**b**) Recovery of MMP 24 h after photoactivation. Normal RA and GIN27 GBM cells successfully recovered their normal MMP 24 h after photoactivation. Loss of MMP in other GBM cells persisted after 24 h. N: represents the number of independent experiments. 15+ cells were examined in each experiment. (*) p value < 0.0001, (ns) p value > 0.9999 (not significant).

3.2. GBM Cells Failed to Recover Their MMP 24 h after Photodynamic Treatment, in Contrast to Normal RA

We wanted to assess whether light-induced MMP depolarization was reversible. To this end, we re-loaded cells with TMRM 24 h after light application and measured TMRM fluorescence intensity. Note, that in this series, we did not calculate the ratio as in the previous section because we were interested in the absolute intensity values rather than the dynamics of the process. As shown in Figure 2b, the mitochondria remained depolarized in all human GBM lines, with the exception of GIN27. Importantly, mitochondria in RA fully recovered their membrane potential, evident by normal TMRM loading after 24 h.

3.3. Photodynamic Activation of TMRM Decreased GBM Survival

To study the effect of TMRM-PDT on GBM cell survival, cells were loaded with TMRM (300 nM) and exposed to green light. Three days later the density of the DAPI-positive nuclei was strongly reduced in wells subjected to TMRM-PDT compared to controls (see Figure 3). Curiously, this was also seen for the GIN27 line which seemed to be less affected by PDT in previous experiments (Figures 1 and 2).

3.4. Milder Treatment Regimes Help Achieve a Preferential Effect on GBM Cell Lines

Given that GBM mitochondria were generally hyperpolarized, we sought to determine whether this could lead to a preferential effect of PDT on GBM, using milder treatment. This was only tested on UP lines for operational reasons.

Thus, 30 s, 60 s, or 90 s (1.4 mW/mm^2) and a lower concentration of TMRM (100 nM) were evaluated. As shown in Figure 4, the number of DAPI-positive nuclei 3 days after photoactivation was significantly reduced in GBM lines but not in RA following milder treatment regimens.

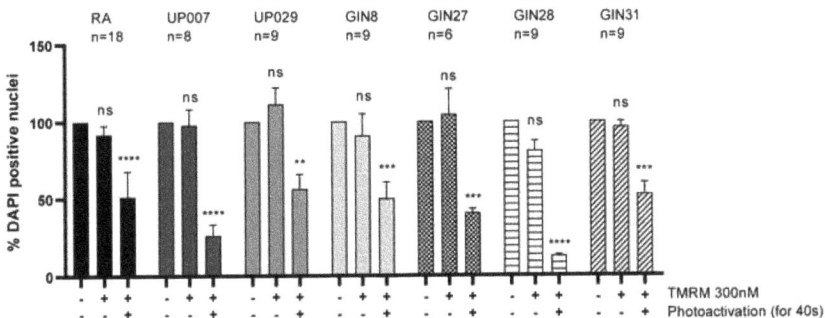

Figure 3. Three days after TMRM-PDT (300 nM; 40 s; 1.06 mW/mm^2), density of cells was reduced. N is the total number of repeats from 7 independent experiments for RA, 2 for GIN27 and 3 for the other GBM cells. (**) p value < 0.003, (***) p value < 0.001, (****) p value < 0.0001. ns—not significant.

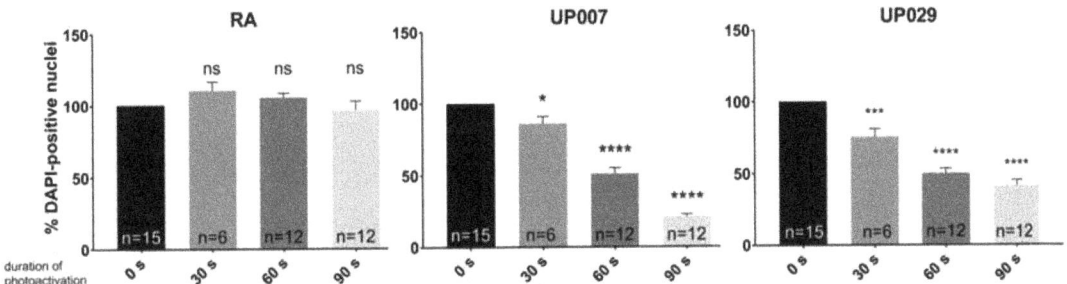

Figure 4. Dependence of TMRM-PDT (100 nM; 0 s, 30 s, 60 s, 90 s; 1.4 mW/mm^2)) on the duration of illumination. N is the total number of repeats from 4 independent experiments. (*) p value < 0.05, (***) p value < 0.001, (****) p value < 0.0001. ns—not significant.

3.5. Effect of TMRM Is Concentration Dependent

In order to better demonstrate the dependence of the TMRM effect on its concentration, we applied different concentrations while using a slightly shortened duration of illumination (30 s) in order to preserve at least some cells in stimulated wells—which was important for counting purposes. The number of DAPI-positive nuclei was not affected with TMRM loading at 100 nM while 800 nM significantly affected all tested cell types (Figure 5). In fact, the effect on both GBM cell lines was much greater than on RA ($p < 0.001$ in both cases).

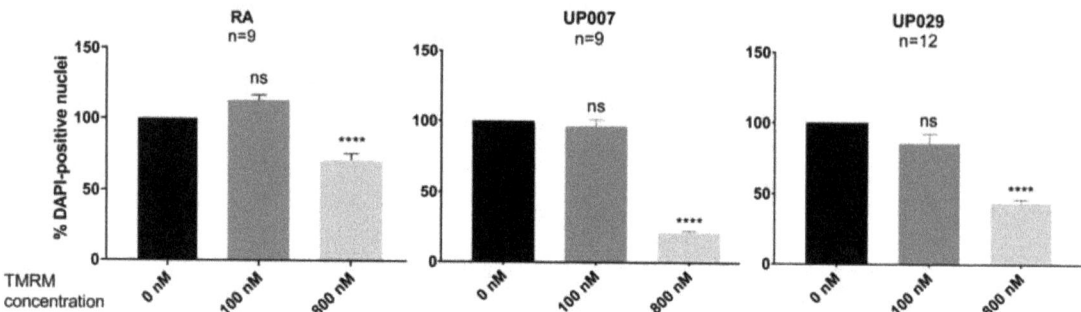

Figure 5. The dependence of TMRM-PDT (0 nM, 100 nM and 800 nM for 30 s; 1.4 mW/mm^2) on TMRM concentration. N is the total number of datapoints from 4 independent experiments. (****) p value < 0.001. Differences between the effect of 800 nM on RA (relative decrease in cell density) and either of the GBM cell lines were highly significant ($p < 0.01$ in either case). ns—not significant.

3.6. TMRM-PDT with Preloading of the Dye

Mitochondrial membranes of GBM cells are generally more polarized relative to normal cells such as RA (Figure 2a). Thus, TMRM should theoretically accumulate and remain in the mitochondria longer in GBM cells, making them more vulnerable to TMRM-PDT. Indeed, TMRM-PDT applied to cells preloaded with TMRM for 40 min, 24 h before application of the light, had a preferential effect on the GBM lines compared to RA (Figure 6, Supplementary Figure S2).

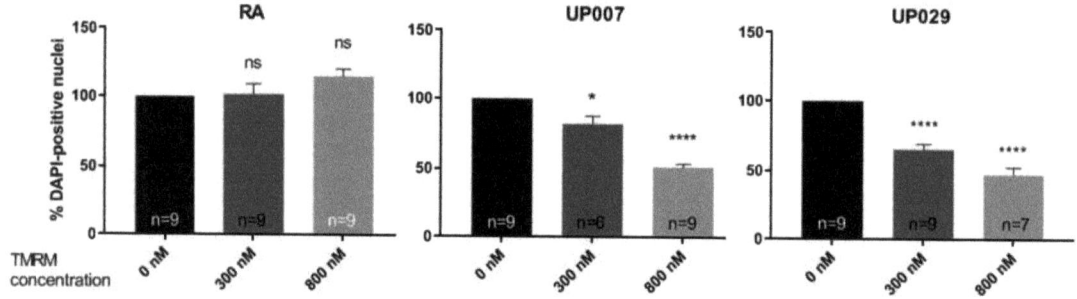

Figure 6. Delayed photoactivation of TMRM enables selective effect on GBM cells. Cells were loaded with TMRM, 300 nM or 800 nM which was then removed from the media. Twenty-four hours later, light was applied for 30 s (1.4 mW/mm^2). When counted 3 days later, the number of remaining GBM but not RA was strongly decreased. This specificity was achieved by preferential retention of TMRM in GBM cells. N is the total number of datapoints from 3 independent experiments. (*) p value < 0.05, (****) p value < 0.0001. ns—not significant.

3.7. TMRM or Green Light Is Not Toxic to GBM Cells or RA

We controlled for the detrimental effects of TMRM without light application (dark toxicity) for RA and all GBM lines. Cells were loaded with different concentrations of TMRM for 40 min and later tested with the LDH-assay. No cytotoxicity of TMRM was observed with all five concentrations used (Figure 7).

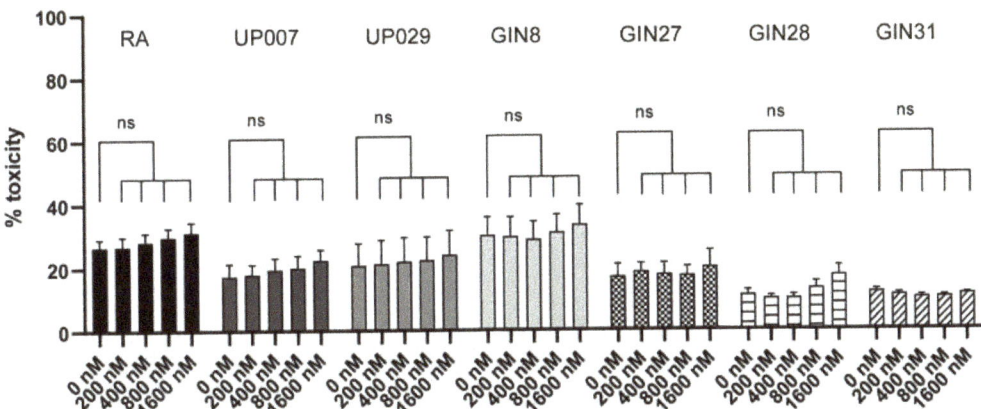

Figure 7. Control tests for TMRM dark toxicity. TMRM dark toxicity in the absence of illumination assessed using LDH assay. No statistically significant difference in toxicity between any of the 5 concentrations used in this experiment compared to the controls. N = 9: is the total number of datapoints for each condition from 3 independent experiments. ns—not significant.

Moreover, we increased the time of incubation with TMRM up to 48 h without light application (dark toxicity) for the RA and two GBM lines (UP007 and UP029). Incubation for 48 h with TMRM at concentrations between 50 nM and 300 nM had no significant effect on the proliferation of either of the two GBM lines or the RA, while 800 nM had some effect on UP007 and RA (Figure 8a). For the control of the light effect, illumination was carried out for 60 s and 120 s (1.4 mW/mm^2) which are harsher conditions than in any other series, but this had no effect on either type of cells (Figure 8b).

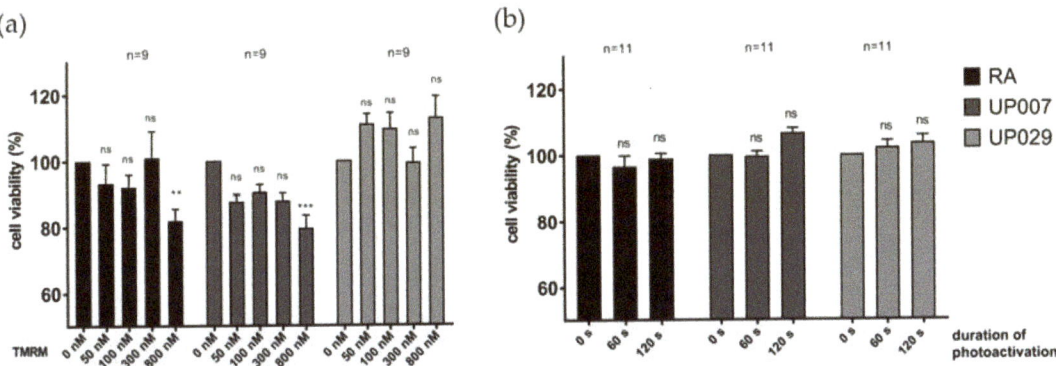

Figure 8. Further control experiments to assess the dark toxicity of TMRM and the effect of green light. (**a**) Prolonged incubation with TMRM for 48 h with no photoactivation had a minimal effect on GBM or RA cell density as measured using MTT assay. (**b**) When applied to unloaded cells, green light 1.4 mW/mm^2 on its own, had no effect on the survival of GBM cell lines or RA (PrestoBlue assay). N: is the total number of datapoints for each condition from 3 independent experiments (6 for RA in panel A.). (**) $p < 0.01$, (***) $p < 0.001$. ns—not significant.

3.8. PDT Effect on Viability of GBM Cells Is Long Lasting

Even though PDT resulted in a rapid loss of many GBM cells, a few were still visible in the wells after 10 days of culturing post PDT. We therefore compared their viability using the PrestoBlue assay which can be performed on the same batch of cells longitudinally and reports the metabolic health status of the cells. As shown in Figure 9a,b, UP007 and UP029 cell lines after 2, 5 and 10 days had a severely compromised metabolic status. We assumed that the main mechanism of cell death after TMRM-PDT is apoptosis. In order to visualize this process, we used a genetically encoded Caspase sensor CA-GFP as listed in the Methods. Lentiviral transduction of the cell lines was performed to generate stably expressing clones. Ten days after TMRM-PDT for 60 s (1.06 mW/mm^2), photoactivation green fluorescence was clearly visible in most surviving cells in both cell lines, but not in the untreated controls (Supplementary Figure S1).

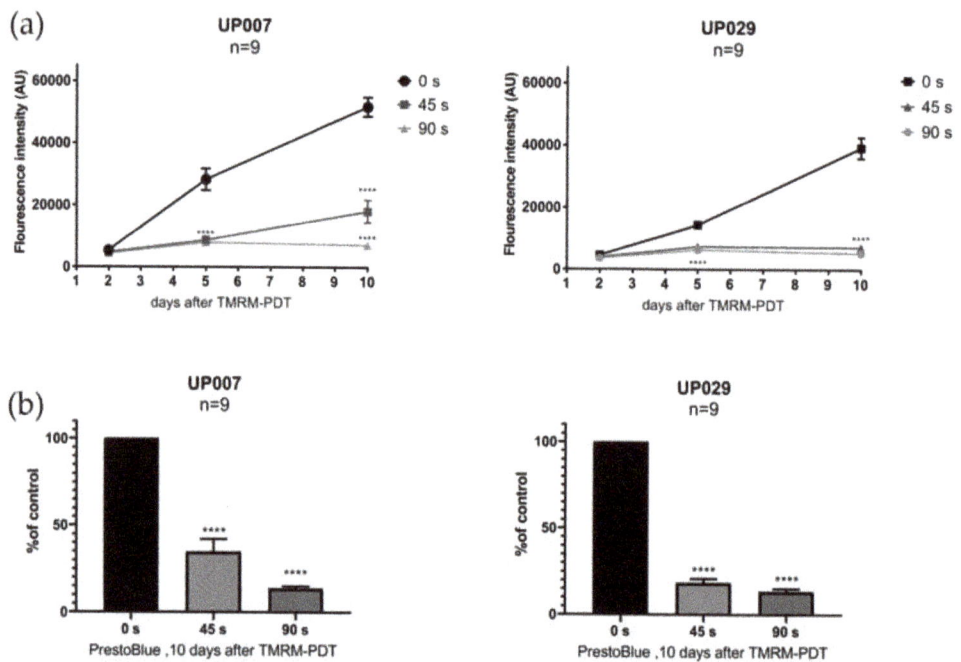

Figure 9. Lasting effects of TMRM-PDT. (**a**) Single episode of TMRM-PDT permanently affected the viability of GBM cell lines (PrestoBlue assay). GBM lines were photoactivated for 0 s, 45 s or 90 s after being loaded with 300 nM TMRM. N: is the total number of datapoints from 3 independent experiments. (****) p value < 0.0001. Data are given as the mean ± SEM. (**b**) Effect of varying light exposure on cell viability assessed 10 days after TMRM-PDT, Presto Blue assay. (****) p value < 0.0001.

3.9. NKH477—But Not Clotrimazole—Enhances the Effect of PDT in Several GBM Cell Lines

Perfect illumination of target areas and equal TMRM loading of the cells is much harder to achieve in a surgical theatre than in the research laboratory. Therefore, it is always desirable to develop additional strategies to potentiate the effect of PDT. Elevating cAMP levels in GBM cells has been implicated in multiple studies as a mechanism which could counter GBM aggressiveness and improve survival [16]. GBM cells were therefore incubated with 10 μM of adenylate cyclase activator NKH477 for 24 h before a sub-optimal TMRM-PDT regime was applied. We found that the dual targeting of GBM cells with a sub-lethal dose of NKH477 and low-intensity PDT (20 s illumination) resulted in the decreased viability of some GBM cell lines. This difference was statistically significant compared to either one of the treatments alone and to negative controls (Figure 10). Glycolysis inhibition with clotrimazole was also attempted to further drain glycolytic energy source after TMRM-PDT, which theoretically compromises mitochondrial functions, but this dual treatment protocol did not result in any significant additive effect (Figure 10).

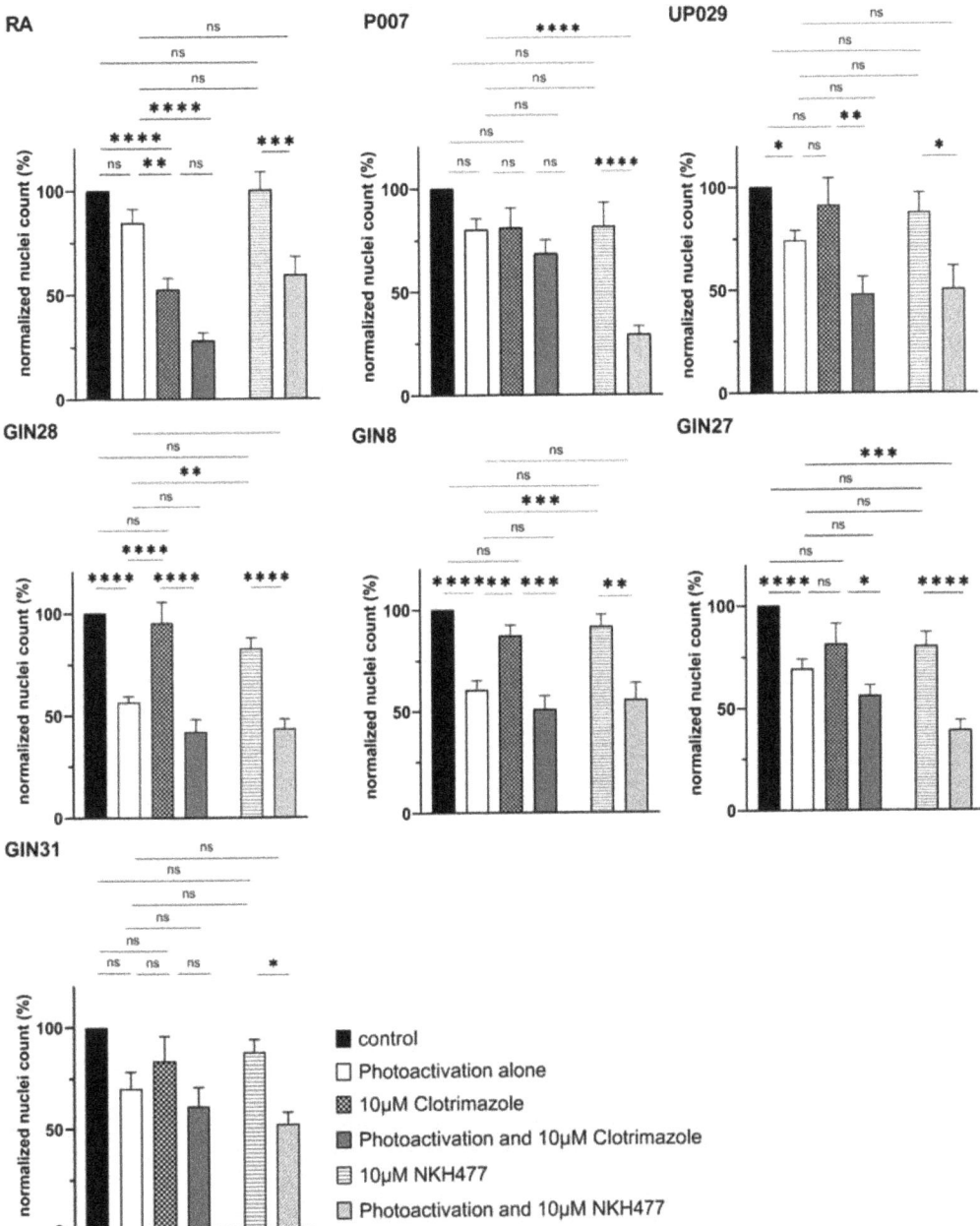

Figure 10. Synergistic effect of a low-dose NKH477 pre-treatment plus sub-lethal photoactivation (20 s) of TMRM-loaded GBM cells resulted in a significant decrease in the viability of some GBM cell lines (in UP007 and GIN27) compared to the controls or treatment with NKH477 alone or TMRM-PDT alone. No significant effect of clotrimazole after TMRM-PDT was observed. The number of independent experiments is: 5 for RA, 4 for UP007, UP029, GIN8, and GIN28 cells and 3 for GIN27 and GIN31 cells—all in duplicates. (ns) $p > 0.05$, (*) $p < 0.033$, (**) $p < 0.002$, (***) $p < 0.0002$, (****) $p < 0.0001$, alpha = 0.05. ns—not significant.

4. Discussion

We here re-evaluated the potential of PDT to therapeutically target the infiltration of residual GBM disease within the brain parenchyma adjacent to the area of surgical resection, with the aim of reducing the number and viability of surviving tumor cells, and thus, improve patient prognosis. Controversies surround the use of 5ALA as a photosensitizer for PDT. First, the main peak of its excitation is 405 nm–420 nm, but this wavelength essentially does not spread in brain tissue. Furthermore, the wavelengths > 600 nm which were attempted for PDT with 5ALA may penetrate deeper into the tissues, but they are not efficient for 5ALA excitation. Second, 5ALA has a low ROS yield, meaning that it generates a small amount of free radicals upon photoactivation, and this becomes a major issue when long wavelength light is used [6].

In this study, we demonstrated the application of the MMP-driven dye TMRM as a photosensitizer for PDT targeting GBM cells. TMRM is a member of the rhodamine family and is commonly used to measure MMP in cells [17]. Changes of MMP directly correlate with changes in TMRM florescence intensity [18]. TMRM is highly mobile and instantly leaves the mitochondria if not retained by the MMP. It has also been reported to have minimal non-specific (non-mitochondrial) accumulation and interference with mitochondrial respiration compared to other commonly used rhodamine derivatives [19]. Moreover, TMRM has peak excitation/emission wavelengths of 548 nm/573 nm, respectively. Thus, TMRM can be effectively excited by a light of green/yellow spectrum. In comparison with the 405 nm–420 nm peak for 5ALA, this must increase the efficiency of PDT due to the better tissue penetration of these wavelengths.

We found that TMRM-PDT is effective in compromising the viability/survival of the GBM cells, as shown in Figure 3. Unfortunately, the effect was also seen on normal RA. However, by carefully tweaking the protocol in terms of TMRM loading concentration and illumination times, we were able to achieve significant cytotoxic selectivity to GBM cells over RA (Figure 4). Possibly, using lower concentrations of TMRM in vivo might help to achieve a selective suppressant effect on GBM infiltrating cells. The ability of GBM mitochondria to accumulate more TMRM and better retain it matches with the generally known tendency of tumor cells to have hyperpolarized mitochondria [20,21]. We believe that greater selectivity can be achieved with the protocol where photoactivation takes place after the cells are allowed to dissipate the TMRM initially loaded into them. In our experiment, this was demonstrated using 48 h delay (Figure 6). We assume that the selective suppression of the GBM cells was due to the retention of the dye in their mitochondria because of the hyperpolarized MMP. This could and should make the clearance of the dye out of normal cells more efficient than in tumor cells. From a clinical perspective, this protocol would require a preloading of the tissue with TMRM prior to light application which should follow after a delay. One needs to take into account that, unless the molecules are actively retained in brain cells in vivo, they are going to be very quickly washed away into the general circulation. Thus, in the living brain, it might only take 1–2 h for the healthy cells to release TMRM while the GBM cell could still have it concentrated in their mitochondria.

In this work, we did not study the potential impact of PDT on neurons, but this is a particularly difficult task in vitro. Essentially all experiments on cultured rodent neurons employ cells from embryos which have a completely different metabolic profile compared to the mature neurons in the brain in vivo. We do not believe that such cultures would be a suitable model for this type of work. Instead, it may be better to test whether TMRM strongly affects neurons in rodent studies in vivo, as we hope to do in future studies.

We were also able to show that TMRM is not toxic without light illumination at concentrations up to 3.2 µM, which is consistent with previous data [18]. Further, it requires comparatively low power to elicit specific cytotoxicity which decreases the chances for light-related tissue damage (see [6] for further discussion).

We attempted to enhance the efficacy of TMRM-PDT by employing a sub-lethal PDT regimen combined with NKH477 or clotrimazole. Clotrimazole is an inhibitor of phosphofructokinase, one of the key enzymes in glycolysis [22]. It has previously been tested on GBM cells and has resulted in the blockade of the cell cycle and consequently cell death. We reasoned that TMRM-PDT would perturb mitochondrial energy production and the addition of a glycolysis inhibitor would further compromise cellular energy sources and induce cell death. Unfortunately, clotrimazole at the low concentration we used (10 µM) was enough to affect RA. Moreover, no additive effect was detected on GBM cells (Figure 10). However, a combination with NKH477 has shown some promising results. NKH477 is a water-soluble forskolin hydrochloride derivative that can directly stimulate adenylate cyclase, the generator of cAMP [23]. cAMP elevation is known to cause detrimental effects on GBM cells [24–26]. Moreover, it has been documented that an elevated cAMP level in GBM leads to hyperpolarization of mitochondria [25] and would theoretically lead to the greater accumulation of TMRM in GBM cells and enhance the PDT effect. Interestingly, NHK477 significantly potentiated the effect of TMRM-PDT only for UP007 and GIN27 GBM cells (Figure S4). A trend was noted with other cell lines, but differences were not statistically significant (Figure 10). Heterogenous responses of GBM lines to this approach are not surprising because these tumors are characterized by a non-uniform molecular makeup and biological behavior. A hypothetical explanation for the effect of NKH477 is that it changes gene expression in GBM cells and via yet poorly defined mechanisms leads to the further hyperpolarization of their mitochondria, as illustrated by Supplementary Figure S5.

5. Conclusions

There is an urgent need for more innovative and less invasive therapeutic modalities to treat GBM. The major source for GBM recurrences is that of the infiltrating GBM cells that are left after surgical resection for which local therapy modalities could be used to efficaciously target residual disease cells.

Its proposed topical application of TMRM may raise some of the usual concerns, such as liver or kidney toxicity, but might be less problematic because the overall dose delivered into the brain will be fairly small, especially because only a periphery of the postoperative cavity needs to be impregnated with it. As a first step, one could start by testing the consequences of injecting TMRM into the brain of experimental animals and then checking for signs of pathology and inflammation.

We envision a treatment protocol for GBM where, following surgery, the walls of the cavity and ~2 cm of the surrounding parenchyma are infiltrated with TMRM, and after a delay to allows healthy brain cells to expel the photosensitizer, light is directly delivered into the brain parenchyma where disease infiltrations are suspected.

Light delivery systems for this type of surgery are already being developed [27] and our early findings encourage continued enthusiasm in this research area.

Supplementary Materials: The following are available online at https://www.mdpi.com/article/10.3390/biomedicines9101453/s1: Figure S1: Activation of caspase reporter in surviving UP007 cells 10 days after TMRM-PDT; Figure S2: Images of GBM cells and RA taken 24 h after 40 min loading with different concentrations of TMRM; Figure S3: Loss of MMP in GBM cells persists 24 h after photodynamic treatment; Figure S4: Hypothetical mechanism of action of the combined NKH477 and TMRM-PDT regimen; Figure S5: Schematic representation of the mechanism of delayed TMRM-PDT.

Author Contributions: A.V. and R.S. (equal contributions) performed the experiments, evaluated results, generated figures and wrote parts of the manuscript; S.J.S. generated and provided GIN cell lines; R.R. edited the manuscript; A.G.T. edited the text and figures and provided guidance for some of the experiments; S.K. led the study, wrote parts of the manuscript and edited the figures. All authors have read and agreed to the published version of the manuscript.

Funding: A.G.T. and S.K. are in receipt of British Heart Foundation funding (PG/18/8/33540 and RG/19/5/34463). A.V. was in receipt of the Fellowship of the President of Russian Federation (2019, №558). R.S. was supported by the scholarship from King Abdul-Aziz University, Kingdom of Saudi Arabia.

Institutional Review Board Statement: RA in the UK were obtained using regulations set by the Home Office in accordance with the Animal Welfare Act 2006 and the guidelines of the Declaration of Helsinki (Russian Federation), and approved by the Institutional Review Board.

Informed Consent Statement: Not applicable.

Acknowledgments: A.V. is a recipient of the Presidential Fellowship of the Russian Federation. R.S. is a recipient of a scholarship from King Abdul-Aziz University, Kingdom of Saudi Arabia. We gratefully acknowledge the use of MicroManager software (Mark Tsuchida at the Laboratory for Optical and Computational Instrumentation at the University of Wisconsin, Madison, with help from Nico Stuurman from the laboratory of Ron Vale at the University of California, San Francisco).

Conflicts of Interest: The authors declare no conflict of interest.

References

1. Yao, M.; Li, S.; Wu, X.; Diao, S.; Zhang, G.; He, H.; Bian, L.; Lu, Y. Cellular origin of glioblastoma and its implication in precision therapy. *Cell. Mol. Immunol.* **2018**, *15*, 737–739. [CrossRef]
2. Wesseling, P.; Capper, D. WHO 2016 Classification of gliomas. *Neuropathol. Appl. Neurobiol.* **2018**, *44*, 139–150. [CrossRef]
3. Stupp, R.; Mason, W.P.; van den Bent, M.J.; Weller, M.; Fisher, B.; Taphoorn, M.J.B.; Belanger, K.; Brandes, A.A.; Marosi, C.; Bogdahn, U.; et al. Radiotherapy plus Concomitant and Adjuvant Temozolomide for Glioblastoma. *N. Engl. J. Med.* **2005**, *352*, 987–996. [CrossRef]
4. Lara-Velazquez, M.; Al-Kharboosh, R.; Jeanneret, S.; Vazquez-Ramos, C.; Mahato, D.; Tavanaiepour, D.; Rahmathulla, G.; Quinone-Hinojosa, A. Advances in brain tumor surgery for glioblastoma in adults. *Brain Sci.* **2017**, *7*, 166. [CrossRef] [PubMed]
5. Hadjipanayis, C.G.; Stummer, W. 5-ALA and FDA approval for glioma surgery. *J. Neurooncol.* **2019**, *141*, 479–486. [CrossRef] [PubMed]
6. Vasilev, A.; Sofi, R.; Rahman, R.; Smith, S.J.; Teschemacher, A.G.; Kasparov, S. Using Light for Therapy of Glioblastoma Multiforme (GBM). *Brain Sci.* **2020**, *10*, 75. [CrossRef]
7. Stepp, H.; Beck, T.; Pongratz, T.; Meinel, T.; Kreth, F.-W.; Tonn, J.C.; Stummer, W. ALA and malignant glioma: Fluorescence-guided resection and photodynamic treatment. *J. Environ. Pathol. Toxicol. Oncol.* **2007**, *26*, 157–164. [CrossRef] [PubMed]
8. Olzowy, B.; Hundt, C.S.; Stocker, S.; Bise, K.; Reulen, H.J.; Stummer, W. Photoirradiation therapy of experimental malignant glioma with 5-aminolevulinic acid. *J. Neurosurg.* **2002**, *97*, 970–976. [CrossRef] [PubMed]
9. Johansson, A.; Faber, F.; Kniebühler, G.; Stepp, H.; Sroka, R.; Egensperger, R.; Beyer, W.; Kreth, F.W. Protoporphyrin IX fluorescence and photobleaching during interstitial photodynamic therapy of malignant gliomas for early treatment prognosis. *Lasers Surg. Med.* **2013**, *45*, 225–234. [CrossRef]
10. Beck, T.J.; Kreth, F.W.; Beyer, W.; Mehrkens, J.H.; Obermeier, A.; Stepp, H.; Stummer, W.; Baumgartner, R. Interstitial photodynamic therapy of nonresectable malignant glioma recurrences using 5-aminolevulinic acid induced protoporphyrin IX. *Lasers Surg. Med.* **2007**, *39*, 386–393. [CrossRef] [PubMed]
11. Juzenas, P.; Juzeniene, A.; Kaalhus, O.; Iani, V.; Moan, J. Noninvasive fluorescence excitation spectroscopy during application of 5-aminolevulinic acid in vivo. *Photochem. Photobiol. Sci.* **2002**, *1*, 745–748. [CrossRef] [PubMed]
12. Schwake, M.; Nemes, A.; Dondrop, J.; Schroeteler, J.; Schipmann, S.; Senner, V.; Stummer, W.; Ewelt, C. In-Vitro Use of 5-ALA for Photodynamic Therapy in Pediatric Brain Tumors. *Neurosurgery* **2018**, *83*, 1328–1337. [CrossRef] [PubMed]
13. Liu, B.; Mosienko, V.; Vaccari Cardoso, B.; Prokudina, D.; Huentelman, M.; Teschemacher, A.G.; Kasparov, S. Glio- and neuroprotection by prosaposin is mediated by orphan G-protein coupled receptors GPR37L1 and GPR37. *Glia* **2018**, *66*, 2414–2426. [CrossRef] [PubMed]
14. Nicholls, S.B.; Chu, J.; Abbruzzese, G.; Tremblay, K.D.; Hardy, J.A. Mechanism of a genetically encoded dark-to-bright reporter for caspase activity. *J. Biol. Chem.* **2011**, *286*, 24977–24986. [CrossRef]
15. Hewinson, J.; Paton, J.F.R.; Kasparov, S. Viral gene delivery: Optimized protocol for production of high titer lentiviral vectors. *Methods Mol. Biol.* **2013**, *998*, 65–75. [CrossRef]
16. Grbovic, O.; Jovic, V.; Ruzdijic, S.; Pejanovic, V.; Rakic, L.; Kanazir, S. 8-Cl-cAMP affects glioma cell-cycle kinetics and selectively induces apoptosis. *Cancer Invest.* **2002**, *20*, 972–982. [CrossRef]
17. Scaduto, R.C.; Grotyohann, L.W. Measurement of mitochondrial membrane potential using fluorescent rhodamine derivatives. *Biophys. J.* **1999**, *76*, 469–477. [CrossRef]
18. Monteith, A.; Marszalec, W.; Chan, P.; Logan, J.; Yu, W.; Schwarz, N.; Wokosin, D.; Hockberger, P. Imaging of Mitochondrial and Non-Mitochondrial Responses in Cultured Rat Hippocampal Neurons Exposed to Micromolar Concentrations of TMRM. *PLoS ONE* **2013**, *8*, e58059. [CrossRef]
19. Zorova, L.D.; Popkov, V.A.; Plotnikov, E.Y.; Silachev, D.N.; Pevzner, I.B.; Jankauskas, S.S.; Babenko, V.A.; Zorov, D.B.; Balakireva, A.V.; Juhaszova, M.; et al. Mitochondrial membrane potential. *Anal. Biochem.* **2018**, *552*, 50–59. [CrossRef]
20. Zhang, B.; Wang, D.; Guo, F.; Xuan, C. Mitochondrial membrane potential and reactive oxygen species in cancer stem cells. *Fam. Cancer* **2015**, *14*, 19–23. [CrossRef]

21. Forrest, M.D. Why cancer cells have a more hyperpolarised mitochondrial membrane potential and emergent prospects for therapy. *bioRxiv* **2015**, 1–42. [CrossRef]
22. Penso, J.; Beitner, R. Clotrimazole decreases glycolysis and the viability of lung carcinoma and colon adenocarcinoma cells. *Eur. J. Pharmacol.* **2002**, *451*, 227–235. [CrossRef]
23. Morinobu, S.; Fujimaki, K.; Okuyama, N.; Takahashi, M.; Duman, R. Stimulation of adenylyl cyclase and induction of brain-derived neurotrophic factor and TrkB mRNA by NKH477, a novel and potent forskolin derivative. *J. Neurochem.* **1999**, *72*, 2198–2205. [CrossRef] [PubMed]
24. Lv, P.; Wang, W.; Cao, Z.; Zhao, D.; Zhao, G.; Li, D.; Qi, L.; Xu, J. Fsk and IBMX inhibit proliferation and proapoptotic of glioma stem cells via activation of cAMP signaling pathway. *J. Cell. Biochem.* **2019**, *120*, 321–331. [CrossRef]
25. Xing, F.; Luan, Y.; Cai, J.; Wu, S.; Mai, J.; Gu, J.; Zhang, H.; Li, K.; Lin, Y.; Xiao, X.; et al. The Anti-Warburg Effect Elicited by the cAMP-PGC1α Pathway Drives Differentiation of Glioblastoma Cells into Astrocytes. *Cell Rep.* **2017**, *18*, 468–481. [CrossRef]
26. Daniel, P.M.; Filiz, G.; Mantamadiotis, T. Sensitivity of GBM cells to cAMP agonist-mediated apoptosis correlates with CD44 expression and agonist resistance with MAPK signaling. *Cell Death Dis.* **2016**, *7*. [CrossRef]
27. Schipmann, S.; Müther, M.; Stögbauer, L.; Zimmer, S.; Brokinkel, B.; Holling, M.; Grauer, O.; Molina, E.S.; Warneke, N.; Stummer, W. Combination of ALA-induced fluorescence-guided resection and intraoperative open photodynamic therapy for recurrent glioblastoma: Case series on a promising dual strategy for local tumor control. *J. Neurosurg.* **2021**, *134*, 426–436. [CrossRef]

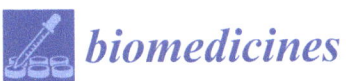

Article

DNA Hypermethylation Involves in the Down-Regulation of Chloride Intracellular Channel 4 (CLIC4) Induced by Photodynamic Therapy

Pei-Chi Chiang [1,†], Pei-Tzu Li [1,†], Ming-Jen Lee [2] and Chin-Tin Chen [1,*]

1. Department of Biochemical Science and Technology, College of Life Science, National Taiwan University, Taipei 10617, Taiwan; peggier309@gmail.com (P.-C.C.); peitzuli@gmail.com (P.-T.L.)
2. Department of Neurology and Medical Genetics, National Taiwan University Hospital, Taipei 10012, Taiwan; mjlee@ntu.edu.tw
* Correspondence: chintin@ntu.edu.tw
† The first two authors contributed equally to this work.

Abstract: The altered expression of chloride intracellular channel 4 (CLIC4) was reported to correlate with tumor progression. Previously, we have shown that the reduced cellular invasion induced by photodynamic therapy (PDT) is associated with suppression of CLIC4 expression in PDT-treated cells. Herein, we attempted to decipher the regulatory mechanisms involved in PDT-mediated CLIC4 suppression in A375 and MDA-MB-231 cells in vitro. We found that PDT can increase the expression and enzymatic activity of DNA methyltransferase 1 (DNMT1). Bisulfite sequencing PCR further revealed that PDT can induce hypermethylation in the *CLIC4* promoter region. Silencing DNMT1 rescues the PDT-induced CLIC4 suppression and inhibits hypermethylation in its promoter. Furthermore, we found tumor suppressor p53 involves in the increased DNMT1 expression of PDT-treated cells. Finally, by comparing CLIC4 expression in lung malignant cells and normal lung fibroblasts, the extent of methylation in *CLIC4* promoter was found to be inversely proportional to its expression. Taken together, our results indicate that CLIC4 suppression induced by PDT is modulated by DNMT1-mediated hypermethylation and depends on the status of p53, which provides a possible mechanistic basis for regulating CLIC4 expression in tumorigenesis.

Keywords: CLIC4; DNA methylation; oxidative stress; PDT

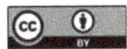

1. Introduction

Photodynamic therapy (PDT) has been developed as an alternative approach for cancer treatment [1]. PDT is based on the administration of exogenous photosensitizer followed by selective light irradiation onto tissue lesion to trigger the production of reactive oxygen species (ROS) [2]. The tumoricidal action of PDT involves the cancer cell killing, disruption of tumor vasculature with the following local inflammation. There are many studies conducted to investigate the molecular mechanisms involved in PDT-mediated cell death [3–5]. In addition to cell death, a few other studies reported that the primary tumor treated by PDT exhibits a decreased incidence of distant metastasis [6–8]. Our previous findings further revealed that the reduced invasiveness of PDT-treated cells relates to the decreased expression of chloride intracellular channel 4 (CLIC4) [9]. However, the molecular mechanisms involved in regulating the expression of CLIC4 by PDT-induced oxidative stress remain elusive.

The family of chloride intracellular channel (CLIC) proteins are ubiquitously expressed in various tissues and implicated in diverse physiologic functions [10,11]. CLIC4 is the most studied member in the CLIC family and found in soluble and membrane bound forms [12,13]. The biological functions of CLIC4 are found to be involved in regulating cell cycle arrest, apoptosis, metabolic stress, cytoskeletal organization, cell differentiation, and morphogenesis [14]. Knockdown CLIC4 in cultured cells can reduce cell proliferation and migration ability as well as induce apoptosis [14,15]. Expressing antisense CLIC4 in tumors derived from transplanting these cells into nude mice may further demonstrate the role of CLIC4 in tumor progression. Down-regulation of CLIC4 in tumors inhibits tumor growth, increases tumor apoptosis and reduces tumor cell proliferation [14]. In addition, loss of CLIC4 in tumor cells as well as gain in tumor stroma cells have been identified in multiple human cancers, which represents the malignant progression [11,16]. Up-regulation of CLIC4 in tumor stroma enhances the growth of cancer xenografts and significantly involves in the process of the transforming growth factor (TGF)-β-mediated myofibroblast conversion, which is a hallmark of a nurturing tumor microenvironment [17–19]. Recently, CLIC4 has been found to have broad prospects as a serum/tissue biomarker and therapeutic target for epithelial ovarian cancer. Compared with normal and benign controls, the level of CLIC4 protein was significantly increased in serum from ovarian cancer patients. Increased CLIC4 expression is considered a negative indicator of patient survival [20]. Although CLIC4 was reported to be implicated in tumorigenesis, no mutation or deletion of the *CLIC4* gene was found in tumor tissues with different stage of pathological condition [11]. Therefore, the molecular mechanisms underlying the regulation of CLIC4 expression are still not clear.

The absence of mutations in the *CLIC4* gene during tumorigenesis implies that epigenetic or post-translational modifications may be involved in its expression control. The GC-rich in the *CLIC4* promoter region suggests that DNA methylation may play a role in mediating CLIC4 transcription. DNA methylation is one category of epigenetics, which has been defined as the study of stable and heritable alterations of chromatin states and dynamics as well as in gene expression potential but do not attributable to mutations in the primary DNA sequence [21,22]. DNA methylation occurs via covalently adding of a methyl group to cytosine residue in CpG dinucleotides, which are concentrated in a short stretch of DNA called CpG island. CpG island is defined as a region with at least 200 bp, the proportion of GC content greater than 50%, and observed to expected CpG ratio (O/E) greater than 0.6 [23]. The CpG islands usually locate in the 5' end of the candidate genes and nearly 60% of them are in the promoter region [24,25]. Hypomethylation of regulatory sequences, in general, tends to correlate with an increased gene expression, while hypermethylation is typically associated with transcriptional silencing [26]. Growing evidences demonstrate that aberrant promoter methylation of genes can be induced by reactive oxygen species [27,28]. As mentioned, ROS are the major cytotoxic agents responsible for cellular damage induced by PDT [29–31]. Although it has been shown that oxidative stress can promote hypermethylation and further suppress gene expression, there are few studies regarding whether PDT-induced oxidative stress may affect DNA methylation. Demyanenko et al. found that 5-aminilevulinic acid (ALA)-mediated PDT alters expression of proteins involved in epigenetic regulation in the mouse cerebral cortex [32]. However, whether there is any change in DNA methylation in PDT-treated cells remains unknown.

In the present study, we investigated the status and the associated molecular mechanisms of DNA methylation in the promoter region of *CLIC4* gene in PDT-treated cells. Our results indicate that suppression of CLIC4 expression by PDT-induced oxidative stress is modulated by DNA methylation in a DNA methyltransferases 1 (DNMT1)-dependent manner and relies on the status of tumor suppressor protein p53. Furthermore, analyzing the methylation status of *CLIC4* promoter in lung malignant cells and normal lung fibroblast cell lines reveal that the extent of methylation status in *CLIC4* promoter is inversely proportional to its expression level. This work provides an insight into a new mechanism by which PDT induces molecular alterations through DNA methylation and suggests a possible regulatory mechanism of CLIC4 during tumorigenesis.

2. Materials and Methods

2.1. Cell Culture and Photodynamic Treatment

Human melanoma A375 cells and lung adenocarcinoma epithelial A549 cells were cultured in Dulbecco's modified Eagle's medium (DMEM) supplemented with 10% (v/v) fetal bovine serum (FBS). Human breast adenocarcinoma MDA-MB-231 cells, lung adenocarcinoma CL1-0 cells, non-small cell lung cancer H1299 cells and large cell lung cancer H460 cells were cultured in RPMI1640 medium supplemented with 10% (v/v) FBS. Human lung fibroblast MRC-5 cells were cultured in Eagle's minimum essential medium (MEM) supplemented with 10% (v/v) FBS. All cells were grown at 37 °C under 5% CO_2. MRC-5 was obtained from American Type Culture Collection (ATCC, Manassas, VA, USA). A375, MDA-MB-231, A549, H1299, H460 and PC3 were obtained from The National Health Research Institutes (NHRI) Cell Bank (Taipei, Taiwan). Both cell lines of A375 and MDA-MB-231 were authenticated using the PromegaGenePrint 10 System (Promega, Madison, WI, USA) and analyzed by ABI PRISM 3730 GENETIC ANALYZER and GeneMapper software V3.7 (Applied Biosys-tems, Carlsbad, CA, USA). CL1-0 was a kind gift from Dr. Pan-Chyr Yang's Lab. (Department of Internal Medicine, National Taiwan University Hospital, Taipei, Taiwan) [33]. For photodynamic treatment, cells were incubated with 1 mM ALA (Sigma-Aldrich, St. Louis, MO, USA) in serum free medium for 3 h and then exposed to specific dose of light as indicated that corresponds to LD_{50}. Light source for ALA-PDT is a home-made high-power LED array with the wavelength centered at 635 ± 5 nm. Immediately after light irradiation, cells were cultured in complete medium until further analysis.

2.2. Western Blotting

Immunoblot analysis was carried out as described previously [34]. Briefly, cell lysates were separated by SDS-PAGE gel. Protein samples were transferred to a nitrocellulose membrane, blocked with 5% (w/v) skim milk, and probed with specific primary antibodies. The primary antibodies used are anti-CLIC4 antibody (Abcam, Cambridge, UK), anti-p53 antibody (Cell Signaling Technology, Beverly, MA, USA) and anti-DNMT1 antibody (Epitomics, Burlingame, CA, USA). The horseradish peroxidase (HRP)-conjugated secondary antibody was used and the immunocomplex was visualized by Chemiluminescence Reagent Plus (Blossom Biotechnology Inc., Boston, MA, USA). Chemiluminescence detection was measured directly by a Biospectrum 810 Imaging System (UVP, Upland, CA, USA). For the loading control, the membranes were further stripped and re-probed with anti-GAPDH antibody (GeneTex, Irvine, CA, USA) and anti-Tubulin antibody (Cell signaling, Boston, MA, USA). The origin immunoblots and the replicated data in this study are shown in Supplementary Figure S7 online. Band blots for each protein were from the same set of samples. Before hybridizing with each antibody, according to the expected molecular weight of target proteins, blots were cropped from different sections of the same whole blot to conserve reagents and avoid signal fading caused by striping and re-probing. However, we did not retain the full-length photograph of the blot when experiments were performed.

2.3. Reverse Transcription-PCR Analysis

To assess gene expression, total RNA from cells was extracted by using Trizol reagent (Invitrogen, Carlsbad, CA, USA) according to the manufacturer's instructions. The obtained RNA was reverse transcribed with SuperScript II reverse transcriptase (Invitrogen, Carlsbad, CA, USA) based on the manufacturer's protocol. The primer sequences used for PCR are as follows: CLIC4, 5′-gCAgTgATggTgAAAgCATAg-3′ (forward) and 5′-TATAAATggTgggTgggTCC-3′ (reverse); DNMT1, 5′-ACCgCTTCTACTTCCTCgAggCCTA-3′ (forward) and 5′-gTTgCAgTCCTCTgTgAACACTgTgg-3′ (reverse); p53, 5′-TTggATCCATgTTTTgCCAACTggCC-3′ (forward) and 5′-TTgAATTCAggCTCCCCTTT-CTTgCg-3′ (reverse); β-actin, 5′-TggACTTCgAgCAAgAgATgg-3′ (forward) and 5′-ATCTCCTTCTgCATCCTgTCg-3′ (reverse); GAPDH, 5′-gACCACAgTCCATgCCATCA-3′ (forward) and 5′-gTCCACCACCCTgTTgCTgTA-3′ (reverse). RT-PCR was performed as previously described [34].

The PCR products were resolved on a 2% (w/v) non-denaturing agarose gel and analyzed using EtBr staining. The original images of electrophoresis gels in this study are shown in Supplementary Figure S8 online. The band intensities of PCR products were measured by analyzing the gel images on the ImageJ software. The mRNA expression level of each gene was normalized to β-actin and GAPDH for RT-PCR and real-time PCR, respectively. To assess mRNA expression, cDNA product was also used as a template for real-time PCR analysis using ABI Fast SYBR Green Master Mix Kit (Thermo Fisher Scientific, Waltham, MA, USA) with ABI StepOne system (Thermo Fisher Scientific, Waltham, MA, USA). Results were expressed as fold change over the controls.

2.4. RNA Interference

shRNA vectors were obtained from the National RNAi Core Facility (Academia Sinica, Taipei, Taiwan). The target sequence for DNMT1 and p53 shRNAs were as follows: shDNMT1#1, 5′-CCgggCCCAATgAgACTgACATCAACTCgAgTTgATgTCATCTCATTgggCTTTTT-3′; shDNMT1#2, 5′-CCggCgACTACATCAAAggCAgCAACTCgAgTTgCTgCCTTTgATgTAgTCgTTTTT-3′; shp53#1, 5′-CCggCACCATCCACTACAACTACATCTCgAgATgTAgTTgTAgTggATggTgTTTTT-3′; shp53#2, 5′-CCggCggCgCACAgAggAAgAgAATCTCgAgATTCTCTTCCTCTgTgCgCCgTTTTT-3′; shp53#3, 5′-CCgggAgggATgTTTgggAgATgTACTCgAgTACATCTCCCAAACATCCCTCTTTTT-3′. Templates were inserted into lentiviral plasmids (pLKO.1-puro). Cells were transiently transfected with a validated empty vector, DNMT1 or p53 shRNA using Lipofectamine 2000 (Invitrogen, Carlsbad, CA, USA). After six hours of transfection, the cells were replaced with fresh medium and incubated at 37 °C for another 72 h. On the following day, the treated cells were harvested and used for further analysis.

2.5. DNA Methyltransferases Activity

The sampled cells were harvested, and the nuclear protein samples were prepared with the nuclear extraction reagent (Panomics Inc., Fremont, CA, USA). The DNMT enzymatic activity assay was measured using DNMT Activity/Inhibition Assay Kit (Active Motif Inc., Carlsbad, CA, USA) according to the manufacturer's instruction. All the assays were performed in duplicate in three sets of independent experiments. Background levels were determined in assays in which the template DNA was excluded.

2.6. Bisulfite Genomic Sequencing

Methylation status of the CLIC4 promoter was assessed by bisulfite sequencing. Genomic DNA was extracted from the sampled cells by the Quick-gDNA MicroPrep (Zymo Research Inc., Irvine, CA, USA) and subjected to bisulfite conversion using EZ DNA Methylation Kit (Zymo Research Inc., Irvine, CA, USA) according to the manufacturer's recommendations. For each conversion, 0.5 µg of genomic DNA was used. PCR was performed for amplifying the promoter CpG island from the *CLIC4* gene. The primer sequences are as follows: BSP #1 (forward), 5′-TTTTTTAgAggATTTgggAAAT-3′; BSP #1 (reverse), 5′-CTTAACAACCAACATATTCACAAA-3′; BSP #2 (forward), 5′-TAgTTATTTgggAggTTgAgg-3′; BSP #2 (reverse), 5′-ACRCCCCACAACTAATAAA-3′; BSP #3A (forward), 5′-TgAgTTTTggggTgTTg-3′; BSP #3A (reverse), 5′-AAAAAATTCCCCAAAAACC-3′; BSP #3B (forward), 5′-TgTTAggTTYgggTTTTT-3′; BSP #3B (reverse), 5′-AACCRAAAAAAAACCTCT-3′; BSP #3C (forward), 5′-gggYgTYgTAgAggTT-3′; BSP #3C (reverse), 5′-CRCCRAAAACRAAAC-3′; BSP #3D (forward), 5′-gAgAgTTTYgAggYgT-3′; BSP #3D (reverse), 5′-ACCACRACTTCAACTCCT-3′; BSP #4 (forward), 5′-gTgTTgAggAgTTgAAgTYgT-3′; BSP #4 (reverse), 5′-TACCCAAAACAAAAAAACACAA-3′. The amplified fragments were subcloned into the pCR4-TOPO vector by TA cloning (Invitrogen, Carlsbad, CA, USA) and the colony PCR products were submitted for nucleotide sequencing.

2.7. Statistical Analysis

All experiments were performed and repeated at least three times. Data in bar graphs are expressed as the mean and standard deviation from 3 independent experiments. The statistical significance of experimental data was evaluated by two-tailed Student's t-test and considered statistically significant with * $p < 0.05$, ** $p < 0.01$ and *** $p < 0.001$.

3. Results

3.1. Inhibition of DNA Methylation Restores PDT-Induced Reduction of CLIC4 Expression

Previously, we have shown that PDT can induce chromatin modification by regulating the expression and activity of histone acetyltransferase p300 (p300HAT) [31], suggesting epigenetic modifications may play an important role in PDT-mediated gene regulation. To examine whether epigenetic modifications involve in regulating PDT-induced suppression of CLIC4 expression, we first used a DNMT inhibitor and a histone deacetylase (HDAC) inhibitor, 5-azacytidine (5AZA) and Trichostatin A (TSA), to block DNA methylation and histone acetylation before PDT treatment. As shown in Figure 1a, 5AZA can significantly restore the mRNA expression level of CLIC4 in PDT-treated A375 and MDA-MB-231 cells. The effect of 5AZA was shown in a dose-dependent manner in reversing the decreased levels of CLIC4 mRNA (Figure 1b) and protein (Figure 1c) expression in PDT-treated cells. Pre-treatment of 5AZA did not affect the viability of PDT-treated cells (see Supplementary Figure S1 online), indicating that CLIC4 expression restored by 5AZA treatment was not accompanied by a change in cell viability. Meanwhile, we also found that the mRNA expression level of CLIC4 after PDT was not affected by TSA (see Supplementary Figure S2 online). These results indicate that the regulatory mechanisms involved in the suppressed expression of CLIC4 may relate to the DNA methylation in PDT-treated cells.

3.2. Oxidative Stress Mediated by PDT Increases the Expression and Activity of DNMT1

Among the DNMT protein family, DNMT1 is the most abundant one in mammalian cells, which plays a role in methylating newly replicated DNA [35]. In addition, alterations of DNMT1 induced by oxidative stress have been observed in hydrogen peroxide-treated cells [36,37]. To examine whether PDT-mediated alteration of DNA methylation is due to the activation of DNMT1, we first analyzed the DNMT1 mRNA expression level in PDT-treated A375 and MDA-MB-231 cells. As shown in Figure 2a, the DNMT1 mRNA expression level was significantly elevated in a time-dependent manner following PDT, which was related to the increase of DNMT1 enzymatic activity (Figure 2b). Moreover, pre-treatment of A375 and MDA-MB-231 cells with the ROS scavenger, N-acetyl cysteine (NAC), could reverse the PDT-induced up-regulation of DNMT1 and suppression of CLIC4 expression (Figure 3). These results indicate that PDT-induced oxidative stress can up-regulate the expression and activity of DNMT1, which may further down-regulate the CLIC4 expression via DNA methylation.

(a)

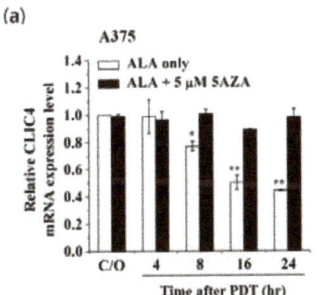 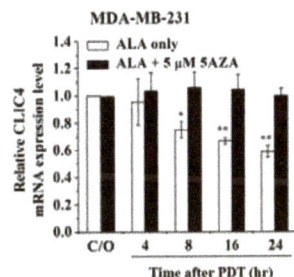

Figure 1. Cont.

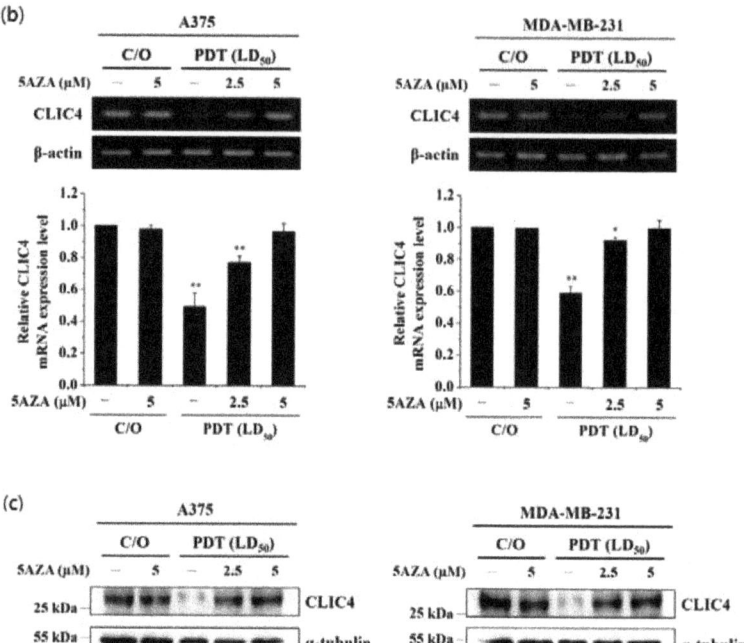

Figure 1. Inhibition of DNA methylation relieves the suppression of CLIC4 expression induced by PDT-mediated oxidative stress. Cells were pre-incubated with 5AZA for 2 h prior to light irradiation. For ALA-PDT, cells were pre-incubated with 1 mM ALA for 3 h and then exposed to specific wavelength (635 ± 5 nm) of light, 2 J/cm^2 and 4 J/cm^2 for A375 (left panel) and MDA-MB-231 (right panel) cells, respectively. To verify the mRNA expression level of CLIC4, total RNA samples were isolated (**a**) from PDT-treated cells at the time indicated (4, 8, 16 and 24 h after ALA-PDT) with or without pre-incubation of 5 µM 5AZA, and (**b**) from PDT-treated cells at 24 h as indicated with or without pre-incubation of 2.5 and 5 µM 5AZA. The relative mRNA expression level of each gene was measured by RT-PCR and normalized to β-actin; (**c**) The protein expression level of CLIC4 was analyzed by Western blotting, and α-tubulin was used as an internal control. The control group was cells only treated with ALA w/o light irradiation. For electrophoretic gels, the same volume of each PCR product was loaded, and band blots for each gene were cropped from different gels. For immunoblots, equal volume of each sample with the same concentration was loaded into each well, and the blots were cropped from different sections of the same gel. Data represent from three independent experiments. Each bar shown is the mean fold change relative to control ± SD. Results are considered to be statistically significant at * $p < 0.05$ and ** $p < 0.01$.

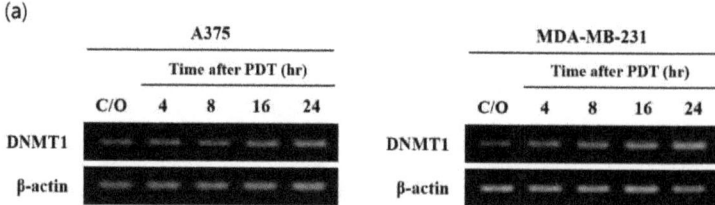

Figure 2. *Cont.*

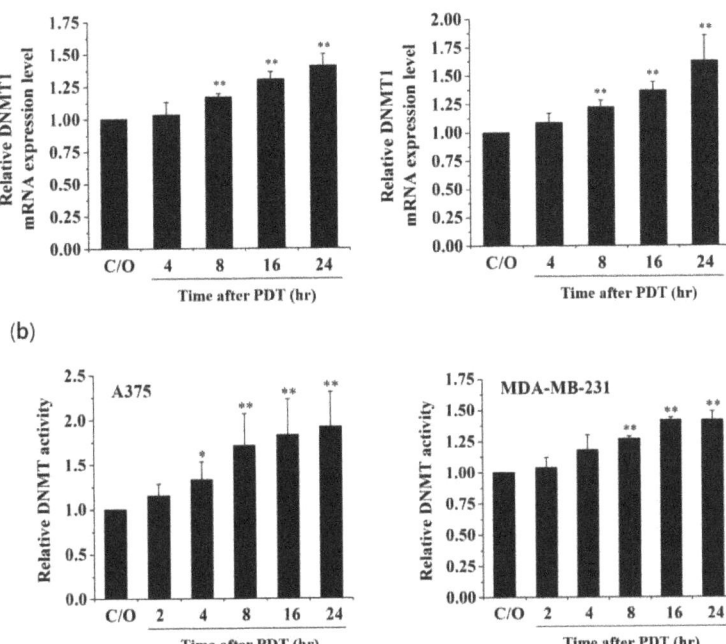

Figure 2. Increase of mRNA expression level and enzymatic activity of DNMT1 in PDT-treated cancer cells. (a) RT-PCR was performed to analyze the mRNA expression level of DNMT1 in A375 (left panel) and MDA-MB-231 (right panel) cells at the time indicated after ALA-PDT. The light dose for A375 and MDA-MB-231 cells is 2 J/cm^2 and 4 J/cm^2, respectively. The relative mRNA expression level of each gene was measured by RT-PCR and normalized to β-actin. The same volume of each PCR product was loaded, and band blots for each gene were cropped from different gels; (b) Nuclear protein samples were extracted from PDT-treated cells. 5 μg protein of each sample was used for analyzing the DNMT activity assay. The control group was cells only treated with ALA w/o light irradiation. Data represent from three independent experiments. Each bar shown is the mean fold change relative to control ± SD. Results are considered to be statistically significant at * $p < 0.05$ and ** $p < 0.01$.

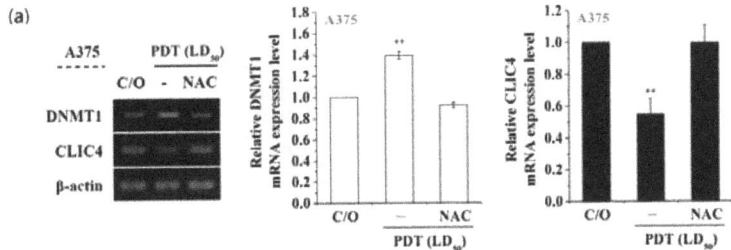

Figure 3. Cont.

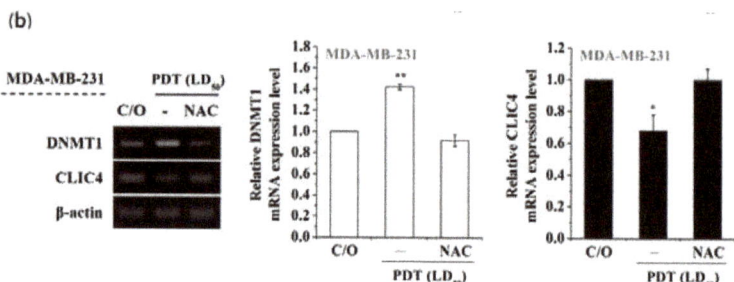

Figure 3. Scavenging ROS production suppresses the PDT-induced increase of DNMT1 and constrains the following CLIC4 suppression. Cells were co-incubated with both 1 mM ALA and 5 mM NAC for 3 h and then exposed to specific wavelength (635 ± 5 nm) of light, 2 J/cm^2 and 4 J/cm^2 for (a) A375 and (b) MDA-MB-231 cells, respectively. Total RNA samples were isolated from PDT-treated cells 24 h after ALA-PDT to analyze the mRNA expression level. The relative mRNA expression level of each gene was measured by RT-PCR and normalized to β-actin. The control group was cells only treated with ALA w/o light irradiation. The same volume of each PCR product was loaded, and band blots for each gene were cropped from different gels. Data represent from three independent experiments. Each bar shown is the mean fold change relative to control ± SD. Results are considered to be statistically significant at * $p < 0.05$ and ** $p < 0.01$.

3.3. DNMT1 Is Required to Down-Regulate CLIC4 Expression in PDT-Treated Cells

To further verify whether the increased DNMT1 is required for down-regulating CLIC4 in PDT-treated cells, we used two different DNMT1-specific short hairpin RNAs (shRNAs) to knockdown the endogenous DNMT1 followed by assessing the expression of CLIC4. As shown in Figure 4, both shDNMT1 #1 and #2 constructs could effectively reduce the mRNA expression level of DNMT1 in A375 and MDA-MB-231 cells (Figure 4a). The same results were observed in protein expression level analyzed by immunoblotting (Figure 4b). PDT-induced down-regulation of CLIC4 was significantly abrogated in A375 and MDA-MB-231 cells transiently transfected with shDNMT1 but not in cells transfected with the backbone shRNA vector, which indicates a reciprocal change between DNMT1 and CLIC4 expression in the knockdown cells post PDT treatment. These results suggest that DNMT1 is required in PDT-induced CLIC4 suppression.

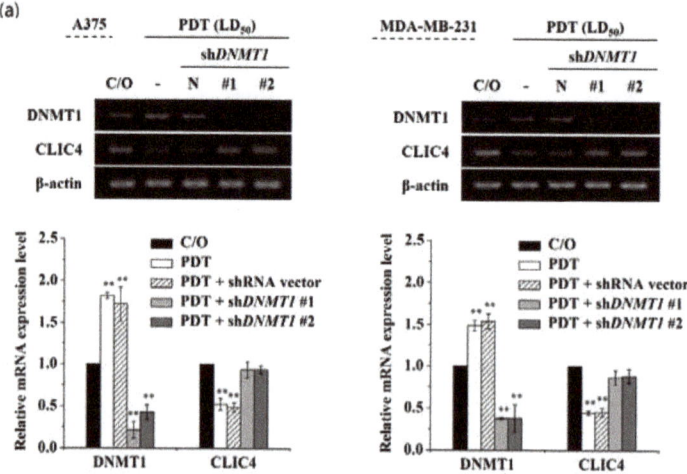

Figure 4. Cont.

(b)

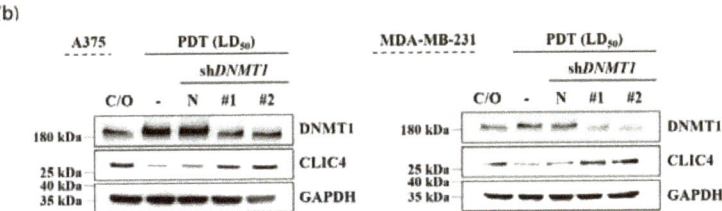

Figure 4. Down-regulation of DNMT1 restored the suppressed expression of CLIC4 in PDT-treated cells. A375 (left panel) and MDA-MB-231 (right panel) cells were transfected with either the shDNMT1 (denoted as shDNMT1 #1 and #2) or an empty shRNA vector (pLKO.1, as negative control). (a) Total mRNA and (b) protein samples were isolated from cells 24 h after ALA-PDT. The light dose for A375 and MDA-MB-231 cells is 2 J/cm^2 and 4 J/cm^2, respectively. The relative mRNA expression level of each gene was measured by RT-PCR and normalized to β-actin. The protein expression levels of DNMT1 and CLIC4 were analyzed by Western blotting, and GAPDH was used as an internal control. The control group was cells only treated with ALA w/o light irradiation. For electrophoretic gels, the same volume of each PCR product was loaded, and band blots for each gene were cropped from different gels. For immunoblots, equal volume of each sample with the same concentration was loaded into each well, and the blots were cropped from different sections of the same gel. Data represent from three independent experiments. Each bar shown is the mean fold change relative to control ± SD. Results are considered to be statistically significant at ** $p < 0.01$.

3.4. The Increased DNMT1 Relates to the Activated p53 in PDT-Treated Cells

It has been shown that DNMT1-mediated methylation is stimulated by the activation of p53 protein [38,39]. On the other hand, PDT-induced up-regulation of p53 has been found in various PDT-treated cells [40,41]. Compared to the cells either untreated or only incubated with ALA, the level of p53 protein indeed was considerably increased following PDT (see Figure S3 online). Therefore, we further addressed whether the DNMT1 up-regulation is associated with the activation of p53 in PDT-treated cells. As shown in Figure 5a,b, the mRNA and protein expression levels of p53 were significantly reduced in three different p53-specific shRNAs transfected cells, which also shows a reciprocal change in mRNA and protein levels between DNMT1 and CLIC4 after PDT. However, knockdown of p53 in cells without PDT treatment would not affect the expression of DNMT1 or CLIC4 (see Figure S4 online). These findings indicate that p53 plays an important role in modulating the increased DNMT1 expression in PDT-treated cells, which may further mediate the suppression of CLIC4 expression by promoting DNA methylation.

3.5. PDT Induces Suppression of CLIC4 Expression by Methylating its Promoter Region in A DNMT1-Dependent Manner

To further explore whether PDT-induced suppression of CLIC4 expression correlates to the DNA hypermethylation, the DNA methylation status of *CLIC4* promoter region in PDT-treated cells was examined. The methylation of CpG islands in the promoter region (−1214 to +795; the transcription start site (TSS) at +1) was assessed by bisulfite sequencing PCR (BSP). Specific primers were used to amplify the region spanning from nucleotide position −1126 to +973, which encompasses 181 CpG sites (Figure 6a). As shown in Figure 6b, compared to the control group, the methylation level at the position between −450 and +250 (containing 62 CpG sites) of *CLIC4* gene showed a substantial increase in PDT-treated cells. The percentage of methylated CpG islands in the assay area is 38.3% for the PDT-treated but only 1.6% for the untreated cells. These results indicate that PDT induces DNA methylation in the promoter region of *CLIC4* may contribute to its suppressed expression. To further investigate whether such a methylation is attributed to the DNMT1 function, the methylation status of *CLIC4* promoter region in A375 cells transfected with DNMT1-specific shRNA was also evaluated. After PDT treatment, there is 15.3% of methylation at the candidate region (nt. −450 to +250) in DNMT1 knockdown cells. These findings suggest that hypermethylation in the *CLIC4* promoter region induced by PDT is mainly DNMT1-dependent.

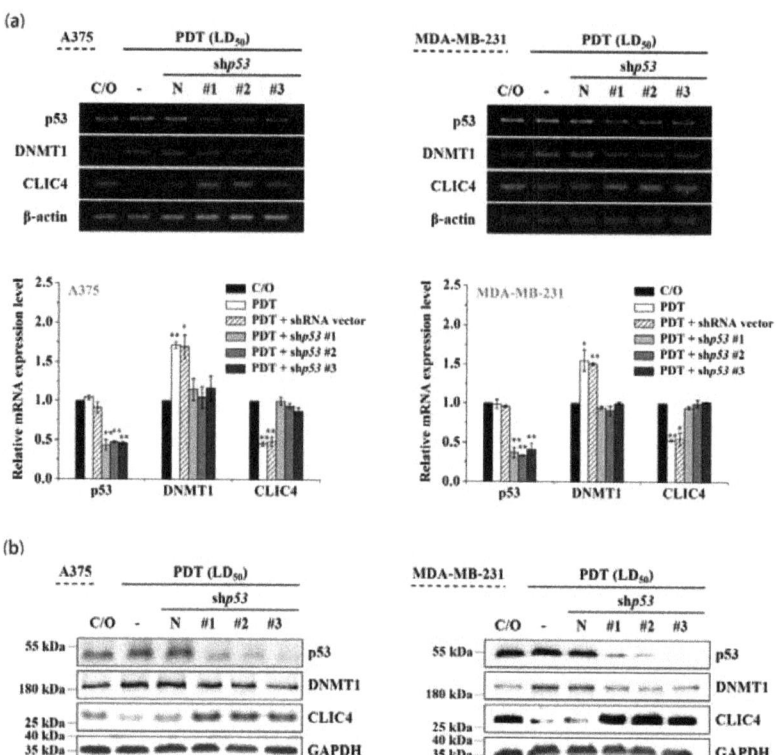

Figure 5. p53 involves in the altered expression of DNMT1 and CLIC4 in PDT-treated cells. A375 (left panel) and MDA-MB-231 (right panel) cells were transfected with either the shp53 (denoted as #1, #2 and #3) or an empty shRNA vector (pLKO.1 as negative control). (**a**) Total mRNA and (**b**) protein samples were isolated from cells 24 h after ALA-PDT. The light dose for A375 and MDA-MB-231 cells is 2 J/cm^2 and 4 J/cm^2, respectively. The relative mRNA expression level of each gene was measured by RT-PCR and normalized to β-actin. The control group was cells only treated with ALA w/o light irradiation. For electrophoretic gels, the same volume of each PCR product was loaded, and band blots for each gene were cropped from different gels. For immunoblots, equal volume of each sample with the same concentration was loaded into each well, and the blots were cropped from different sections of the same gel. Data represent from three independent experiments. Each bar shown is the mean fold change relative to control ± SD. Results are considered to be statistically significant at * $p < 0.05$ and ** $p < 0.01$.

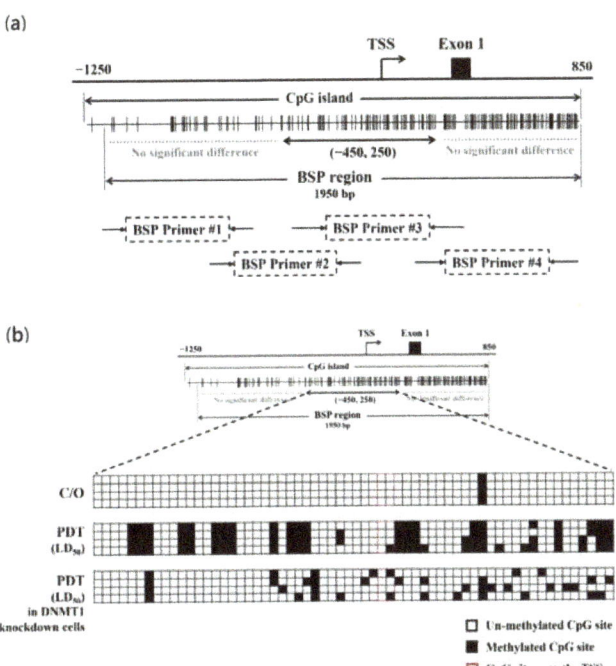

Figure 6. PDT induces the methylation alteration of CLIC4 promoter region in a DNMT1-dependent manner. (**a**) Schematic diagram of the CpG island of CLIC4 promoter. The distribution of CpGs crosses over the promoter and the first exon of CLIC4 gene. The transcriptional start site (TSS) is indicated. Each vertical bar represents the presence of a CpG dinucleotide. BSP1, BSP2, BSP3 and BSP4 represent the regions selected for bisulfite sequencing PCR (marked as BSP region); (**b**) Direct sequencing of bisulfite PCR products was performed in melanoma A375 cells: no-treatment control group, PDT-treated cells, and PDT-treated DNMT1-knockdown cells. Genomic DNA was extracted from cells 24 h after ALA-PDT with the light dose of 2 J/cm^2. Quantification of the bisulfite-sequencing data, shown as the percentage of DNA methylation ($n = 4$) of the region among the CLIC4 gene from position nt. −450 to +250. Methylation status of cytosine is shown as follows: filled square (■), methylated; open square (□), unmethylated.

3.6. CLIC4 Expression Is Regulated by DNA Hypermethylation in Its Promoter Region

The expression of CLIC4 is commonly reduced in many human cancers, including skin, breast, prostate, and lung tumors [11,42]. However, no evidence showed a mutation or deletion in the CLIC4 gene during tumorigenesis. As PDT-mediated CLIC4 suppression is correlated to the induction of methylation in its promoter region, DNA methylation status of the promoter region might contribute to the regulation of CLIC4 expression in cancer cells. In this regard, we first studied the relative mRNA expression level of CLIC4 in different lung cancer cell lines and normal lung fibroblast cell line, MRC-5. As shown in Figure 7a, the mRNA expression level of CLIC4 in normal MRC-5 fibroblasts was significantly higher than the malignant CL1-0, A549 and H460 cancer cells, but similar to that of H1299 cancer cells. Meanwhile, treatment with DNMT inhibitor, 5AZA, resulted in increased level of CLIC4 mRNA expression in CL1-0, A549 and H460 cancer cells (Figure 7a). The bisulfite sequencing analysis revealed that the CpG sites (nt. −450 to +250) are barely methylated and no methylation around the TSS in MRC-5 and H1299 cells, which express the higher level of CLIC4 mRNA (Figure 7b). In contrast, a considerably higher methylation level in the promoter region, especially heavy methylated around the TSS, was found in CL1-0, A549 and H460 cells with lower CLIC4 mRNA expression level. These results suggest that DNA methylation in the promoter region of CLIC4 might relate to the decreased CLIC4 expression during carcinogenesis.

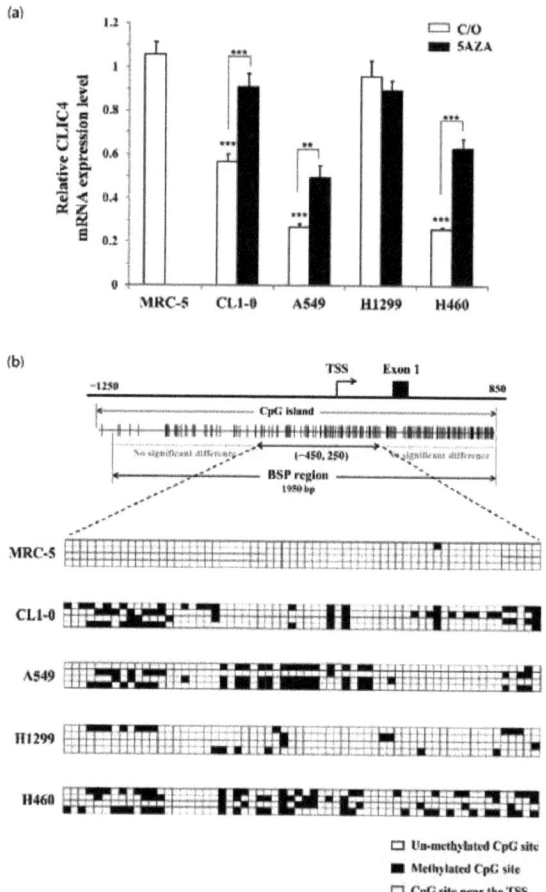

Figure 7. The methylation status of CLIC4 promoter correlates with its mRNA levels in different cell lines. (**a**) The real-time PCR was performed to analyze the mRNA expression level of CLIC4 in normal lung fibroblast cells, MRC-5; and lung cancer cells, CL1-0, A549, H1299, H460. Cells were treated with or without 5 μM 5AZA for 2 h. To compare the mRNA expression level of CLIC4 in different cell line, MRC-5 cells w/o 5AZA treatment were used as a control group. The relative mRNA expression level of each gene was normalized to GAPDH. Data represent from three independent experiments. Each bar shown is the mean fold change relative to control ± SD. Results are considered to be statistically significant at ** $p < 0.01$ and *** $p < 0.001$; (**b**) Direct sequencing of bisulfite PCR products was performed to explore the methylation status of CLIC4 promoter region. Quantification of the bisulfite-sequencing data, shown as the percentage of DNA methylation ($n = 4$) of the region among the *CLIC4* gene from position nt. −450 to +250. Methylation status of cytosine is shown as follows: filled square (°C), methylated; open square (□), unmethylated.

4. Discussion

Our previous study demonstrated that the down-regulation of CLIC4 related to the reduced invasiveness of PDT-treated cells [9]. In this study, we further investigated the regulatory mechanisms involved in PDT-mediated CLIC4 suppression. DNA methylation and histone acetylation are important epigenetic mechanisms involved in transcriptionally regulating gene expression. We have previously demonstrated that the oxidative stress mediated by PDT can significantly up-regulate the activity and expression of p300HAT, which leads to the increased expression of pro-survival molecules such as cyclooxygenase-2 and survivin [31]. However, in this study, we found that the reduced CLIC4 after PDT was not affected by HDAC inhibitor, which indicated that the reduced CLIC4 expression does not relate to the histone acetylation. Demyanenko et al. reported that ALA-PDT can induce the expression of DNA methylation-dependent protein, Kaiso, in the mouse cerebral cortex [32]. Meanwhile, it has been shown that 5AZA can rescue the necrosis of crayfish glial cells induced by photosensitization, indicating DNA methylation may involve in molecular process of PDT-induced cell damage [43]. In this study, we found that the reduced expression of CLIC4 could be reverted in the presence of 5AZA in PDT-treated cells (Figure 1). It has been shown that CLIC4 knockdown can reduce cell proliferation and migration ability as well as induce apoptosis in cultured cells [14,20]. However, we did not find significant difference in the viability of cells pretreated with or without 5AZA after PDT (see Figure S1 online), suggesting the reduced expression of CLIC4 involved in impairing cell migration rather than cell proliferation. In addition, we found that PDT-mediated oxidative stress can up-regulate the expression of DNMT1, and further leads to the suppression of CLIC4 expression through elevating hypermethylation in its promoter region. Altogether, these studies indicate that epigenetic modifications are involved in the regulatory mechanism of PDT-mediated biological consequences, suggesting a treatment modality of combining epigenetic drugs to improve the therapeutic efficacy of photodynamic therapy.

During tumorigenesis, it has been shown that the expression of CLIC4 was down-regulated in tumor cells but up-regulated in stromal cells [11,16]. In addition, up-regulation of CLIC4 involves in the TGF-β–mediated myofibroblast conversion, suggesting its role in malignant progression [18,19]. Previously, we have shown that the reduced invasiveness of PDT-treated cells relates to the decreased CLIC4 expression [9]. In this study, we further found that PDT can up-regulate the expression of DNMT1, leading to the suppression of CLIC4 expression. In this regard, we speculate that the clinical advantages of PDT might not only exert its therapeutic effects at tumor tissues but also reduce the CLIC4 expression in surviving tumor cells and stromal cells to suppress the malignant progression.

p53, a tumor suppressor gene, is frequently inactivated in many cancers. p53 protein plays a decisive role of cell fate upon stress stimuli. With different cell lines and photosensitizers, growing evidences demonstrate that p53 activation contributes to cell killing upon PDT [44–47]. Here, we reported that up-regulation of p53 following PDT relates to the increased DNMT1 expression, leading to hypermethylation of the *CLIC4* promoter region. This epigenetic modification resulted in the decrease of CLIC4 expression in PDT-treated cells. Although p53 is considered as the upstream activator of CLIC4, restoring expression of p53 does not increase CLIC4 expression in cutaneous squamous cell lines [42]. Correspondingly, we also found that silencing of p53 expression in untreated cancer cells would not affect DNMT1 and CLIC4 expression (see Figure S4 online). To clarify the relationship between p53 and CLIC4 under PDT-mediated oxidative stress, we used the following cancer cell lines for further analysis: A375 (wild-type p53), MDA-MB-231 (stabilized mutant p53), and PC3 (p53-null) cancer cell lines [48]. We found that up-regulation of p53 following PDT relates to the increased DNMT1 expression, leading to hypermethylation of the CLIC4 promoter region in A375 cells with wild-type p53. In contrast, PDT did not significantly increase the p53 expression in MDA-MB-231 cell line which has an endogenously high level of the mutant p53. But knockdown of p53 in PDT-treated MDA-MB-231 cells can still prevent the up-regulation of DNMT1 and restore the down-regulation of CLIC4 (Figure 5). For p53-null PC3 prostate cancer cells, PDT can still induce the expression of DNMT1 with further decrease in CLIC4 expression (see Figure S5 online). Therefore, the expression level of p53 might not be the only factor for the expression of DNMT1 and CLIC4 in response to PDT-mediated oxidative stress. In fact, there are two other protein members of the p53 family, p63 and p73, existed in the p53-null PC3 cells [44]. We speculated that in addition to p53, the p53 isoforms might also conduce to the DNMT1-dependent CLIC4 regulation. In fact, as shown in Figure S6 online, PDT significantly increased the mRNA expression levels of p73 and *DNMT1* in the p53-null PC3 cells. Altogether, these results indicate that the p53 family may play an important role in modulating the increased expression of DNMT1 and the following suppressed expression of CLIC4 by promoting DNA methylation in PDT-treated cells. It is noteworthy that PDT did not significantly increase the p53 expression in MDA-MB-231 cell line which has a high level of the mutant p53 (unpublished data). However, the silencing of p53 expression in PDT-treated MDA-MB-231 cells can still prevent the up-regulation of DNMT1 and restore the down-regulation of CLIC4 (Figure 5). These findings suggest that, in addition to p53, other regulatory mechanisms may also be involved in regulating DNMT1-mediated CLIC4 expression in PDT responses.

Considerable evidences implicate that the distribution of CLIC4 expression in many human neoplasms directly correlates with cancer pathogenesis [49,50]. The Yuspa et al. demonstrated that the suppression of CLIC4 expression is not resulting from the gene mutations and suggested other changes such as epigenetic modification may be responsible for the regulation of CLIC4 [11,20]. The promoter region of *CLIC4* shows a high frequency of CpG sites, suggesting the possibility of promoter silencing by methylation. In this study, we employed the direct bisulfite sequencing PCR to examine the methylation status and demonstrated that PDT-induced oxidative stress can suppress the CLIC4 expression by methylating in its promoter, particularly at the region spanning from position nt. −450 to 250. Furthermore, comparing among the different lung cancer cells and the normal fibroblasts, the DNA methylation status of this region was found to be correlated to the mRNA expression level of *CLIC4* (Figure 7). These findings imply that DNA methylation of the promoter region may be a regulatory mechanism of CLIC4 expression in malignant tumor progression.

In summary, this study demonstrated that the down-regulation of CLIC4 after PDT is mediated by the hypermethylation of its promoter region. The regulatory mechanism involves in the increased expression of p53 and following DNMT1, which further induce hypermethylation in the promoter region of *CLIC4*. Exploration of the methylation status of *CLIC4* promoter and its transcribed mRNA level in malignant lung cancer and normal fibroblast cells revealed the highly methylated status in the malignant cells expressing lower mRNA levels of *CLIC4*. In the future, it is worthwhile to further address whether modulating the DNMT1 activity to regulate the CLIC4 expression could become a novel approach to inhibit the tumor malignancy.

Supplementary Materials: The following are available online at https://www.mdpi.com/article/10.3390/biomedicines9080927/s1, Figure S1: Cell viability in PDT-treated cells with 5-azacytidine (5AZA) pre-treatment. Figure S2: Inhibition of histone deacetylase (HDAC) activity by Trichostatin A (TSA) cannot suppress the PDT-induced reduction of CLIC4, Figure S3: p53 activation following PDT in A375 cells, Figure S4: *DNMT1* and *CLIC4* mRNA expression levels in p53-knockdown A375 cells, Figure S5: PDT induced DNMT1 expression and further suppressed CLIC4 expression in p53-null PC3 prostate cancer cells, Figure S6: PDT increased *DNMT1* and *p73* expression in p53-null PC3 prostate cancer cells, Figure S7: Original scans of immuno-blots used in main text and supplementary figures, Figure S8: Original scans of electrophoresis gel used in main text and supplementary figures.

Author Contributions: Conceptualization, C.-T.C. and P.-C.C.; Methodology and investigation, P.-C.C. and P.-T.L.; Data analysis and curation, P.-C.C. and P.-T.L. and M.-J.L.; Funding acquisition, C.-T.C.; Writing—original draft preparation, P.-C.C. and P.-T.L.; Writing—review and editing, P.-C.C. and C.-T.C.; Supervision and project administration, C.-T.C. All authors have read and agreed to the published version of the manuscript.

Funding: This research was supported by the Ministry of Science and Technology, Taiwan [grant numbers: NSC 101-2320-B-002-047-MY3, MOST 104-2320-B-002-041, and MOST 107-2314-B-002-057].

Institutional Review Board Statement: Not applicable.

Informed Consent Statement: Not applicable.

Data Availability Statement: The datasets generated during and/or analyzed during the current study are available from the corresponding author on reasonable request.

Conflicts of Interest: The authors declare no conflict of interest.

References

1. Agostinis, P.; Berg, K.; Cengel, K.A.; Foster, T.H.; Girotti, A.W.; Gollnick, S.O.; Hahn, S.M.; Hamblin, M.R.; Juzeniene, A.; Kessel, D.; et al. Photodynamic therapy of cancer: An update. *CA A Cancer J. Clin.* **2011**, *61*, 250–281. [CrossRef]
2. Dolmans, D.E.; Fukumura, D.; Jain, R.K. Photodynamic therapy for cancer. *Nat. Rev. Cancer* **2003**, *3*, 380–387. [CrossRef] [PubMed]
3. Donohoe, C.; Senge, M.O.; Arnaut, L.G.; Gomes-da-Silva, L.G. Cell death in photodynamic therapy: From oxidative stress to anti-tumorimmunity. *BBA-Rev. Cancer* **2019**, *1872*, 188308. [CrossRef] [PubMed]
4. Kessel, D.; Oleinick, N.L. Cell Death Pathways Associated with Photodynamic Therapy: An Update. *Photochem. Photobiol.* **2018**, *94*, 213–218. [CrossRef]
5. Ji, H.-T.; Chien, L.-T.; Lin, Y.-H.; Chien, H.-F.; Chen, C.-T. 5-ALA mediated photodynamic therapy induces autophagic cell death via AMP-activated protein kinase. *Mol. Cancer* **2010**, *9*, 91. [CrossRef] [PubMed]
6. Huang, L.; Lin, H.; Chen, Q.; Yu, L.; Bai, D. MPPa-PDT suppresses breast tumor migration/invasion by inhibiting Akt-NF-κB-dependent mMP-9 expression via ROS. *BMC Cancer* **2019**, *19*, 1159. [CrossRef] [PubMed]
7. Momma, T.; Hamblin, M.; Wu, H.C.; Hasan, T. Photodynamic therapy of orthotopic prostate cancer with benzoporphyrin derivative: Local control and distant metastasis. *Cancer Res.* **1998**, *58*, 5425.
8. Schreiber, S.; Gross, S.; Brandis, A.; Harmelin, A.; Rosenbach-Belkin, V.; Scherz, A.; Salomon, Y. Local photodynamic therapy (PDT) of rat C6 glioma xenografts with Pd-bacteriopheophorbide leads to decreased metastases and increase of animal cure compared with surgery. *Int. J. Cancer* **2002**, *99*, 279–285. [CrossRef] [PubMed]
9. Chiang, P.C.; Chou, R.H.; Chien, H.F.; Tsai, T.; Chen, C.T. Chloride intracellular channel 4 involves in the reduced inva-siveness of cancer cells treated by photodynamic therapy. *Lasers Surg Med.* **2013**, *45*, 38–47. [CrossRef]
10. Littler, D.; Harrop, S.J.; Goodchild, S.; Phang, J.M.; Mynott, A.V.; Jiang, L.; Valenzuela, S.; Mazzanti, M.; Brown, L.; Breit, S.N.; et al. The enigma of the CLIC proteins: Ion channels, redox proteins, enzymes, scaffolding proteins? *FEBS Lett.* **2010**, *584*, 2093–2101. [CrossRef] [PubMed]
11. Suh, K.S.; Crutchley, J.M.; Koochek, A.; Ryscavage, A.; Bhat, K.; Tanaka, T.; Oshima, A.; Fitzgerald, P.; Yuspa, S.H. Reciprocal Modifications of CLIC4 in Tumor Epithelium and Stroma Mark Malignant Progression of Multiple Human Cancers. *Clin. Cancer Res.* **2007**, *13*, 121–131. [CrossRef] [PubMed]
12. Edwards, J.C. A novel p64-related Cl- channel: Subcellular distribution and nephron segment-specific expression. *Am. J. Physiol. Content* **1999**, *276*, F398–F408. [CrossRef]
13. Littler, D.R.; Assaad, N.N.; Harrop, S.J.; Brown, L.J.; Pankhurst, G.J.; Luciani, P.; Aguilar, M.-I.; Mazzanti, M.; Berryman, M.A.; Breit, S.N.; et al. Crystal structure of the soluble form of the redox-regulated chloride ion channel protein CLIC4. *FEBS J.* **2005**, *272*, 4996–5007. [CrossRef]
14. Suh, K.S.; Mutoh, M.; Gerdes, M.; Yuspa, S.H. CLIC4, an Intracellular Chloride Channel Protein, Is a Novel Molecular Target for Cancer Therapy. *J. Investig. Dermatol. Symp. Proc.* **2005**, *10*, 105–109. [CrossRef]
15. Abdul-Salam, V.B.; Russomanno, G.; Chen, C.N.; Mahomed, A.S.; Yates, L.A.; Wilkins, M.R.; Zhao, L.; Gierula, M.; Dubois, O.; Schaeper, U.; et al. CLIC4/Arf6 Pathway. *Circ. Res.* **2019**, *124*, 52–65. [CrossRef]
16. Suh, K.S.; Malik, M.; Shukla, A.; Yuspa, S.H. CLIC4, skin homeostasis and cutaneous cancer: Surprising connections. *Mol. Carcinog.* **2007**, *46*, 599–604. [CrossRef]
17. Shukla, A.; Edwards, R.; Yang, Y.; Hahn, A.; Folkers, K.; Ding, J.; Padmakumar, V.C.; Cataisson, C.; Suh, K.S.; Yuspa, S.H. CLIC4 regulates TGF-β-dependent myofibroblast differentiation to produce a cancer stroma. *Oncogene* **2013**, *33*, 842–850. [CrossRef]
18. Yao, Q.; Qu, X.; Yang, Q.; Good, D.A.; Dai, S.; Kong, B.; Wei, M.Q. Blockage of transdifferentiation from fibroblast to myofibroblast in experimental ovarian cancer models. *Mol. Cancer* **2009**, *8*, 78. [CrossRef] [PubMed]
19. Yao, Q.; Qu, X.; Yang, Q.; Wei, M.; Kong, B. CLIC4 mediates TGF-beta1-induced fibroblast-to-myofibroblast transdifferen-tiation in ovarian cancer. *Oncol. Rep.* **2009**, *22*, 541–548. [PubMed]
20. Singha, B.; Harper, S.L.; Goldman, A.R.; Bitler, B.; Aird, K.M.; Borowsky, M.E.; Cadungog, M.G.; Liu, Q.; Zhang, R.; Jean, S.; et al. CLIC1 and CLIC4 complement CA125 as a diagnostic biomarker panel for all subtypes of epithelial ovarian cancer. *Sci. Rep.* **2018**, *8*, 1–14. [CrossRef]
21. Goldberg, A.; Allis, C.D.; Bernstein, E. Epigenetics: A Landscape Takes Shape. *Cell* **2007**, *128*, 635–638. [CrossRef]
22. Jaenisch, R.; Bird, A. Epigenetic regulation of gene expression: How the genome integrates intrinsic and environmental signals. *Nat. Genet.* **2003**, *33*, 245–254. [CrossRef]
23. Gardiner-Garden, M.; Frommer, M. CpG Islands in vertebrate genomes. *J. Mol. Biol.* **1987**, *196*, 261–282. [CrossRef]
24. Suzuki, M.M.; Bird, A. DNA methylation landscapes: Provocative insights from epigenomics. *Nat. Rev. Genet.* **2008**, *9*, 465–476. [CrossRef]
25. Wang, Y.; Leung, F.C. An evaluation of new criteria for CpG islands in the human genome as gene markers. *Bioinformatics* **2004**, *20*, 1170–1177. [CrossRef] [PubMed]
26. Richardson, B. Impact of aging on DNA methylation. *Ageing Res. Rev.* **2003**, *2*, 245–261. [CrossRef]

27. Bhat, A.V.; Hora, S.; Pal, A.; Jha, S.; Taneja, R. Stressing the (Epi)Genome: Dealing with Reactive Oxygen Species in Cancer. *Antioxid. Redox Signal.* **2018**, *29*, 1273–1292. [CrossRef]
28. Murata, M. Inflammation and cancer. *Environ. Health Prev. Med.* **2018**, *23*, 1–8. [CrossRef]
29. Lan, M.; Zhao, S.; Liu, W.; Lee, C.-S.; Zhang, W.; Wang, P. Photosensitizers for Photodynamic Therapy. *Adv. Health Mater.* **2019**, *8*, e1900132. [CrossRef]
30. Xiong, Y.; Tian, X.; Ai, H.-W. Molecular Tools to Generate Reactive Oxygen Species in Biological Systems. *Bioconjug. Chem.* **2019**, *30*, 1297–1303. [CrossRef]
31. Tsai, Y.J.; Tsai, T.; Peng, P.C.; Li, P.T.; Chen, C.T. Histone acetyltransferase p300 is induced by p38MAPK after photo-dynamic therapy: The therapeutic response is increased by the p300HAT inhibitor anacardic acid. *Free Radic. Biol. Med.* **2015**, *86*, 118–132. [CrossRef]
32. Demyanenko, S.; Uzdensky, A.; Sharifulina, S.; Lapteva, T.; Polyakova, L. PDT-induced epigenetic changes in the mouse cerebral cortex: A protein microarray study. *Biochim. Biophys. Acta (BBA) Gen. Subj.* **2014**, *1840*, 262–270. [CrossRef]
33. Yang, P.-C.; Luh, K.-T.; Wu, R.; Wu, C.-W. Characterization of the Mucin Differentiation in Human Lung Adenocarcinoma Cell Lines. *Am. J. Respir. Cell Mol. Biol.* **1992**, *7*, 161–171. [CrossRef]
34. Tsai, T.; Ji, H.T.; Chiang, P.-C.; Chou, R.-H.; Chang, W.-S.W.; Chen, C.-T. ALA-PDT results in phenotypic changes and decreased cellular invasion in surviving cancer cells. *Lasers Surg. Med.* **2009**, *41*, 305–315. [CrossRef] [PubMed]
35. Leonhardt, H.; Page, A.W.; Weier, H.-U.; Bestor, T.H. A targeting sequence directs DNA methyltransferase to sites of DNA replication in mammalian nuclei. *Cell* **1992**, *71*, 865–873. [CrossRef]
36. Lim, S.-O.; Gu, J.-M.; Kim, M.S.; Kim, H.-S.; Park, Y.N.; Park, C.K.; Cho, J.W.; Jung, G. Epigenetic Changes Induced by Reactive Oxygen Species in Hepatocellular Carcinoma: Methylation of the E-cadherin Promoter. *Gastroenterology* **2008**, *135*, 2128–2140.e8. [CrossRef] [PubMed]
37. Zhang, R.; Kang, K.A.; Kim, K.C.; Na, S.-Y.; Chang, W.Y.; Kim, G.Y.; Kim, H.S.; Hyun, J.W. Oxidative stress causes epigenetic alteration of CDX1 expression in colorectal cancer cells. *Gene* **2013**, *524*, 214–219. [CrossRef] [PubMed]
38. Estève, P.O.; Chin, H.G.; Pradhan, S. Human maintenance DNA (cytosine-5)-methyltransferase and p53 modulate expres-sion of p53-repressed promoters. *Proc. Natl. Acad. Sci. USA* **2005**, *102*, 1000–1005. [CrossRef]
39. Qin, W.; Leonhardt, H.; Pichler, G. Regulation of DNA methyltransferase 1 by interactions and modifications. *Nucleus* **2011**, *2*, 392–402. [CrossRef] [PubMed]
40. Gracia-Cazaña, T.; Mascaraque, M.; Lucena, S.R.; Vera-Álvarez, J.; Gonzalez, S.; Gilaberte, Y. Biomarkers of basal cell carcinoma resistance to methyl-aminolevulinate photodynamic therapy. *PLoS ONE* **2019**, *14*, e0215537. [CrossRef]
41. Zawacka-Pankau, J.; Krachulec, J.; Grulkowski, I.; Bielawski, K.P.; Selivanova, G. The p53-mediated cytotoxicity of pho-todynamic therapy of cancer: Recent advances. *Toxicol. Appl. Pharmacol.* **2008**, *232*, 487–497. [CrossRef] [PubMed]
42. Suh, K.; Malik, M.; Shukla, A.; Ryscavage, A.; Wright, L.; Jividen, K.; Crutchley, J.M.; Dumont, R.A.; Fernandez-Salas, E.; Webster, J.D.; et al. CLIC4 is a tumor suppressor for cutaneous squamous cell cancer. *Carcinogenesis* **2012**, *33*, 986–995. [CrossRef]
43. Sharifulina, S.; Komandirov, M.; Uzdensky, A. Epigenetic regulation of death of crayfish glial cells but not neurons induced by photodynamic impact. *Brain Res. Bull.* **2014**, *102*, 15–21. [CrossRef]
44. Acedo, P.; Zawacka-Pankau, J. p53 family members—important messengers in cell death signaling in photodynamic therapy of cancer? *Photochem. Photobiol. Sci.* **2015**, *14*, 1390–1396. [CrossRef] [PubMed]
45. Li, L.; Chen, Y.; Wang, X.; Feng, X.; Wang, P.; Liu, Q. Comparison of protoporphyrin IX produced cell proliferation inhibition between human breast cancer MCF-7 and MDA-MB-231 cells. *Die Pharm.* **2014**, *69*, 621–628.
46. O'Connor, A.E.; Mc Gee, M.M.; Likar, Y.; Ponomarev, V.; Callanan, J.J.; O'Shea, D.F.; Byrne, A.T.; Gallagher, W.M. Mechanism of cell death mediated by a BF2-chelated tetraaryl-azadipyrromethene photodynamic therapeutic: Dissection of the apoptotic pathway in vitro and in vivo. *Int. J. Cancer* **2011**, *130*, 705–715. [CrossRef]
47. Song, J.; Wei, Y.; Chen, Q.; Xing, D. Cyclooxygenase 2-mediated apoptotic and inflammatory responses in photodynamic therapy treated breast adenocarcinoma cells and xenografts. *J. Photochem. Photobiol. B Biol.* **2014**, *134*, 27–36. [CrossRef] [PubMed]
48. Carroll, A.G.; Voeller, H.J.; Sugars, L.; Gelmann, E.P. p53 oncogene mutations in three human prostate cancer cell lines. *Prostate* **1993**, *23*, 123–134. [CrossRef] [PubMed]
49. Peretti, M.; Angelini, M.; Savalli, N.; Florio, T.; Yuspa, S.H.; Mazzanti, M. Chloride channels in cancer: Focus on chloride intracellular channel 1 and 4 (CLIC1 AND CLIC4) proteins in tumor development and as novel therapeutic targets. *Biochim. Biophys. Acta (BBA)-Biomembr.* **2015**, *1848*, 2523–2531. [CrossRef]
50. Leanza, L.; Biasutto, L.; Managò, A.; Gulbins, E.; Zoratti, M.; Szabò, I. Intracellular ion channels and cancer. *Front Physiol.* **2013**, *4*, 227. [CrossRef] [PubMed]

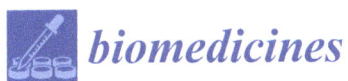

Article

Target-Oriented Synthesis of Marine Coelenterazine Derivatives with Anticancer Activity by Applying the Heavy-Atom Effect

Carla M. Magalhães [1], Patricia González-Berdullas [1], Diana Duarte [2,3], Ana Salomé Correia [2,3], José E. Rodríguez-Borges [4], Nuno Vale [2,3], Joaquim C. G. Esteves da Silva [1,2] and Luís Pinto da Silva [1,5,*]

1. Chemistry Research Unit (CIQUP), Faculty of Sciences, University of Porto, Rua do Campo Alegre 687, 4169-007 Porto, Portugal; up201201533@edu.fc.up.pt (C.M.M.); patricia.berdullas@fc.up.pt (P.G.-B.); jcsilva@fc.up.pt (J.C.G.E.d.S.)
2. OncoPharma Research Group, Center for Health Technology and Services Research (CINTESIS), Rua Doutor Plácido da Costa, 4200-450 Porto, Portugal; dianaduarte29@gmail.com (D.D.); anncorr07@gmail.com (A.S.C.); nunovale@med.up.pt (N.V.)
3. Department of Community Medicine, Health Information and Decision (MEDCIDS), Faculty of Medicine, University of Porto, Alameda Professor Hernâni Monteiro, 4200-319 Porto, Portugal
4. LAQV/REQUIMTE, Department of Chemistry and Biochemistry, Faculty of Sciences, University of Porto, Rua do Campo Alegre 697, 4169-007 Porto, Portugal; jrborges@fc.up.pt
5. LACOMEPHI, GreenUPorto, Department of Geosciences, Environment and Territorial Planning, Faculty of Sciences, University of Porto, Rua do Campo Alegre 697, 4169-007 Porto, Portugal
* Correspondence: luis.silva@fc.up.pt

Citation: Magalhães, C.M.; González-Berdullas, P.; Duarte, D.; Correia, A.S.; Rodríguez-Borges, J.E.; Vale, N.; Esteves da Silva, J.C.G.; Pinto da Silva, L. Target-Oriented Synthesis of Marine Coelenterazine Derivatives with Anticancer Activity by Applying the Heavy-Atom Effect. Biomedicines 2021, 9, 1199. https://doi.org/10.3390/biomedicines9091199

Academic Editor: Stefano Bacci

Received: 26 July 2021
Accepted: 8 September 2021
Published: 11 September 2021

Publisher's Note: MDPI stays neutral with regard to jurisdictional claims in published maps and institutional affiliations.

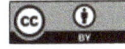

Copyright: © 2021 by the authors. Licensee MDPI, Basel, Switzerland. This article is an open access article distributed under the terms and conditions of the Creative Commons Attribution (CC BY) license (https://creativecommons.org/licenses/by/4.0/).

Abstract: Photodynamic therapy (PDT) is an anticancer therapeutic modality with remarkable advantages over more conventional approaches. However, PDT is greatly limited by its dependence on external light sources. Given this, PDT would benefit from new systems capable of a light-free and intracellular photodynamic effect. Herein, we evaluated the heavy-atom effect as a strategy to provide anticancer activity to derivatives of coelenterazine, a chemiluminescent single-molecule widespread in marine organisms. Our results indicate that the use of the heavy-atom effect allows these molecules to generate readily available triplet states in a chemiluminescent reaction triggered by a cancer marker. Cytotoxicity assays in different cancer cell lines showed a heavy-atom-dependent anticancer activity, which increased in the substituent order of hydroxyl < chlorine < bromine. Furthermore, it was found that the magnitude of this anticancer activity is also dependent on the tumor type, being more relevant toward breast and prostate cancer. The compounds also showed moderate activity toward neuroblastoma, while showing limited activity toward colon cancer. In conclusion, the present results indicate that the application of the heavy-atom effect to marine coelenterazine could be a promising approach for the future development of new and optimized self-activating and tumor-selective sensitizers for light-free PDT.

Keywords: photodynamic therapy; cancer; coelenterazine; chemiluminescence; heavy-atom effect; triplet chemiexcitation; self-activating photosensitizers

1. Introduction

Photodynamic therapy (PDT) is a clinically approved cancer treatment with great potential due to its minimally invasive nature, fewer side effects, and fast healing rate of healthy tissues [1,2]. PDT consists of the irradiation of a tumor site, in which a photosensitizer is accumulated, with light of a specific wavelength. Upon photoexcitation, the photosensitizer will be excited from its ground state (S_0) to its lowest singlet excited state (S_1) and will undergo intersystem crossing (ISC) to triplet states (T_1), now capable of sensitizing the highly cytotoxic singlet oxygen after reacting with triplet oxygen [1,3]. Unfortunately, the low penetration of light into biologic tissues limits this therapy to the treatment of superficial tumors or tumors on the outer lining of internal organs and cavities [4,5]. Furthermore, PDT is also unable to treat metastatic tumors due to these localization-based limitations [5]. Given this, the development of novel tumor-selective photosensitizers capable of intracellular activation without an external light source is essential for eliminating PDT restrictions regarding tumor size and localization [4,6].

Theoretically, triplet excited states can be generated in a light-free and tumor-selective way, by using the chemiluminescent reaction of marine coelenterazine (Clz) (Scheme 1a) [6,7]. Chemiluminescence consists of the conversion of thermal energy into excitation energy due to a chemical reaction, without an excitation source [6]. For Clz, specifically, the chemiluminescent reaction consists of its oxidation into an unstable cyclic peroxide intermediate (dioxetanone), which rapidly decomposes into the light-emitter, coelenteramide. The chemiluminescence of Clz has the advantage of being triggered solely by superoxide anion, a reactive oxygen species (ROS) typically overexpressed in cancer cells, without requiring any catalyst/cofactor (Scheme 1b) [8]. The key step for chemiexcitation is the decomposition of dioxetanone, during which S_0 becomes degenerated with both T_1 and S_1 states [9]. However, for Clz, the $S_0 \rightarrow T_1$ ISC pathway is generally thought of as inefficient, as this system is only known for its efficient generation of singlet excited states [10,11].

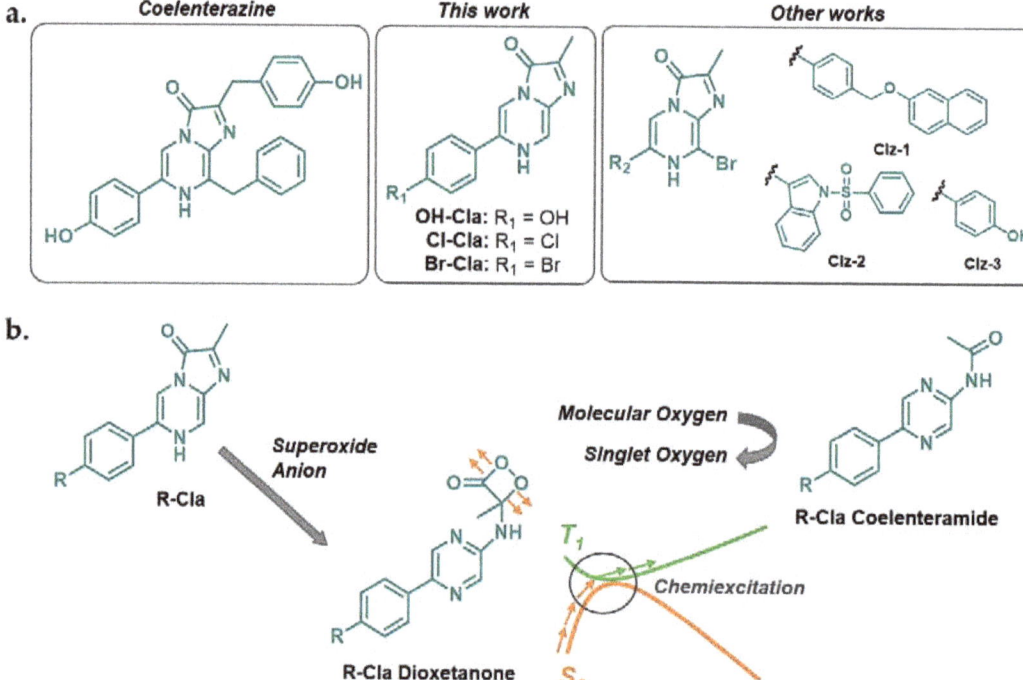

Scheme 1. Chemical structures of coelenterazine and derivatives (**a**). Schematic representation of the proposed tumor-selective and self-activating photodynamic therapy based on the chemiluminescent reaction of R-Cla (**b**).

Enhancing the $S_0 \rightarrow T_1$ ISC pathway can then enable the use of the chemiluminescent reaction of Clz as a self-excitation mechanism to directly generate triplet states able to sensitize singlet oxygen, thus leading to a light-free intracellular reaction exclusively triggered by a cancer marker (superoxide anion). One of the most effective strategies to enhance the efficiency of ISC pathways is through the heavy-atom effect (e.g., introduction of halogen atoms) [3]. Accordingly, we recently synthesized 6-(4-bromophenyl)-2-methylimidazo [1, 2−a] pyrazin-3(7H)-one (Br-Cla) (Scheme 1a), a brominated Clz derivative in which the hydroxyl of the phenol group was substituted by bromine, and the *p*-cresol and benzyl moieties of Clz were replaced by a methyl group and a hydrogen atom, respectively [12]. Br-Cla showed superoxide-triggered singlet oxygen sensitization and presented anticancer activity toward prostate and breast cancer without inducing toxicity toward noncancer cells [12,13]. Given the promising results and the interesting profile of tumor-selectivity, we continued our research focus and reported the synthesis of three other brominated Clz derivatives (Clz-1, Clz-2, and Clz-3) (Scheme 1a) [13]. These novel compounds showed potential for superoxide-induced generation of triplet states via a CL reaction, while also presenting relevant anticancer activity toward breast and prostate cancer.

Thus, studies with Br-Cla and the remaining brominated Clz derivatives (Scheme 1) provided results indicating that these compounds possess significant potential as prototypical light-free and self-activating single-molecule photosensitizers. However, as all developed derivatives bore a bromine heteroatom, it is not clear if the resulting anticancer activity results from the heavy-atom effect on the CL reaction or if it results from an intrinsic activity related to the imidazopyrazinone core (common to all). Such information is essential to understand if we are indeed in the presence of prototypical light-free and self-activating photosensitizers or in the presence of new potential chemotherapeutic drugs with tumor-selectivity characteristics [12,13].

To further understand the true potential of these Clz derivatives as novel anticancer compounds, it is also important to know how they behave toward different cancer types and assess their spectrum of application. So far, our knowledge in this regard is limited to their application to prostate and breast cancer [12,13].

Herein, we aimed to clarify these topics by employing a target-oriented approach. Specifically, we report the synthesis of three Cla derivatives (OH-, Cl-, and Br-substituted Cla, Scheme 1a), with the rationale that the substitution with halogen atoms of increasing size should enhance the heavy-atom effect into the studied system. If successful, this should increase the ISC rate of the $S_0 \rightarrow T_1$ pathway present in the chemiluminescent reaction of these compounds and, hence, favor T_1 chemiexcitation in the increasing order of OH < Cl < Br. If the reported anticancer activity of the compounds is indeed related to the intracellular superoxide-triggered T_1 chemiexcitation, this should lead to heavy-atom-dependent enhancement of their cytotoxicity in the increasing order of OH < Cl < Br. Thus, these three derivatives were subjected to a detailed and in-depth luminometry, photophysical, and theoretical characterization of their chemiluminescent reactions, focused on the possible superoxide-induced generation of triplet excited states. Subsequently, their cytotoxicity was also evaluated for the first time toward neuroblastoma and colon cancer cell lines, with the resulting performance compared with that obtained for breast and prostate cancer. With this approach, we will be able to understand if the heavy-atom effect is indeed responsible for the anticancer activity of these molecules, supporting their identification as prototypical light-free and self-activating photosensitizers, and to understand the scope of their cytotoxicity toward different cancer types.

2. Materials and Methods

2.1. In Silico Modeling

The S_0 geometry optimization and frequency calculations for OH-Cla dioxetanone were performed with the ωB97XD functional [14] and the 6-31G(d,p) basis set, as well as with an open-shell (U) and broken-symmetry approach. Intrinsic reaction coordinate (IRC) calculations were carried out to assess if the obtained transition state (TS) connects the desired reactants and products. The energies of the S_0 IRC-obtained structures were re-evaluated by single-point calculations with the same functional but using the 6-31 + G (d,p) basis set. The T_1 state was calculated by performing single-point calculations at the same level of theory, on top of the S_0 IRC-obtained structures. ωB97XD is a long-range-corrected hybrid exchange-correlation functional, which provides quite good estimates for $\pi \rightarrow \pi^*$ and $n \rightarrow \pi^*$ local excitation, as well as charge transfer and Rydberg states [15]. Geometry optimizations, frequency calculations, and IRC calculations were made in vacuo, while single-point calculations were made in implicit water using a polarizable continuum model (IEFPCM). All calculations were made using the Gaussian 09 program package [16]. This approach has been used with success before in the study of the chemiexcitation of dioxetanones [9,17].

2.2. Synthesis of the Compounds

Br-Cla was prepared following the procedure described in [12], while OH- and Cl-Cla were synthesized through the same synthetic pathway with some modifications (Scheme S1). The detailed synthetic procedure is available in the Supplementary Materials. Briefly, these compounds were obtained through an initial Suzuki-Miyaura cross-coupling between 5-bromopyrazin-2-amine and the corresponding arylboronic acid derivative (Scheme S1). Condensation of the resulting precursor with methyl glyoxal in acid medium yielded the desired reaction product (Scheme S1). High-performance liquid chromatography coupled to a diode array detector (HPLC-DAD), Fourier-transform infrared (FT-IR), and UV-Vis spectroscopy data, as well as details for all compounds, are presented in the Supplementary Materials. ^{1}H-NMR and high-resolution mass spectra (HR-MS) for OH-/Cl-Cla are also available in the Supplementary Materials, whereas they were presented in [12] for Br-Cla.

2.3. Luminometric and Photophysical Characterization

Chemiluminescence kinetic measurements were performed in a homemade luminometer using a Hamamatsu HC135-01 photomultiplier tube. All reactions took place at room temperature at least in sextuplicate. The light-emitting reactions took place at room temperature at least in sextuplicate and were carried out in either N,N-dimethylformamide (DMF)-acetate buffer pH 5.14 (0.68%) or methanol in the presence of a superoxide anion source (potassium superoxide, KO_2). The steady-state chemiluminescent and fluorescent spectra of the three Cla derivatives were measured using a Horiba Jovin Fluoromax 4 spectrofluorimeter, with an integration time of 0.1 s. Slit widths of 5 nm were used for both the excitation and emission monochromators when obtaining fluorescent spectra. Chemiluminescent spectra were obtained with a slit of 29 nm for the emission monochromators. Quartz cells with a 10 mm path length were used.

The light-emitting reactions took place at ambient temperature at least in sextuplicate and were carried out in DMF-acetate buffer pH 5.14 (0.68%) or methanol (in the presence of potassium superoxide (KO_2)) The chemiluminescent and fluorescent spectra were obtained in 2 mL DMF-acetate buffer pH 5.14 (0.68%) solutions and measured using a Horiba Jovin Fluoromax 4 spectrofluorimeter (The detailed procedure is available in the Supplementary Materials).

2.4. Cellular Assays

2.4.1. Cell Lines and Culture

The HT-29 and SH-SY5Y cell lines were obtained from ATCC. The human colon cancer HT-29 cell line was cultured at 37 °C and 5% CO_2 in McCoy's 5a Medium Modified supplemented with 10% fetal bovine serum, 100 U/mL penicillin G, and 100 µg/mL streptomycin. Cells were maintained in the logarithmic growth phase and the medium was changed every 3 days. Cells were trypsinized with 0.25% trypsin-EDTA and subcultured in the same medium. SH-SY5Y human neuroblastoma cells were cultured in Dulbecco's modified Eagle medium (DMEM), supplemented with 100 U/mL penicillin/100 µg/mL streptomycin, and 10% heat-inactivated fetal bovine serum (FBS), incubated at 37 °C in a humidified atmosphere of 95% air and 5% CO_2. For cell culture maintenance, cells were subcultured once a week and the cell medium was renewed every 2 days. Both the human prostate (PC-3) and the breast (MCF-7) cancer cell lines were cultured in DMEM supplemented with 10% fetal bovine serum (FBS) and 1% antibiotics/antimycotics (complete medium), and they were incubated in a 5% CO_2 incubator at 37 °C.

2.4.2. Cell Treatment

Before each treatment, HT-29, SH-SY5Y, PC-3, and MCF-7 cells were seeded in 96-well plates in triplicate with the following densities: 5000 cells/well for PC-3 and MCF-7, 15,000 cells/well for HT-29, and 20,000 cells/well for SH-SY5Y. For assays involving HT-29 and SH-SY5Y lines, cells were treated with OH-, Cl-, and Br-Cla (in DMSO) at 0.01, 0.1, 1, 10, 20, 30, 50, 75, or 100 µM for 48 h. During the experimental period, cells were maintained at 37 °C with 5% CO_2. Controls were composed of DMSO 0.1% v/v. Cells were exposed to the different treatments for 48h. For assays involving PC-3 and MCF-7 lines, cells were treated with Br-Cla at 0.1, 1, 10, 25, 50, and 75 µM (in methanol) for 72 h [13]. The control was methanol at a maximum final concentration of 0.1% v/v. The half-maximal inhibitory concentration (IC_{50}) value was determined for the different assays by MTT viability assay.

2.4.3. MTT Cytotoxicity Assays

After cell treatment with the Cla derivatives, mitochondrial function was evaluated since mitochondrial dehydrogenases of living cells can reduce the MTT (yellow) to formazans, which are purple compounds. At the end of incubation, the cell medium was removed and 100 µL of MTT solution (0.5 mg/mL in PBS) was added to each well. Cells were then incubated for 3 h, protected from light. After this period, the MTT solution was removed, and DMSO (100 µL/well) was added to solubilize the formazan crystals. Absorbance was measured at 570 nm using an automated microplate reader (Tecan Infinite M200, Tecan Group Ltd., Männedorf, Switzerland). All conditions were performed in triplicate.

2.4.4. Data Analysis and Statistical Analysis

GraphPad Prism 8 (GraphPad Software Inc., San Diego, CA, USA) was used to produce concentration-response curves by nonlinear regression analysis. MTT results are presented as the mean ± SEM for n experiments performed. All data were assessed in three independent experiences. Statistical comparisons between control and treatment groups were performed with one-way ANOVA test. Statistical significance was accepted at a p-value < 0.05.

2.4.5. Cell Morphology

Cell morphology was assessed on a Leica DMI 6000B microscope equipped with a Leica DFC350 FX camera and then analyzed with the Leica LAS X imaging software v3.7.4 (Leica Microsystems, Wetzlar, Germany).

3. Results and Discussion

3.1. In Silico Characterization of R-Cla Derivatives

It is important to verify if all the proposed R-Cla derivatives have an intrinsically available pathway for T_1 chemiexcitation during their chemiluminescent reaction, which can be enhanced by the heavy-atom effect, before their synthesis and characterization. Thus, we calculated the potential energy curves for both the S_0 and T_1 states during the thermolysis of OH-Cla (Scheme 1 and Figure 1), with a density functional theory (DFT) approach [11,17]. Similar calculations were previously performed for Br-Cla dioxetanone [12] (Figure 1). Therefore, OH-Cla dioxetanone was chosen to be studied as a reference, since OH-Cla and Br-Cla are on opposite sides regarding the expected enhancement of ISC rate due to the heavy-atom effect.

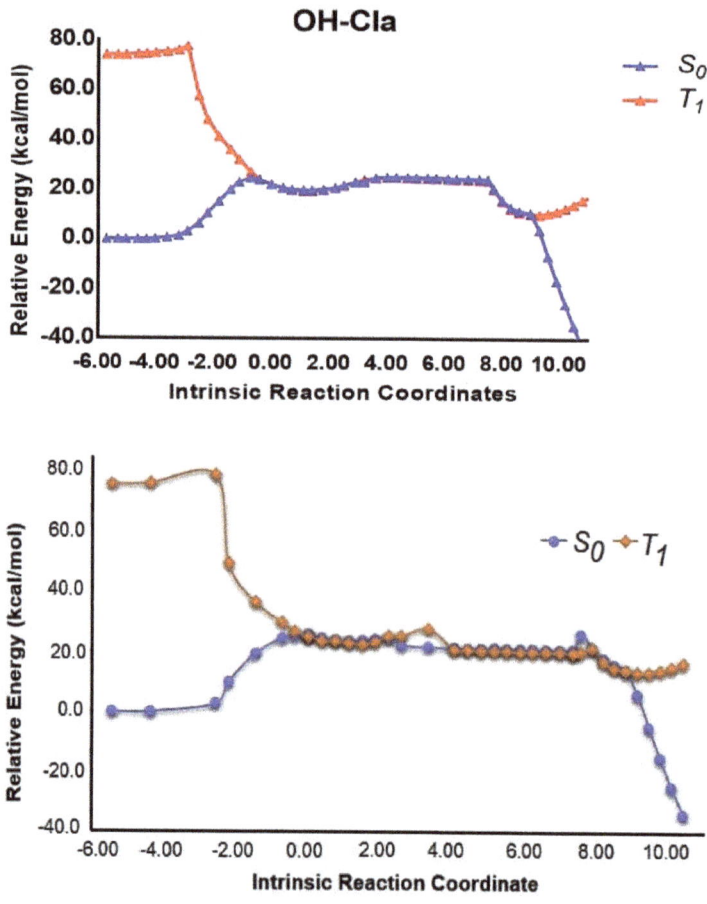

Figure 1. Potential energy curves (in kcal·mol^{-1}) for the S_0 and T_1 states during the thermolysis of OH-Cla (top) and Br-Cla dioxetanones (bottom), as a function of intrinsic reaction coordinates (in amu$^{1/2}$ bohr). Calculations were made with the ωB97XD density functional in implicit water. The bottom figure is reprinted with permission from [12]. Copyright Elsevier 2019.

As consistent with previous reports for different dioxetanones (including Br-Cla) [6,9,11,12,17], the S_0 thermolysis of OH-Cla dioxetanone proceeds via a stepwise biradical mechanism that involves the cleavage of two bonds of the peroxide ring: first by the breaking of the O-O bond, followed by C-C bond cleavage. The S_0 activation energy for the thermolysis reaction of OH-Cla dioxetanone is 24.7 kcal·mol^{-1}, only 0.8 kcal·mol^{-1} lower than that of Br-Cla (25.5 kcal mol^{-1}) [12]. The interplay between S_0 and T_1 states during the thermolysis reaction (Figure 1) is more important. While, for both dioxetanones, the $S_0 - T_1$ energy gap is significant at the beginning of the reaction (~75 kcal·mol^{-1}), when reaching the TS and onward, both states become degenerated in a large and flat region of the potential energy surface (PES).

This indicates that both chemiluminescent reactions possess an intrinsic pathway for T_1 chemiexcitation, in line with previous studies for this type of system [9,11,12,18]. However, as ISC is a spin-forbidden process, the $S_0 \to T_1$ chemiexcitation pathway for OH-Cla is not expected to be efficient [19]. Given the identical energetic profiles found for OH-Cla and Br-Cla (Figure 1), the addition of halogen atoms of increasing size in Cl-Cla and Br-Cla should only enhance the rate of the ISC process, due to the heavy-atom effect.

Thus, this substitution appears to be ideal to assess solely the heavy-atom effect on the possible anticancer activity of these molecules.

It should be noted that an efficient ISC is not the only parameter determining the performance of a photosensitizer in singlet oxygen generation, as it should also have a T_1 state with an energy higher than 0.98 eV (the required energy to convert molecular oxygen into singlet oxygen) [20]. We modeled the adiabatic $S_0 - T_1$ energy gap of OH-Cla coelenteramide and found a value of 2.78 eV. Furthermore, this value is identical to what was found by us previously for Br-Cla [12]. Thus, both OH-Cla and Br-Cla compounds possess enough energy to generate singlet oxygen. It should be noted that this value was obtained with the M06-2X functional and the 6-31 + G (d,p) basis set, in implicit water, using the SMD model. This approach was used to ensure consistency between studies, as this was the approach used before to calculate the $S_0 - T_1$ energy gap of Br-Cla coelenteramide [12].

3.2. Synthesis of Cla Derivatives

Given that the in silico modeling results indicate that the chemiluminescent reactions of these Cla derivatives present intrinsic pathways for light-free generation of triplet states capable of sensitizing singlet oxygen, we then proceeded to the synthesis of OH-Cla, Cl-Cla, and Br-Cla (Scheme S1). The introduction of heteroatoms with increasing size should enhance the ISC rate due to the heavy-atom effect, thereby allowing us to obtain model molecules with different efficiencies of triplet state generation.

The structures of these compounds were confirmed with ^{1}H-NMR spectroscopy (Figures S1–S4) and HR-MS spectrometry (Figures S5–S8) [12]. Complementary analyses by FT-IR spectroscopy showed that the compounds share an intense band in the N-H/C-H stretching region, compatible with highly conjugated heteroaromatics, as well as several bands in the C=C/C=N/C=O bending region. For OH-Cla, minor differences (attributable to the OH moiety) can be observed in the stretching region (Figures S9–S11). HPLC-DAD further confirmed the high purity of these compounds (Figures S12–S14). Analysis by UV-Vis spectroscopy (Figures S15–S17) revealed quite similar absorbance spectra for all compounds, with three bands at ~280 nm, ~350 nm, and ~450 nm. The similarity is expected given that all derivatives present identical molecular structures. Nevertheless, an interesting substitution-related trend was observed, as the relative intensity of the band at ~450 nm (in comparison with the one at ~350 nm) decreased in a relevant manner in the following order: OH > Cl > Br (Figures S15–S17).

3.3. Luminometric and Photophysical Characterization

After synthesizing the target derivatives and completing their structural characterization, it is essential to perform their luminometric and photophysical characterization. Specifically, before assessing the potential role of the heavy-atom effect in the anticancer properties of these compounds, it is required to find out if the introduction of heteroatoms of increasing size enhances the T_1 chemiexcitation of these compounds. Thus, we subjected these compounds to a detailed luminometric and photophysical characterization.

First, we measured the chemiluminescent output of the three Cla derivatives in an aprotic solvent (DMF) with addition of buffer (acetate buffer, pH 5.14), conditions in which Clz and derivates are known to readily generate chemiluminescence by reacting with dissolved oxygen [17]. All compounds emitted chemiluminescence (Figure 2a and Figure S18) with the typical kinetic profile, with a quick rise in light emission on the millisecond timescale and subsequent decay to basal levels (all within 600 ms). Interestingly, there is a clear halogen substitution effect in which the light emitted by Cl- and Br-Cla is significantly lower than that emitted by OH-Cla. Furthermore, among halogenated compounds, the light output decreases in the order of OH > Cl > Br. In solution, triplet states are generally more easily quenched than singlet excited states, thereby not leading to light emission in solution at room temperature. Thus, the quite lower light output of halogenated Cla compounds is indicative of the halogen's ability to enhance ISC during dioxetanone's thermolysis, by increasing the triplet-to-singlet product ratio of the studied chemiluminescent reactions [19,21].

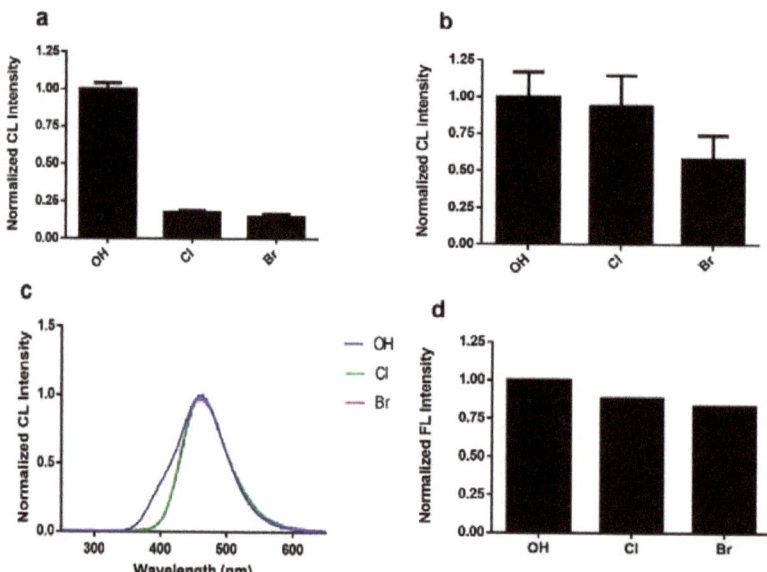

Figure 2. (**a**) Normalized chemiluminescence output of OH-, Cl-, and Br-Cla in DMF-acetate buffer pH 5.14 (0.68%). (**b**) Chemiluminescence intensity of OH-, Cl-, and Br-Cla in the presence of 20 mg of KO_2 in methanol. (**c**) Normalized chemiluminescence spectra of OH-, Cl-, and Br-Cla in DMF-acetate buffer pH 5.14 (0.68%). (**d**) Normalized fluorescence intensity of spent chemiluminescent reactions of OH-, Cl-, and Br-Cla coelenteramide after 30 min of reaction.

One other possible explanation for these variations in intensity could be that the introduction of the halogen atoms decreased the energetic favorability of the S_0 reaction. However, in our previous study of Br-Cla [12], we already found that bromination does not impede the reaction, as it is still highly exothermic (-97.1 kcal·mol^{-1}). Furthermore, the S_0 energetics for the thermolysis of OH-Cla and Br-Cla dioxetanones are identical (Figure 1), which means that halogenation should not affect the efficiency of the S_0 chemiluminescent reaction.

Further support for this conclusion was obtained by analyzing the chemiluminescent kinetic profiles of these compounds (Figure S18). There were no significant differences between compounds, with the kinetic profiles showing identical rises and subsequent decay of light emission in the same timeframe, showing that halogenation does not affect the kinetics of the reaction. The steady-state chemiluminescent spectra (measured during the chemiluminescent reaction in a spectrofluorometer, without the use of an excitation source) were identical for all R-Cla compounds (Figure 2c), with emission maxima at ~480 nm. Lastly, we also measured the 2D excitation-emission matrices (EEMs) for the spent reaction mixtures (30 min after addition to aprotic solvents) of the three compounds (Figure 3). The resulting EEMs were quite similar to each other, with just one emissive center with an excitation wavelength maximum at ~280 nm. The main difference is only a small blue-shift of ~25 nm in the emission maxima between OH-Cla (~425 nm) and Cl-/Br-Cla (~400 nm). Given this high similarity between EEMs for the spent reaction mixtures, we can conclude that halogenation does not affect the outcome of the chemiluminescent reaction in terms of obtained products.

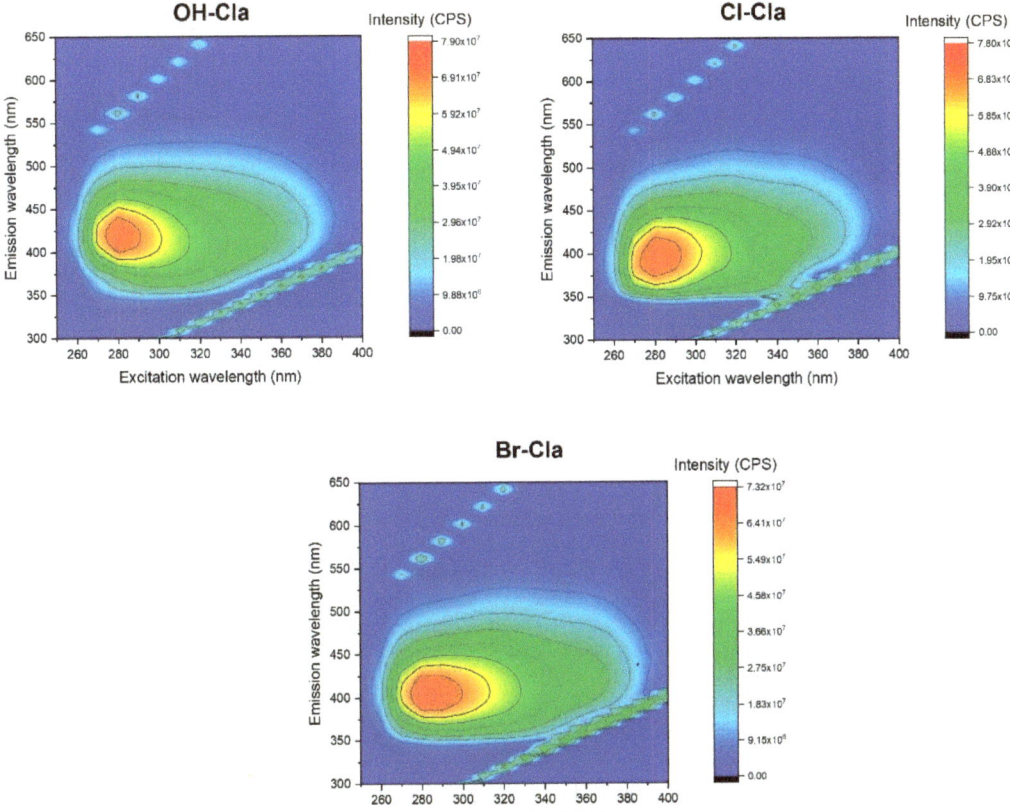

Figure 3. The 2D excitation-emission matrices (EEMs) of spent chemiluminescent reactions of OH-, Cl-, and Br-Cla after 30 min of reaction in DMSO-acetate buffer pH 5.14 (0.68%) solution.

Lastly, a possible explanation for the lower light output, other than the increase in T_1 chemiexcitation, could be that halogenation decreases the singlet emission efficiency of the resulting chemiluminophore (coelenteramide). To verify this hypothesis, we also measured the fluorescence intensity of the spent reaction mixtures (after 30 min of reaction) in an aprotic solvent (Figures 2d and 3). There is indeed a small decrease in emission intensity of the reaction product that correlates with halogen substitution. However, for one, this decrease is significantly lower than that found for the chemiluminescent output (Figure 2a). Furthermore, given that the decrease in emission intensity occurs in the order of OH > Cl > Br, this also indicates a heavy-atom effect. More specifically, this observation is consistent with fluorescence quenching due to ISC enhancement, during the photo-excitation process. Thus, these results also support the conclusion that the decrease in chemiluminescent light output is due to the heavy-atom effect, which enhances the T_1 chemiexcitation and increases the resulting triplet-to-singlet product ratio.

Having demonstrated that the addition of halogens enhances the production of triplet states, it is also important to assess the ability of the superoxide anion to trigger the chemiluminescent reaction of the studied molecules. This type of ROS is overexpressed in cancer cells [22,23]; thus, it could be thought of as a cancer marker inducing chemiluminescence and a tumor-selectivity profile to our molecules. It should be noted that we previously demonstrated our compounds as having selectivity for breast cancer, as Br-Cla induced significant toxicity toward breast cancer cell lines without affecting non-cancer cell lines in the same concentration range [12].

The ability of superoxide anions to trigger the chemiluminescent reaction of these compounds was demonstrated by measuring their chemiluminescent output, after KO_2 addition (a known superoxide anion source) in methanol. Interestingly, all compounds responded to the addition of KO_2 with immediate emission of light and subsequent decay to basal levels (Figure S19). The kinetics of this reaction is significantly quicker than in aprotic solvents, but this difference can be attributed to the instability of KO_2 in solution. The more relevant result is that all compounds responded similarly to superoxide anion, meaning that they can be activated by a cancer marker. It should also be pointed out that the measured chemiluminescent output showed a substitution-induced effect, in the order OH > Cl > Br (Figure 2b). Once again, this points to halogen substitution increasing the triplet-to-singlet ratio.

3.4. In Vitro Cytotoxic Activity of R-Cla

The next step of this study was the evaluation of the in vitro anticancer activity of these compounds. Both the in silico modeling and the luminometric/photophysical characterization showed that the introduction of halogens enhances the superoxide anion-triggered generation of triplet states (with enough energy to sensitize singlet oxygen), without affecting the chemiluminescent reaction. Thus, if the anticancer activity found before for this type of molecules [12,13] is indeed related to a light-free and self-activating photodynamic effect, we should see a halogen-dependent effect on their anticancer activity.

Given this, the potential anticancer activity of the three R-Cla compounds was evaluated in both colon cancer (HT-29) and neuroblastoma (SH-SY5Y) cell lines with a standard MTT assay for exposure times of 48h, along with changes in cell morphology analyzed by microscopy.

OH-Cla did not have any effect on the viability of colon cancer cells (Figure 4) and did not cause any changes in their morphology (Figure 5b). This indicates that OH-Cla has no anticancer activity toward these cells, which is expected since, without the heavy-atom effect introduced by the halogens, there is no reason for efficient T_1 chemiexcitation. Interestingly, while Cl-Cla induced virtually no anticancer effect in these cells, there was a statistically significant difference at a concentration of 100 µM (Figure 4). In addition, microscopic analysis at the two highest concentrations indicated that the cells were rounder and in lesser number, without the formation of aggregates (Figure 5c). As for Br-Cla, there was a relevant decrease in cellular viability at the highest concentration (100 µM) (Figure 4), with the morphological analysis showing a clear decrease in the number of cells at the highest concentration, as well as a change in the size and shape of the cells, which were smaller and rounder (Figure 5d).

These results are interesting because the observed anticancer activity toward HT-29 cell lines was low, while we could observe a distinct halogen-dependent effect. Specifically, OH-Cla did not present any activity, while Cl-Cla and Br-Cla presented increasing activity. This is a first demonstration of the heavy-atom effect, which indicates that this anticancer activity is indeed related to a light-free and self-activating photodynamic effect.

It should also be noted that a positive control test was performed by exposing these cells to an antineoplastic drug commonly used in colon cancer therapy, 5-fluorouracil (5-FU), in the same concentration range as R-Cla (Figure S20). This drug induced a significant decrease in cell viability for all concentrations, while microscopic evaluation revealed that all cells appeared to be morphologically changed (Figure S21a–c).

In neuroblastoma cells (Figures 6 and 7), the results were similar and neither OH-Cla nor Cl-Cla altered cell viability in a relevant manner. On the contrary, Br-Cla (Figures 6 and 7d) induced a significant decrease in cell viability, although not as marked as for 5-FU (Figures S20b and S22), which was also used as a positive control for neuroblastoma cells. This compound induced a sharp decrease in cell viability. The cell viability results were consistent with microscopic evaluation (Figures 7 and S22).

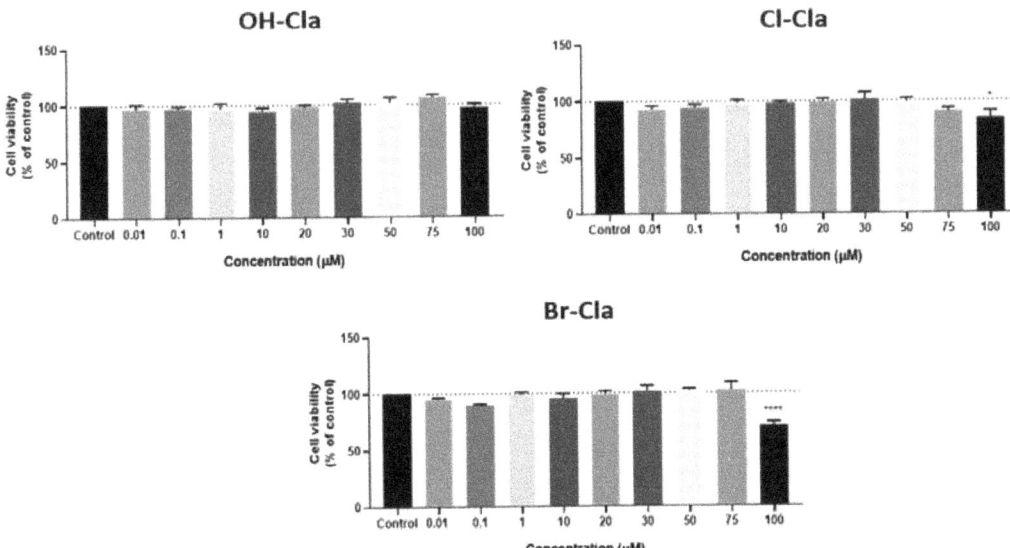

Figure 4. Effect of OH-, Cl-, and Br-Cla on HT-29 cell viability. Cells were cultured in the presence of increasing concentrations of each compound. After 48 h, an MTT assay was performed to measured cellular viability. Results are presented as mean ± SEM. * Statistically significant vs. control at $p < 0.05$; **** statistically significant vs. control at $p < 0.0001$.

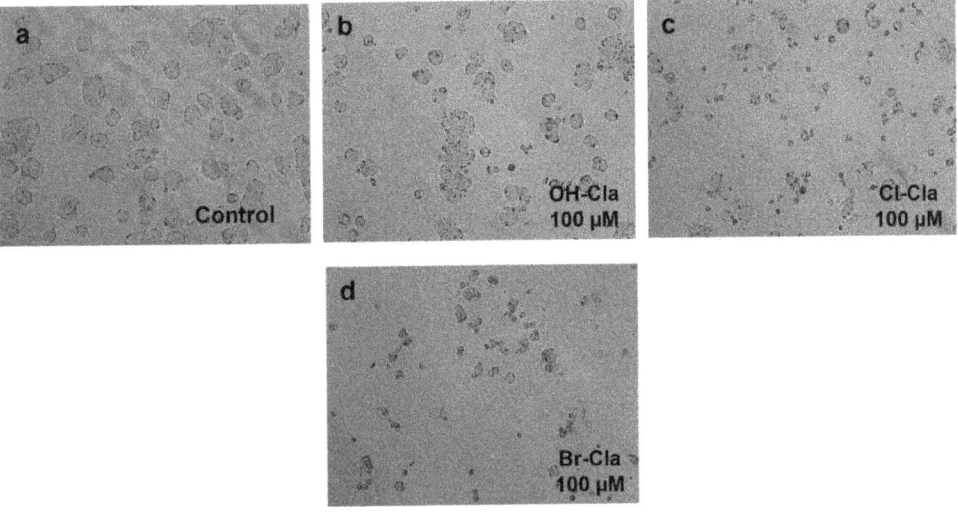

Figure 5. Microscopic cellular visualization of HT-29 cells after 48 h of incubation with cell medium and (**a**) 0.1% DMSO (control), (**b**) OH-Cla, (**c**), Cl-Cla, or (**d**) Br-Cla. Representative images were obtained with a high contrast brightfield objective (10×) (LionHeart FX Automated Microscope), from three independent experiments.

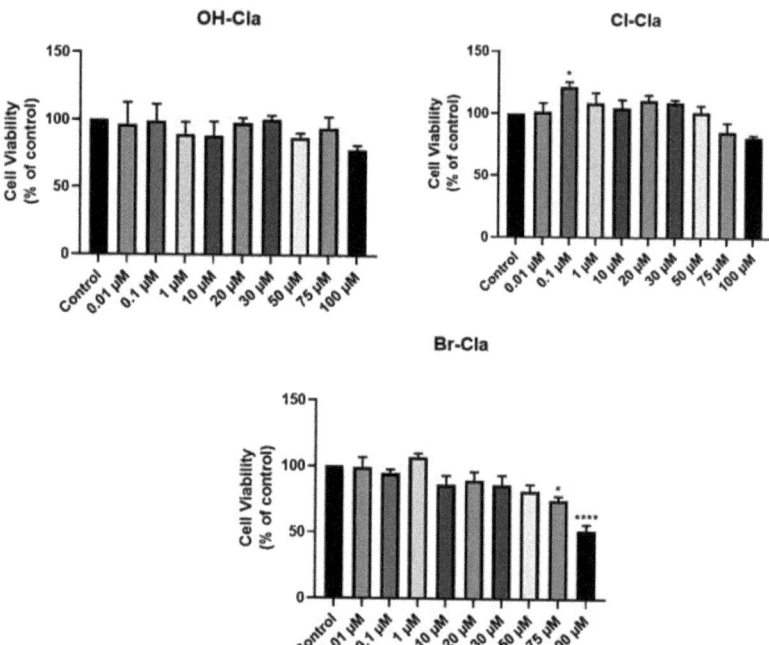

Figure 6. Effects of OH-, Cl-, and Br-Cla on SH-SY5Y cellular viability. Cells were cultivated in the presence of increasing concentrations of each compound. After 48 h, an MTT assay was performed to measured cellular viability. Results are presented as mean ± SEM. * Statistically significant vs. control at $p < 0.05$; **** statistically significant vs. control at $p < 0.0001$.

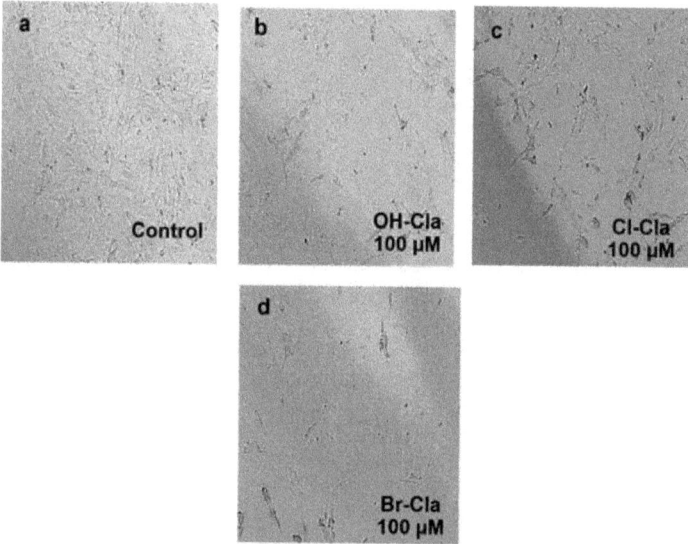

Figure 7. Microscopic cellular visualization of SH-SY5Y cells after 48 h of incubation with cell medium and (**a**) 0.1% DMSO (control), (**b**) OH-Cla, (**c**), Cl-Cla, or (**d**) Br-Cla. Representative images were obtained with a high contrast brightfield objective (10×) (LionHeart FX Automated Microscope), from three independent experiments.

Given this, it is clear that there was a halogen-dependent effect on the anticancer activity of these compounds for both cancer cell lines. This is in line with our proposition that the addition of halogens to Clzs will provide them with anticancer activity, by enhancing T_1 chemiexcitation and the subsequent intracellular generation of triplet states capable of sensitizing singlet oxygen [12,13]. In conclusion, our results indicate that the anticancer activity of our Clz derivatives [12,13] is indeed related to the heavy-atom-induced triplet state generation during their chemiluminescent reaction. Therefore, it appears that we can consider our compounds as prototypical single-molecule-photosensitizers capable of an intracellular and self-activating photodynamic effect, which is triggered by a cancer marker.

Having said that, it is also important to note that the intrinsic anticancer activity of the studied compounds (including Br-Cla) might not be as high as desired toward neuroblastoma and colon cancer cell lines, especially when compared to 5-FU. Given this, it is important to determine whether the magnitude of the obtained anticancer activity is similar across different cancer types or if it is dependent on the studied cell line.

To clarify this topic, we calculated for the first time the IC_{50} of Br-Cla for different cell lines. Br-Cla was chosen for its consistent toxicity in this study, contrary to OH-Cla and Cl-Cla. IC_{50} values were determined for neuroblastoma SH-SY5Y, prostate PC-3, and breast MCF-7 cancer cell lines (Table 1). We did not include assays with the HT-29 cancer cell line, due to the limited toxicity of Br-Cla toward it (Figure 4). We included assays with PC-3 and MCF-7 cell lines due to previous promising results of Br-Cla and other Clz derivatives toward them [12,13]. For the assays with these two cell lines, we maintained the conditions employed before for consistency purposes [13].

Table 1. IC_{50} (in µM) values for Br-Cla in neuroblastoma SH-SY5Y, prostate PC-3, and breast MCF-7 cancer cell lines. Assays were performed with either 48 (SH-SY5Y) or 72 h (PC-3 and MCF-7) [13].

Molecule	SH-SY5Y	PC-3	MCF-7
Br-Cla	50.92	24.28	21.56 (33.84) [1]

[1] The value within parentheses refers to 24 h treatment.

The impact of treatment with Br-Cla on the cellular viability of PC-3 and MCF-7 cell lines can be found in Figure 8. The anticancer activity of Br-Cla was improved in these two cell lines; in breast MCF-7 cancer cell lines, there was a noticeable decrease in cell viability from 10 µM onward, whereas, in prostate PC-3 cancer cells, Br-Cla decreased the cell viability from 25 µM onward, achieving toxicity values higher than 50% at a concentration of 75 µM. This improved efficiency was confirmed by the determined IC_{50} values (Table 1). More specifically, for SH-SY5Y, the obtained IC_{50} was more than double the values found for the other cell lines. Interestingly, the IC_{50} values found for PC-3 and MCF-7 cells were similar, although slightly lower for the latter cell line. Furthermore, to discard the hypothesis that these differences could be related to the different duration of treatment with Br-Cla, we also determined the IC_{50} for the MCF-7 cell line with 24 h treatment (Table 1). This value (33.84 µM) was found to be significantly higher than that found for 72 h treatment (21.56 µM), which indicates that increasing the incubation time increased the obtained IC_{50}. More important is that the IC_{50} found for SH-SY5Y (50.92 µM) was still significantly higher than the IC_{50} found for MCF-7, irrespective of the duration of treatment with Br-Cla.

Thus, the results indicate that it is safe to state that the magnitude of the anticancer activity of Br-Cla is dependent on the cancer cell type, being higher for prostate and breast cancer than for neuroblastoma and colon cancer. Further studies are required to assess if these differences arise from (among other possibilities) higher resistance of HT-29 and SH-SY5Y cell lines to the photodynamic effect, lower efficiency of internalization of R-Cla compounds into these cell lines, or a lower generation of superoxide anion in these cells.

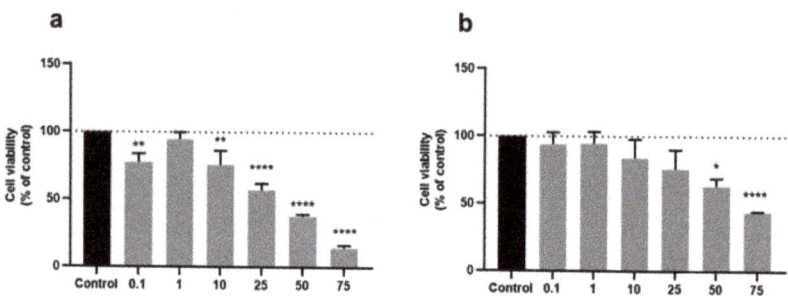

Figure 8. Relative viabilities of (**a**) MCF-7 and (**b**) PC-3 cells after 72 h incubation with several concentrations of Br-Cla, always without light irradiation. Results are presented as mean ± SEM. * Statistically significant vs. control at $p < 0.05$; ** statistically significant vs. control at $p < 0.01$; **** statistically significant vs. control at $p < 0.0001$.

4. Conclusions

In conclusion, we reported the target-oriented synthesis of three Clz derivatives (OH-Cla and its halogenated Cl- and Br- derivatives), to provide anticancer activity to this class of compounds through the heavy-atom effect. On the basis of this strategy, we developed novel compounds able to directly generate readily available triplet excited states with enough energy to sensitize singlet oxygen, in a chemiluminescent reaction triggered by a cancer marker. This was achieved by the introduction of the heavy-atom effect into this system, which enhanced the ISC rate of available $S_0 \rightarrow T_1$ chemiexcitation pathways. The anticancer activity of these compounds was evaluated toward different cancer cell lines, and a clear halogen effect was observed with Cl-Cla and Br-Cla presenting increasing toxicities. Furthermore, it was found that the magnitude of the anticancer activity of these types of compounds is dependent on the cancer cell line, being more relevant in prostate and breast cancer than in neuroblastoma and colon cancer. Thus, the results indicate that applying the heavy-atom effect to marine Clz would be a promising strategy for designing self-activating and light-free photosensitizers. With this design strategy, the Clz system appears to be a prototypical system for optimized photosensitizers to be used in PDT strategies not limited by the need for external light sources.

5. Patents

Patent PCT/IB2019/053642 (pending)—chemiluminescent imidazopyrazinone-based photosensitizers with available singlet and triplet excited states.

Supplementary Materials: The following are available online at https://www.mdpi.com/article/10.3390/biomedicines9091199/s1: Scheme S1. General synthetic procedure for the synthesis of the coelenterazine analogs; Figure S1. 1H-NMR spectrum of 2a in CDCl3; Figure S2. 1H-NMR spectrum of 2b in CDCl3; Figure S3. 1H-NMR spectrum of OH-Cla in MeOH d4; Figure S4. 1H-NMR spectrum of Cl-Cla in MeOH d4; Figure S5. ESI-MS (+) spectrum of 2a; Figure S6. ESI-MS (+) spectrum of 2b; Figure S7. HR-MS ESI (−) spectrum of OH-Cla; Figure S8. HR-MS ESI (+) spectrum of Cl-Cla; Figure S9. FT-IR spectrum of OH-Cla; Figure S10. FT-IR spectrum of Cl-Cla; Figure S11. FT-IR spectrum of Br-Cla; Figure S12. HPLC chromatogram and DAD-UV/Vis spectrum of OH-Cla; Figure S13. HPLC chromatogram and DAD-UV/Vis spectrum of Cl-Cla; Figure S14. HPLC chromatogram and DAD-UV/Vis spectrum of Br-Cla; Figure S15. Absorbance spectra of OH-Cla in MeOH:CH3CN (1:1) and CH3CN:water:formic acid (3:2:0.1); Figure S16. Absorbance spectra of Cl-Cla in MeOH:CH3CN (1:1) and CH3CN:water:formic acid (3:2:0.1); Figure S17. Absorbance spectra of Br-Cla in MeOH:CH3CN (1:1) and CH3CN:water:formic acid (3:2:0.1); Figure S18. Normalized chemiluminescence profiles of OH-, Cl-, and Br-Cla in DMF-acetate buffer pH 5.14 (0.68%); Figure S19. Normalized chemiluminescence profiles of OH-, Cl-, and Br-Cla in the presence of 15 mg of KO_2 in methanol; Figure S20. Cellular viability assays of HT-29 (a) and SH-SY5Y (b) cells after 48 h of incubation with 5-FU; Figure S21. Microscopic cellular visualization of HT-29 cells after 48 h of incubation with 5-FU at (a) 0.01 µM, (b) 20 µM, and (c) 100 µM; Figure S22. Microscopic cellular visualization of SH-SY5Y cells after 48 h of incubation with 5-FU at (a) 10 µM and (b) 100 µM.

Author Contributions: Conceptualization, L.P.d.S.; investigation, C.M.M., P.G.-B., D.D., A.S.C. and L.P.d.S.; writing—original draft preparation, C.M.M., P.G.-B. and L.P.d.S.; writing—review and editing, L.P.d.S., N.V., J.E.R.-B. and J.C.G.E.d.S.; supervision, L.P.d.S. and N.V.; funding acquisition, L.P.d.S. and N.V. All authors have read and agreed to the published version of the manuscript.

Funding: The Portuguese "Fundação para a Ciência e Tecnologia" (FCT) is acknowledged for funding the project PTDC/QUI-QFI/2870/2020, the framework in which this work was conducted. FCT is also acknowledged for funding this research within the following R&D Units: CIQUP (project UIDB/00081/2020), GreenUPorto (project UIDB/05748/2020), CINTESIS (project UIDB/4255/2020), and LAQV/REQUIMTE (UIDB/50006/2020). L. Pinto da Silva acknowledges funding from FCT under the Scientific Employment Stimulus (CEECIND/01425/2017). Nuno Vale thanks FCT for supporting these studies in the framework of project IF/00092/2014/CP1255/CT0004. Patricia González-Berdullas acknowledges funding for her postdoctoral position, in the framework of project PTDC/QUI-QFI/2870/2020. Carla Magalhães acknowledges FCT for her PhD grant (SFRH/BD/143211/2019). Diana Duarte acknowledges FCT for funding her PhD grant (SFRH/BD/140734/2018). Ana Correia acknowledges FCT for funding her PhD grant (SFRH/BD/146093/2019).

Acknowledgments: The Laboratory of Computational Modeling of Environmental Pollutant-Human Interactions (LACOMEPHI) and the Materials Centre of the University of Porto (CEMUP) are acknowledged.

Conflicts of Interest: The authors declare no conflict of interest.

References

1. Li, Y.; Wang, C.; Zhou, L.; Wei, S. A 2-pyridone modified zinc phthalocyanine with three-in-one multiple functions for photodynamic therapy. *Chem. Commun.* **2021**, *57*, 3127–3130. [CrossRef]
2. Li, X.; Shi, Z.; Wu, J.; Wu, J.; He, C.; Hao, X.; Duan, C. Lighting up metallohelices: From DNA binders to chemotherapy and photodynamic therapy. *Chem. Commun.* **2020**, *56*, 7537–7548. [CrossRef]
3. Xiao, Y.-F.; Chen, J.-X.; Chen, W.-C.; Zheng, X.; Cao, C.; Tan, J.; Cui, X.; Yuan, Z.; Ji, S.; Lu, G.; et al. Achieving high singlet-oxygen generation by applying the heavy-atom effect to thermally activated delayed fluorescent materials. *Chem. Commun.* **2021**, *57*, 4902–4905. [CrossRef]
4. Fan, W.; Huang, P.; Chen, X. Overcoming the Achilles' heel of photodynamic therapy. *Chem. Soc. Rev.* **2016**, *45*, 6488–6519. [CrossRef]
5. Yano, S.; Hirohara, S.; Obata, M.; Hagiya, Y.; Ogura, S.-I.; Ikeda, A.; Kataoka, H.; Tanaka, M.; Joh, T. Current states and future views in photodynamic therapy. *J. Photochem. Photobiol. C Photochem. Rev.* **2011**, *12*, 46–67. [CrossRef]
6. Magalhães, C.M.; Esteves da Silva, J.C.G.; Pinto da Silva, L. Chemiluminescence and Bioluminescence as an Excitation Source in the Photodynamic Therapy of Cancer: A Critical Review. *ChemPhysChem* **2016**, *17*, 2286–2294. [CrossRef] [PubMed]
7. Jiang, T.; Du, L.; Li, M. Lighting up bioluminescence with coelenterazine: Strategies and applications. *Photochem. Photobiol. Sci.* **2016**, *15*, 466–480. [CrossRef]
8. Bronsart, L.L.; Stokes, C.; Contag, C.H. Multimodality Imaging of Cancer Superoxide Anion Using the Small Molecule Coelenterazine. *Mol. Imaging Biol.* **2016**, *18*, 166–171. [CrossRef] [PubMed]
9. Pinto da Silva, L.; Magalhaes, C.M.; Esteves da Silva, J.C.G. Interstate Crossing-Induced Chemiexcitation Mechanism as the Basis for Imidazopyrazinone Bioluminescence. *ChemistrySelect* **2016**, *1*, 3343–3356. [CrossRef]
10. Kaskova, Z.M.; Tsarkova, A.S.; Yampolsky, I.V. 1001 lights: Luciferins, luciferases, their mechanisms of action and applications in chemical analysis, biology and medicine. *Chem. Soc. Rev.* **2016**, *45*, 6048–6077. [CrossRef]
11. Magalhães, C.M.; Esteves da Silva, J.C.G.; Pinto da Silva, L. Study of coelenterazine luminescence: Electrostatic interactions as the controlling factor for efficient chemiexcitation. *J. Lumin.* **2018**, *199*, 339–347. [CrossRef]
12. Pinto da Silva, L.; Núñez-Montenegro, A.; Magalhães, C.M.; Ferreira, P.J.O.; Duarte, D.; González-Berdullas, P.; Rodríguez-Borges, J.E.; Vale, N.; Esteves da Silva, J.C.G. Single-molecule chemiluminescent photosensitizer for a self-activating and tumor-selective photodynamic therapy of cancer. *Eur. J. Med. Chem.* **2019**, *183*, 111683. [CrossRef]
13. Pinto da Silva, L.; Magalhães, C.M.; Núñez-Montenegro, A.; Ferreira, P.J.O.; Duarte, D.; Rodríguez-Borges, J.E.; Vale, N.; Esteves da Silva, J.C.G. Study of the Combination of Self-Activating Photodynamic Therapy and Chemotherapy for Cancer Treatment. *Biomolecules* **2019**, *9*, 384. [CrossRef]
14. Chai, J.D.; Head-Gordon, M. Long-range corrected hybrid density functionals with damped atom-atom dispersion corrections. *Phys. Chem. Chem. Phys.* **2008**, *10*, 6615–6620. [CrossRef] [PubMed]
15. Adamo, C.; Jacquemin, D. The calculations of excited-state properties with time-dependent density functional theory. *Chem. Soc. Rev.* **2013**, *42*, 845–856. [CrossRef] [PubMed]
16. Frisch, M.J.; Trucks, G.W.; Schlegel, H.B.; Scuseria, G.E.; Robb, M.A.; Cheeseman, J.R.; Scalmani, G.; Barone, V.; Petersson, G.A.; Nakatsuji, H.; et al. *Gaussian 09, Revision D.01*; Gaussian, Inc.: Wallingford, CT, USA, 2016.

17. Magalhães, C.M.; Esteves da Silva, J.C.G.; Pinto da Silva, L. Comparative study of the chemiluminescence of coelenterazine, coelenterazine-e and Cypridina luciferin with an experimental and theoretical approach. *J. Photochem. Photobiol. B Biol.* **2019**, *190*, 21–31. [CrossRef] [PubMed]
18. Pinto da Silva, L.; Magalhães, C.M. Mechanistic insights into the efficient intramolecular chemiexcitation of dioxetanones from TD-DFT and multireference calculations. *Int. J. Quantum Chem.* **2018**, *119*, e25881. [CrossRef]
19. Vacher, M.; Fdez Galván, I.; Ding, B.W.; Schramm, S.; Berraud-Pache, R.; Naumov, P.; Ferré, N.; Liu, Y.J.; Navizet, I.; Roca-Sanjuán, D.; et al. Chemi- and Bioluminescence of Cyclic Peroxides. *Chem. Rev.* **2018**, *118*, 6927–6974. [CrossRef] [PubMed]
20. Schweitzer, C.; Schmidt, R. Physical mechanisms of generation and deactivation of singlet oxygen. *Chem. Rev.* **2003**, *103*, 1685–1757. [CrossRef]
21. Adam, W.; Baader, W.J. Effects of Methylation on the Thermal Stability and Chemiluminescence Properties of 1,2-Dioxetanes. *J. Am. Chem. Soc.* **1985**, *107*, 410–416. [CrossRef]
22. Dakubo, G.D. Mitochondrial reactive oxygen species and cancer. In *Handbook of Free Radicals: Formation, Types and Effects*; Kozyrev, D., Slutsky, V., Eds.; Nova Science Pub. Inc.: Hauppauge, NY, USA, 2010; pp. 99–116.
23. Figueira, T.R.; Barros, M.H.; Camargo, A.A.; Castilho, R.F.; Ferreira, J.C.B.; Kowaltowski, A.J.; Sluse, F.E.; Souza-Pinto, N.C.; Vercesi, A.E. Mitochondria as a Source of Reactive Oxygen and Nitrogen Species: From Molecular Mechanisms to Human Health. *Antioxid. Redox Signal.* **2013**, *18*, 2029–2074. [CrossRef] [PubMed]

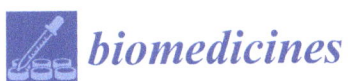

Article

Amphiphilic Protoporphyrin IX Derivatives as New Photosensitizing Agents for the Improvement of Photodynamic Therapy

Stéphane Desgranges [1], Petras Juzenas [2], Vlada Vasovic [2], Odrun Arna Gederaas [3], Mikael Lindgren [3], Trond Warloe [2], Qian Peng [2,4,*] and Christiane Contino-Pépin [1,*]

1. Equipe Chimie Bioorganique et Systèmes Amphiphiles, Avignon Université, 84000 Avignon, France; stephane.desgranges@univ-avignon.fr
2. Department of Pathology, Oslo University Hospital, 0379 Oslo, Norway; petras.juzenas@rr-research.no (P.J.); vlada.vasovic@rr-research.no (V.V.); trond.warloe@gmail.com (T.W.)
3. Department of Physics, Faculty of Natural Sciences, Norwegian University of Science and Technology, 7491 Trondheim, Norway; odrun.gederaas@ntnu.no (O.A.G.); mikael.lindgren@ntnu.no (M.L.)
4. Department of Optical Science and Engineering, School of Information Science and Technology, Fudan University, Shanghai 200433, China
* Correspondence: qian.peng@rr-research.no (Q.P.); christine.pepin@univ-avignon.fr (C.C.-P.)

Abstract: Photodynamic therapy (PDT) is a non-invasive therapeutic modality based on the interaction between a photosensitive molecule called photosensitizer (PS) and visible light irradiation in the presence of oxygen molecule. Protoporphyrin IX (PpIX), an efficient and widely used PS, is hampered in clinical PDT by its poor water-solubility and tendency to self-aggregate. These features are strongly related to the PS hydrophilic–lipophilic balance. In order to improve the chemical properties of PpIX, a series of amphiphilic PpIX derivatives endowed with PEG_{550} headgroups and hydrogenated or fluorinated tails was synthetized. Hydrophilic–lipophilic balance (HLB) and log *p*-values were computed for all of the prepared compounds. Their photochemical properties (spectroscopic characterization, photobleaching, and singlet oxygen quantum yield) were also evaluated followed by the in vitro studies of their cellular uptake, subcellular localization, and photocytotoxicity on three tumor cell lines (4T1, scc-U8, and WiDr cell lines). The results confirm the therapeutic potency of these new PpIX derivatives. Indeed, while all of the derivatives were perfectly water soluble, some of them exhibited an improved photodynamic effect compared to the parent PpIX.

Keywords: photodynamic therapy; protoporphyrin IX; amphiphiles; photochemical properties; photocytotoxicity

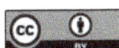

1. Introduction

Photodynamic therapy (PDT) is an emerging relatively non-invasive clinical modality, which is increasingly used to treat malignant or non-malignant diseases [1–3]. PDT combines two individually non-toxic components of a photosensitive molecule called "photosensitizer" (PS) and light, that can induce tissue damage in the presence of molecular oxygen [4]. PDT requires light with appropriate wavelengths of 600–800 nm (absorbed by the photosensitizer) that undergoes an inter-crossing system from the excited singlet state to the excited triplet state [5]. This PS excited triplet state can exchange an electron or a hydrogen atom with a neighboring substrate, such as cell membrane or organic molecule (Type I photochemical reaction) or transfer energy to ground state molecular oxygen (Type II photochemical reaction). The type I reaction leads to dangerous reactive oxygen species (ROS), among which are superoxide anion radical, hydrogen peroxide, and hydroxyl radical. While the type II photochemical reaction generates the singlet molecular oxygen ($^1O_2$), which is a highly reactive form of oxygen that reacts with many biomolecules including lipids, proteins, and nucleic acids [6]. Both types of photochemical reactions can occur simultaneously in a ratio depending on the type of PS used, as well as the concentration of organic substrate or oxygen molecule. However, most of the PSs (especially porphyrins) are believed to induce cellular damages through a type II mechanism [2].

Since $^1O_2$ and ROS can only diffuse less than 20 nm within their lifetimes of 10–300 ns in cells [7,8], only the molecules that are proximal to $^1O_2$ and ROS, thus to the subcellular location of the PS, are directly damaged by PDT. Lipophilic PSs, essentially accumulating in lipid bilayers of membrane structures including mitochondria and endoplasmic reticulum, often cause the cell death towards apoptosis. Alternatively, hydrophilic PSs localized largely in endosomes and lysosomes, have been shown to mainly induce necrosis [9–11]. The majority of efficient PSs are hydrophobic, which limits their bioavailability and hampers their systemic administration in vivo with a long retention time in normal tissues of biological systems. For example, a skin accumulation of the FDA approved Photofrin is observed, which constrains patients to avoid sunlight exposure for a prolonged period (up to 2 months) after the PDT treatment. Moreover, hydrophobic PSs tend to aggregate in physiological fluids, which decreases their $^1O_2$ quantum yield [12]. Other ways to reach deeper organs may be through the use of X-rays [13] and harder ionizing irradiation [14].

The effectiveness of PDT depends on the appropriate combination of several factors, such as the nature of the PS, its pharmacokinetics and tumor localization, photoirradiation parameters (wavelength of irradiation, fluence rate) as well as oxygen availability. The prerequisites for an optimal PS include chemical purity, high $^1O_2$ quantum yield, selectivity for targeted tissue and rapid accumulation after administration, activation at wavelengths with optimal tissue penetration (near infrared photons are ideally suited for PS activation since they can penetrate deeply in biological tissues), and rapid clearance from the body [15,16].

To date, most of the PS improvements have focused on their purity profile or on photophysical properties, such as the extension of their wavelength absorption towards the near infrared (NIR) region, enhancement of their excitation coefficient or photochemical yield [15,17]. However, a few groups have dedicated their work to improve their biological properties and particularly their bioavailability [18], through water solubility, better cellular uptake, and devoid of aggregation property [19,20].

Several studies have shown that amphiphilic compounds [15] favor the tumor accumulation, probably due to their dual character, that allows for water solubilization. Therefore, this favors the tissue distribution as well as the capacity to interact with the cell membrane to increase their cellular uptake [21–23]. Moreover, depending on their self-assembling properties, amphiphilic PSs can minimally aggregate intracellularly or disaggregate upon entering the cell, thereby maximizing $^1O_2$ production upon photoirradiation. Among the new generation of PSs we focused on protoporphyrin IX (PpIX) [24], a heme precursor which can be endogenously generated from 5-aminolevulinic acid (ALA). PpIX is a widely used PS exhibiting no dark toxicity and a high triplet state lifetime [25,26]. However, due to its hydrophobic porphyrin skeleton, it is poorly soluble in water and its PDT efficiency suffers from a tendency to form aggregates in vivo [3].

The porphyrin macrocycle itself constitutes an interesting scaffold to design Gemini surfactants with a symmetrical structure [27] that may ensure appropriate lipid-like properties [28,29]. In this study, we have synthetized a series of amphiphilic PpIX derivatives with a variable hydrophilic–lipophilic balance (HLB). In order to perform a well exemplified structure–activity relationship study, various hydrogenated or fluorinated hydrophobic tails of different lengths were conjugated to polyethylene glycol (PEG) hydrophilic moieties on the opposite side of the macrocycle core. The photophysical properties (spectroscopic characterization, photobleaching, and $^1O_2$ quantum yield) of these new amphiphilic PpIX derivatives were evaluated. In addition, their dark toxicity, cellular uptake, subcellular localization, and photocytotoxicity on three different tumor cell lines were studied in vitro and compared to those of the parent PpIX.

2. Materials and Methods

2.1. Chemistry

2.1.1. Chemicals and Reagents

For synthesis, protoporphyrin IX was purchased from porphyrin-systems (Frontier scientific, Halstenbek, Pineberg, Germany). In addition, fluorinated alcohol from Fluorochem (Hadfield, United Kingdom) as well as 1H,1H,2H,2H-perfluorohexanethiol and 1H,1H,2H,2H-perfluorooctanethiol were graciously provided by Atochem (Colombes, Paris, France). All of the reagents were from commercial sources and used as received.

2.1.2. Synthesis and Characterization

The synthetic route leading to PpIX derivatives is a modified procedure, which is derived from the work of Lottner et al. [26].

Briefly, PpIX reacts with a mixture of HBr in acetic acid (33%). Following the removal of HBr and acetic acid, the resulting Bromo-PpIX analogue (**2**) is dissolved in the appropriate alcohol (hydrogenated or fluorinated alcohol of variable lengths) during 16 h, which simultaneously gives the corresponding ether (addition on the two allylic units)/ester (addition on the propionic acid moieties) derivatives **3a–h**. The two ester groups are subsequently saponified with 20 eq of LiOH in a mixture of THF and water (3/1). After the acidic treatment leading to compounds **4a–h**, 1-amino-ω-methoxy-PEG$_{550}$ (compound **1**) is coupled to acid functions using DCC–HOBt as coupling reagents in DMF. Following the removal of the solvent, the final product is purified over LH20 in DCM–MeOH 1/1 to give the final amphiphilic PpIX derivatives **5a–h**. In parallel, the condensation of native PpIX with amino-PEG$_{550}$ (compound **1**), in the presence of DCC–HOBt, led to the PEG$_{550}$-conjugated PpIX (compound **6**).

The synthesis of non-PEGylated intermediates (compounds **2** and **3a–h** to **4a–h**) was confirmed by 1H and 13C-NMR coupled to HRMS analysis, and by 1H-NMR for polymeric derivatives (compounds **6** and **5a–h**) (see NMR spectra and detailed peak assignments in Supplementary Material Section).

2.2. Biological Testing

2.2.1. PDT of Tumor Cells with PpIX Derivatives

Tumor cells of the three cell lines were cultured as described above. The cells (1.5×10^4) in 100 µL of the medium were seeded in each well of 96-well plastic tissue-culture plates (Nunc, Thermo Fisher Scientific, Roskilde, Denmark) and left for 24 h for proper attachment to the substratum. Then, the cells were washed twice with PBS and incubated with the medium containing one of the PpIX derivatives, **5a–h** (amphiphilic derivatives), **6** (PEG$_{550}$-conjugated PpIX) or the parent PpIX at the concentration of 2.5 µM for 24 h prior to irradiation with a blue lamp (fluence rate: 4.88 mW/cm^2) for various exposure times. The lamp consisted of a bank of four fluorescent tubes (model 3026, Applied Photophysics, London, UK) emitting light mainly in the region of 410–500 nm with a maximum around 440 nm. The cell survivals were determined with the MTS cell proliferative assay, a method based on the cellular conversion of a tetrazolium compound by viable cells into a colored formazan product, which is soluble in a cell culture medium and can be detected by 492 nm absorbance. Twenty-four hours after light exposure, 20 µL of MTS (Promega Corporation, Madison, WI, USA) were added to each well and the absorbance of 492 nm was measured after 1-h incubation using a well plate reader (Multiskan Ex, Labsystems, Vantaa, Finland).

2.2.2. Uptake of PpIX Derivatives by Cells In Vitro

Three tumor cells lines of 4T1 murine mammary carcinoma cell line, scc-U8 human head and neck squamous cell carcinoma, and WiDr human colon adenocarcinoma were subcultured in RPMI1640 medium (Gibco, Paisley, Scotland, UK) containing 10% fetal calf serum, 100 U/mL penicillin, 100 µg/mL streptomycin, and 1% glutamine at 37 °C in 5% CO_2 humidified atmosphere. Tumor cells (9.5×10^4) in 400 µL of the medium were seeded in each well of 24-well plastic tissue-culture plates (Nunc) and left for 24 h for proper attachment to the substratum. Then, the cells were washed twice with PBS and incubated with a serum-free medium containing one of the PpIX derivatives, **5a–d, 5f** or parent PpIX at the concentration of 2.5 µM for 24 h in the dark. Thereafter, the cells were washed twice with PBS prior to their addition into a PBS solution by scraping off the cells from the substratum with a Costar cell scraper. The fluorescence of all cell suspensions was determined fluorometrically using a Perkin–Elmer LS50B spectrofluorometer. The excitation wavelength was set at 405 nm and the fluorescent emission was measured at 638 nm using a long-pass cut-off filter (530 nm) on the emission side.

2.2.3. Subcellular Localization of PpIX Derivatives In Vitro

Cells of the three tumor cell lines were grown on Petri dishes with a glass bottom (MatTek Corp., Ashland, MA, USA). Then, they were incubated with the medium containing compounds **5a** and **5b** at the concentration of 2.5 µM for 24 h in the dark. The cells had been washed twice with PBS prior to imaging of the subcellular localization patterns of the fluorescent sensitizers with an Axiovert 40CFL microscope (Carl Zeiss, Jena, Germany) using an oil immersion objective (100 × NA 1.25). A band-pass of 300–400 nm excitation filter was used to detect the PpIX derivatives with a long-pass of 630 nm emission filter.

2.3. Photochemical Properties

2.3.1. Spectroscopic Characterization and Singlet Oxygen Production of PDT Agents

For photophysical measurements, standard 1 cm UV quartz cuvettes (Hellma GmbH & Co. KG, Müllheim, Germany) were employed with Teflon caps that allow for flushing with Argon gas to remove oxygen from the solvent. Herein, THF was used as a solvent. Absorbance spectra were obtained using an U-3010 spectrophotometer (Hitachi, Japan) and the software UV solution. PTI Quantamaster 8075-22 equipped with Double Mono 300 spectrometer chambers for both excitation and emission (Horiba Scientific, Tokyo, Japan). The quantum efficiency (QE) was obtained by exciting samples in the solution (5 µM) at 425 nm and recording the emission spectrum. By dividing the integrated fluorescence signal with the absorbance at the excitation wavelength of 425 nm, one obtains the "single point" QE (Table 1).

Table 1. Octanol–water partition coefficient (log p) and hydrophilic–lipophilic balance (HLB) of porphyrins **6** and **5a–h** computed by the MarvinSketch software. Additionally, the fluorescence quantum efficiencies (QE) of the compounds in THF relative to PpIX (set to 1.0 in column for PpIX) are included (n.d. means 'not determined').

	5a	5b	5c	5d	5e	5f	5g	5h	6	PpIX
Log P	4.23	5.82	7.4	8.99	4.25	5.92	9.26	12.6	3.3	
HLB	18.75	15.28	14.83	14.41	15.34	14.81	13.89	12.14	16.13	
QE	1.2	1.4	1.1	n.d	1.2	1.1	1.1	0.9	n.d	1.0

The singlet oxygen production was demonstrated as the transient singlet oxygen luminescence (1275 nm) of THF solutions with the sample in a standard 90° configuration (excitation and emission path). A tunable OPO laser, NT 342A-SH-10-WW (Ekspla, Vilnius, Lithuania) was used for excitation. For transient recording, a PMT (R5509, Hamamatsu Photonics K.K., Shizuoka, Japan) and interference filter with maximum transmission at 1272.5 nm, as well as a long-pass filter transmitting above 780 nm, were used. An Infiniium BDSU Oscilloscope (Keysight, Santa Rosa, CA, USA) was used to collect the data. Time-gated electronics were used to control the time between laser excitation and the recording of the luminescence transient. The transients were background corrected by subtracting with a signal of the same sample, which was flushed with Argon gas for 10 min. A similar procedure to confirm the singlet oxygen production of Ruthenium complexes for PDT was recently presented in Bogoeva et al. [30].

Shortly, the singlet oxygen yield was estimated by fitting the transient singlet oxygen luminescence to the following expression:

$$I(t) = \frac{C \cdot k_{PS}}{k_{SO} - k_{PS}} \left[e^{-k_{PS}t} - e^{-k_{SO}t} \right] \quad (1)$$

where k_{SO} is the decay rate of the singlet oxygen luminescence and k_{PS} is the decay rate of the photosensitizer triplet. C is a constant proportional to the yield of excited singlet oxygen including instrumental settings, laser power, and number of absorbed PS molecules. Using a set of samples under the same experimental conditions and solvent, it can be taken as proportional to the relative singlet oxygen yield. For more details on the theory and related measurements, see, e.g., Snyder et al. [31] and more recently, Nishimura et al. [32].

The excited triplet state absorbance was measured in samples evacuated from oxygen, using an NT 342B-SH-10-WW laser (Ekspla, Vilnius, Lithuania), array detector (Applied Photophysics, Leatherhead, United Kingdom) and a Xenon flash lamp module (Model L9456-01, 5W, Hamamatsu, Japan) with BWSpec software (B&W Tek, Newark, DE, USA). Transient absorption was obtained by firing the excitation OPO laser and flashlamp using a time-gated electronic accessory for the control of triggers and detectors. Prior to the measurement, the sample was flushed with Argon gas for 10 min in order to remove the oxygen that quenched the triplet signal. The recorded spectra were background corrected by subtracting the spectrum of pure solvent. Since the fluorescence was negligible, the fluorescence emission correction was not required (for details of the set-up and the procedure of further analyzing triplet state absorption data, see Glimsdal et al.) [33].

2.3.2. Photobleaching of PpIX Derivatives, **5b** and **5c**, in WiDr Cells after Blue Light Exposure

Light Source for In Vitro Cell Experiments

For blue light exposure, the culture dishes (Ø = 6 cm, Nunc, Roskilde, Denmark) were illuminated (from below, at room temperature) using a LumiSource® blue light box (PCI Biotech AS, Oslo, Norway), consisting of four Osram tubes (18 W, peak wavelength 435 nm). The light intensity at the level of the cells was 13 mW/cm^2, measured with an Optometer UDT model 161, radiometer-photometer (united Detector Technology, Culver City, CA, USA) giving a total light dose of 3.1 J/cm^2 at the cell level during a 4 min illumination period.

Cell Culture

The cell line WiDr was cultured in RPMI 1640 medium containing 10% (v/v) FCS, L-glutamine (80 mg/L), streptomycin (100 U/mL), and grown in an atmosphere of 95% air and 5% CO$_2$ at 37 °C, subcultured approximately twice a week.

Fluorescence Measurements and Photobleaching Experiments

WiDr cells were seeded in culture dishes (2.0 × 10^6 cells per dish) and grown for 24 h before incubation with compound **5b**, **5c** or native protoporphyrin IX (2.5 µM, 24 h). Following incubation, the cells were washed three times (PBS) and blue light illuminated (in PBS) by LumiSource® (435 nm, 0–7.74 J/cm^2). The cells were detached by accutase (1 mL, 500–720 U/mL, Sigma-Aldrich, 37 °C) for 3–10 min (depending on the light dose) prior to centrifugation (1500 rpm, 5 min) and resuspension in PBS. By manual counting (Bürcher chamber, Merck, Darmstadt, Germany), a final cell concentration of 1 million/mL in PBS was prepared. The cell suspensions (2 mL) were immediately transferred to quartz cuvettes for fluorescence measurements recorded employing a PTI Quantamaster as described in 2.3.1 at Ex: 410 nm and Em: 550–780 nm. As a control, the fluorescence spectra of three different cell samples incubated with PpIX (2.5 µM, 24 h) were analyzed using Ex: 405 nm. All of the samples including the control cells ("no light" and "no photosensitizer") were protected from light by aluminum foil during the experimental set-up.

2.4. Software Employed

The software MarvinSketch (version 21.9.0, calculation module developed by ChemAxon, http://www.chemaxon.com/marvin/sketch/index.php, accessed on 13 December 2021), using the VG function based on the atomic log p increments method, was used to predict the log p-values [34]. The log p-value is a quantitative descriptor of lipophilicity or hydrophobicity. The same MarvinSketch software was also used to assess the HLB of PpIX derivatives by applying the Davies' method [35]. The latter method, with a scale from 0 to 20, is based on the chemical groups of the molecule, where 0 indicates a completely hydrophobic molecule, while 20 indicates a completely hydrophilic molecule. According to Fung, a value from 8–12 indicates an oil–water emulsifier, a value from 13–16 is typical of detergents, and a value from 15–20 indicates a hydrotropic behavior [36].

3. Results and Discussion

3.1. Synthesis and Characterization

Porphyrins belong to the tetrapyrrole family, whose chemistry, photo-properties, and supra-molecular properties are extensively reviewed [24,37]. In our effort to produce an efficient synthesis of amphiphilic PSs, PpIX was chosen as a starting material to prepare the Gemini-like analogues. Indeed, PpIX exhibits two different functions on opposite sides of the porphyrin macrocycle, namely two propionic acid moieties at positions 13 and 17 and two vinyl groups at positions 3 and 8 (Scheme 1). A non-ionic polar headgroup was grafted to the acidic functions through an amide bond, more specifically a flexible PEG chain with a number of 12 repeating ethylene glycol units (i.e., PEG$_{550}$ moiety). The PEG chain length remained constant, as it was long enough to ensure the final water solubility of the macromolecule. Hydrophobic chains of variable lengths, hydrogenated or fluorinated, were incorporated at the vinyl site to study the impact of hydrophobicity on subcellular localization and cytotoxic efficiency. Fluorinated tails were introduced to limit the detergency of the resulting amphiphilic PpIX analogues due to the dual hydrophobic and lipophobic nature of fluoroalkyl chains. The length of hydrocarbon chains varies from 4 to 10 carbons (compounds **5a–5d**), while the fluorinated tails length varies from 1 to 6 fluorinated carbons (compounds **5e–5h**). In addition, an ethylene spacer group is only located near the alcohol function to avoid synthetic issues related to the CF$_2$ electron-withdrawing effect. Moreover, as the tetrapyrrole core is hydrophobic itself, we also synthetized a PEG$_{550}$-conjugated PpIX analogue (compound **6**) bearing only two PEG$_{550}$ moieties, in order to evaluate the impact of hydrophobic tails on the photophysical properties, as well on the cellular uptake and cytotoxicity of PpIX derivatives.

The synthetic pathway was efficient and straight forward, since the final products were obtained in four steps with overall yields ranging from 32.2% to 65.3%. Our approach was to use native PpIX as a central core and to modify the propionic and vinylic groups in an orthogonal manner. The amino-PEG$_{550}$ (**1**) used in the synthesis was easily obtained in three steps from the commercially available monomethyl-PEG$_{550}$ alcohol with an overall yield of 62%. Briefly, the PEG-alcohol was converted into its mesylate derivative, which then underwent a nucleophilic substitution with NaN$_3$ to give the corresponding azido-PEG$_{550}$ derivative. The latter was reduced by LiAlH$_4$ to give the final amino-PEG$_{550}$ compound (**1**).

The vinyl groups can undergo several types of reaction, such as reduction, oxidation, substitution, elimination, electrocyclic reactions, and olefin metathesis [2,37]. The well-known hydrobromination procedure for the functionalization of porphyrin vinyl groups was applied. In addition, the reaction was performed using the HBr–AcOH system to quantitatively yield the corresponding dibromo analogue (**2**). Then, the introduction of hydrophobic chains through ether bonds by the reacting compound (**2**) with the suitable alcohol [2,23] led to the expected ethers. In the meantime, esterification of the two carboxylic acid groups afforded the tetra-substituted PpIX series (**3a–h**) with yields ranging from 63% to 100%. The simultaneous esterification is due to the presence of the two protonated pyrrole rings, which act as catalysts [38]. The hydrolysis of the ester bond of compounds **3a–h** with LiOH in a mixture of water and THF, followed by an acidic treatment, led to compounds **4a–h**, with yields ranging from 76% to 100%. The amino-PEG$_{550}$ hydrophilic moiety **1** was finally introduced via the conventional peptidic coupling method using DCC–HOBt as a coupling reagent to yield the amphiphilic PpIX analogues, **5a–h**. The final compounds were purified by LH20 in MeOH with yields ranging from 32% to 65%. The PEG$_{550}$-conjugated PpIX (**6**) was readily obtained by coupling native PpIX with amino-PEG$_{550}$ (**1**) in the presence of DCC–HOBt in 50.3% yield.

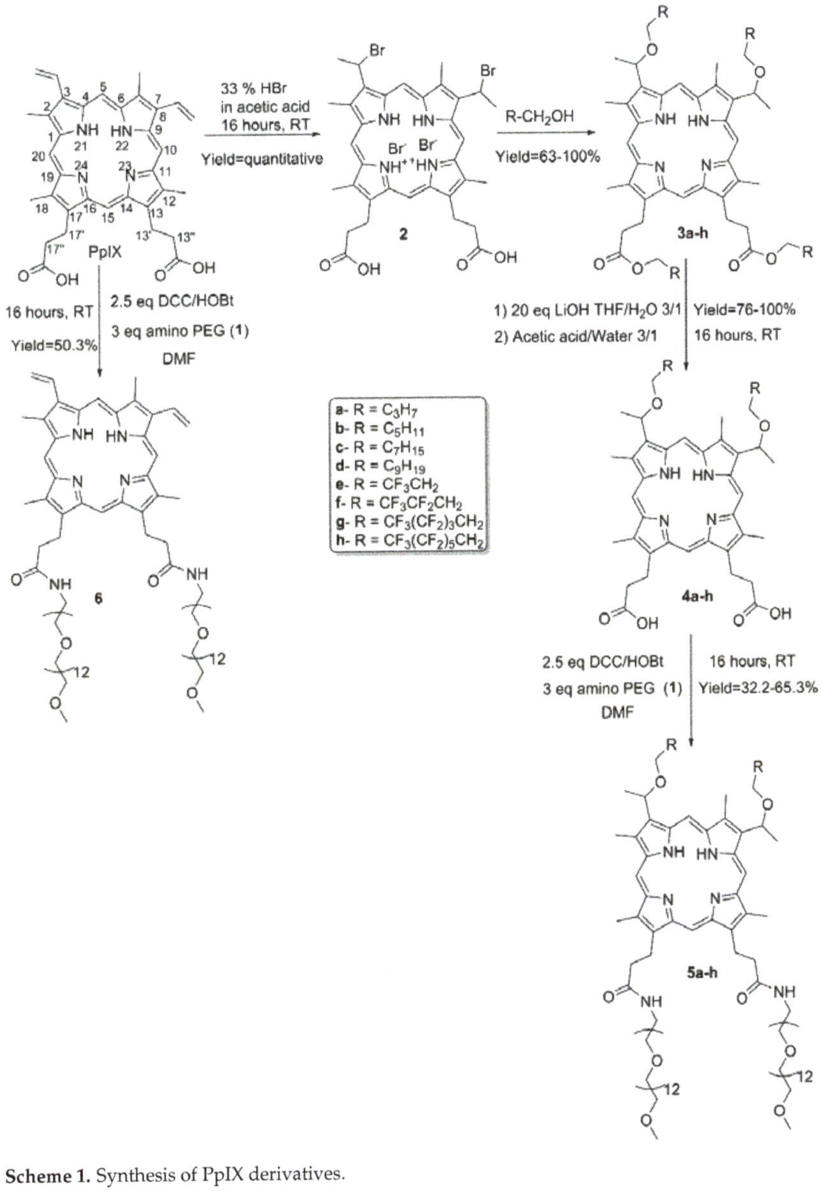

Scheme 1. Synthesis of PpIX derivatives.

The octanol–water partition coefficient (log p) is a suitable descriptor to predict the intracellular localization of compounds, according to their hydrophilic–lipophilic properties. For example, a better affinity towards biological membranes is correlated with the compound's higher hydrophobicity [7,39]. The MarvinSketch software of ChemAxon was used to calculate the HLB and log p of all final PpIX derivatives (listed in Table 1) in order to compare them in terms of hydrophobicity. With regards to all of the series, except for compound **6** which lacks the hydrophobic tail, the HLB and log p are inversely correlated. The compounds have calculated HLB values ranging from 12.14 to 18.75, indicating that they are all perfectly water soluble. Most of the PpIX derivatives possess an HLB between 13 and 16 relative to the detergency properties, according to Fung [36]. In parallel, their log p ranges from 3.3 for compound **6**, which lacks hydrophobic chains to 12.6 for compound **5h**, which comprises two perfluorinated chains of six carbons. As expected, for the same tail length, fluorinated derivatives exhibit higher log p-values than the hydrogenated analogues [40]. For example, compound **5c** endowed with two C_8 hydrocarbon chains (C_8H_{17}) has a log p of 7.4, while for the same tail length, compound **5h** endowed with two C_8 hemifluorinated chains ($C_2H_4C_6F_{13}$) has a log p of 12.6.

3.2. Biological Assays

3.2.1. PDT of Tumor Cells with PpIX Derivatives

Figure 1 shows the cell survivals after PDT with PpIX or PpIX derivatives **5a–h** (amphiphilic derivatives) and **6** (PEG_{550}-PpIX) as a function of light exposure times in the tumor cell lines of 4T1, scc-U8, and WiDr. The cell survivals were decreased with increasing light exposure times during PDT with PpIX, as well as compounds **5b** and **5c** in all of the three cell lines studied. With a 60-s light exposure, the PDT killed almost all of the 4T1 and scc-U8 cells and about 70% of the WiDr cells. Both compounds **5b** and **5c** had a considerable PDT efficiency to the parent PpIX in all of the three cell lines. Similarly, the compound **5f**-mediated PDT killed 70–100% of the cells in both scc-U8 and WiDr cell lines, but significantly less than compounds **5b** and **5c**, as well as PpIX in the 4T1 cells. The PDT killing effect of the other PpIX derivatives was lower than PpIX in all of the cell lines. In general, lipophilic photosensitizers have a stronger photodynamic effect than the hydrophilic dyes on killing cells in vitro due to the localization of cell membranous structures [7]. However, the hydrophobic dyes are not water soluble and cannot be used for the drug administration in the in vivo biological models, due to the fact that they are easily aggregated in water with reduced photodynamic efficiency. Water soluble amphiphilic sensitizers with a relatively long C-chain hydrophobic tail may be suitable for use in biological systems in vivo. Among the currently proposed PpIX derivatives, it seems that the "limit" forms of the series, compounds **5h** (endowed with the longer fluorinated chains, log p = 12.6) and **6** (lacking hydrophobic tails, log p = 3.3) are indeed totally inactive (both are inactive on 4T1 cells or compound **6** is inactive on the WiDr cell line) or exhibit a low cell killing effect (for compound **5h** on scc-U8 and WiDr cells). The stronger photodynamic effects were obtained by compounds **5b** and **5c** with log p-values between 5.82 and 7.4 and endowed with C6- and C8-chains, respectively. Of note, compound **5f** bearing two C4 hemifluorinated chains ($C_2H_4C_2F_5$) but with a log p-value of 5.92, has a photodynamic effect which is comparable to compounds **5b** and **5c** on the scc-U8 and WiDr cell lines. While compound **5a**, which is endowed with two C4 hydrogenated chains (C_4H_9) and a log p-value of 4.23, has a low killing effect on the 4T1 and WiDr cells. These results show that a fine-tuning of the amphiphilic coating of PpIX might improve its photodynamic effect independently of the cell line, although the mechanism of action of each resulting PpIX derivative is probably complex and cell specific [41]. This may be due to the fact that amphiphilic dyes are localized in multiple cellular structures, and thus target several cellular structures to generate an effective damage to the cells after light irradiation.

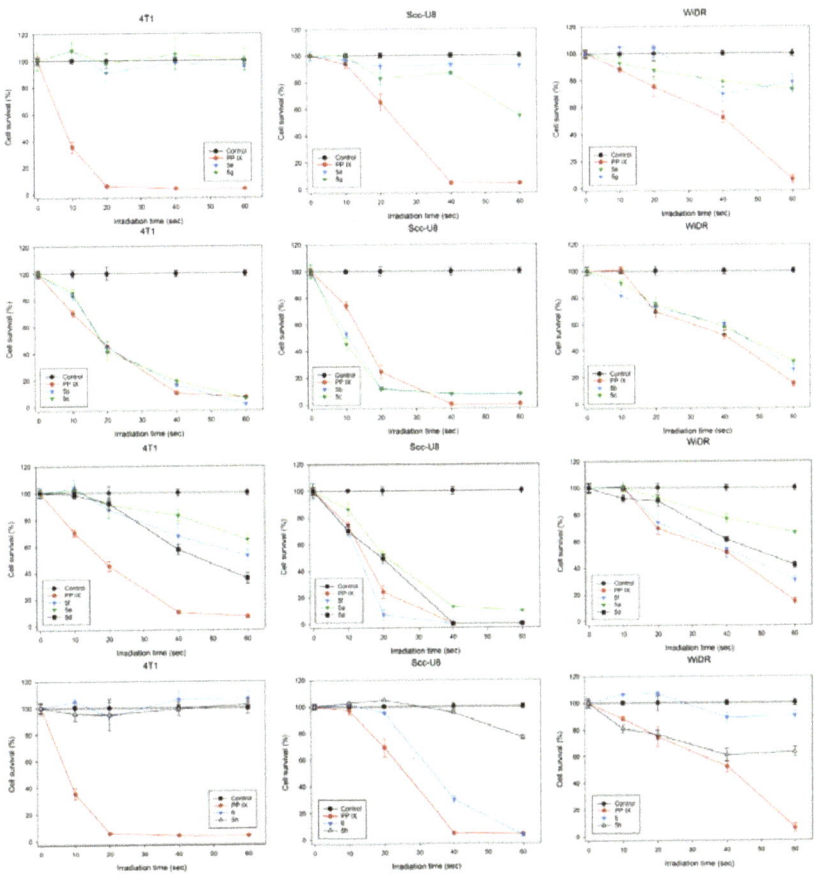

Figure 1. PDT of tumor cells with native PpIX and PpIX derivatives, **5a–h** and **6**.

3.2.2. Uptake of PpIX Derivatives by Cells In Vitro

Figure 2 shows the uptake of **5a–d**, **5f**, and parent PpIX (both at 2.5 µM) by the tumor cell lines of 4T1, scc-U8, and WiDr in vitro. The compounds were studied at very low concentrations (2.5 µM) to avoid aggregation. Of note, a dynamic light scattering (DLS) analysis showed that at this concentration, all of the PpIX derivatives were under a monomeric form (see DLS data in Supplementary Material) [42]. In general, the results show that there is an individual variation of cellular uptake of the five PpIX derivatives within a single cell line and also among the three cell lines. The cellular uptake of the PpIX derivatives is similar to the parent PpIX in the 4T1 and scc-U8 cell lines, while significantly more than the parent PpIX in the WiDr cells (p-values = 0.013 for **5b**, <0.001 for **5c**, 0.002 for **5f**, 0.015 for **5a**, and <0.001 for **5d**). Compounds **5c** and **5f** appeared to be taken up significantly more by the cell lines than the other PpIX derivatives, except for the 4T1 cells where only compound **5c** was more internalized. Of note, the two PpIX derivatives, **5c** and **5f**, have very close HLB values of 14.83 and 14.81, respectively. The WiDr cells of the five PpIX derivatives were taken up more than the other two cell lines. These results show that according to the cell line, the uptake can be significantly different. Moreover, it should be mentioned that PBS was used to measure the amount of PpIX and its derivatives, **5a–d** and **5f**, which are all water soluble in the cells. Furthermore, due to the limited solubility of the parent PpIX in the buffer, its cellular uptake was probably underestimated.

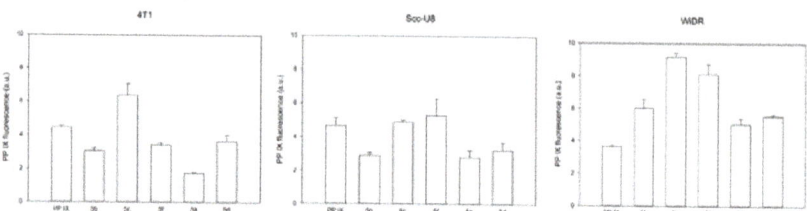

Figure 2. Cellular uptake of PpIX and PpIX derivatives, **5a–d** and **5f**.

3.2.3. Subcellular Localization of PpIX Derivatives In Vitro

Two PpIX derivatives, **5a** and **5b**, with different lipophilic properties (log p-values of 4.23 and 5.82, respectively) were chosen to study the subcellular localization in the three cell lines of 4T1, Scc-U8, and WiDr. Compound **5b**, with a relatively higher lipophilicity, demonstrated both diffuse and granular patterns in all of the three cell lines studied (Figures 3 and 4), suggesting that it was localized in both biomembrane structures and lysosomes. Compound **5a**, with a lower lipophilic character, showed only the lysosomal localization as a granular pattern (Figures 3 and 4). In general, these results are consistent with previous reports that hydrophilic dyes in the lysosomes and amphiphilic are located in both membranous structures and lysosomes, while hydrophobic sensitizers are mainly localized in the cellular membranous structures [7]. Compound **5b** is esterified with a C6-chain aliphatic alcohol, while compound **5a** is esterified with a C4-chain aliphatic alcohol. A longer C-chain anchored to the porphyrin core displays a relatively more hydrophobic behavior, as illustrated by the log p-values. Therefore, this favors a subcellular localization in the cell membranous structures.

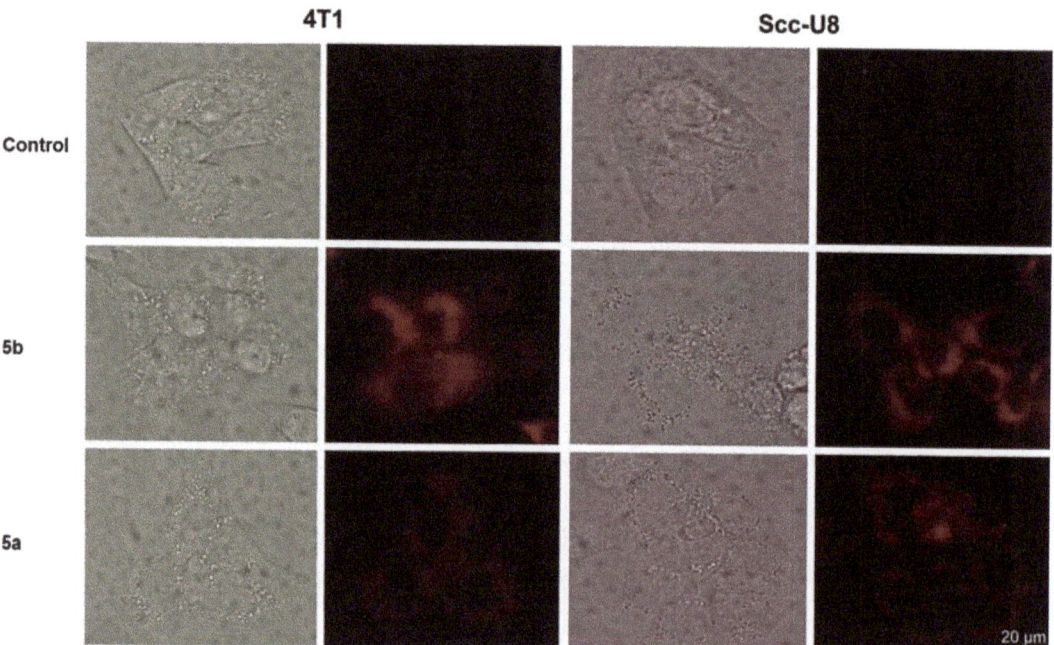

Figure 3. Cellular localization of PpIX derivatives, **5a** and **5b**, in 4T1 and Scc-U8 cells. Scale bar = 20 μm.

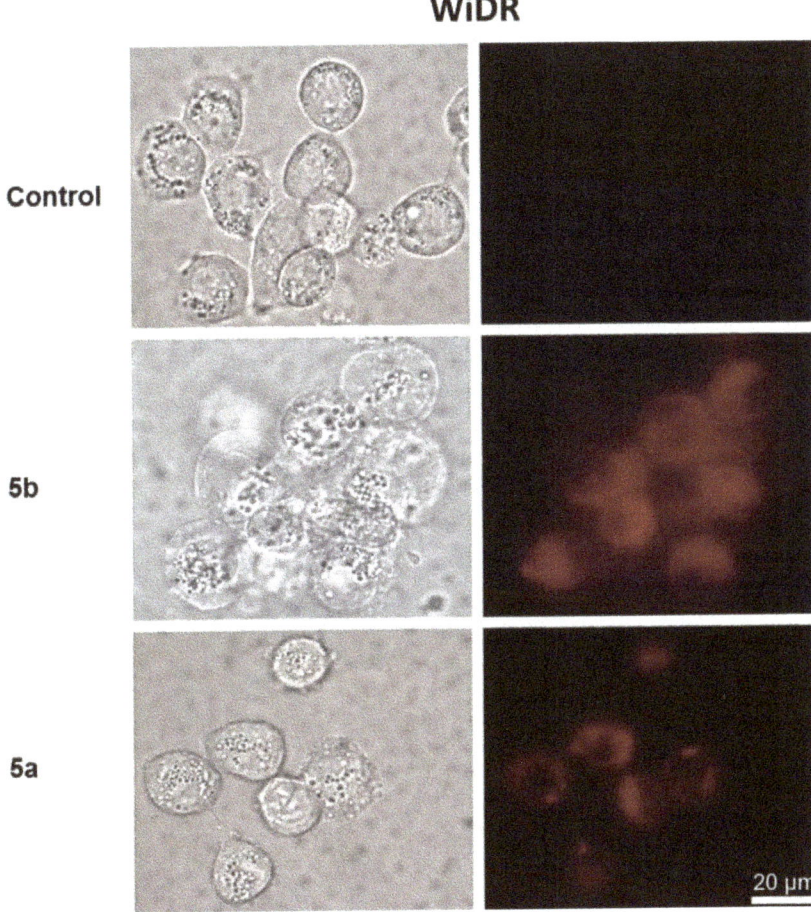

Figure 4. Cellular localization of PpIX derivatives, **5a** and **5b**, in WiDR cells. Scale bar = 20 μm.

3.3. Photochemical Properties

3.3.1. Results of Photophysical Properties

The absorbance and fluorescence spectra of **5a–h** compounds, which are recorded using water as a solvent, are displayed in Figure 5. The absorption shows the characteristic Q-bands in the wavelength range of 490–650 nm, which is indeed very similar for all of the compounds studied. Similar splitting of the Q-bands can be seen in most free-base porphyrin forms, such as in dendrimer substituted tetra-phenyl porphyrins [43]. The splittings are caused by a vibrational substructure of several vibrational modes of the ring structure around 1600 cm^{-1}, and can be assigned to 1-0, 0-0 (Q_y) and 1-0, 0-0 (Q_x) vibrational substructure for the transitions at approximately at 500, 535, 570, and 620 nm (Figures 5 and S3), where x is taken as the direction along the N–H bond [44]. Interestingly, for the porphyrins investigated here, there are also some additional bands resolved towards the IR side. The quantum efficiencies (QE) relative to PpIX were obtained using THF as a solvent and are presented in Table 1.

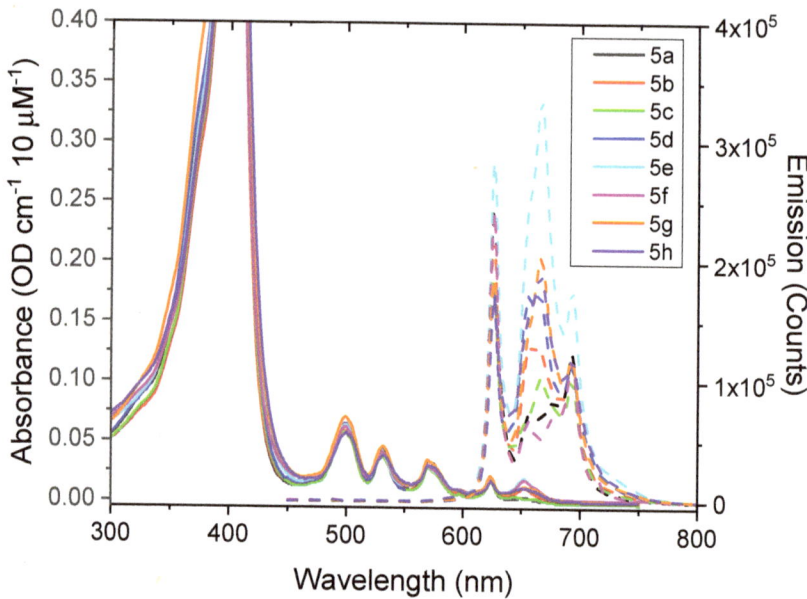

Figure 5. Absorbance (solid lines) and emission (dashed) spectra of compounds dissolved in H_2O (10 µM). Herein, the vertical scale of the absorbance is adjusted to focus on the Q-bands in the 500–650 nm range. The dashed curves are fluorescence emission spectra upon excitation at 425 nm.

It is logical to observe similar spectral characteristics in all of the amphiphilic compounds since they all have undergone the same chemical reaction. Moreover, only the periphery of PpIX was modified. It is well known that the modification of the PpIX core significantly affects its photophysical properties [45]. However, the spectral properties are slightly affected, which seems to be associated with the anchoring of the PEG moiety through the amide bond, since similar spectra are observed between the PEG_{550}-conjugated PpIX and amphiphilic PpIX derivatives, which are presented here.

It was not possible to directly detect a singlet oxygen from the water solvents of these compounds, owing to the low solubility of oxygen in water in combination with the strong quenching of triplet states that usually occur in water. On the other hand, organic solvents are known to have approximately an order of magnitude higher oxygen solubility than more polar solvents, such as water, methanol, and DMSO [46,47]. There are also less strong vibrations from the solvent molecules that can quench the intermediate triplet state. Therefore, THF was used for the demonstration of triplet state formation and energy transfer to form a singlet oxygen in these compounds. In order to confirm the production of singlet oxygen of PpIX derivatives, the triplet excited state absorption (TESA) recorded for UV excitation (lex = 355 nm), as well as the direct transient singlet oxygen luminescence at 1275 nm upon excitation at 425 nm, were investigated (Figure S3 of the Supplementary Materials).

The linear absorption spectra recorded for the 5 µM THF solutions used for TESA all have a ground state absorbance in the range between OD 0.1–0.2 at 355 and 425 nm (data not shown). Therefore, there are no issues with self-absorption at these wavelengths. In order to prove the existence of triplet states, the excited state absorption was measured by exciting an Argon gas flushed sample with a ns laser pulse at 355 nm, and recording the full spectrum with a broad band flash lamp and a gated detector, a few microseconds after the excitation pulse. In Figure S3 (left panel), these spectra are shown as broad features covering the region in the range 300–480 nm. In addition, there are sharper peaks, showing up as depleted (negative) absorption bands, overlayed onto the broad triplet absorption, notably the Q-bands in the range 490–650 nm (for details on how to interpret these spectra, see Glimsdal et al. [33]). By repeating the procedure for a sample that contains oxygen, the triplet absorption signal is strongly quenched and diminished (data not shown).

A singlet oxygen yield is difficult to quantify accurately. Moreover, it strongly depends on the solvent, solvent oxygen content, and many factors (see [32,48] for detailed studies of substituted PpIX variants). Here, it was estimated from the transient luminescence of singlet oxygen that has a characteristic line-shape, as shown in Figure 6. For clarity, we only show the results for compound **5d** using air-saturated THF as a solvent. Herein, the transient signal has been background corrected with the signal from the same sample bubbled with Argon gas for 10 min, to remove the oxygen dissolved in the solvent. The time-trace was fitted to a double exponential function giving two characteristic time decays. In this case, the rise time was determined as 3.0 ± 0.02 μs and the decay as 24.4 ± 0.08 μs using Equation (1) (Experimental Section). The former represents the decay of the triplet state of the sensitizer, whereas the longer decay is very characteristic for the singlet oxygen itself, strongly depending on the solvent, e.g., [31,49]. The results of six representative compounds along with the fitted parameters are shown in Supplementary Material (Figure S3 (right panel, Table S1)). The substituted derivatives of PpIX all show a similar or slightly higher singlet oxygen yield than the bare original PpIX molecule. The latter points to an efficient inter-system that crosses to triplet states. However, these triplet states are dark and did not appear as phosphorescence in the oxygen evacuated samples. Taken together, the transient absorption and singlet oxygen luminescence experiments confirmed the energy transfer from the ground state absorption via the triplet state to the proximate dissolved oxygen molecules in order to obtain the singlet oxygen. The singlet oxygen yield is similar to or better than the PpIX itself.

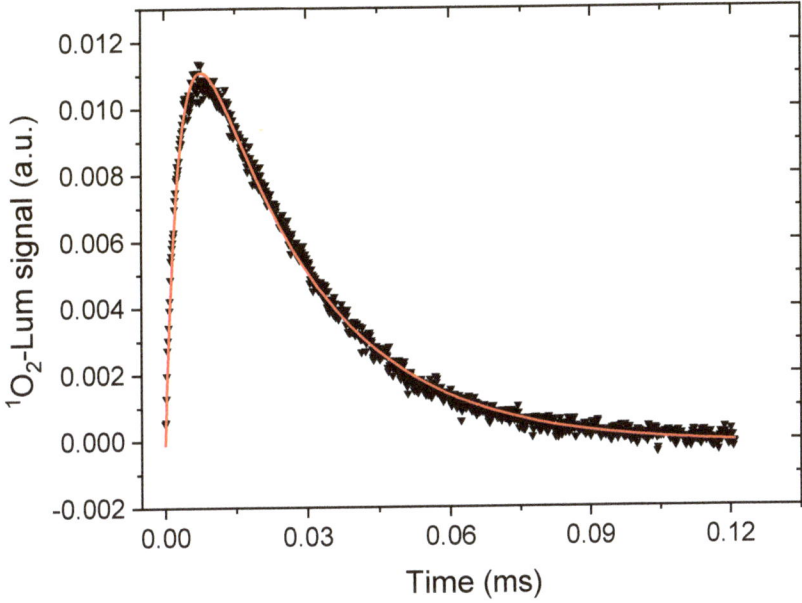

Figure 6. Transient singlet oxygen luminescence at 1275 nm upon excitation of compound **5d** at 425 nm in THF. The solid red curve is fit to a double exponential, as described in the text.

3.3.2. Photobleaching of PpIX Derivatives, 5b and 5c, in WiDr Cells after Blue Light Exposure

Based on the promising in vitro results (especially to the phototoxicity assays) on the three lines of human cancer cells, the more potent PpIX derivatives, **5b** and **5c**, were studied with respect to the photobleaching processes, as described by Gederaas et al. [50] using four different blue light doses (0.39–7.74 J/cm^2) on WiDr human colon adenocarcinoma cells. All of the bleaching experiments were performed in parallel with the native PpIX (2.5 µM, 24 h) under similar instrumental settings. Control cells as "no light" and "no photosensitizer" were also included.

The fluorescence spectra from representative experiments for compounds **5b** and **5c** are shown in Figure 7. In addition, the bleaching spectra including all of the measurements from 4–5 independent experiments are shown in Figure 8. The photobleaching properties of **5b**- and **5c**-incubated WiDr cells illustrate a reduction in the photobleaching of **5b**, to a large extent as 81.2% and 74.2% for compound **5c** after blue light exposure, from 0–7.74 J/cm^2 (0–600 s). As a control, the fluorescence of PpIX cell suspensions (n = 3) was compared to the fluorescence measurements using Ex: 405 nm [51], which results in a reduction of 13.3% compared to the excitation at 410 nm. From these data, it was concluded that fluorescence measurements at Ex: 410 nm were sufficient for compounds **5b**, **5c**, and native PpIX-incubated WiDr cells in the same experiment. Of note, the fluorescence of PpIX-incubated cells without light was about 50 times less compared to the fluorescence of **5b**- and **5c**-incubated cells without light, using an excitation wavelength of 410 nm.

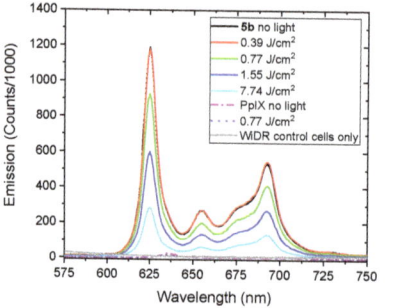
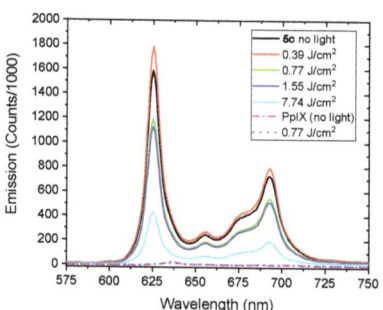

Figure 7. Representative fluorescence spectra of compounds **5b** (**Left**) and **5c** (**Right**) blue light doses. Spectra are averages of 3–5 experiments except for control experiments with PpIX and cells only.

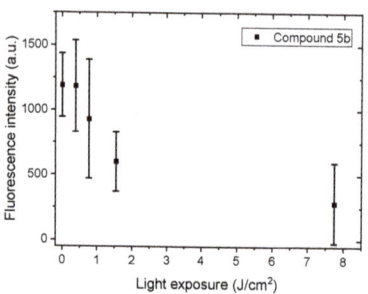
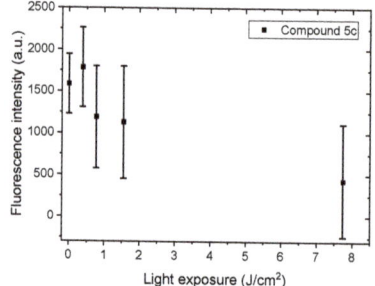

Figure 8. Bleaching data of compounds **5b**- (**Left**) and **5c**- (**Right**) incubated WiDr cells. The standard deviations are based on 3–5 experiments from data presented in Figure 7.

The bleaching curves were given by the generic formula:

$$F(t) = A * \exp(-k * t) \qquad (2)$$

then, the fitted rates (k) and amplitude factors A were stated for each case.

By comparing the photobleaching data in this study with the published results on the tetrapyrrole photosensitizer TPCS$_{2a}$ (Amphinex^R), on the same cell line [50], a relatively fast photobleaching process was observed for both compounds **5b** and **5c**, and possibly faster by compound **5b**. Moreover, based on the 5-aminolevulinic-based photobleaching studies, using confocal scanning microscopy on single rat bladder cancer cells (AY27), a dramatic decrease in PpIX fluorescence was observed the first 20 s of continuous light exposure. The fluence rate in the AY27 study corresponded to a light dose of 45 J/cm^2 after 0.5 s [52]. Depending on the photosensitizer and actual light dose, the rapid photobleaching may cause incomplete tumor destruction. For an optimizing illumination with respect to the cell type, light intensity, and exposure time, further experiments are necessary.

The photobleaching process of protoporphyrin IX derivatives, **5b** and **5c**, were studied in WiDr cells using four different blue light doses and compared with the bleaching of native protoporphyrin IX in the same experiments. The present results document a greater photobleaching in WiDr cells of the less lipophilic PpIX derivative, compound **5b** ($\log p = 5.82$) compared to compound **5c** ($\log p = 7.4$).

4. Conclusions

A novel class of amphiphilic PpIX derivatives was synthesized, bearing two PEG$_{550}$ headgroups (ensuring hydrophilicity) and two hydrogenated or hemifluorinated tails (ensuring hydrophobicity) of different lengths (e.g., containing 4 to 10 carbons). Their synthesis was straight forward by taking advantage of the four anchoring points of the porphyrin core to afford Gemini-like surfactants with a PpIX central scaffold. The resulting amphiphilic PpIX derivatives were fully characterized by NMR analysis, and their hydrophilic–lipophilic balance (HLB) and partition coefficient ($\log p$) were computed using the MarvinSketch software of ChemAxon. The photochemical properties (spectroscopic characterization, photobleaching, and singlet oxygen quantum yield) were evaluated followed by in vitro assays to assess their cellular uptake, subcellular localization, and phototoxic efficiency on three tumor cell lines (4T1, scc-U8, and WiDr cell lines). Although further investigation is needed to build a structure–activity relationship, our results confirm the therapeutic potency of this new family of PpIX derivatives. Furthermore, all of these derivatives are not only water soluble, but some of them also exhibit a higher photodynamic effect than the native PpIX.

Supplementary Materials: The following supporting information can be downloaded at: http://www.mdpi.com/xxx/s1. Figures S1 and S2: DLS data. Figure S3: Spectral data of triplet excited state absorption (left) and transient singlet oxygen luminescence (right); Table S1: Summary of fitting parameters to transient singlet oxygen luminescence; Figures S4–S71: 1H and 13C-NMR spectra of all PpIX derivatives.

Author Contributions: Conceptualization, S.D., Q.P. and C.C.-P.; methodology S.D., P.J., V.V., O.A.G., M.L., Q.P. and C.C.-P.; software, S.D., P.J., V.V., O.A.G. and M.L.; validation, S.D., P.J., V.V., O.A.G., M.L., Q.P. and C.C.-P.; formal analysis, S.D., P.J., V.V., O.A.G., M.L., Q.P. and C.C.-P.; investigation, S.D., P.J., V.V., O.A.G., M.L., T.W., Q.P. and C.C.-P.; resources, Q.P., O.A.G., M.L. and C.C.-P.; data curation, S.D., P.J., V.V., O.A.G. and M.L.; writing—original draft preparation, S.D., O.A.G., M.L., Q.P. and C.C.-P.; writing—review and editing, S.D., O.A.G., M.L., Q.P. and C.C.-P.; visualization, S.D., P.J., V.V., O.A.G., M.L., Q.P. and C.C.-P.; supervision, Q.P. and C.C.-P.; project administration, Q.P. and C.C.-P.; funding acquisition, Q.P. and C.C.-P. All authors have read and agreed to the published version of the manuscript.

Funding: This research was funded by ERANET EuroNanoMed-II program (Project SonoTherag, ANR-13-ENM2-0005-01) (The Research Council of Norway, Project No. 236189).

Institutional Review Board Statement: Not applicable.

Informed Consent Statement: Not applicable.

Data Availability Statement: The authors agree with MDPI Research Data Policies.

Acknowledgments: The authors acknowledge Pierre Guillet for his assistance in computing the HLB and log p-values with the MarvinSketch software. The authors also thank Tom Andre Hansen, NTNU for his technical assistance.

Conflicts of Interest: The authors declare no conflict of interest.

References

1. Dougherty, T.J.; Gomer, C.J.; Henderson, B.W.; Jori, G.; Kessel, D.; Korbelik, M.; Moan, J.; Peng, Q. Photodynamic Therapy. *J. Natl. Cancer Inst.* **1998**, *90*, 889–905. [CrossRef] [PubMed]
2. Agostinis, P.; Berg, K.; Cengel, K.A.; Foster, T.H.; Girotti, A.W.; Gollnick, S.O.; Hahn, S.M.; Hamblin, M.R.; Juzeniene, A.; Kessel, D.; et al. Photodynamic therapy of cancer: An update. *CA A Cancer J. Clin.* **2011**, *61*, 250–281. [CrossRef] [PubMed]
3. Oniszczuk, A.; Wojtunik-Kulesza, K.A.; Oniszczuk, T.; Kasprzak, K. The potential of photodynamic therapy (PDT)—Experimental investigations and clinical use. *Biomed. Pharmacother.* **2016**, *83*, 912–929. [CrossRef] [PubMed]
4. Dolmans, D.E.J.G.J.; Fukumura, D.; Jain, R.K. Photodynamic therapy for cancer. *Nat. Rev. Cancer* **2003**, *3*, 380–387. [CrossRef]
5. Robertson, C.A.; Evans, D.H.; Abrahamse, H. Photodynamic therapy (PDT): A short review on cellular mechanisms and cancer research applications for PDT. *J. Photochem. Photobiol. B Biol.* **2009**, *96*, 1–8. [CrossRef]
6. Wang, S.; Gao, R.; Zhou, F.; Selke, M. Nanomaterials and singlet oxygen photosensitizers: Potential applications in photodynamic therapy. *J. Mater. Chem.* **2004**, *14*, 487–493. [CrossRef]
7. Peng, Q.; Moan, J.; Nesland, J.M. Correlation of subcellular and intratumoral photosensitizer localization with ultrastructural features after photodynamic therapy. *Ultrastruct. Pathol.* **1996**, *20*, 109–129. [CrossRef]
8. Moan, J.; Berg, K. The photodegradation of porphyrins in cells can be used to estimate the lifetime of singlet oxygen. *Photochem. Photobiol.* **1991**, *53*, 549–553. [CrossRef]
9. Kessel, D.; Antolovich, M.; Smith, K.M. The Role of the Peripheral Benzodiazepine Receptor in the Apoptotic Response to Photodynamic Therapy. *Photochem. Photobiol.* **2001**, *74*, 346–349. [CrossRef]
10. Plaetzer, K.; Kiesslich, T.; Verwanger, T.; Krammer, B. The Modes of Cell Death Induced by PDT: An Overview. *Med. Laser Appl.* **2003**, *18*, 7–19. [CrossRef]
11. Oleinick, N.L.; Morris, R.L.; Belichenko, I. The role of apoptosis in response to photodynamic therapy: What, where, why, and how. *Photochem. Photobiol. Sci.* **2002**, *1*, 1–21. [PubMed]
12. Master, A.M.; Livingston, M.; Oleinick, N.L.; Sen Gupta, A. Optimization of a nanomedicine-based silicon phthalocyanine 4 photodynamic therapy (Pc 4-PDT) strategy for targeted treatment of EGFR-overexpressing cancers. *Mol. Pharm.* **2012**, *9*, 2331–2338. [CrossRef] [PubMed]
13. Wang, G.D.; Nguyen, H.T.; Chen, H.; Cox, P.B.; Wang, L.; Nagata, K.; Hao, Z.; Wang, A.; Li, Z.; Xie, J. X-Ray Induced Photodynamic Therapy: A Combination of Radiotherapy and Photodynamic Therapy. *Theranostics* **2016**, *6*, 2295–2305. [CrossRef]
14. Cline, B.; Delahunty, I.; Xie, J. Nanoparticles to mediate X-ray-induced photodynamic therapy and Cherenkov radiation photodynamic therapy. *WIREs Nanomed. Nanobiotechnol.* **2019**, *11*, e1541. [CrossRef]
15. Allison, R.R.; Sibata, C.H. Oncologic photodynamic therapy photosensitizers: A clinical review. *Photodiagn. Photodyn. Ther.* **2010**, *7*, 61–75. [CrossRef] [PubMed]
16. Mazzone, G.; Russo, N.; Sicilia, E. Theoretical investigation of the absorption spectra and singlet-triplet energy gap of positively charged tetraphenylporphyrins as potential photodynamic therapy photosensitizers. *Can. J. Chem.* **2013**, *91*, 902–906. [CrossRef]
17. Ethirajan, M.; Chen, Y.; Joshi, P.; Pandey, R.K. The role of porphyrin chemistry in tumor imaging and photodynamic therapy. *Chem. Soc. Rev.* **2011**, *40*, 340–362. [CrossRef]
18. Josefsen, L.B.; Boyle, R.W. Unique Diagnostic and Therapeutic Roles of Porphyrins and Phthalocyanines in Photodynamic Therapy, Imaging and Theranostics. *Theranostics* **2012**, *2*, 916–966. [CrossRef]
19. Uchoa, A.F.; de Oliveira, K.T.; Baptista, M.S.; Bortoluzzi, A.J.; Iamamoto, Y.; Serra, O.A. Chlorin photosensitizers sterically designed to prevent self-aggregation. *J. Org. Chem.* **2011**, *76*, 8824–8832. [CrossRef]
20. Quartarolo, A.D.; Pérusse, D.; Dumoulin, F.; Russo, N.; Sicilia, E. Hydrophilic annulated dinuclear zinc(II) phthalocyanine as Type II photosensitizers for PDT: A combined experimental and (TD)-DFT investigation. *J. Porphyr. Phthalocyanines* **2013**, *17*, 980–988. [CrossRef]
21. Cauchon, N.; Tian, H.; Langlois, R.; La Madeleine, C.; Martin, S.; Ali, H.; Hunting, D.; van Lier, J.E. Structure−photodynamic activity relationships of substituted zinc trisulfophthalocyanines. *Bioconjugate Chem.* **2005**, *16*, 80–89. [CrossRef] [PubMed]
22. Wiehe, A.; Shaker, Y.M.; Brandt, J.C.; Mebs, S.; Senge, M.O. Lead structures for applications in photodynamic therapy. Part 1: Synthesis and variation of m-THPC (Temoporfin) related amphiphilic A2BC-type porphyrins. *Tetrahedron* **2005**, *61*, 5535–5564. [CrossRef]
23. Woooburn, K.W.; Vardaxis, N.J.; Hill, J.S.; Kaye, A.H.; Reiss, J.A.; Phillips, D.R. Evaluation of porphyrin characteristics required for photodynamic therapy. *Photochem. Photobiol.* **1992**, *55*, 697–704. [CrossRef] [PubMed]

24. Pavlov, V.Y. Modern aspects of the Chemistry of protoporphyrin IX. *Russ. J. Org. Chem. C/C Zhurnal Org. Khimii* **2007**, *43*, 1–34. [CrossRef]
25. Takemura, T.; Ohta, N.; Nakajima, S.; Sakata, I. Critical importance of the triplet lifetime of photosensitizer in photodynamic therapy of tumor. *Photochem. Photobiol.* **1989**, *50*, 339–344. [CrossRef]
26. Topkaya, D.; Lafont, D.; Poyer, F.; Garcia, G.; Albrieux, F.; Maillard, P.; Bretonniere, Y.; Dumoulin, F. Design of an amphiphilic porphyrin exhibiting high in vitro photocytotoxicity. *New J. Chem.* **2016**, *40*, 2044–2050. [CrossRef]
27. Galstyan, A.; Riehemann, K.; Schafers, M.; Faust, A. A combined experimental and computational study of the substituent effect on the photodynamic efficacy of amphiphilic Zn(ii)phthalocyanines. *J. Mater. Chem. B* **2016**, *4*, 5683–5691. [CrossRef]
28. Singh, S.; Aggarwal, A.; Bhupathiraju, N.V.S.D.K.; Arianna, G.; Tiwari, K.; Drain, C.M. Glycosylated Porphyrins, Phthalocyanines, and Other Porphyrinoids for Diagnostics and Therapeutics. *Chem. Rev.* **2015**, *115*, 10261–10306. [CrossRef]
29. Pisarek, S.; Maximova, K.; Gryko, D. Strategies toward the synthesis of amphiphilic porphyrins. *Tetrahedron* **2014**, *70*, 6685–6715. [CrossRef]
30. Bogoeva, V.; Siksjø, M.; Sæterbø, K.G.; Melø, T.B.; Bjørkøy, A.; Lindgren, M.; Gederaas, O.A. Ruthenium porphyrin-induced photodamage in bladder cancer cells. *Photodiagn. Photodyn. Ther.* **2016**, *14*, 9–17. [CrossRef]
31. Snyder, J.W.; Skovsen, E.; Lambert, J.D.C.; Poulsen, L.; Ogilby, P.R. Optical detection of singlet oxygen from single cells. *Phys. Chem. Chem. Phys.* **2006**, *8*, 4280–4293. [CrossRef] [PubMed]
32. Nishimura, T.; Hara, K.; Honda, N.; Okazaki, S.; Hazama, H.; Awazu, K. Determination and analysis of singlet oxygen quantum yields of talaporfin sodium, protoporphyrin IX, and lipidated protoporphyrin IX using near-infrared luminescence spectroscopy. *Lasers Med. Sci.* **2020**, *35*, 1289–1297. [CrossRef] [PubMed]
33. Glimsdal, E.; Dragland, I.; Carlsson, M.; Eliasson, B.; Melø, T.B.; Lindgren, M. Triplet Excited States of Some Thiophene and Triazole Substituted Platinum(II) Acetylide Chromophores. *J. Phys. Chem. A* **2009**, *113*, 3311–3320. [CrossRef] [PubMed]
34. Viswanadhan, V.N.; Ghose, A.K.; Revankar, G.R.; Robins, R.K. Atomic physicochemical parameters for three dimensional structure directed quantitative structure-activity relationships. 4. Additional parameters for hydrophobic and dispersive interactions and their application for an automated superposition of certain naturally occurring nucleoside antibiotics. *J. Chem. Inf. Comput. Sci.* **1989**, *29*, 163–172.
35. Davies, J. A quantitative kinetic theory of emulsion type, I. Physical chemistry of the emulsifying agent. In Proceedings of the International Congress of Surface Activity, London, UK, 8–13 April 1957; pp. 6–438.
36. Fung, H.-K.; Wibowo, C.; Ng, K.M. Chapter 8–Product-centered Process Synthesis and Development: Detergents. In *Computer Aided Chemical Engineering*; Ng, K.M., Gani, R., Dam-Johansen, K., Eds.; Elsevier: Amsterdam, The Netherlands, 2007; Volume 23, pp. 239–274.
37. Bhosale, S.V.; Bhosale, S.V.; Shitre, G.V.; Bobe, S.R.; Gupta, A. Supramolecular Chemistry of Protoporphyrin IX and Its Derivatives. *Eur. J. Org. Chem.* **2013**, *2013*, 3939–3954. [CrossRef]
38. Lottner, C.; Bart, K.C.; Bernhardt, G.; Brunner, H. Hematoporphyrin-derived soluble porphyrin-platinum conjugates with combined cytotoxic and phototoxic antitumor activity. *J. Med. Chem.* **2002**, *45*, 2064–2078. [CrossRef]
39. Stamati, I.; Kuimova, M.K.; Lion, M.; Yahioglu, G.; Phillips, D.; Deonarain, M.P. Novel photosensitisers derived from pyropheophorbide-a: Uptake by cells and photodynamic efficiency in vitro. *Photochem. Photobiol. Sci.* **2010**, *9*, 1033–1041. [CrossRef]
40. Krafft, M.P.; Riess, J.G. Chemistry, Physical Chemistry, and Uses of Molecular Fluorocarbon–Hydrocarbon Diblocks, Triblocks, and Related Compounds—Unique "Apolar" Components for Self-Assembled Colloid and Interface Engineering. *Chem. Rev.* **2009**, *109*, 1714–1792. [CrossRef]
41. Gederaas, O.A.; Schønberg, S.A.; Ramstad, S.; Berg, K.; Johnsson, A.; Krokan, H.E. Cell specific effects of polyunsaturated fatty acids on 5-aminolevulinic acid based photosensitization. *Photochem. Photobiol. Sci.* **2005**, *4*, 383–389. [CrossRef]
42. Topel, Ö.; Çakır, B.A.; Budama, L.; Hoda, N. Determination of critical micelle concentration of polybutadiene-block-poly(ethyleneoxide) diblock copolymer by fluorescence spectroscopy and dynamic light scattering. *J. Mol. Liq.* **2013**, *177*, 40–43. [CrossRef]
43. Vestberg, R.; Nyström, A.; Lindgren, M.; Malmström, E.; Hult, A. Porphyrin-Cored 2,2-Bis(methylol)propionic Acid Dendrimers. *Chem. Mater.* **2004**, *16*, 2794–2804. [CrossRef]
44. Minaev, B.; Lindgren, M. Vibration and Fluorescence Spectra of Porphyrin-Cored 2,2-Bis(methylol)-propionic Acid Dendrimers. *Sensors* **2009**, *9*, 1937–1966. [CrossRef] [PubMed]
45. Sternberg, E.D.; Dolphin, D.; Brückner, C. Porphyrin-based photosensitizers for use in photodynamic therapy. *Tetrahedron* **1998**, *54*, 4151–4202. [CrossRef]
46. Franco, C.; Olmsted, J. Photochemical determination of the solubility of oxygen in various media. *Talanta* **1990**, *37*, 905–909. [CrossRef]
47. Sato, T.; Hamada, Y.; Sumikawa, M.; Araki, S.; Yamamoto, H. Solubility of Oxygen in Organic Solvents and Calculation of the Hansen Solubility Parameters of Oxygen. *Ind. Eng. Chem. Res.* **2014**, *53*, 19331–19337. [CrossRef]
48. Nifiatis, F.; Athas, J.; Don, K.; Gunaratne, D.; Gurung, Y.; Monette, K.; Shivokevich, P. Substituent Effects of Porphyrin on Singlet Oxygen Generation Quantum Yields. *Open Spectrosc. J.* **2011**, *5*, 1–12. [CrossRef]
49. Callaghan, S.; Vindstad, B.E.; Flanagan, K.J.; Melø, T.B.; Lindgren, M.; Grenstad, K.; Gederaas, O.A.; Senge, M.O. Structural, Photophysical, and Photobiological Studies on BODIPY-Anthracene Dyads. *ChemPhotoChem* **2021**, *5*, 131–141. [CrossRef]

50. Gederaas, O.A.; Johnsson, A.; Berg, K.; Manandhar, R.; Shrestha, C.; Skåre, D.; Ekroll, I.K.; Høgset, A.; Hjelde, A. Photochemical internalization in bladder cancer–Development of an orthotopic in vivo model. *Photochem. Photobiol. Sci.* **2017**, *16*, 1664–1676. [CrossRef]
51. Johansson, J.; Berg, R.; Svanberg, K.; Svanberg, S. Laser-induced fluorescence studies of normal and malignant tumour tissue of rat following intravenous injection of δ-amino levulinic acid. *Lasers Surg. Med.* **1997**, *20*, 272–279. [CrossRef]
52. Gederaas, O.A.; Husebye, H.; Johnsson, A.B.; Callaghan, S.; Brunsvik, A. In vitro and in vivo effects of HAL on porphyrin production in rat bladder cancer cells (AY27). *J. Porphyr. Phthalocyanines* **2019**, *23*, 813–820. [CrossRef]

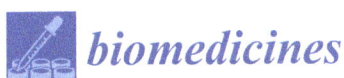

Article

Photodynamic Inactivation of Antibiotic-Resistant and Sensitive *Aeromonas hydrophila* with Peripheral Pd(II)- vs. Zn(II)-Phthalocyanines

Vanya N. Mantareva [1,*], Vesselin Kussovski [2], Petya Orozova [3], Lyudmila Dimitrova [2], Irem Kulu [4], Ivan Angelov [1], Mahmut Durmus [4] and Hristo Najdenski [2]

[1] Institute of Organic Chemistry with Centre of Phytochemistry, Bulgarian Academy of Sciences, 1113 Sofia, Bulgaria; ipangelov@gmail.com
[2] The Stephan Angeloff Institute of Microbiology, Bulgarian Academy of Sciences, 1113 Sofia, Bulgaria; vkussovski@gmail.com (V.K.); lys22@abv.bg (L.D.); hnajdenski@gmail.com (H.N.)
[3] National Diagnostic Research Veterinary Institute, 1000 Sofia, Bulgaria; Nrl-fmcd@bfsa.bg
[4] Department of Chemistry, Gebze Technical University, Gebze 41400, Kocaeli, Turkey; iremkulu@gtu.edu.tr (I.K.); durmus@gtu.edu.tr (M.D.)
* Correspondence: Vanya.Mantareva@orgchm.bas.bg

Abstract: The antimicrobial multidrug resistance (AMR) of pathogenic bacteria towards currently used antibiotics has a remarkable impact on the quality and prolongation of human lives. An effective strategy to fight AMR is the method PhotoDynamic Therapy (PDT). PDT is based on a joint action of a photosensitizer, oxygen, and light within a specific spectrum. This results in the generation of singlet oxygen and other reactive oxygen species that can inactivate the pathogenic cells without further regrowth. This study presents the efficacy of a new Pd(II)- versus Zn(II)-phthalocyanine complexes with peripheral positions of methylpyridiloxy substitution groups (pPdPc and ZnPcMe) towards Gram-negative bacteria *Aeromonas hydrophila* (*A. hydrophila*). Zn(II)-phthalocyanine, ZnPcMe was used as a reference compound for *in vitro* studies, bacause it is well-known with a high photodynamic inactivation ability for different pathogenic microorganisms. The studied new isolates of *A. hydrophila* were antibiotic-resistant (R) and sensitive (S) strains. The photoinactivation results showed a full effect with 8 µM pPdPc for S strain and with 5 µM ZnPcMe for both R and S strains. Comparison between both new isolates of *A. hydrophila* (S and R) suggests that the uptakes and more likely photoinactivation efficacy of the applied phthalocyanines are independent of the drug sensitivity of the studied strains.

Keywords: antimicrobial multidrug resistance (AMR); photodynamic therapy (PDT); palladium and zinc phthalocyanines; antibiogram of bacterial isolates; *Aeromonas hydrophila*

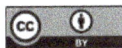

1. Introduction

Among the most harmful bacterial pathogens for human health is *Aeromonas hydrophila*, with the characteristics of a foodborne pathogen of emergent status [1]. The genus *Aeromonas* is characterized as a waterborne and food-developed opportunistic Gram-negative bacteria [2]. The species has been considered as causing a wide spectrum of human diseases, such as wound infections, bacteremia and septicemia, and persistent infections in immunocompromised patients [3]. *A. hydrophila* has the ability to grow at cold temperatures, which may be a negative aspect concerning the safety of human lives. Moreover, observations showed that *A. hydrophila* causes infections in humans with a low capability for inactivation with the clinically approved treatments [4–6]. The scientific curiosity about this species has increased because of the following reasons: (i) the fast distribution of *Aeromonas* all over the world, (ii) the trials for the correct identification and sorting of pathogenic *Aeromonas* species, (iii) the incidence of strains with antimicrobial resistance, and (iv) the ability of some strains to remain alive after the conventional wastewater treatments [5]. Poor water quality, the ubiquitous nature and rapid spreading of harmful pathogens, environmental adverse conditions, and high stocking densities are important factors that contribute to the wide-spreading of infections [6]. These characteristics, together with the rising resistance in common pathogenic bacteria to the known drugs, are what make disease prevention a difficult mission. The determination of the natural horizontal gene transfer showed that *Aeromonas* sp. can acquire mobile genetic elements protecting antimicrobial resistance [7]. An example is the plasmid-mediated quinolone resistance (e.g., qnrS and aac (60)-Ib-cr), carbapenemase (e.g., blaKPC, blaNDM, blaGES, blaIMP, blaVIM, and blaOXA-48), and aminoglycosides-encoding genes (e.g., rmtD), typical for *Aeromonas* species [8].

Photodynamic therapy (PDT) with porphyrinoids features as a more effective alternative strategy, which is under intensive interest to keep under control the pathogenic bacterial species causing acute infections [9,10]. Lately, PDT has been well-accepted as an emergency, low-cost antimicrobial treatment for local infections without other therapeutic options [11]. After the Golden age of antibiotics, PDT method has been of scientific interest because of the fast development of AMR and the fast increase in cases with lethal outcomes due to this resistance [12]. Antimicrobial PDT has been recently well-accepted as a potential preferable choice over the traditional antibiotics because of the lack of side effects, pathogenicity reversal, and further regrowth of the pathogenic species after the treatment [13]. Studies described aPDT as a method with a lack of development of resistance with a fast response after a single application [14,15].

Phthalocyanines (Pcs) are recognized as second-generation photosensitizers for PDT after the porphyrin derivatives, which are well-accepted as appropriate for anticancer PDT [16,17]. Presently, the studies with phthalocyanine derivatives for the inactivation of pathogens are more in the experimental stage than in clinical practice [18]. Most of the known metallophthalocyanines (MPcs) have been considered for aPDT studies because of their suitable photo-physicochemical properties, such as intensive far-red or near-infrared absorption (>670 nm) and high triplet state quantum yields with a preferable singlet oxygen generation [19]. The water-soluble and cationic MPcs coordinated with different metals and semi-metals were obtained via quaternization reaction of N-attached substitution groups [16–19]. These phthalocyanines have been well-documented as proper photosensitizers for PDT applications [20].

Palladium phthalocyanine complexes with different substitution groups are known to have promising photophysical, photochemical, and photobiological properties [21,22]. The effect of an open-shell metal ion, such as palladium (Pd^{2+}), in the Pc-ligand molecule leads to an increase in the triplet state and the further singlet oxygen production with relatively high quantum yields of the recently studied Pd(II)-phthalocyanine [22]. Our previous study with Pd(II)-phthalocyanine with four non-peripheral methylpyridiloxy groups (nPdPc) suggested a promising photodynamic inactivation capacity of multidrug-resistant *Staphylococcus aureus* (MRSA) but a low efficiency for *A. hydrophila* drug-resistant strain [22].

In the present study, two new isolates of Gram-negative bacterium *A. hydrophila* as antibiotic- resistant (R) and sensitive (S) strains were characterized for their susceptibility to common antibiotics (antibiograms). The photodynamic efficiency of a newly synthesized peripheral methylpyridiloxy-substituted Pd(II)-phthalocyanine (pPdPc) was studied in comparison to the well-known similar compound Zn(II)-phthalocyanine (ZnPcMe) on both *A. hydrophila* strains. The new palladium phthalocyanine pPdPc was tested for the uptake behavior on these pathogenic bacterial strains. In addition, the cytotoxicity studies on representative model cell lines were performed. The obtained results suggested very promising properties of the studied phthalocyanines as photosensitizers for PDT of Gram-negative *A. hydrophila* strains.

2. Material and Methods

2.1. Phthalocyanines

The phthalocyanines of palladium (pPdPc) and zinc (ZnPcMe) were prepared and further studied as a mixture of positional isomers (Figure 1). The synthesis was carried out according to the previously published synthetic procedures which were used with slight modifications [22,23].

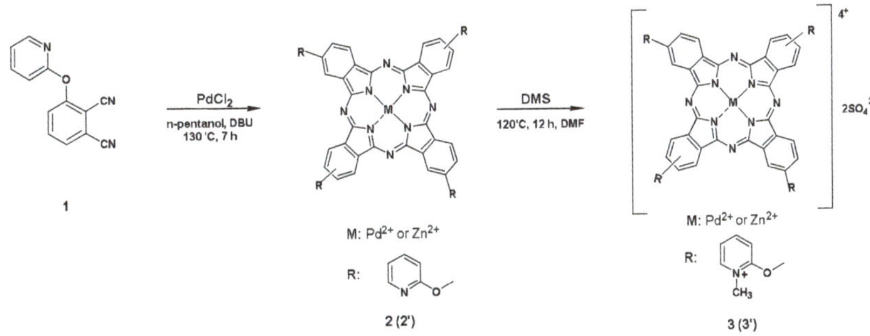

Figure 1. Synthesis of tetra-methylpyridiloxy-substituted Pd(II)- and Zn(II)-phthalocyanines.

2.1.1. Synthesis of 2,(3),9(10),16(17),23(24)-Tetrakis-[(2-pyridyloxy) phthalocyaninato] Palladium (II), (2)

A mixture of anhydrous palladium (II) chloride (0.179 g, 1 mmol), 4-pyridyloxyphthalonitrile (0.442 g, 2 mmol), DBU (3.32 mL, 2 mmol), and n-pentanol (5 mL), was stirred at 130 °C for 7 h under a nitrogen atmosphere. After cooling, the solution was dropped in n-hexane. The green solid product was precipitated and collected by filtration and washed with n-hexane. After washing, the crude product was purified by column chromatography (SiO$_2$) using a CH$_2$Cl$_2$-MeOH (50:1) solvent system. The results were as follows: Yield: 0.86 g (52%). IR [v_{max}/cm^{-1}]: 3092 (Ar-CH), 1657 (C=C), 1576, 1532, 1500, 1399, 1327, 1287, 1258, 1127, 1109 (C-O-C), 1045, 805, and 744. ^{1}H-NMR (CDCl$_3$): δ, ppm 7.31–7.96 (14H, m, Pc-H, and Pyridyl-H) and 6.00–6.90 (14H, m, Pc-H and Pyridyl-H). MALDI-TOF-MS m/z: Calc. 991.28 for C$_{52}$H$_{28}$N$_{12}$O$_4$Pd; Found [M]$^+$ 991.38, 1014.82 [M+Na]$^+$.

2.1.2. Synthesis of 2,(3),9(10),16(17),13(24)-Tetrakis-{[(2-(N-methyl)pyridyloxy]phthalocyaninato} Palladium (II) Sulphate, (3)

Phthalocyanine 2 (100 mg, 0.1mmol) was heated (120 °C) in freshly distilled DMF (0.5 mL), and dimethyl sulphate (0.2 mL) was added dropwise. The mixture was stirred at 120 °C for 12 h. After this time, the mixture was cooled to room temperature, and the product was precipitated with hot acetone and collected by filtration. The green solid product was washed successively with hot ethanol, ethyl acetate, THF, chloroform, n-hexane, and diethyl ether. The resulting hygroscopic product dried over phosphorous pentoxide. The results were as follows: Yield: 0.11 g (73%). IR [v_{max}/cm^{-1}]: 3064 (Ar-CH), 1655, 1578 (C=C), 1533, 1476, 1329, 1230 (S=O), 1182, 1110 (S=O), 1030 (C-O-C), 935, 837, 767, and 662 (S-O). ^{1}H-NMR (DMSO-d_6): δ, ppm 7.42–8.01 (28H, m, Pc-H and Pyridyl-H) and 3.86–4.44 (12H, m, CH$_3$). UV/Vis (DMSO), λ$_{max}$, nm (log ε): 318 (4.57), 623 (4.13), and 662 (4.27). MALDI-TOF-MS m/z: Calc. 1243.54 for C$_{56}$H$_{40}$N$_{12}$O$_{12}$S$_2$Pd; Found 311.741 [(M+4)/4]$^+$.

2.2. Bacterial Strains

Two strains of *A. hydrophila* as multidrug-resistant (R) and drug-sensitive (S) strains were recently isolated from local water resources. They were tested and confirmed as *A. hydrophila* strains by the classical microbiological tests and MALDI-TOF mass spectrometry analysis (Bruker, Munich, Germany). Trypticase soy agar (TSA) (Difco) was used for the cultivation of *A. hydrophila*. The strains were aerobically cultivated on nutrient media for 24 h at 28 °C. Cells were harvested and suspended in sterile phosphate-buffered saline (PBS) of pH 7.4. Suspensions were diluted to a cell density of ~10^6 CFU·mL^{-1}. The viable cells in the suspensions were counted by plating the serial dilutions on solid culture media. The number of visible colonies (colonies forming units, CFU) present on an agar plate was multiplied by the dilution factor to provide the values in CFU·mL^{-1}.

2.3. Photodynamic Inactivation Study

The stock solutions of the studied phthalocyanines (~2 mM) were freshly prepared in dimethylsulphoxide (DMSO, Uvasol) and kept in a dark place during the experiments. The preparative glassware and vials were covered with aluminium foil and flushed with argon in order to prevent photobleaching of the experimental solutions. The absorption spectra were recorded on a Shimadzu UV–vis 3000 apparatus (Osaka, Japan) to control the exact concentrations before the experiments. All solids and solvents were purchased through Sigma-Aldrich (FOT, Sofia, Bulgaria).

Both strains were grown aerobically at 28 °C overnight. Then cells were harvested by centrifugation and were suspended in sterile phosphate-buffered solutions (pH 7.4). The absorbances of the cell suspensions were measured as having an optical density of 0.490 at 600 nm using a spectrophotometer Unico 2100UV, which corresponded to 10^9 CFU·mL^{-1}. Prior to each experiment, the cell suspensions were diluted to the bacterial density of 10^6 CFU·mL^{-1}. The cell suspensions were incubated with the tested phthalocyanine in the concentration range from 0.04 µM to 20 µM for 15 min. The portions of suspension (200 µL) were placed in a standard 96-well polystyrene plate, and light was applied. Four groups of bacterial cells were collected: (1) only cells (no light and no Pc); (2) dark control—with PS, but without light; (3) light control—without any PS, but with light irradiation; and (4) the PDI treated groups. The cells were exposed to an LED at 665 nm (ELO Ltd., Sofia, Bulgaria) with a power density of 100 mW·cm^{-2} and light dose of 50 J·cm^{-2}. A portion of 0.1 mL was taken off and diluted (10-fold) with a buffer. Aliquots (0.025 mL) were spread over Trypticase® Soy agar with 0.5% yeast extract. The obtained results are presented as numbers of CFU of bacteria developed for 48 h incubation (28 °C) on the agar dishes.

2.4. Uptake Study

In the present study, the bacterial suspensions of *A. hydrophila* as multidrug-resistant (R) and drug-sensitive (S) strains with a range of cell density (10^5–10^8 CFU·mL^{-1}) were incubated with pPdPc with concentration 5 µM. The chemical extraction was carried out with a mixture tetrahydrofuran–sodiumdodecyl sulfate (THF: SDS, 1:1). The new phthalocyanine is water-soluble but aggregated in water media. Prior experiments, the cell suspensions were prepared by serial dilutions in phosphate buffered solutions. The applied procedure included a chemical extraction of pPdPc and fluorescence measurements (exc: 610 nm). The used protocol was previously published for non-peripheral palladium phthalocyanine, nPdPc [22].

2.5. Statistics

The experiments were carried out in triplicate. The collected data were presented as a mean value ± standard deviation (SD), and the difference between two means was compared by an unpaired Student's test. $P < 0.05$ was considered as significant.

3. Results

Palladium and zinc phthalocyanine complexes with peripheral methylpyridiloxy substitution groups (pPdPc and ZnPcMe) were synthesized according to the Refs [22,23]. The bacterial strains, *A. hydrophila*, antibiotic-resistant (R) and *A. hydrophila*, sensitive (S), were isolated and used in the photodynamic inactivation studies with Pd(II)- and Zn(II)-phthalocyanines. The antibiotic susceptibility profiles of these bacterial strains were obtained (Table 1). The results showed the following order of resistance and sensitivity: (1) the strain *A. hydrophila* (R)—resistant to Ampicillin, Ceftiofur, Florfenicol, Enrofloxacin,

Co-Trimoxazol, Doxycycline, and Sparfloxacin; (2) the strain *A. hydrophila* (S)—sensitive to Ceftiofur, Florfenicol, Enrofloxacin, Co-Trimoxazol, Doxycycline, and Sparfloxacin, and resistant to Ampicillin.

Table 1. Antibiotic-resistant (R) and sensitive (S) strains of *A. hydrophila*.

Aeromonas hydrophila (R)			*Aeromonas hydrophila* (S)		
Antimicrobial Agent	Disk Content (μg)	Sensitivity	Antimicrobial Agent	Disk Content (μg)	Sensitivity
Ampicillin	10	R	Ampicillin	10	R
Ceftiofur	30	R	Ceftiofur	30	S
Florfenicol	30	R	Florfenicol	30	S
Enrofloxacin	5	R	Enrofloxacin	5	S
Cotrimo-xazol	25	R	Cotrimo-xazol	25	S
Doxycyclin	30	R	Doxycyclin	30	S
Sparfloxacin	5	R	Sparfloxacin	5	S

Zn(II)-phthalocyanine was tested before on a number of pathogenic strains that were susceptible to the applied PDT protocol with ZnPcMe [24,25]. The peripherally substituted pPdPc, which was a new compound in this study, showed full photoinactivation ability at a concentration of 8 μM for the sensitive *A. hydrophila* strain (Figure 2). By increasing the concentrations up to 20 μM, this compound showed dark toxicity for both tested *A. hydrophila* strains (S and R). At lower concentrations (<2 μM), pPdPc showed no phototoxicity on either *A. hydrophila* S or on R strains. Comparison of the inactivation ability of pPdPc on the used *A. hydrophila* R and S strains showed log 3.32 for the R strain and resp. 5.47 log for the S strain (8 μM of pPdPc). Photodynamic inactivation with 5 μM of pPdPc was obtained with values of 2.34 log and 3.17 log toward R and S strains, respectively. In the studied concentrations, the dark toxicity was not observed. By a specific light spectrum of irradiation (665 nm), photodynamic inactivation was achieved, with slightly high results for concentrations of 5 and 8 μM for the tested antibiotic-sensitive strain of *A. hydrophila*.

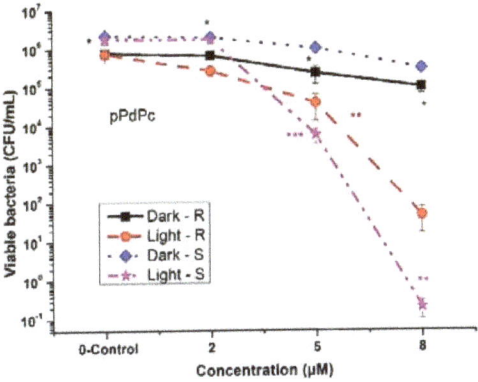

Figure 2. Photodynamic inactivation of *A. hydrophila* (R and S) planktonic cultured with peripheral Pd(II)-phthalocyanine (pPdPc) and an LED at 665 nm irradiation. * $p < 0.005$; ** $p < 0.008$, and *** $p < 0.01$.

The new cationic phthalocyanine pPdPc was evaluated for the uptake into both bacterial *A. hydrophila* strains (Figure 3). As can be seen, the uptakes showed similarity for the studied suspensions with different cell densities. The highest uptakes were obtained for the complexes incubated in more diluted suspensions in comparison to the high-density cell suspensions without the influence of the characteristics of the strain. As is well-studied, the bacterial wall of the Gram (−) species is more complicated, which additionally increases the resistance. The cationic phthalocyanines are well-studied as being more favorable for antibacterial PDT because of the proper electrostatic interaction of these compounds with cell membranes [26].

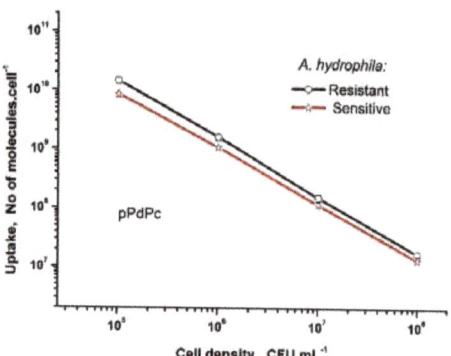

Figure 3. Uptake of Pd(II)-phthalocyanine (pPdPc) in *A. hydrophila* (R and S) strains as suspensions with different cell densities as obtained by fluorescence measurements.

The well-explored compound, tetra-methylpyridiloxy Zn(II)-phthalocyanine (Zn-PcMe), was also tested in the present study. ZnPcMe was studied with promising photoinactivation efficacy towards pathogenic bacteria, fungus, and viruses [24,25]. For concentrations up to 5 µM, ZnPcMe was examined without dark toxicity on both tested strains (Figure 4). The full photodynamic inactivation result (~log 6) was determined for 5 µM of ZnPcMe but with low efficiency (<log 3) at lower concentrations. These observations confirm the previous studies with ZnPcMe, with photoinactivation capacity at lower concentrations [26]. Considering the structures of both peripherally substituted complexes, the phototoxic effect of ZnPcMe was higher than that of pPdPc (Figures 2 and 4). However, the new pPdPc showed a strong photoinactivation ability at a concentration of 8 µM, which was higher than the concentration observed in the previous study with nPdPc on another resistant *A. hydrophila* [22]. The results demonstrated that the effect of aPDT treatment is strongly dependent on the characteristics of the strain. Additionally, in vitro studies on cell cultures were carried out and showed that Pd(II)-phthalocyanines with different positions of substituents had a lack of cytotoxicity on cell cultures, such as chick embryo fibroblasts, calf trachea cell lines, Vero cell lines, and MDBK cell lines.

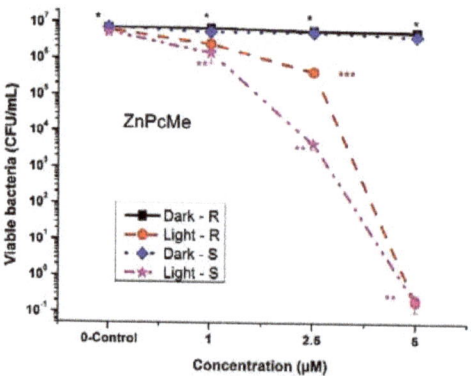

Figure 4. Photodynamic inactivation of *A. hydrophila* (R and S) planktonic cultured with Zn(II)-phthalocyanine (ZnPcMe) and an LED at 665 nm irradiation. * $p < 0.005$; ** $p < 0.008$, and *** $p < 0.01$.

4. Discussion

Aeromonas species are widely spread in water, water habitats, and in many food products, such as seafood; raw foods of animal origin, such as poultry, ground meat, and raw milk; and raw vegetables. *Aeromonas*-associated illnesses are usually caused by stress and unpredicted changes in environmental conditions. Fresh water quality, overcrowding of social communities in poor countries, undesirable changes in temperature, low oxygen and a very high amount of CO_2 in the air, and the increase in nitrite or ammonia saturation, are considered as predisposing aspects for acute infections. *Aeromonas spp.* are known to be intrinsically resistant to many b-lactams, due to the production of multiple inducible, chromosomally encoded b-lactamases [27]. The spectrum of diseases includes gastroenteritis, septicemia, and traumatic and aquatic wound infections.

The fast development of drug resistance towards the variety of antibiotics features the emergency need of an effective approach, such as PDT, to keep harmful pathogens under control [28,29]. Previous studies to inactivate the drug-resistant *A. hydrophila*, which is a ubiquitous Gram-negative bacterium causing diseases in reptiles, amphibians, farm fish, and humans, showed that the drinking water isolate of this bacterium, as well as the native counterparts, are liable to PDT treatment with cationic phthalocyanine complexes, with different hydrocarbon chains as substituents [28]. The experimental photodynamic studies with *Aeromonas* sp. suggested that they are susceptible to PDT, but with different success of inactivation, in dependence on the structure of the photosensitizer and the applied irradiation conditions [22,28]. It was found that the cationic nature and optimal physico-chemical properties of the phthalocyanines correlate with the uptakes and the efficiency of aPDT towards pathogenic bacteria [30,31]. Referring to the uptake of phthalocyanines by *A. hydrophila*, as was studied before, there was a noticeable inverse dependence on the cell density of suspension [28]. *A. hydrophila* cells incubated with Zn(II)-phthalocyanines with different lengths of hydrocarbon chains showed that an approx. 10-fold increase in cell density has resulted in a significant decrease in the uptake behavior of at least one order of magnitude [28]. The phenomenon was explained by the sterical hindrance between molecules at high bacterial density, which results in the decrease in the number of attached molecules per bacterial cell [32]. Our previous results with ZnPcMe (3 µM) showed a complete photoinactivation at a lower light dose of $30 \: J \cdot cm^{-2}$. The advantage of the aPDT method is also presented with the current experiments with two isolates *A. hydrophila*, which showed significant photoinactivations (>5 log) with the applied phthalocyanines.

This study suggests that both phthalocyanines, which differ in the coordinated metal ions palladium (pPdPc) and zinc (ZnPcMe), have comparable and slightly higher photoinactivation efficacy for ZnPcMe. The full phototoxic effect was observed with complex ZnPcMe, which is known as a highly effective photosensitizer in the photodynamic inactivation of pathogenic species, including viruses [24,25]. The results with *A. hydrophila* support the role of zinc as a proper metal ion for PDT photosensitizers [26,28]. Lately, it was reported that cationic photosensitizers have a high impact on the antimicrobial efficiency because of the binding ability and the charge density distribution of cationic groups [33]. In comparison with the routine antibiotic treatment, which usually requires long-term drug usage to have a result, the PDT procedure is non-toxic to the whole human body, with a single local application of the photosensitizer and a short time of irradiation. As was reported for other pathogenic strains, the short incubation time of the photosensitizer and the mild light doses within a specific spectrum of irradiation are sufficient to kill bacteria in a single treatment, with a fast response after the procedure [34]. Meanwhile, the promising in vivo results were obtained with the Zn(II)-phthalocyanine ZnPcMe studied for the inflammatory reaction of biological tissue for applications in clinical dental practice [35,36]. These observations concluded that the photodynamic method with phthalocyanines can be considered as promising for the inactivation of pathogenic bacteria associated with acute infections in dentistry. This study showed an excellent biocompatibility with a laser at 665 nm irradiation, which was observed on experimental animals by means of histopathology [36]. In vivo examination suggested that the used in the present study ZnPcMe did not lead to damaging tissue reactions either as was compared to Fotosan™. This proper biocompatibility is a basis to recommend ZnPcMe for safe administration and the approval certifications for application in clinical practice.

5. Conclusions

The new isolates of Gram-negative bacteria *Aeromonas hydrophila* were analyzed for their susceptibility towards common antibiotics. The obtained antibiograms were for two bacterial strains of *A. hydrophila*: antibiotic-resistant (R) and sensitive (S). Both strains were used to study the photodynamic efficacy of a new palladium phthalocyanine with peripheral methylpyridiloxy groups (pPdPc). In comparison, an effective photosensitizer, such as the zinc phthalocyanine complex (ZnPcMe), was investigated. In vitro studies with the new pPdPc showed similar efficacy for both strains of *A. hydrophila* at concentrations above 5 µM by irradiation with a 665 nm light source. The novelty in the uptake study is that the bacterial cells incubated with pPdPc accumulated similar values independently on the bacterial strain—resistant (R) or sensitive (S). This indicates the ability of an analogous inactivation capacity towards the studied strains. The non-specificity of the PDT action towards both strains with similar photocytotoxicity was also shown. In this study, it was shown that the new isolates of the Gram-negative *A. hydrophila* species, while are challenging for inactivation with antibiotics, are susceptible to PDT with Pd(II)- and Zn(II)-phthalocyanine complexes.

Author Contributions: Conceptualization, V.N.M. and V.K.; bacterial analysis, P.O. and V.K.; investigations, I.K., V.K. and L.D.; data curation, I.A. and V.N.M.; writing—original draft preparation, V.N.M., I.K. and V.K.; writing—review and editing, V.N.M., V.K., M.D. and H.N.; supervision, V.N.M., M.D. and H.N.; project administration, V.N.M. and I.A.; Funding acquisition, V.N.M. All authors have read and agreed to the published version of the manuscript.

Funding: This research study was supported by project KP-06-H29/11, 2018 and KP-06-H23/8, 2018 of the National Science Fund, Bulgaria.

Institutional Review Board Statement: Not applicable.

Informed Consent Statement: Not applicable.

Data Availability Statement: Not applicable.

Conflicts of Interest: The authors declare no conflict of interest. The funder had no role in the design of the study; in the collection, analyses, or interpretation of data; in the writing of the manuscript; or in the decision to publish the results.

References

1. Berendonk, T.U.; Manaia, C.M.; Merlin, C.; Fatta-Kassinos, D.; Cytryn, E.; Walsh, F.; Buergmann, H.; Sørum, H.; Norström, M.; Pons, M.-N.; et al. Tackling antibiotic resistance: The environmental framework. *Nat. Rev. Microbiol.* **2015**, *13*, 310–317. [CrossRef] [PubMed]
2. Conte, D.; Palmeiro, J.K.; Bavaroski, A.A.; Rodrigues, L.S.; Cardozo, D.; Tomaz, A.P.; Camargo, J.O.; Dalla-Costa, L.M. Antimicrobial resistance in Aeromonas species isolated from aquatic environments in Brazil. *J. Appl. Microbiol.* **2021**, *131*, 169–181. [CrossRef] [PubMed]
3. Varela, A.R.; Nunes, O.; Manaia, C.M. Quinolone resistant Aeromonas spp. as carriers and potential tracers of acquired antibiotic resistance in hospital and municipal wastewater. *Sci. Total Environ.* **2016**, *542*, 665–671. [CrossRef] [PubMed]
4. Skwor, T.; Shinko, J.; Augustyniak, A.; Gee, C.; Andraso, G. Aeromonas hydrophila and Aeromonas veronii Predominate among Potentially Pathogenic Ciprofloxacin- and Tetracycline-Resistant Aeromonas Isolates from Lake Erie. *Appl. Environ. Microbiol.* **2013**, *80*, 841–848. [CrossRef]
5. Navarro, A.; Martinez-Murcia, A. Phylogenetic analyses of the genus Aeromonas based on housekeeping gene sequencing and its influence on systematics. *J. Appl. Microbiol.* **2018**, *125*, 622–631. [CrossRef]
6. Scarafile, G. Antibiotic resistance: Current issues and future strategies. *Rev. Heal. Care* **2016**, *7*, 3–16. [CrossRef]
7. Baron, S.; Granier, S.A.; Larvor, E.; Jouy, E.; Cineux, M.; Wilhelm, A.; Gassilloud, B.; Le Bouquin, S.; Kempf, I.; Chauvin, C. Aeromonas Diversity and Antimicrobial Susceptibility in Freshwater—An Attempt to Set Generic Epidemiological Cut-Off Values. *Front. Microbiol.* **2017**, *8*, 503–509. [CrossRef]

8. Moura, Q.; Fernandes, M.R.; Cerdeira, L.; Santos, A.C.M.; de Souza, T.A.; Ienne, S.; Pignatari, A.C.C.; Gales, A.C.; Silva, R.M.; Lincopan, N. Draft genome sequence of a multidrug-resistant *Aeromonas hydrophila* ST508 strain carrying rmtD and blaCTX-M-131isolated from a bloodstream infection. *J. Glob. Antimicrob. Resist.* **2017**, *10*, 289–290. [CrossRef] [PubMed]
9. Sobotta, L.; Skupin-Mrugalska, P.; Piskorz, J.; Mielcarek, J. Porphyrinoid photosensitizers mediated photodynamic inactivation against bacteria. *Eur. J. Med. Chem.* **2019**, *175*, 72–106. [CrossRef]
10. Almeida-Marrero, V.; González-Delgado, J.A.; Torres, T. Emerging Perspectives on Applications of Porphyrinoids for Photodynamic Therapy and Photoinactivation of Microorganisms. *Macroheterocycles* **2019**, *12*, 8–16. [CrossRef]
11. Wainwrigh, M.; Maisch, T.; Nonell, S.; Plaetzer, K.; Almeida, A.; Tegos, G.P.; Hamblin, M.R. Photoantimicrobials—are we afraid of the light? *Lancet Infect. Dis.* **2017**, *17*, 49. [CrossRef]
12. Nasrin, S.; Hegerle, N.; Sen, S.; Nkeze, J.; Sen, S.; Permala-Booth, J.; Choi, M.; Sinclair, J.; Tapia, M.D.; Johnson, J.K.; et al. Distribution of serotypes and antibiotic resistance of invasive Pseudomonas aeruginosa in a multi-country collection. *BMC Microbiol.* **2022**, *22*, 1–12. [CrossRef]
13. Prochnow, E.P.; Martins, M.R.; Campagnolo, C.B.; Santos, R.C.; Villetti, M.A.; Kantorski, K.Z. Antimicrobial photodynamic effect of phenothiazinic photosensitizers in formulations with ethanol on Pseudomonas aeruginosa biofilms. *Photodiagnosis Photodyn. Ther.* **2015**, *13*, 291–296. [CrossRef] [PubMed]
14. Paronyan, M.H.; Koloyan, H.O.; Avetisyan, S.V.; Aganyants, H.A.; Hovsepyan, A. Study of the possible development of bacterial resistance to photodynamic in- activation. *Biol. J. Armen.* **2019**, *71*, 17–22.
15. Pedigo, L.A.; Gibbs, A.J.; Scott, R.J.; Street, C.N. Absence of bacterial resistance following repeat exposure to photodynamic therapy. In: Photodynamic Therapy: Back to the Future. *Int. Soc. Opt. Photonics* **2009**, *7380*, 73803.
16. Galstyan, A. Turning Photons into Drugs: Phthalocyanine-Based Photosensitizers as Efficient Photoantimicrobials. *Chem. Eur. J.* **2020**, *27*, 1903–1920. [CrossRef]
17. Spesia, M.B.; Durantini, E.N. Evolution of Phthalocyanine Structures as Photodynamic Agents for Bacteria Inactivation. *Chem. Rec.* **2022**, e202100292. [CrossRef] [PubMed]
18. Li, X.; Zheng, B.-D.; Peng, X.-H.; Li, S.-Z.; Ying, J.-W.; Zhao, Y.; Huang, J.-D.; Yoon, J. Phthalocyanines as medicinal photosensitizers: Developments in the last five years. *Coord. Chem. Rev.* **2019**, *379*, 147–160. [CrossRef]
19. Sen, P.; Mack, J.; Nyokong, T. Indium phthalocyanines: Comparative photophysicochemical properties and photodynamic antimicrobial activities against Staphylococcus aureus and Escherichia coli. *J. Mol. Struct.* **2021**, *1250*, 131850. [CrossRef]
20. Ogunsipe, A.; Nyokong, T. Photophysical and photochemical studies of sulphonated non-transition metal phthalocyanines in aqueous and non-aqueous media. *J. Photochem. Photobiol. A Chem.* **2005**, *173*, 211–220. [CrossRef]
21. Karanlık, C.C.; Atmaca, G.Y.; Erdoğmuş, A. Improved Singlet Oxygen Yields of New Palladium Phthalocyanines Using Sonochemistry and Comparisons with Photochemistry. *Polyhedron* **2021**, *206*, 115351. [CrossRef]
22. Kulu, I.; Mantareva, V.; Kussovski, V.; Angelov, I.; Durmuş, M. Effects of metal ion in cationic Pd(II) and Ni(II) phthalocyanines on physicochemical and photodynamic inactivation properties. *J. Mol. Struct.* **2021**, *1247*, 131288. [CrossRef]
23. Wöhrle, D.; Iskander, N.; Graschew, G.; Sinn, H.; Friedrich, E.A.; Maierborst, W.; Stern, M. Synthesis of positively charged phthalocyanines and their activity in the photodynamic therapy of cancer cells. *Photochem. Photobiol.* **1990**, *51*, 351–356. [CrossRef]
24. Remichkova, M.; Mukova, L.; Nikolaeva-Glomb, L.; Nikolova, N.; Doumanova, L.; Mantareva, V.; Angelov, I.; Kussovski, V.; Galabov, A.S. Virus inactivation under the photodynamic effect of phthalocyanine zinc(II) complexes. 2016, 72, 123–128. *Zeitschrift für Naturforschung C* **2016**, *72*, 123–128.
25. Nikolaeva-Glomb, L.; Mukova, L.; Nikolova, N.; Kussovski, V.; Doumanova, L.; Mantareva, V.; Angelov, I.; Wöhrle, D.; Galabov, A.S. Photodynamic Effect of some Phthalocyanines on Enveloped and Naked Viruses. *Acta Virol.* **2017**, *61*, 341–346. [CrossRef]
26. Mantareva, V.; Angelov, I.; Syuleyman, M.; Kussovski, V.; Eneva, I.; Avramov, L.; Borisova, E. Phthalocyanines Structure Versus Photodynamic Effectiveness towards Pathogenic Microorganisms: Our Recent Experience. *J. Biomed. Photonics Eng.* **2021**, *7*, 040202. [CrossRef]
27. Goni-Urriza, M.; Pineau, L.; Capdepuy, M.; Roques, C.; Caumette, P.; Quentin, C. Antimicrobial resistance of mesophilic *Aeromonas* spp. isolated from two European rivers. *J. Antimicrob. Chemoth.* **2000**, *46*, 297–301. [CrossRef] [PubMed]
28. Kussovski, V.; Mantareva, V.; Angelov, I.; Orozova, P.; Wöhrle, D.; Schnurpfeil, G.; Borisova, E.; Avramov, L. Photodynamic inactivation of Aeromonas hydrophila by cationic phthalocyanines with different hydrophobicity. *FEMS Microbiol. Lett.* **2009**, *294*, 133–140. [CrossRef] [PubMed]
29. Ribeiro, P.S.C.; Lourenço, M.O.L. Overview of cationic phthalocyanines for effective photoinactivation of pathogenic microorganisms. *J. Photochem. Photobiol. C Photochem. Rev.* **2021**, *48*, 100422. [CrossRef]
30. Le Guern, F.; Ouk, T.S.; Yerzhan, I.; Nurlykyz, Y.; Arnoux, P.; Frochot, C.; Leroy-Lhez, S.; Sol, V. Photophysical and Bactericidal Properties of Pyridinium and Imidazolium Porphyrins for Photodynamic Antimicrobial Chemotherapy. *Molecules* **2021**, *26*, 1122. [CrossRef]
31. Kwiatkowski, S.; Knap, B.; Przystupski, D.; Saczko, J.; Kędzierska, E.; Knap-Czop, K.; Kotlińska, J.; Michel, O.; Kotowski, K.; Kulbacka, J. Photodynamic therapy–Mechanisms, photosensitizers and combinations. *Biomed. Pharmacother.* **2018**, *106*, 1098–1107. [CrossRef]
32. Mantareva, V.; Kussovski, V.; Angelov, I. Cationic Metal Phthalocyanines as Effective Photosensitizers Towards Pathogenic Microorganisms. In *Photosensitizers: Types, Uses and Selected Research*; Withmire, C., Ed.; Nova Science Publishing Inc.: New York, NY, USA, 2016; p. 115.

33. Heredia, D.A.; Durantini, J.E.; Ferreyra, D.D.; Reynoso, E.; Gonzalez Lopez, E.J.; Durantini, A.M.; Milanesio, E.M.; Durantini, E.N. Charge density distribution effect in pyrrolidine-fused chlorins on microbial uptake and antimicrobial photoinactivation of microbial pathogens. *J. Photochem. Photobiol. B Biol.* **2021**, *225*, 11232. [CrossRef] [PubMed]
34. Rapacka-Zdończyk, A.; Woźniak, A.; Michalska, K.; Pierański, M.; Ogonowska, P.; Grinholc, M.; Nakonieczna, J. Factors Determining the Susceptibility of Bacteria to Antibacterial Photodynamic Inactivation. *Front. Med.* **2021**, *8*. [CrossRef] [PubMed]
35. Dogandzhiyska, V.; Dimitrov, S.L.; Angelov, I.; Mantareva, V.; Gueorgieva, T. Investigation of biocompatibility of Zn- and Ga-based Metal phthalocyanine and FotoSan ™ Photosensitizers, activated by laser light. *SYLWAN* **2021**, *165*, 151–163.
36. Gueorgieva, T.; Dimitrov, S.L.; Angelov, I.; Mantareva, V.; Dogandzhiyska, V. In Vivo study of the inflammatory reaction against three different laser light activated photosensitizers. *SYLWAN* **2021**, *165*, 126–136.

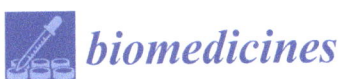

Article

N-Doped Graphene Quantum Dots/Titanium Dioxide Nanocomposites: A Study of ROS-Forming Mechanisms, Cytotoxicity and Photodynamic Therapy

Pravena Ramachandran [1], Boon-Keat Khor [2], Chong Yew Lee [2], Ruey-An Doong [3], Chern Ein Oon [4], Nguyen Thi Kim Thanh [5,6,*] and Hooi Ling Lee [1,7,*]

1. Nanomaterials Research Group, School of Chemical Sciences, Universiti Sains Malaysia (USM), Gelugor 11800, Penang, Malaysia; pravena@ioioleo.com
2. School of Pharmaceutical Sciences, Universiti Sains Malaysia (USM), Gelugor 11800, Penang, Malaysia; khorboonkeat@student.usm.my (B.-K.K.); chongyew@usm.my (C.Y.L.)
3. Institute of Analytical and Environmental Sciences, National Tsing Hua University, Hsinchu 30013, Taiwan; radoong@mx.nthu.edu.tw
4. Institute for Research in Molecular Medicine (INFORMM), Universiti Sains Malaysia (USM), Gelugor 11800, Penang, Malaysia; chern.oon@usm.my
5. Biophysics Group, Department of Physics and Astronomy, University College London, Gower Street, London WC1E 6BT, UK
6. UCL Healthcare Biomagnetics and Nanomaterials Laboratories, 21 Albemarle Street, London W1S 4BS, UK
7. School of Chemistry, The University of Sydney, Sydney, NSW 2006, Australia
* Correspondence: ntk.thanh@ucl.ac.uk (N.T.K.T.); hllee@usm.my (H.L.L.)

Citation: Ramachandran, P.; Khor, B.-K.; Lee, C.Y.; Doong, R.-A.; Oon, C.E.; Thanh, N.T.K.; Lee, H.L. N-Doped Graphene Quantum Dots/Titanium Dioxide Nanocomposites: A Study of ROS-Forming Mechanisms, Cytotoxicity and Photodynamic Therapy. *Biomedicines* **2022**, *10*, 421. https://doi.org/10.3390/biomedicines10020421

Academic Editors: Kyungsu Kang and Stefano Bacci

Received: 6 December 2021
Accepted: 9 January 2022
Published: 10 February 2022

Publisher's Note: MDPI stays neutral with regard to jurisdictional claims in published maps and institutional affiliations.

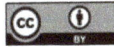

Copyright: © 2022 by the authors. Licensee MDPI, Basel, Switzerland. This article is an open access article distributed under the terms and conditions of the Creative Commons Attribution (CC BY) license (https://creativecommons.org/licenses/by/4.0/).

Abstract: Titanium dioxide nanoparticles (TiO_2 NPs) have been proven to be potential candidates in cancer therapy, particularly photodynamic therapy (PDT). However, the application of TiO_2 NPs is limited due to the fast recombination rate of the electron (e^-)/hole (h^+) pairs attributed to their broader bandgap energy. Thus, surface modification has been explored to shift the absorption edge to a longer wavelength with lower e^-/h^+ recombination rates, thereby allowing penetration into deep-seated tumors. In this study, TiO_2 NPs and N-doped graphene quantum dots (QDs)/titanium dioxide nanocomposites (N-GQDs/TiO_2 NCs) were synthesized via microwave-assisted synthesis and the two-pot hydrothermal method, respectively. The synthesized anatase TiO_2 NPs were self-doped TiO_2 (Ti^{3+} ions), have a small crystallite size (12.2 nm) and low bandgap energy (2.93 eV). As for the N-GQDs/TiO_2 NCs, the shift to a bandgap energy of 1.53 eV was prominent as the titanium (IV) tetraisopropoxide (TTIP) loading increased, while maintaining the anatase tetragonal crystal structure with a crystallite size of 11.2 nm. Besides, the cytotoxicity assay showed that the safe concentrations of the nanomaterials were from 0.01 to 0.5 mg mL^{-1}. Upon the photo-activation of N-GQDs/TiO_2 NCs with near-infrared (NIR) light, the nanocomposites generated reactive oxygen species (ROS), mainly singlet oxygen ($^1O_2$), which caused more significant cell death in MDA-MB-231 (an epithelial, human breast cancer cells) than in HS27 (human foreskin fibroblast). An increase in the N-GQDs/TiO_2 NCs concentrations elevates ROS levels, which triggered mitochondria-associated apoptotic cell death in MDA-MB-231 cells. As such, titanium dioxide-based nanocomposite upon photoactivation has a good potential as a photosensitizer in PDT for breast cancer treatment.

Keywords: titanium dioxide; N-doped graphene quantum dots; photodynamic therapy; near-infrared light; reactive oxygen species; apoptosis

1. Introduction

In recent years, scientists have focused on nanoparticle research in the biomedical field, particularly in cancer therapies. Nanoparticles offer numerous advantages as they can easily penetrate tissues, cross cellular barriers, preferentially localize and accumulate at tumor sites and are able to overcome instant clearance by the lymphatic system [1]. Nanoparticles can play multiple roles, as they can be used for diagnosis and therapy simultaneously. Metal or metal oxide nanoparticles can generate ROS in the presence of light illumination to induce cell death [2,3]. Acting as a photosensitizer or nanocarrier, metal oxides exhibit relatively good stability when compared to existing organic nanoparticles (liposomes, dendrimers, polymer-based NPs), with regard to temperature and pH change [4,5].

An optical irradiation-induced generation of ROS by a photosensitizer that promotes cell killing is known as photodynamic therapy (PDT). PDT is an emerging non-invasive, clinically approved and localized therapy for several diseases, including cancers. PDT surpasses existing traditional cancer treatments as it can be specifically targeted, is non-invasive, causes negligible drug resistance and is highly effective with fewer adverse side effects [6].

The efficacy of PDT depends on the type of photosensitizing agents employed. Numerous inorganic and organic materials such as cadmium selenide (CdSe), chlorin e6 (Ce6), hypocrellin A (HA), inorganic [7] and porphyrin-based materials and organic materials [8], were explored as photosensitizing agents in PDT for cancer treatments. However, most of these materials have drawbacks including poor water dispersibility and photostability, as well as the inability to absorb at longer wavelengths (>700 nm), which restricts light penetration leading to the imprecision of their cell-killing potential. This leads to undesirable toxicity, potentially causing damage to both cancer and non-cancerous cells/tissues.

The application of metal oxide nanoparticles as a photosensitizer has been extensively studied due to the limitations of existing porphyrin-based photosensitizers. Upon administration via tumoral injection, nanoparticle-based drugs are preferentially taken up and accumulate at the tumor sites due to the enhanced permeability and retention (EPR) effect, a condition where tumors possess unusually leaky blood vessels and an impaired lymphatic system [9]. Thus, it offers an effective method to precisely locate and cause tumor cell destruction simultaneously, preventing overdose of photosensitizers with controllable treatment duration.

Among the existing metal oxide nanoparticles, TiO_2 NPs have attracted considerable research interest due to their unique photocatalytic properties that can be utilized to kill cancer cells upon illumination. When TiO_2 NPs are irradiated with an energy equal to or greater than the bandgap of TiO_2 (3.2 eV), the electrons (e^-) in the valence band (VB) of TiO_2 are excited to the conduction band (CB), creating positive holes (h^+) in the VB. This occurrence leads to a redox reaction on the surface of these semiconductor nanoparticles resulting in the generation of ROS, comprising of superoxide anions ($O_2^{-\bullet}$), hydroxyl radicals ($^\bullet OH$) and hydrogen peroxide (H_2O_2) [10,11].

Meanwhile, as an inorganic photosensitizer, TiO_2 is more stable than classic photosensitizers in performing PDT. This trait is attributed to the nanoscale size and anti-photodegradable stability of TiO_2. It has been reported that TiO_2 NPs were used as a PDT agent in various types of cancer cells, such as human hepatocellular carcinoma cell line (HepG2) [12], leukemia cells (K592) [13], cervical cancer cells (HeLa) [14], breast epithelial cells (MCF7 and MDA-MB-468) [15], as well as non-small cell lung cancer (NSCLC) [16]. Despite their excellent performance as photosensitizers, their potential toxicity is still an obstacle to their application in PDT [17,18]. Furthermore, the activation of pristine TiO_2 is triggered upon shorter wavelength UV light irradiation to generate ROS.

To overcome the shortcomings of TiO_2, depositing quantum dots onto TiO_2 has received the utmost attention due to their distinctive properties. Modifying the surface properties of TiO_2 with QDs will assist in extending the light absorption properties of TiO_2 to longer wavelengths. Therefore, this will allow deeper penetration into tissues. TiO_2 modified with transition metals (Cu, Zn) and metal oxides (ZnO, NiO) often induce additional ROS generation in the absence of light irradiation. Moreover, incorporating noble metals such as Ag and Pt is considered to be more effective due to their high stability and anti-cancer activity, but their high cost restricts the application [19–24]. Generally, in PDT, QDs possess a dual-function nature as an energy transducer and as carriers of photosensitizers [25]. Sensitizing TiO_2 with metal chalcogenides quantum dots such as

CdSe, cadmium sulfide (CdS), lead sulfide (PbS), cadmium telluride (CdTe) and copper oxide (CuO) inevitably impede their benefits [26–30]. Most of these QDs of group II–VI contain highly toxic heavy metals that are unstable and induce toxicity, which causes environmental hazards. Thus, incorporating TiO_2 with carbonaceous-material-based QDs has been identified as a potential approach. Therefore, the utilization of N-GQDs to modify TiO_2 surfaces has great research interest. Besides, heteroatom doping (N atom) of GQDs results in high quantum yield, good stability, and higher catalytic activity, by tuning their electrochemical properties [31]. Good biocompatibility properties of N-GQDs will help to reduce the toxicity of TiO_2 in the absence of light illumination, which warrants further exploration in PDT as a photosensitizer [32]. Furthermore, as a carrier, N-GQDs ensure precise localization of the potential N-GQDs/TiO_2 NCs at the site of the tumor and, therefore, avoid harm to non-cancerous cells. Thus, the incorporation of TiO_2 with N-GQDs holds great promise in PDT.

Herein, in this study, TiO_2 NPs and TiO_2 conjugated with N-GQDs (N-GQDs/TiO_2 NCs) were synthesized via microwave-assisted synthesis and two-pot hydrothermal method, respectively. Their corresponding in vitro cytotoxicity was studied using the MDA-MB-231 Triple-negative breast cancer (TNBC) breast cancer cell line and HS27 human fibroblast cell line to evaluate the cellular response towards the nanostructures. TNBC is an aggressive subtype with a poor prognosis. In order to assess the impact of the nanocomposite, we have chosen a more aggressive type than the conventional MCF-7 cells. Although chemotherapy remains the mainstay for the treatment of TNBC, systemic toxicity and adverse effects associated with chemotherapy highlight the need for an alternative theory. As such, MDA-MB-231 TNBC (mentioned as MDA-MB-231 from now onward) was employed as the cell model to be evaluated in the current proposed photodynamic therapy. The photodynamic activity of the near-infrared light active-N-GQDs/TiO_2 NCs was evaluated by monitoring the in vitro photokilling effects on the cells under light irradiation and the mechanisms where the nanocomposites possessed photokilling properties were investigated.

2. Materials and Methods

2.1. Materials

Citric acid-1-hydrate (Bendosen, Laboratory Chemicals, Johor Bahru, Malaysia); ethylenediamine; glycerol; ethanol, 98%; hydrochloric acid, HCl 37%; phosphate-buffered saline (PBS) (QREC, Grade AR, (Asia) Sdn. Bhd, Rawang, Selangor, Malaysia); titanium(IV) tetraisopropoxide, TTIP ≥ 97% purity; commercial pure anatase, ≥99%; sodium pyruvate; dimethyl sulfoxide, DMSO; 1,4-benzoquinone (Sigma-Aldrich, Co., St. Louis, MO, USA); phosphate buffered saline (PBS) (Sigma-Aldrich, Co., Taufkirchen, Germany); Dulbecco's modified Eagle's medium, DMEM; penicillin-streptomycin solution, 10,000 units/mL (Nacalai Tesque, Nakagyo-ku, Kyoto, Japan); fetal bovine serum (FBS) (TICO Europe, DJ, Amstelveen, The Netherlands); CellTiter 96® AQueous One Solution Cell Proliferation Assay (MTS); Caspase-Glo® 3/7 Assay (Promega, Madison, WI, USA); 2′,7′-dichlorofluorescein diacetate (DCFDA, Merck-Millipore, Burlington, MA, USA); tetramethylrhodamine ethyl ester; TMRE-Mitochondrial Membrane Potential Assay Kit (Abcam, Trumpington, Cambridge CB2 0AX, UK) were used as purchased without any further purification.

2.2. Synthesis of TiO_2 NPs

The TiO_2 NPs were prepared according to the methodology developed by our laboratory [32]. Briefly, 2 mL of TTIP was hydrolyzed and stirred vigorously at room temperature. The pH of the homogenous mixture was adjusted to 1.3 by adding 37% hydrochloric acid with constant stirring for 30 min. The entire mixture was then transferred to a 100 mL sealed vessel made of high-purity TFM (modified Teflon), which was heated in the commercial microwave digestion system (Multiwave 3000 Anton Paar, Graz, Austria) at 600 W for 20 min. The resulting precipitate was washed with distilled water for several cycles and isolated through centrifugation (8500 rpm, 10 min), followed by drying in the oven at 50 °C for 24 h. The dried TiO$_2$ NPs were annealed at 500 °C for 2 h.

2.3. Synthesis of N-GQDs/TiO$_2$ NCs

The N-GQDs/TiO$_2$ NCs were synthesized using the methodology developed previously [32]. Briefly, 3 mL of TTIP in 50 mL distilled water was continuously stirred for 30 min before transferring into a Teflon-lined stainless-steel autoclave (capacity = 100 mL). The mixture in the stainless hydrothermal reactor was heated in the oven at 160 °C for 24 h. The obtained sol was washed in distilled water and placed in a beaker containing 50 mL distilled water. Then, citric acid and ethylenediamine were added simultaneously into the magnetically stirred sol for 30 min, followed by hydrothermal treatment at 180 °C for 4 h. The obtained precipitate was washed, centrifuged and dried in a vacuum oven at 60 °C overnight.

2.4. Characterizations

The powder X-ray diffraction (XRD) technique was used to analyze the crystallographic structure, crystallinity and phase purity of the synthesized samples. The XRD patterns were recorded on a PW 3040/60 X'PERT PRO, PANalytical using CuKα (1.5406 Å) radiation in the range 2θ = 10–90°. Besides, X-ray photoelectron spectroscopy (XPS) was used to identify the surface composition of the synthesized materials. A High-Resolution Multi Technique X-Ray Spectrometer (Axis Ultra DLD XPS, Kratos) with monochromatic Al Kα (1486.6 eV), X-ray radiation (15 kV and 10 mA) and equipped with a hemispherical analyzer which operated at 150 W was used to analyses the materials. Curve fitting was accomplished using OriginPro (version 8.5), whereby all the obtained binding energy (BE) was calibrated using the C 1s line at 284.6 eV. Meanwhile, a Perkin Elmer Lamda 35 was used to record ultraviolet-visible diffuse reflectance (UV-Vis DRS) spectra of the samples.

2.5. Cell Culture and the Conditions

MDA-MB-231 was obtained from Dr. Chern Ein Oon (INFORMM, USM); meanwhile, HS27 was obtained from the Centre for Drug Research, USM. The MDA-MB-231 and HS27 cells were cultured in DMEM medium and DMEM high glucose medium, respectively, were then supplemented with 10% FBS and 1% penicillin–streptomycin, and incubated at 37 °C with 5% CO$_2$ and 90% humidity.

2.6. Cytotoxicity Assay

The in vitro cytotoxicity assay of nanomaterials was performed using an MTS assay following the manufacturer's protocol. The cells were seeded in 96-well plate (10,000 cells/well) and treated with cell culture medium containing different concentrations of nanomaterials (0.01, 0.05, 0.1, 0.5 and 1.0 mg mL^{-1}) for 24 h. Then, the MTS solution was added to each well, followed by incubation for 4 h. The absorbance of each well at 490 nm was recorded using a Multiskan Go UV microplate reader (ThermoFisher Scientific, Waltham, MA, USA). The cells that were incubated with cell culture medium without any treatment were referred to as the control group. The results are expressed in mean ± standard deviation (SD) as a percentage compared to control. The cell viability was calculated according to the following Equation (1).

$$\text{Percentage of viable cells (\%)} = \frac{\text{Absorbance (Treated)} - \text{Absorbance (Blank)}}{\text{Absorbance (Untreated)} - \text{Absorbance (Blank)}} \times 100\% \quad (1)$$

2.7. Photokilling Effects of N-GQDs/TiO$_2$ NCs on MDA-MB-231 and HS27 Cells

To study the photokilling effects, cells seeded in 96-well plates were incubated with a medium containing 0.05–0.5 mg mL^{-1} N-GQDs/TiO$_2$ NCs for 3 h in the dark. Then, the cells were washed with PBS and re-suspended in a fresh medium. The cells were irradiated with 20 W tungsten halogen lamp with an ultraviolet and visible cut-off filter eliminating UV-Vis light λ < 700 nm, resulting in NIR (700–900 nm) at 55 mW cm^{-2}, which then resulted in light energies of 16.5, 33 and 66 J cm^{-2} for 5, 10 and 20 min, respectively. The light intensity was measured using a Solar Light PMA2100 Dual-Input Data Logging Radiometer. The irradiated cells were then incubated in the dark for 24 h. After the incubation period, the cell viability was determined using the MTS assay. The results are expressed in mean ± SD as a percentage compared to control.

2.8. Measurement of Reactive Oxygen Species (ROS) Level

2.8.1. Measurement of Intracellular ROS Levels

The intracellular levels of ROS were measured by exposing the cells to different concentrations of N-GQDs/TiO$_2$ NCs for 3 h, were washed with PBS and then re-suspended in a fresh DMEM medium. The cells were then irradiated for 20 min and incubated at 37 °C for 4 h. Five mM of DCFDA was used as a stock, then 5 µL of 5 mM DCFDA was further diluted in 5 mL medium to make up the final concentration of 5 µM. After the incubation, the medium was replaced with 100 µL of 5 µM DCFDA solution and incubated at 37 °C for 1 h. Then, the DCFDA solution was removed, washed with PBS before incubating with 1% Triton-X lysis buffer (100 µL) for 30 min. Thereafter, lysed cells were centrifuged at 10,000 rpm for 15 min. The suspension was harvested and placed into 96-well plates. Clean lysis buffer acted as a blank control and was prepared in parallel with samples. The fluorescent intensity was measured using a Plate Chameleon™ Multitechnology plate reader at excitation and emission wavelengths of 485 nm and 535 nm, respectively. The data are expressed in mean ± SD as a percentage compared to control.

2.8.2. Measurement of Specific Types of ROS

To evaluate the specific types of ROS generated by N-GQDs/TiO$_2$ NCs with light irradiation, several ROS quenchers for specific ROS were used, including sodium pyruvate, DMSO, 1,4-benzoquinone and glycerol for the detection of H_2O_2, $^{\bullet}OH$, $O_2^{-\bullet}$ and $^1O_2/O_2^{-\bullet}$, respectively. First, 100 µL of 0.5 mg mL^{-1} N-GQDs/TiO$_2$ NCs in PBS were mixed with 50 µL DCFDA (without quenchers) and irradiated with light. The fluorescent intensities of DCFDA were recorded, and a linear plot of intensity versus time was plotted with a slope noted as S_{ref}. Then, several specific ROS quenchers (10 mM sodium pyruvate, 0.28 M DMSO, 10 mM 1,4-benzoquinone and 5 vol % glycerol) were respectively added into the sample solution containing DCFDA before irradiation [33–35]. For the light-irradiated sample solutions, the level of ROS generated in the presence of quenchers was measured with an interval of 5 min for 20 min using a Plate Chameleon TM Multitechnology plate reader at excitation and an emission wavelength of 485 nm and 535 nm, respectively. The slope of the linear line plotted based on the results obtained is expressed as S_q. The results are expressed in mean ± SD as a percentage compared to control. Thus, the specific ROS percentage was calculated according to the following Equation (2).

$$\text{ROS generated (\%)} = \left(1 - \frac{S_q}{S_{ref}}\right) \times 100\% \qquad (2)$$

2.9. Measurement of Caspase-3/7 Activity

Caspase-3/7 activity in the cells was assessed using Caspase-Glo® 3/7 reagent following the manufacturer's protocol. The treated and non-treated MDA-MB-231 cells were washed with PBS and re-suspended in a fresh DMEM medium. Thereafter the light irradiation, the cells were incubated for 24 h. A 100 µL of Caspase-Glo® 3/7 reagent was added to each well, followed by 3 h incubation at room temperature in the dark. Non-treatment cells were used as a control in this assay. The luminescence readings were then measured using the M5 multi-detection microplate reader. The data were expressed in mean ± SD as percentage compared to control.

2.10. Measurement of Mitochondrial Activity

To further study the mitochondrial activity of the cells after the PDT treatment, a tetramethylrhodamine ethyl ester (TMRE) assay was used following the manufacturer's protocol. Briefly, 1 µM TMRE (100 µL) was added to each well of the control and PDT-treated MDA-MB-231 cells. Then, the fluorescent readings were then measured using the M5 multi-detection microplate reader at excitation and an emission wavelength of 544 nm and 590 nm, respectively. The data are expressed in mean ± SD as percentage compared to control.

2.11. Statistical Analysis

The data are presented as the mean ± SD of two independent experiments, each performed in triplicate. The statistically significant differences in cell viability ($p < 0.05$) were analyzed using an ANOVA by GraphPad Prism 5.0 software, California. The ANOVA test is carried out to compare the statistical differences among different cell groups (control cells, HS27 and MDA-MB-231 cells).

3. Results and Discussion

3.1. X-ray Powder Diffraction

The XRD analysis was executed to study the crystallographic properties of pure TiO_2 NPs and N-GQDs/TiO_2 NCs. The XRD patterns of TiO_2 NPs and N-GQDs/TiO_2 NCs are depicted in Figure 1. The Figure 1 shows the reflection of (101), (004), (200), (105), (211), (204), (116), (220), (215) and (224) peaks at 2θ values of 25.27°, 37.79°, 48.21°, 54.40°, 55.06°, 62.56°, 68.85°, 70.25°, 75.16° and 82.88°, respectively, which correspond to the formation of the pure single-phase of anatase TiO_2 NPs with tetragonal structure (space group, I41/amd, lattice parameter, a = b = 0.378 nm and c = 0.951 nm), which are indexed based on ICSD 01-071-1166. Similarly, the diffraction peaks of TiO_2 incorporated with N-GQDs were in good agreement with the typical diffraction pattern of anatase phase TiO_2 (ICSD 01-071-1166) and the obtained XRD pattern matched well with as-synthesized TiO_2 NPs. The (101) planes, prominently reflected in the XRD pattern of the nanomaterials, were in good agreement with the measured lattice spacing of 0.351 nm, as reported in our previous work [32]. The obtained findings suggest that the structure and phase purity of TiO_2 remained intact, as N-GQDs were incorporated on the surface of the TiO_2, and not into the TiO_2 lattice. Moreover, no additional peaks attributed to the N-GQDs were observed in all the nanocomposite samples. This observation could be due to the lower concentration of N-GQDs and relatively low diffraction intensity of graphene (2θ ~ 25.60°) in the nanocomposites, thus, these might be shielded by the major peak in the anatase phase TiO_2 (2θ = 25.26°) [36]. Besides, it can be observed that the intensity of the diffraction peaks' height declined with the incorporation of N-GQDs, due to the low crystalline nature of the N-GQDs [37].

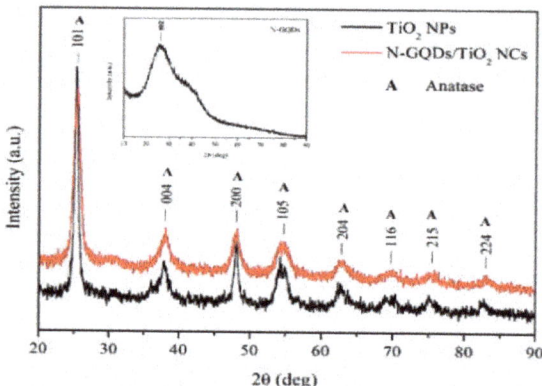

Figure 1. X-ray diffractograms synthesized TiO_2 NPs and N-GQDs/TiO_2 NCs. The inset shows the X-ray diffractograms of N-GQDs.

Table S1 presents the crystallite size, lattice parameters and lattice strain calculated from XRD data obtained for both samples. The obtained results depict that the average crystallite size (Scherrer equation) of N-GQDs/TiO$_2$ NCs decreased when compared to the pure TiO$_2$ NPs, which can be attributed to the confinement effect of graphene sheets that were ascribed to the size change in the sp^2 domains, similar to the reported studies [38,39]. The obtained results are further supported by the average particle size obtained based on the high resolution transmission electron microscopic (HRTEM) analysis (TiO$_2$ NPs = 11.46 ± 2.8 nm, N-GQDs/TiO$_2$ NCs = 9.16 ± 2.4 nm) [32]. Moreover, the lattice parameters a and c correspond to the respective XRD patterns of the TiO$_2$ NPs, and N-GQDs/TiO$_2$ NCs were in accordance with the reference data of the anatase tetragonal structure (ICSD 01-071-1166). The incorporation of N-GQDs onto the surface of TiO$_2$ poses no influence on the lattice parameters. Meanwhile, the calculated lattice strain of N-GQDs/TiO$_2$ NCs was higher than that of TiO$_2$ NPs, due to the smaller crystallite size and a lower degree of crystallinity, ascribed to the lower crystalline nature of N-GQDs in the nanocomposite [40]. Thus, conjugation of N-GQDs into TiO$_2$ lowers the crystallinity and particle size, which induces additional strain without altering the lattice parameter values.

3.2. UV-Visible Diffuse Reflectance Spectroscopy (UV-Vis DRS)

The calculated bandgap curves of TiO$_2$ NPs and N-GQDs/TiO$_2$ NCs are shown in Figure 2. The spectrum of anatase TiO$_2$ is also shown for better comparison. The bandgaps were obtained based on the Kubelka-Munk rule by plotting $(khv)^{1/2}$ versus photon energy (hv). Based on the results obtained, it was found that all N-GQDs incorporated into TiO$_2$ recorded lower bandgap energies than that of synthesized TiO$_2$ (2.91 eV) and commercial pure anatase TiO$_2$ (3.20 eV). The reduction in the bandgap of the as-synthesized TiO$_2$ NPs is attributed to surface defects due to the presence of surface oxygen vacancies and Ti^{3+} self-doping, which was further confirmed by XPS analysis in Section 3.3. Moreover, the bandgap value of TiO$_2$ NPs reflects that it can be activated upon the visible light source. Besides, as no Ti^{3+} environment was found in the Ti 2p spectra of the nanocomposite (Section 3.3), therefore the significant blue-shift in the bandgap energy of the N-GQDs/TiO$_2$ NCs is attributed to the existence of Ti-O-C bonding between N-GQDs and TiO$_2$ [41,42]. This interaction facilitates an efficient interfacial charge transfer process between TiO$_2$ and N-GQDs. This phenomenon further ensures the prolonged lifetime of the excited states due to the improved charge separation in the nanocomposites. This observation implies that the introduction of N-GQDs onto the surface of TiO$_2$ has shifted the optical bandgap, which enables the nanocomposite to generate e^-/h^+ pairs even though they have been irradiated with longer, non-toxic NIR light.

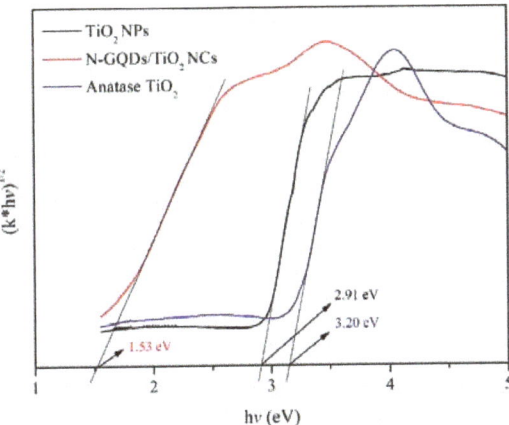

Figure 2. The bandgap of synthesized TiO$_2$ NPs, N-GQDs/TiO$_2$ NCs and anatase TiO$_2$.

3.3. X-ray Photoelectron Spectroscopy (XPS)

XPS was employed to study the surface composition and chemical states of TiO_2 NPs and N-GQDs/TiO_2 NCs. The resulting high-resolution XPS spectra depict Ti 2p, O 1s and C 1s states for both samples. Meanwhile, an additional XPS spectrum of N 1s was recorded for N-GQDs/TiO_2 NCs. The Ti 2p spectrum of both samples show two prominent peaks at ~458.0 eV and ~464.0 eV, assigned to Ti $2p_{3/2}$ and Ti $2p_{1/2}$ spin-orbital splitting photoelectrons, respectively (Figure 3a,b). It was found that there was a blue-shift of 0.3 eV in both Ti^{4+} $2p_{3/2}$ (458.3 eV) and Ti^{4+} $2p_{1/2}$ (464.0 eV) peaks in the N-GQDs/TiO_2 NCs when compared with those in the synthesized TiO_2 spectrum (Ti^{4+} $2p_{3/2}$ = 458.6 eV and Ti^{4+} $2p_{1/2}$ = 464.3 eV). This shifting might be due to the formation of Ti-O-C bonds [43,44]. Besides, further deconvolution of Ti 2p of TiO_2 NPs resulted in another two peaks which are Ti^{3+} $2p_{3/2}$ (458.0 eV) and Ti^{3+} $2p^{1/2}$ (463.3 eV), while no Ti^{3+} state was observed in N-GQDs/TiO_2 NCs. With the appearance of the Ti^{3+} state, it suggests the as-synthesized TiO_2 NPs are self-doped TiO_2. Enhanced microwave power irradiation could lead to the conversion of Ti^{4+} to Ti^{3+} by forming oxygen vacancies. Generally, microwave energy can increase the heating rate. Thus, conducting the reaction at higher microwave power will result in a higher rate of hydrolysis and condensation of the TTIP precursor [45]. Besides, as the condensation rate increased, it increases the formation of oxygen vacancy and Ti^{3+} ions by removing more surface oxygen. Meanwhile, the excess electrons from oxygen vacancies are trapped on Ti^{4+} ions to form Ti^{3+} species. The proposed formation mechanism of oxygen vacancies and Ti^{3+} ions is shown in Figure S1.

Whereas, for the O 1s spectra (Figure 3c,d), it was found that several chemical states of oxygen were present in the samples. Both samples exhibited the main peak centered at 529.0 eV, assigned to the lattice oxygen (Ti-O-Ti). Another peak, observed at 531.1 eV for TiO_2 NPs, corresponds to the hydroxyl group that adsorbed on the surface of the TiO_2 [45,46]. Additionally, a peak at 531.5 eV is assigned to the Ti-O-C bonds in N-GQDs/TiO_2 NCs, suggesting that the N-GQDs and TiO_2 were probably coupled via Ti-O-C bonds, which could promote interfacial electron transfer [47,48].

Meanwhile, the C 1s spectra of TiO_2 NPs and N-GQDs/TiO_2 NCs (Figure 3e,f) were deconvoluted and fitted with two and four peaks, respectively. A strong peak at 284.6 eV and a shoulder peak at 285.6 eV in TiO_2 NPs are attributed to the adventitious carbon of the carbon tape attached to the sample holder and residual carbon that was associated with the carbon residues from the TTIP precursor, respectively [43,49]. Furthermore, the peak at 284.7 eV in N-GQDs/TiO_2 NCs was assigned to sp^2 hybridized carbon atoms (C=C) in the honeycomb lattice structure of N-GQDs.

Moreover, three peaks, centered at 285.5 eV, 286.1 eV and 288.8 eV, were ascribed to a C-N bond with sp^2 orbital, C-OH (hydroxyl carbon) and O-C=O (carboxylate carbon), respectively. There was no Ti-C carbide bond-related peak (~282 eV) observed in the C 1s spectrum of N-GQDs/TiO_2 NCs [50]. This finding further implies the anchoring of N-GQDs on the surface of TiO_2 via Ti-O-C bond formation.

Furthermore, an additional N 1s spectrum was observed for N-GQDs/TiO_2 NCs and it was fitted into two peaks (Figure 3g). The main peak at 400.3 eV is attributed to the pyrrolic N and the peak at 401.1 eV corresponds to graphitic N within the graphene lattice [37,51]. The absence of a Ti-N bond (~396 eV) in the N 1s spectrum indicates that TiO_2 was not doped with N atoms, while it reaffirms the presence of N atoms doped into the graphene lattice [52].

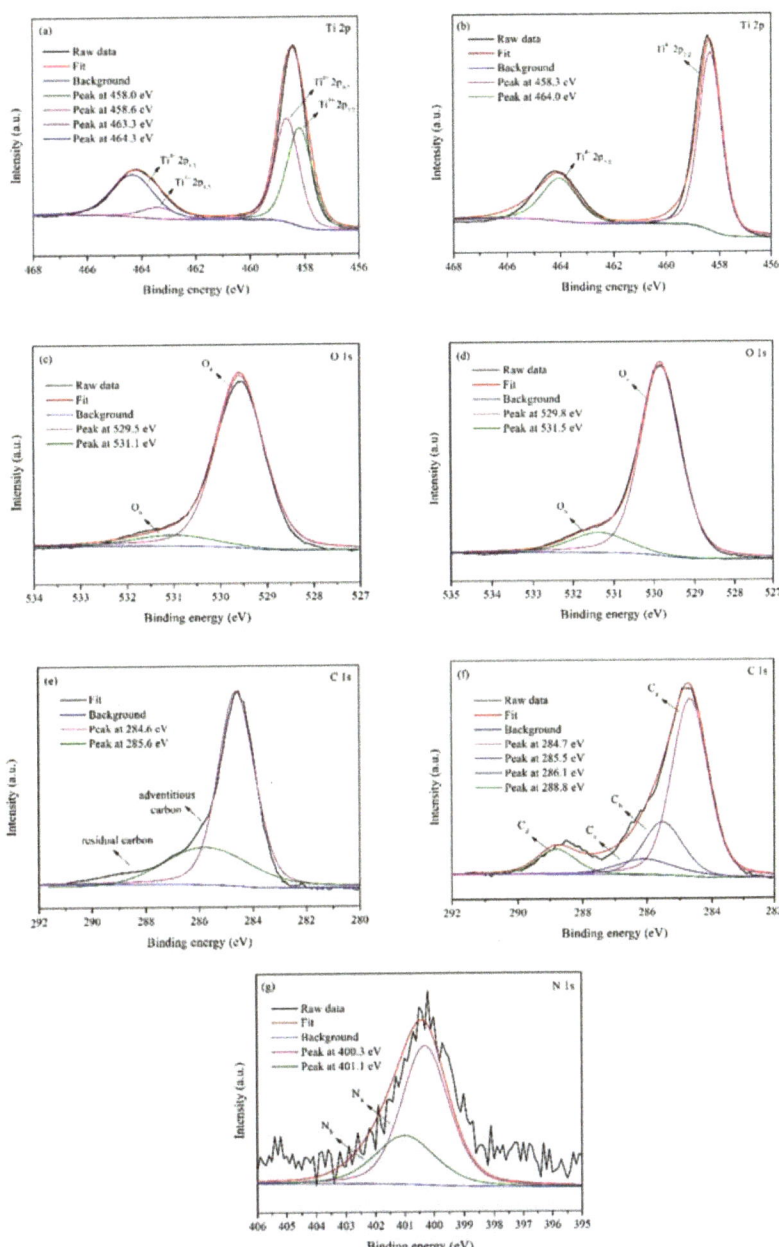

Figure 3. High-resolution XPS spectra of Ti 2p of synthesised (**a**) TiO_2 NPs and (**b**) N-GQDs/TiO_2 NCs, O 1s of synthesized (**c**) TiO_2 NPs and (**d**) N-GQDs/TiO_2 NCs, C 1s of synthesised (**e**) TiO_2 NPs and (**f**) N-GQDs/TiO_2 NCs, (**g**) N 1s of synthesized N-GQDs/TiO_2 NCs.

3.4. Characterisation of the Nanomaterials in Cell Culture Treatment, Their In Vitro Cytotoxicity Assessment and Photodynamic Therapy

The behavior of the nanomaterials in the cell culture environment and their interaction with biological substrates were studied by determining their respective hydrodynamic size and zeta potential in the deionized water (DI water) and cell culture medium (Supplementary Figure S2). Overall, nanomaterials dispersed in DMEM without any dispersing agent resulted in a higher hydrodynamic size than in DI water, due to higher ionic strength content in the cell culture medium. Meanwhile, there was a significant decrease in the hydrodynamic size of the nanomaterials dispersed in complete cell culture medium (DMEM + 1% FBS). This effect is attributed to the formation of protein corona, which provides electrostatic repulsion between particles. These findings are in good agreement with previously reported works [13,20]. Furthermore, hydrodynamic sizes of 0.1 mg mL^{-1} N-GQDs/TiO$_2$ NCs (49.2 $\pm$ 4.5 nm) dispersed in complete cell culture medium were observed to be smaller than for TiO$_2$ NPs (51.1 $\pm$ 3.3 nm). Consistent with the obtained hydrodynamic size, the zeta potential values of 0.1 mg mL^{-1} N-GQDs/TiO$_2$ NCs (-23.2 ± 2.1 mV) in a medium containing 1% FBS were more negatively charged than for TiO$_2$ NPs (-21.5 ± 1.6 mV), suggesting nanocomposite disaggregation. Moreover, N-GQDs (0.1 mg mL^{-1}) dispersed in complete cell culture medium have the smallest hydrodynamic size (11.8 $\pm$ 5.2 nm) and a large negative value of zeta potential (-30.0 ± 2.7 mV), which leads to good dispersion of the quantum dots. These properties of N-GQDs improve the dispersibility of the TiO$_2$ in the nanocomposite [32].

In this study, the in vitro cytotoxicity of TiO$_2$ NPs and N-GQDs/TiO$_2$ NCs (0.01, 0.05, 0.1, 0.5 and 1.0 mg mL^{-1}) were evaluated using MDA-MB-231 and HS27 cells for 24 h.

The reason we conducted the PDT reaction for 24 h was due to the significant drop in the cell viability after 48 h treatment when compared to 24 h without light irradiation, based on our previous study [32]. Cytotoxicity of nanocomposites in the absence of light is a critical property before PDT treatment. Similarly, other work also studied the 24 h PDT of TiO$_2$ that was conjugated with reduced graphene oxide [12]. The MDA-MB-231 cells were used as a cancer cell model, while HS27 represented a non-cancerous cell, control model to test the cytotoxicity of the nanomaterials. As shown in Figure 4a,b, the viability of the cells after 24 h incubation was not significantly altered as the concentration of TiO$_2$ NPs increased from 0.05 to 0.5 mg mL^{-1}, then, at 1.0 mg mL^{-1}, there was a 29% and 23% decrease in viability of MDA-MB-231 and HS27 cells, respectively. Moreover, when compared to the control group, the lower concentrations of nanoparticles (0.05–0.1 mg mL^{-1}) did not exhibit a significant growth inhibitory effect in the cell viability of both cell lines. Moreover, the cell viability trend of the synthesized nanocomposites was similar to that of TiO$_2$ NPs at lower concentrations (0.01–0.1 mg mL^{-1}). However, it increased significantly at 0.5 and 1.0 mg mL^{-1} when compared to TiO$_2$ NPs in both cell lines. Furthermore, this observation indicates that TiO$_2$ NPs exhibit a more prominent toxicity level than the nanocomposites (0.5 mg mL^{-1} ($p < 0.01$) & 1.0 mg mL^{-1} ($p < 0.001$)), which is attributed to their distinct characteristics (particle size, crystallinity and composition) in both cell lines [53,54]. Meanwhile, as for the nanocomposite, good biocompatibility characteristics of N-GQDs (0.5 mg mL^{-1} ($p < 0.05$) & 1.0 mg mL^{-1} ($p < 0.01$)) after 24 h post-treatment helps to mitigate the toxicity effects of TiO$_2$ (Supplementary Figure S3). Based on the obtained results, it has been proven that incorporating N-GQDs into TiO$_2$ did not render any additional toxicity to the nanocomposite when compared to TiO$_2$ NPs after 24 h post-treatment [32]. The initial cell viability study presents the safe concentration from 0.01 mg mL^{-1} to 0.5 mg mL^{-1}, as viability decreased prominently at 1.0 mg mL^{-1}. Overall, the synthesized nanomaterials induced toxicity in a dose- and time-dependent manner.

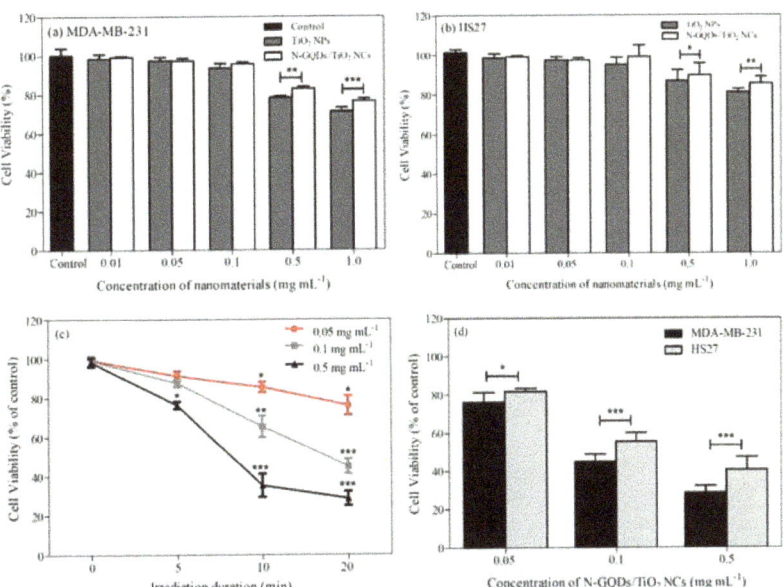

Figure 4. Cell viability of (**a**) MDA-MB-231 and (**b**) HS27 cells, (**c**) MDA-MB-231 cells treated with different concentrations of N-GQDs/TiO$_2$ NCs (0.05–0.5 mg mL^{-1}), then irradiated with various doses of NIR light (5–20 min) and (**d**) MDA-MB-231 and HS27 cells treated with different concentrations of N-GQDs/TiO$_2$ NCs (0.05–0.5 mg mL^{-1}), then irradiated with NIR light for 20 min. The cell viability was estimated at 24 h after irradiation. Data are presented as the mean ± SD of two independent experiments made in three replicates (n = 6). Significant difference was tested using one and two-way ANOVA followed by the Tukey's (**a**,**b**,**d**) and Bonferroni post-hoc tests (**c**), respectively * (p < 0.05), ** (p < 0.01) and *** (p < 0.001).

The 'safe concentrations' of the nanocomposite that were identified from the cytotoxicity assay were used to determine their photokilling properties on MDA-MB-231. The cell-killing effects were measured under irradiation of near-infrared (NIR) light for 5, 10 and 20 min resulting in light energies of 16.5, 33 and 66 J cm^{-2}, respectively, as shown in Figure 4c. A low-power (20 W) lamp was used in this study to minimize the effect of temperature. The nanocomposite led to a slight decrease in cell viability at lower concentrations (0.05 mg mL^{-1}) and short irradiation duration (5 min) when compared to the control cells. However, a substantial decrease in cell viability with the highest photokilling effect was observed at nanocomposite doses of 0.1 and 0.5 mg mL^{-1} under the irradiation of NIR light for 20 min. Irradiation of nanocomposites (0.05–0.5 mg mL^{-1}) for 20 min resulted in a 24, 65 and 72% reduction in cell viability, respectively, when compared to control cells as determined after 24 h of incubation. It is noteworthy that, unlike carcinogenic UV light, NIR light is generally considered safe to humans, without inducing adverse side effects such as tissue damage, severe skin aging or oxidative stress [55]. Besides, the application of longer wavelength NIR light is more effective in PDT than UV and visible light as it has a greater ability to penetrate the human skin, and reaches the subcutaneous tissues (e.g., deeper-seated tumor), the capillaries and other major components of living tissues such as water, hemoglobin in blood and proteins [56]. The obtained results indicated that both the applied concentration of N-GQDs/TiO$_2$ NCs and light irradiation duration, as well the intensity, regulate the induction of cell death. Moreover, the anti-cancer effects of N-GQDs/TiO$_2$ NCs are light exposure-dependent.

The efficacy of the treatment for cancer cells mainly depends on cellular selectivity and inducing photodamage to the targeted cancer cells when compared to normal cells.

To test the selectivity of the treatment, a comparative study was carried out on the HS27 cell line, since the human skin will be the first to be exposed to the light-based PDT treatment before deep penetration into the breast cancer cells (Figure 4d). Similar to the results obtained in the cytotoxicity assay, a lower concentration (0.05 mg mL^{-1}) of nanocomposites had no significant influence on the photokilling effects on HS27. When nanocomposite concentrations of 0.1 and 0.5 mg mL^{-1} were used, a 45 and 60% reduction in HS27 cells were observed, respectively. Nevertheless, the obtained finding of HS27 cells was less than the 65% and 72% reduction seen in the cell viability of MDA-MB-231 cells at the respective concentrations of the nanocomposite. The phototoxic effect of PDT was observed in both non-cancerous and cancer cells, however, synthesized N-GQDs/TiO$_2$ NCs selectively induced more photodamage in the cancerous MDA-MB-231 cells than HS27 cells. The selective toxicity of the nanocomposite might be associated with the difference in the morphology [57], as well as structural and functional differences, of the mitochondria [58,59] between cancer and normal cells.

3.5. Production of Reactive Oxygen Species (ROS)

The major cause of PDT cytotoxicity is the induction of oxidative stress through the direct production of ROS. The effects of N-GQDs/TiO$_2$ NCs as a photosensitizer on ROS generation were evaluated by measuring the intracellular ROS levels using DCFDA staining of the MDA-MB-231 and HS27 cells (Figure 5a). The analysis of the dichlorofluorescein (DCF) intensity indicated that the ROS generated increased as a function of the concentration of nanocomposite (0.05–0.5 mg mL^{-1}). The ROS assay carried out provides a clear view of the differential effects of N-GQDs/TiO$_2$ NCs-based therapy on MDA-MB-231 and HS27 cells. Minimal fluorescent signals were recorded for HS27 cells. In contrast, MDA-MB-231 registered higher fluorescent intensity, which corresponds with the obtained cell viability of the MDA-MB-231 cells after the PDT treatment. Generally, cancer cells have increased levels of ROS, as they have higher basal ROS levels than in normal cells, which are associated with the abnormal and aggressive growth of cancer cells [60]. However, the reduction–oxidation (redox) balance within cancer cells is maintained by a marked endogenous antioxidant capacity. An excessive amount of ROS can lead to oxidative damage to all components of the cell (lipids, proteins and DNA). Therefore, maintaining ROS homeostasis is vital for cell survival and growth. Contrary to normal/non-cancerous counterparts, cancer cells with increased oxidative stress induced by exogenous agents are more vulnerable to cellular death. This phenomenon reflects the disruption of redox homeostasis, following either elevation of ROS generation or decrease in ROS-scavenging capacity, due to impaired antioxidant system in the cancer cells [61]. Meanwhile, non-cancerous cells with lower levels of basal ROS levels have the capability of maintaining redox homeostasis via the antioxidant defense system, which mainly consists of antioxidants (glutathione) and enzymes (superoxide dismutase, catalase, glutathione peroxidase and glutathione S-transferase). This defense system can scavenge excessive ROS and stabilize the ROS levels under physiological conditions [62,63]. Thus, an increased ROS level was observed in MDA-MB-231 cells when compared to HS27 cells. As the photo-killing effects and intracellular ROS in MDA-MB-231 cells were significantly higher than that of HS27, thus, further study on cellular apoptosis and mitochondrial activity assays were carried out using MDA-MB-231 cells only.

To elucidate a link between oxidative stress and the observed cellular outcomes induced by different PDT doses, four ROS scavengers, sodium pyruvate, DMSO, 1,4-benzoquinone and glycerol as effective scavengers of H_2O_2, $^\bullet OH$, $O_2^{-\bullet}$ and $^1O_2/O_2^{-\bullet}$ quenchers, were used, respectively. The amount of a particular type of ROS generated by the nanocomposite in the presence of a specific ROS quencher was monitored by the quenching in the fluorescent intensity of DCF. Then, the resulting percentage of ROS was calculated by comparing the decrease in the fluorescent intensity with the measured intensity in the absence of the scavenger (Figure 5b), and the obtained results are listed in Table 1. The calculated results depict that overall, the nature of ROS formed is mainly

$^1O_2$ instead of $O_2^{-\bullet}$, H_2O_2 and $^\bullet OH$, which were responsible for the PDT cytotoxicity that killed the cancer cells. The obtained results were also supported by the reported N-TiO$_2$ and ZnO NPs that were applied in PDT as a photosensitizer [35,64]. Besides, based on the literature, it has been stated that singlet oxygen is the major cytotoxic agent that plays a significant role in photobiological activity [65].

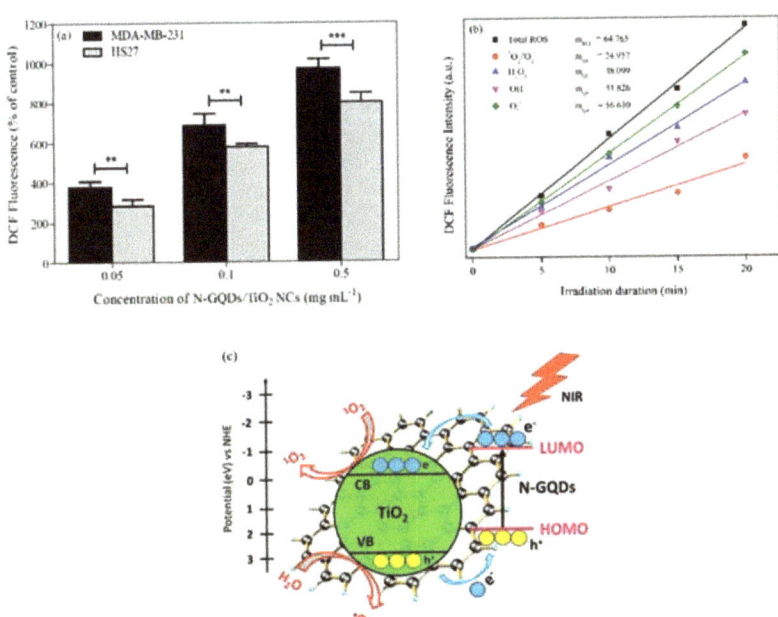

Figure 5. (a) ROS levels of MDA-MB-231 and HS27 cells were treated with different concentrations of N-GQDs/TiO$_2$ NCs (0.05–0.5 mg mL^{-1}) and were irradiated with NIR light for 20 min. Data are presented as the mean ± SD of two independent experiments made in three replicates ($n = 6$) and normalized to control. Significant difference was tested using a two-way ANOVA followed by a Bonferroni post-hoc test and compared to MDA-MB-231, ** ($p < 0.01$) and *** ($p < 0.001$), (b) Comparison of photo-induced ROS generated by N-GQDs/TiO$_2$ NCs under irradiation of NIR light as a function of irradiation time and (c) A proposed possible mechanism of ROS generation by N-GQDs/TiO$_2$ NCs upon NIR light irradiation.

Table 1. Proportion of different ROS (%) generated by N-GQDs/TiO$_2$ NCs (0.5 mg mL^{-1}) under irradiation of NIR light for 20 min.

Types of ROS	Percentage
$^1O_2/O_2^{-\bullet}$	61.5 ± 1.8
H_2O_2	25.7 ± 1.7
$^\bullet OH$	30.9 ± 0.9
$O_2^{-\bullet}$	12.6 ± 1.6

Data are presented as the mean ± SD of two independent experiments made in three replicates ($n = 6$).

Furthermore, Figure 5c shows a proposed possible mechanism of ROS generation by N-GQDs/TiO$_2$ NCs upon NIR light irradiation. In the synthesized nanocomposites, N-GQDs with discrete electronic levels serve as a light absorber, generate electrons and enable donor–acceptor contact with TiO$_2$, which facilitates direct contact with the TiO$_2$ surface. When p-type N-GQDs and n-type TiO$_2$ form a p-n heterojunction, free electrons in TiO$_2$ are transferred to N-GQDs and thus, create holes in the valence band (VB) of TiO$_2$

(Equation (3)) [66]. Upon NIR light irradiation, the N-GQDs absorb the light, leading to the excitation of electrons from the highest occupied molecular orbital (HOMO) to the lowest unoccupied molecular orbital (LUMO), as shown in Equation (4). Then, the electrons are transferred to the CB of TiO$_2$ (Equation (5)). Based on the literature, the LUMO level of GQDs is located in the range of −0.5 to −1.0 eV (with respect to normal hydrogen electrode, NHE), and additionally doping with electron-rich N atoms could further lower the work function of the GQDs [67,68]. Moreover, based on our previous work, TiO$_2$ NPs synthesized employing the hydrothermal method has a bandgap of 3.00 eV, thus, the position of the conduction band (CB) of anatase TiO$_2$ is at −0.18 eV (with respect to NHE), whereby, the LUMO of the N-GQDs is located above the CB of anatase TiO$_2$. Therefore, theoretically, the electron transfer from the LUMO of the N-GQDs to CB of the TiO$_2$ is thermodynamically favorable, while the generated holes accumulate in the HOMO of N-GQDs. This results in efficient charge separation and greatly suppresses the rate of recombination of e$^-$/h$^+$ pairs. TiO$_2$ accepts the electrons, and the excited electrons reduce the molecular oxygen to generate singlet oxygen molecules (^{1}O$_2$) (Equations (6) and (7)). According to the energy band positioning profile, the holes in the HOMO (~1.9 eV) is above a threshold of •OH/H$_2$O (~2.5 eV). Hence, it would not be able to split the water molecules and produce the hydroxyl radicals (•OH) [69]. The holes in the VB of TiO$_2$ (2.82 eV) could act as oxidants to oxidize the water molecules into •OH and H$^+$ as minor products (Equation (8)). Based on the ROS quenching study, it was found that singlet oxygen molecules are major products formed during the photodynamic process. Therefore, in this case, TiO$_2$ served as the catalytic reaction activating region, meanwhile, N-GQDs functioned as a good electron transport medium.

$$TiO_2(e^-) + N-GQDs \rightarrow TiO_2(h^+) + N-GQDs(e^-) \quad (3)$$

$$N-GQDs + h\nu \rightarrow N-GQDs(e^- + h^+) \quad (4)$$

$$N-GQDs(e^-) + TiO_2 \rightarrow N-GQDs(h^+) + TiO_2(e^-) \quad (5)$$

$$TiO_2(e^-) + {}^3O_2 \rightarrow TiO_2 + O_2^{-\bullet} \quad (6)$$

$$O_2^{-\bullet} + H^+ + e^- \rightarrow {}^1O_2 + H_2O_2 \quad (7)$$

$$TiO_2(h^+) + H_2O \rightarrow TiO_2 + {}^\bullet OH + H^+ \quad (8)$$

3.6. Mechanism of Photokilling Properties on MDA-MB-231 Cells

In this work, Caspase Glo-3/7 was employed to study the types of cell death pathways that may occur. Based on Figure 6a, an increase in the nanocomposite concentrations led to an increase in the caspase 3/7 activity and release of caspases. Therefore, successful activation of Caspase Glo-3/7 indicates N-GQDs/TiO$_2$-mediated PDT induces the apoptosis-based cell death pathway in MDA-MB-231 cells. The activated executioner caspase (caspase-3 and -7) can result in cleavage of the cellular substrates and eventually leads to the cellular changes observed in apoptotic cells. Once activated, nuclear lamins are cleaved and this is followed by condensation of chromatin and shrinkage of nuclear material [70]. Besides, it also activates the cleavage of Caspase-activated DNase (CAD), which leads to DNA fragmentation [71]. Moreover, cell fragmentation and the formation of apoptotic bodies are caused by cleaved cytoskeletal proteins. This apoptosis signaling pathways are directly involved in inducing cancer cell death.

Generally, apoptosis can be initiated via either activation of death receptors or mitochondrial release of cytochrome c, known as extrinsic and intrinsic apoptosis, respectively [72]. To further study the apoptotic pathway, tetramethylrhodamine ethyl ester (TMRE) was used to label active mitochondria. Based on Figure 6b, exposure to N-GQDs/TiO$_2$ NCs in the presence of NIR light irradiation for 20 min altered the mitochondrial membrane potential in the MDA-MB-231 cells by reducing it (decreasing TMRE fluorescence intensity) significantly in a concentration-dependent manner, as accessed with the TMRE assay, which was identified as the early apoptotic signal. Generally, the generated exogenous ROS targets the organelle membrane [73]. The increased production of highly reactive ROS will cause damage to the mitochondrial membranes. This obtained result indicates the collapse of the mitochondrial membrane potential, which triggers mitochondrial outer membrane permeabilization (MOMP). The vast array of cellular stress signals, including MOMP, activates mitochondrial-dependent apoptosis, leading to the release of intermembrane protein, cytochrome c, from the inner membrane of mitochondria into the cytosol, inducing chromatin condensation and the formation of apoptotic bodies [74]. Moreover, the decline in the mitochondria membrane potential level might also be accompanied by the significant drop in adenosine triphosphate (ATP) generation, which consequently leads to initiation of apoptosis (cellular death) due to insufficient energy for cell survival [75]. The findings further imply that exogenous ROS could precede to the mitochondrial dysfunction, which is the critical event of apoptosis, indicating N-GQDs/TiO$_2$-mediated PDT induces mitochondrial-dependent apoptosis.

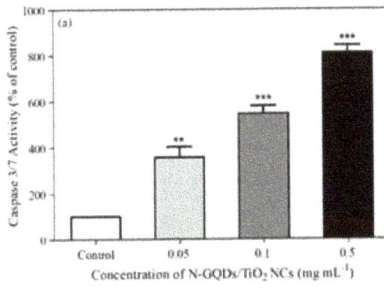
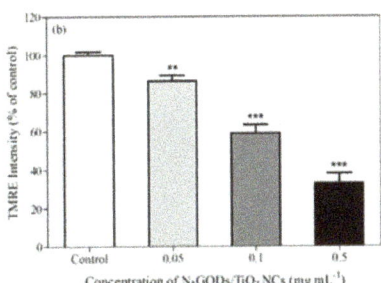

Figure 6. (a) Induction of apoptosis, (b) Measurement of the mitochondrial membrane potential of MDA-MB-231 cells treated with different concentrations of N-GQDs/TiO$_2$ NCs (0.05–0.5 mg mL^{-1}) and were irradiated with NIR light for 20 min. Data are presented as the mean ± SD of three replicates (n = 3) Significant difference was tested using a one-way ANOVA followed by the Tukey's post-hoc test as compared to control ** ($p < 0.01$) and *** ($p < 0.001$).

4. Conclusions

This work reports the successful synthesis of TiO$_2$ conjugated with N-GQDs via the two-pot hydrothermal method through the formation of Ti-O-C on the surface of the TiO$_2$. Besides, the light absorption edge of the anatase phase nanocomposite is extended to a longer, non-toxic NIR light region by narrowing down the bandgap to 1.53 eV, which could improve the penetrability of the nanocomposite when administered in deeper locations in the breast tissue. Unlike most metal oxides, the TiO$_2$-nanocomposite with N-GQDs did not induce significant toxicity in the absence of light when compared to TiO$_2$ NPs, which is a critical property in designing PDT photosensitizers. Under NIR light irradiation, nanocomposite doses (0.1 and 0.5 mg mL^{-1}) induced significantly higher cell death in MDA-MB-231 cells than in HS27 cells due to the increased ROS levels, particularly singlet oxygen ($^1O_2$), observed in the cancer cells. The development of this titanium dioxide-based nanocomposite in the current study could be a potential alternative photosensitizer with the ability to effect mitochondrial-dependent apoptosis in the cells. Thus, the incorporation of N-GQDs in TiO$_2$ can be a promising candidate for photosensitizer in PDT combined with NIR light activation.

Supplementary Materials: The following supporting information can be downloaded at: https://www.mdpi.com/article/10.3390/biomedicines10020421/s1, Figure S1: The possible formation mechanism of oxygen vacancies and Ti^{3+} ions; Figure S2: Hydrodynamic size and zeta potential of N-GQDs, TiO_2 NPs, N-GQDs/TiO_2 NCs in cell culture medium (mean $\pm$ SD, n = 3). The nanomaterials were dispersed in water or medium with or without FBS (1%, v/v), then sonicated, vortexed and hydrodynamic size and zeta; Figure S3: Cell viability of MDA-MB-231 and HS27 cells after 24 h post-treatment. Data are presented as the mean $\pm$ SD of two independent experiments made in three replicates (n = 6) and normalized to control. Significant difference was tested using two-way ANOVA followed by Bonferroni post-hoc test as compared to control * (p < 0.05) and ** (p < 0.01); Table S1: Crystallite size, lattice parameters and lattice strain of TiO_2 NPs and N-GQDs/TiO_2 NCs.

Author Contributions: Conceptualization: P.R. and H.L.L.; data acquisition and analysis: P.R., B.-K.K., H.L.L., C.Y.L. and N.T.K.T; writing-original draft: P.R.; writing-reviewing and editing: H.L.L., C.Y.L., R.-A.D., C.E.O. and N.T.K.T.; supervision: H.L.L. and C.Y.L.; funding acquisition: H.L.L. and N.T.K.T. All authors have read and agreed to the published version of the manuscript.

Funding: This research was financially supported by USM Research University Individual (RUI) Grant (1001/PKimia/8011086), Royal Society of Chemistry (RSC) International Mobility Grant (M19-2989) and EPSRC.

Institutional Review Board Statement: Not applicable.

Informed Consent Statement: Not applicable.

Data Availability Statement: Not applicable.

Acknowledgments: The authors wish to thank the USM Research University Individual (RUI) Grant (1001/PKimia/8011086) for the funding obtained in this project. H.L.L. and N.T.K.T. would like to acknowledge the Research Mobility Grant (M19-2989) awarded by the Royal Society of Chemistry (RSC); N.T.K.T. thanks EPSRC. The authors also wish to thank Vikneswaran Murugaiyah from the School of Pharmaceutical Sciences, USM for his assistance and discussion in this project.

Conflicts of Interest: The authors declare no conflict of interest.

References

1. Blanco, E.; Shen, H.; Ferrari, M. Principles of nanoparticle design for overcoming biological barriers to drug delivery. *Nat. Biotechnol.* **2015**, *33*, 941–951. [CrossRef] [PubMed]
2. Duman, F.D.; Sebek, M.; Thanh, N.T.K.; Loizidou, M.; Shakib, K.; MacRobert, A.J. Enhanced photodynamic therapy and fluorescence imaging using gold nanorods for porphyrin delivery in a novel: In vitro squamous cell carcinoma 3D model. *J. Mater. Chem. B* **2020**, *8*, 5131–5142. [CrossRef]
3. Wang, S.; Gao, R.; Zhou, F.; Selke, M. Nanomaterials and singlet oxygen photosensitizers: Potential applications in photodynamic therapy. *J. Mater. Chem.* **2004**, *14*, 487–493. [CrossRef]
4. Rui, L.L.; Cao, H.L.; Xue, Y.D.; Liu, L.C.; Xu, L.; Gao, Y.; Zhang, W.A. Functional organic nanoparticles for photodynamic therapy. *Chin. Chem. Lett.* **2016**, *27*, 1412–1420. [CrossRef]
5. Abrahamse, H.; Kruger, C.A.; Kadanyo, S.; Mishra, A. Nanoparticles for Advanced Photodynamic Therapy of Cancer. *Photomed. Laser Surg.* **2017**, *35*, 581–588. [CrossRef]
6. Li, W.-T. Nanoparticles for photodynamic therapy. In *Handbook of Biophotonic*; Popp, J., Tuchin, V.V., Chiou, A., Heinemann, S., Eds.; Wiley-VCH Verlag GmbH & Co. KGaA: Weinheim, Germany, 2013; Volume 2, pp. 321–336.
7. Zheng, H. A review of progress in clinical photodynamic therapy. *Technol. Cancer Res. Treat.* **2005**, *4*, 283–293.
8. Lin, Y.; Zhou, T.; Bai, R.; Xie, Y. Chemical approaches for the enhancement of porphyrin skeleton-based photodynamic therapy. *J. Enzyme Inhib. Med. Chem.* **2020**, *35*, 1080–1099. [CrossRef] [PubMed]
9. Maeda, H.; Nakamura, H.; Fang, J. The EPR effect for macromolecular drug delivery to solid tumors: Improvement of tumor uptake, lowering of systemic toxicity, and distinct tumor imaging in vivo. *Adv. Drug Deliv. Rev.* **2013**, *65*, 71–79. [CrossRef]
10. Linsebigler, A.L.; Lu, G.; Yates, J.T. Photocatalysis on TiO_2 Surfaces: Principles, mechanisms, and selected results. *Chem. Rev.* **1995**, *95*, 735–758. [CrossRef]
11. Kang, X.; Liu, S.; Dai, Z.; He, Y.; Song, X.; Tan, Z. Titanium dioxide: From engineering to applications. *Catalysts* **2019**, *9*, 191. [CrossRef]
12. Shang, H.; Han, D.; Ma, M.; Li, S.; Xue, W.; Zhang, A. Enhancement of the photokilling effect of TiO_2 in photodynamic therapy by conjugating with reduced graphene oxide and its mechanism exploration. *J. Photochem. Photobiol. B Biol.* **2017**, *177*, 112–123. [CrossRef] [PubMed]

13. Moosavi, M.A.; Sharifi, M.; Ghafary, S.M.; Mohammadalipour, Z.; Khataee, A.; Rahmati, M.; Hajjaran, S.; Łos, M.J.; Klonisch, T.; Ghavami, S. Photodynamic N-TiO$_2$ nanoparticle treatment induces controlled ROS-mediated autophagy and terminal differentiation of leukemia cells. *Sci. Rep.* **2016**, *6*, 34413. [CrossRef] [PubMed]
14. Li, Z.; Pan, X.; Wang, T.; Wang, P.N.; Chen, J.Y.; Mi, L. Comparison of the killing effects between nitrogen-doped and pure TiO$_2$ on HeLa cells with visible light irradiation. *Nanoscale Res. Lett.* **2013**, *8*, 96. [CrossRef] [PubMed]
15. Lagopati, N.; Tsilibary, E.P.; Falaras, P.; Papazafiri, P.; Pavlatou, E.A.; Kotsopoulou, E.; Kitsiou, P. Effect of nanostructured TiO$_2$ crystal phase on photoinduced apoptosis of breast cancer epithelial cells. *Int. J. Nanomed.* **2014**, *9*, 3219–3230.
16. Wang, Y.; Cui, H.; Zhou, J.; Li, F.; Wang, J.; Chen, M.; Liu, Q. Cytotoxicity, DNA damage, and apoptosis induced by titanium dioxide nanoparticles in human non-small cell lung cancer A549 cells. *Environ. Sci. Pollut. Res.* **2015**, *22*, 5519–5530. [CrossRef]
17. Ghosh, M.; Bandyopadhyay, M.; Mukherjee, A. Genotoxicity of titanium dioxide (TiO$_2$) nanoparticles at two trophic levels: Plant and human lymphocytes. *Chemosphere* **2010**, *81*, 1253–1262. [CrossRef]
18. Hou, J.; Wang, L.; Wang, C.; Zhang, S.; Liu, H.; Li, S.; Wang, X. Toxicity and mechanisms of action of titanium dioxide nanoparticles in living organisms. *J. Environ. Sci.* **2019**, *75*, 40–53. [CrossRef]
19. Ahmad, J.; Siddiqui, M.; Akhtar, M.; Alhadlaq, H.; Alshamsan, A.; Khan, S.; Wahab, R.; Al-Khadhairy, A.; Al-Salim, A.; Musarrat, J.; et al. Copper doping enhanced the oxidative stress–mediated cytotoxicity of TiO$_2$ nanoparticles in A549 cells. *Hum. Exp. Toxicol.* **2017**, *37*, 496–507. [CrossRef]
20. Ahamed, M.; Khan, M.A.M.; Akhtar, M.J.; Alhadlaq, H.A.; Alshamsan, A. Role of Zn doping in oxidative stress mediated cytotoxicity of TiO$_2$ nanoparticles in human breast cancer MCF-7 cells. *Sci. Rep.* **2016**, *6*, 30196. [CrossRef]
21. Khan, M.M.; Kumar, S.; Khan, M.N.; Ahamed, M.; Al-Dwayyan, A.S. Microstructure and blue-shift in optical band gap of nanocrystalline Al$_x$Zn$_{1-x}$O thin films. *J. Lumin.* **2014**, *155*, 275–281. [CrossRef]
22. Latvala, S.; Hedberg, J.; Bucchianico, S.D.; Möller, L.; Wallinder, I.O.; Elihn, K.; Karlsson, H.L. Nickel release, ROS generation and toxicity of Ni and NiO micro- and nanoparticles. *PLoS ONE* **2016**, *11*, e0159684. [CrossRef] [PubMed]
23. Ahamed, M.; Khan, M.A.M.; Akhtar, M.J.; Alhadlaq, H.A.; Alshamsan, A. Ag-doping regulates the cytotoxicity of TiO$_2$ nanoparticles via oxidative stress in human cancer cells. *Sci. Rep.* **2017**, *7*, 17662. [CrossRef] [PubMed]
24. López, T.; Alvarez, M.; González, R.D.; Uddin, M.J.; Bustos, J.; Arroyo, S.; Sánchez, A. Synthesis, characterization and in vitro cytotoxicity of Pt-TiO$_2$ nanoparticles. *Adsorption* **2011**, *17*, 573–581. [CrossRef]
25. Tabish, T.A.; Scotton, C.J.; Ferguson, D.C.F.; Lin, L.; van der Veen, A.; Lowry, S.; Ali, M.; Jabeen, F.; Winyard, P.G.; Zhang, S. Biocompatibility and toxicity of graphene quantum dots for potential application in photodynamic therapy. *Nanomedicine* **2018**, *13*, 1923–1937. [CrossRef]
26. Guijarro, N.; Lana-Villarreal, T.; Mora-Seró, I.; Bisquert, J.; Gómez, R. CdSe quantum dot-sensitized TiO$_2$ electrodes: Effect of quantum dot coverage and mode of attachment. *J. Phys. Chem. C* **2009**, *113*, 4208–4214. [CrossRef]
27. Wang, H.; Bai, Y.; Zhang, H.; Zhang, Z.; Li, J.; Guo, L. CdS quantum dots-sensitized TiO$_2$ nanorod array on transparent conductive glass photoelectrodes. *J. Phys. Chem. C* **2010**, *114*, 16451–16455. [CrossRef]
28. Ratanatawanate, C.; Tao, Y.; Balkus, K.J. Photocatalytic activity of PbS quantum dot/TiO$_2$ nanotube composites. *J. Phys. Chem. C* **2009**, *113*, 10755–10760. [CrossRef]
29. Yu, X.Y.; Lei, B.X.; Kuang, D.B.; Su, C.Y. Highly efficient CdTe/CdS quantum dot sensitized solar cells fabricated by a one-step linker assisted chemical bath deposition. *Chem. Sci.* **2011**, *2*, 1396–1400. [CrossRef]
30. Reddy, N.L.; Emin, S.; Kumari, V.D.; Venkatakrishnan, S.M. CuO quantum dots decorated TiO$_2$ nanocomposite photocatalyst for stable hydrogen generation. *Ind. Eng. Chem. Res.* **2018**, *57*, 568–577. [CrossRef]
31. Li, M.; Wu, W.; Ren, W.; Cheng, H.M.; Tang, N.; Zhong, W.; Du, Y. Synthesis and upconversion luminescence of N-doped graphene quantum dots. *Appl. Phys. Lett.* **2012**, *101*, 10–13. [CrossRef]
32. Ramachandran, P.; Lee, C.Y.; Doong, R.-A.; Oon, C.E.; Thanh, N.T.K.; Lee, H.L. A titanium dioxide/nitrogen-doped graphene quantum dot nanocomposite to mitigate cytotoxicity: Synthesis, characterization, and cell viability evaluation. *RSC Adv.* **2020**, *10*, 21795–21805. [CrossRef]
33. Talukdar, S.; Dutta, R.K. A mechanistic approach for superoxide radicals and singlet oxygen mediated enhanced photocatalytic dye degradation by selenium doped ZnS nanoparticles. *RSC Adv.* **2015**, *6*, 928–936. [CrossRef]
34. Franco, R.; Panayiotidis, M.I.; Cidlowski, J.A. Glutathione depletion is necessary for apoptosis in lymphoid cells independent of reactive oxygen species formation. *J. Biol. Chem.* **2007**, *282*, 30452–30465. [CrossRef] [PubMed]
35. Pan, X.; Liang, X.; Yao, L.; Wang, X.; Jing, Y.; Ma, J.; Fei, Y.; Chen, L.; Mi, L. Study of the Photodynamic Activity of N-Doped TiO$_2$ Nanoparticles Conjugated with Aluminum Phthalocyanine. *Nanomaterials* **2017**, *7*, 338. [CrossRef] [PubMed]
36. Ghasemi, S.; Esfandiar, A.; Setayesh, S.R.; Yangjeh, A.-H.; Zad, A.I.; Gholami, M.R. Synthesis and characterization of TiO$_2$-graphene nanocomposites modified with noble metals as a photocatalyst for degradation of pollutants. *Appl. Catal. A Gen.* **2013**, *462*, 82–90. [CrossRef]
37. Ou, N.Q.; Li, H.J.; Lyu, B.W.; Gui, B.J.; Sun, X.; Qian, D.J.; Jia, Y.; Wang, X.; Yang, J. Facet-dependent interfacial charge transfer in TiO$_2$/nitrogen-doped graphene quantum dots heterojunctions for visible-light driven photocatalysis. *Catalysts* **2019**, *9*, 345. [CrossRef]
38. Gao, Y.; Pu, X.; Zhang, D.; Ding, G.; Shao, X.; Ma, J. Combustion synthesis of graphene oxide-TiO$_2$ hybrid materials for photodegradation of methyl orange. *Carbon N. Y.* **2012**, *50*, 4093–4101. [CrossRef]

39. Zhang, Q.; Bao, N.; Wang, X.; Hu, X.; Miao, X.; Chaker, M.; Ma, D. Advanced Fabrication of chemically bonded graphene/TiO_2 continuous fibers with enhanced broadband photocatalytic properties and involved mechanisms exploration. *Sci. Rep.* **2016**, *6*, 38066. [CrossRef]
40. Kibasomba, P.M.; Dhlamini, S.; Maaza, M.; Liu, C.P.; Rashad, M.M.; Rayan, D.A.; Mwakikunga, B.W. Strain and grain size of TiO_2 nanoparticles from TEM, Raman spectroscopy and XRD: The revisiting of the Williamson-Hall plot method. *Results Phys.* **2018**, *9*, 628–635. [CrossRef]
41. Zhao, D.; Sheng, G.; Chen, C.; Wang, X. Enhanced photocatalytic degradation of methylene blue under visible irradiation on graphene@TiO_2 dyade structure. *Appl. Catal. B Environ.* **2012**, *111*, 303–308. [CrossRef]
42. Martins, N.C.T.; Ângelo, J.; Girão, A.V.; Trindade, T.; Andrade, L.; Mendes, A. N-doped carbon quantum dots/TiO_2 composite with improved photocatalytic activity. *Appl. Catal. B Environ.* **2016**, *193*, 67–74. [CrossRef]
43. Wang, J.; Gao, M.; Ho, G.W. Bidentate-complex-derived TiO_2/carbon dot photocatalysts: In situ synthesis, versatile heterostructures, and enhanced H_2 evolution. *J. Mater. Chem. A* **2014**, *2*, 5703–5709. [CrossRef]
44. Yu, J.; Zhang, C.; Yang, Y.; Yi, G.; Fan, R.; Li, L.; Xing, B.; Liu, Q.; Jia, J.; Huang, G. Lignite-derived carbon quantum dot/TiO_2 heterostructure nanocomposites: Photoinduced charge transfer properties and enhanced visible light photocatalytic activity. *New J. Chem.* **2019**, *43*, 18355–18368. [CrossRef]
45. Jaafar, N.F.; Jalil, A.A.; Triwahyono, S.; Shamsuddin, N. New insights into self-modification of mesoporous titania nanoparticles for enhanced photoactivity: Effect of microwave power density on formation of oxygen vacancies and Ti^{3+} defects. *RSC Adv.* **2015**, *5*, 90991–91000. [CrossRef]
46. Bharti, B.; Kumar, S.; Lee, H.N.; Kumar, R. Formation of oxygen vacancies and Ti^{3+} state in TiO_2 thin film and enhanced optical properties by air plasma treatment. *Sci. Rep.* **2016**, *6*, 32355. [CrossRef]
47. Umrao, S.; Abraham, S.; Theil, F.; Pandey, S.; Ciobota, V.; Shukla, P.K.; Rupp, C.J.; Chakraborty, S.; Ahuja, R.; Popp, J.; et al. A possible mechanism for the emergence of an additional band gap due to a Ti-O-C bond in the TiO_2-graphene hybrid system for enhanced photodegradation of methylene blue under visible light. *RSC Adv.* **2014**, *4*, 59890–59901. [CrossRef]
48. Rajender, G.; Kumar, J.; Giri, P.K. Interfacial charge transfer in oxygen deficient TiO_2-graphene quantum dot hybrid and its influence on the enhanced visible light photocatalysis. *Appl. Catal. B Environ.* **2018**, *224*, 960–972. [CrossRef]
49. Wang, X.; Zhang, K.; Guo, X.; Shen, G.; Xiang, J. Synthesis and characterization of N-doped TiO_2 loaded onto activated carbon fiber with enhanced visible-light photocatalytic activity. *New J. Chem.* **2014**, *38*, 6139–6146. [CrossRef]
50. Li, H.J.; Ou, N.Q.; Sun, X.; Sun, B.W.; Qian, D.J.; Chen, M.; Wang, X.; Yang, J. Exploitation of the synergistic effect between surface and bulk defects in ultra-small N-doped titanium suboxides for enhancing photocatalytic hydrogen evolution. *Catal. Sci. Technol.* **2018**, *8*, 5515–5525. [CrossRef]
51. Shi, R.; Li, Z.; Yu, H.; Shang, L.; Zhou, C.; Waterhouse, G.I.N.; Wu, L.Z.; Zhang, T. Effect of nitrogen doping level on the performance of N-doped carbon quantum dot/TiO_2 composites for photocatalytic hydrogen evolution. *ChemSusChem* **2017**, *10*, 4650–4656. [CrossRef]
52. Oktay, S.; Kahraman, Z.; Urgen, M.; Kazmanli, K. XPS investigations of tribolayers formed on TiN and (Ti,Re)N coatings. *Appl. Surf. Sci.* **2015**, *328*, 255–261. [CrossRef]
53. Warheit, D.B.; Hoke, R.A.; Finlay, C.; Donner, E.M.; Reed, K.L.; Sayes, C.M. Development of a base set of toxicity tests using ultrafine TiO_2 particles as a component of nanoparticle risk management. *Toxicol. Lett.* **2007**, *171*, 99–110. [CrossRef] [PubMed]
54. Matteis, V.D.; Cascione, M.; Brunetti, V.; Toma, C.C.; Rinaldi, R. Toxicity assessment of anatase and rutile titanium dioxide nanoparticles: The role of degradation in different pH conditions and light exposure. *Toxicol. Vitr.* **2016**, *37*, 201–210. [CrossRef] [PubMed]
55. Bozkurt, A.; Onaral, B. Safety assessment of near infrared light emitting diodes for diffuse optical measurements. *Biomed. Eng. Online* **2004**, *3*, 9. [CrossRef] [PubMed]
56. Banerjee, S.M.; MacRobert, A.J.; Mosse, C.A.; Periera, B.; Bown, S.G.; Keshtgar, M.R.S. Photodynamic therapy: Inception to application in breast cancer. *Breast* **2017**, *31*, 105–113. [CrossRef]
57. Hamblin, M.R.; Newman, E.L. New trends in photobiology. On the mechanism of the tumour-localizing effect in photodynamic therapy. *J. Photochem. Photobiol. B Biol.* **1994**, *23*, 3–8. [CrossRef]
58. Grasso, D.; Zampieri, L.X.; Capelôa, T.; Van de Velde, J.A.; Sonveaux, P. Mitochondria in cancer. *Cell Stress* **2020**, *4*, 114–146. [CrossRef]
59. Jeena, M.T.; Kim, S.; Jin, S.; Ryu, J.H. Recent progress in mitochondria-targeted drug and drug-free agents for cancer therapy. *Cancers* **2020**, *12*, 4. [CrossRef]
60. Kumari, S.; Badana, A.K.; Mohan, G.M.; Shailender, G.; Malla, R.R. Reactive oxygen species: A key constituent in cancer survival. *Biomark. Insights* **2018**, *13*. [CrossRef]
61. Oliveira, M.F.D.; Amoêdo, N.D.; Rumjanek, F.D. Energy and redox homeostasis in tumor cells. *Int. J. Cell Biol.* **2012**, *2012*, 593838. [CrossRef]
62. Toyokuni, S.; Okamoto, K.; Yodoi, J.; Hiai, H. Persistent oxidative stress in cancer. *FEBS Lett.* **1995**, *358*, 593838. [CrossRef]
63. Trachootham, D.; Alexandre, J.; Huang, P. Targeting cancer cells by ROS-mediated mechanisms: A radical therapeutic approach? *Nat. Rev. Drug Discov.* **2009**, *8*, 579–591. [CrossRef] [PubMed]
64. Sardar, S.; Chaudhuri, S.; Kar, P.; Sarkar, S.; Lemmens, P.; Pal, S.K. Direct observation of key photoinduced dynamics in a potential nano-delivery vehicle of cancer drugs. *Phys. Chem. Chem. Phys.* **2015**, *17*, 166–177. [CrossRef]

65. Josefsen, L.B.; Boyle, R.W. Photodynamic therapy and the development of metal-based photosensitizers. *Met. Based. Drugs* **2008**, *2008*, 276109. [CrossRef] [PubMed]
66. Murali, G.; Reddeppa, M.; Reddy, C.S.; Park, S.; Chandrakalavathi, T.; Kim, M.D.; In, I. Enhancing the charge carrier separation and transport via nitrogen-doped graphene quantum dot-TiO$_2$ nanoplate hybrid structure for an efficient NO gas sensor. *ACS Appl. Mater. Interfaces* **2020**, *12*, 13428–13436. [CrossRef] [PubMed]
67. Lin, T.N.; Inciong, M.R.; Santiago, S.R.M.S.; Yeh, T.W.; Yang, W.Y.; Yuan, C.T.; Shen, J.L.; Kuo, H.C.; Chiu, C.H. Photo-induced doping in GaN epilayers with graphene quantum dots. *Sci. Rep.* **2016**, *6*, 23260. [CrossRef]
68. Bian, S.; Zhou, C.; Li, P.; Liu, J.; Dong, X.; Xi, F. Graphene quantum dots decorated titania nanosheets heterojunction: Efficient charge separation and enhanced visible-light photocatalytic performance. *ChemCatChem* **2017**, *9*, 3349–3357. [CrossRef]
69. Bessegato, G.G.; Guaraldo, T.T.; de Brito, J.F.; Brugnera, M.F.; Zanoni, M.V.B. Achievements and trends in photoelectrocatalysis: From environmental to energy applications. *Electrocatalysis* **2015**, *6*, 415–441. [CrossRef]
70. Kivinen, K.; Kallajoki, M.; Taimen, P. Caspase-3 is required in the apoptotic disintegration of the nuclear matrix. *Exp. Cell Res.* **2005**, *311*, 62–73. [CrossRef]
71. Enari, M.; Sakahira, H.; Yokoyama, H.; Okawa, K.; Iwamatsu, A.; Nagata, S. A caspase-activated DNase that degrades DNA during apoptosis, and its inhibitor ICAD. *Nature* **1998**, *391*, 43–50. [CrossRef]
72. Rustin, P. Mitochondria, from cell death to proliferation. *Nat. Genet.* **2002**, *30*, 352–353. [CrossRef]
73. Madkour, H.L. The roles and mechanisms of ros, oxidative stress, and oxidative damage. In *Nanoparticles Induce Oxidative Endoplasmic Reticulum Stress. Nanomedicine Nanotoxicology*; Springer: Cham, Switzerland, 2020; pp. 139–191.
74. Suhaili, S.H.; Karimian, H.; Stellato, M.; Lee, T.H.; Aguilar, M.I. Mitochondrial outer membrane permeabilization: A focus on the role of mitochondrial membrane structural organization. *Biophys. Rev.* **2017**, *9*, 443–457. [CrossRef]
75. Tsujimoto, Y. Apoptosis and necrosis: Intracellular ATP level as a determinant for cell death modes. *Cell Death Differ.* **1997**, *4*, 429–434. [CrossRef]

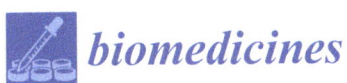

Article

Styrene Maleic Acid Copolymer-Based Micellar Formation of Temoporfin (SMA@ mTHPC) Behaves as A Nanoprobe for Tumor-Targeted Photodynamic Therapy with A Superior Safety

Jun Fang *,†, Shanghui Gao †, Rayhanul Islam, Hinata Nema, Rina Yanagibashi, Niho Yoneda, Natsumi Watanabe, Yuki Yasuda, Naoki Nuita, Jian-Rong Zhou and Kazumi Yokomizo

Faculty of Pharmaceutical Sciences, Sojo University, Ikeda 4-22-1, Kumamoto 860-0082, Japan; gaoshanghui94@gmail.com (S.G.); rayhanulislam88@gmail.com (R.I.); g1651090@m.sojo-u.ac.jp (H.N.); g1651124@m.sojo-u.ac.jp (R.Y.); g1651133@m.ph.sojo-u.ac.jp (N.Y.); g1651134@m.sojo-u.ac.jp (N.W.); g1751126@m.sojo-u.ac.jp (Y.Y.); g1751093@m.sojo-u.ac.jp (N.N.); zhoujr@ph.sojo-u.ac.jp (J.-R.Z.); yoko0514@ph.sojo-u.ac.jp (K.Y.)
* Correspondence: fangjun@ph.sojo-u.ac.jp; Tel.: +81-96-326-4137; Fax: +81-96-326-5048
† Equally contributed to this work.

Abstract: Tumor-targeted photodynamic therapy (PDT) using polymeric photosensitizers is a promising anticancer therapeutic strategy. Previously, we developed several polymeric nanoprobes for PDT using different polymers and PDT agents. In the study, we synthesized a styrene maleic acid copolymer (SMA) micelle encapsulating temoporfin (mTHPC) that is a clinically used PDT drug, SMA@mTHPC, with a hydrodynamic size of 98 nm, which showed high water solubility. SMA@mTHPC maintained stable micelle formation in physiological aqueous solutions including serum; however, the micelles could be disrupted in the presence of detergent (e.g., Tween 20) as well as lecithin, the major component of cell membrane, suggesting micelles will be destroyed and free mTHPC will be released during intracellular uptake. SMA@mTHPC showed a pH-dependent release profile, for which a constant release of ≈20% per day was found at pH 7.4, and much more release occurred at acidic pH (e.g., 6.5, 5.5), suggesting extensive release of free mTHPC could occur in the weak acidic environment of a tumor and further during internalization into tumor cells. In vitro cytotoxicity assay showed a lower cytotoxicity of SMA@mTHPC than free mTHPC; however, similar in vivo antitumor effects were observed by both SMA@mTHPC and free THPC. More importantly, severe side effects (e.g., body weight loss, death of the mice) were found during free mTHPC treatment, whereas no apparent side effects were observed for SMA@mTHPC. The superior safety profile of SMA@mTHPC was mostly due to its micelle formation and the enhanced permeability and retention (EPR) effect-based tumor accumulation, as well as the tumor environment-responsive release properties. These findings suggested SMA@mTHPC may become a good candidate drug for targeted PDT with high safety.

Keywords: EPR effect; polymeric micelles; PDT nanoprobe; tumor targeting; temoporfin

Citation: Fang, J.; Gao, S.; Islam, R.; Nema, H.; Yanagibashi, R.; Yoneda, N.; Watanabe, N.; Yasuda, Y.; Nuita, N.; Zhou, J.-R.; et al. Styrene Maleic Acid Copolymer-Based Micellar Formation of Temoporfin (SMA@ mTHPC) Behaves as A Nanoprobe for Tumor-Targeted Photodynamic Therapy with A Superior Safety. Biomedicines 2021, 9, 1493. https://doi.org/10.3390/biomedicines9101493

Academic Editor: Stefano Bacci

Received: 30 August 2021
Accepted: 14 October 2021
Published: 19 October 2021

Publisher's Note: MDPI stays neutral with regard to jurisdictional claims in published maps and institutional affiliations.

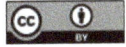

Copyright: © 2021 by the authors. Licensee MDPI, Basel, Switzerland. This article is an open access article distributed under the terms and conditions of the Creative Commons Attribution (CC BY) license (https://creativecommons.org/licenses/by/4.0/).

1. Introduction

Photodynamic therapy is a less invasive therapeutic strategy for cancer, which utilizes photosensitizers (PS) followed by light irradiation [1–3]. Upon light exposure, the PS is excited, and the energy is transferred to molecular oxygen to generate cytotoxic singlet oxygen ($^1O_2$) [3]. $^1O_2$, as an oxygen free radical, rapidly react with biomolecules, i.e., proteins, DNA, and lipid, inducing oxidative damage and apoptosis of the cells [3–5]. Most of the PSs are non-toxic or less toxic agents and they are not harmful without exposure to the light; accordingly, tumor-specific light irradiation will kill cancer cells selectively, without inducing severe side effects to the normal cells, which is an advantage to conventional anticancer chemotherapy. However, conventional PSs are mostly low-molecular weight agents—after systemic administration, they distribute indiscriminately to both tumor tissue and normal tissues, e.g., the skin; ambient light may thus trigger the injury and inflammation of the skin. Actually, in conventional PDT, patients can remain photosensitive for several weeks after treatment, and avoiding excess ambient light is always necessary for patients receiving PDT [4]. In addition, most PSs show poor water-solubility, which hampers their clinical application.

In order for these drawbacks to be overcome, nano-designed PSs have been receiving much attention. Namely, biocompatible polymers, liposome, and antibodies are used to modify PSs resulting in various macromolecular formulations of PSs with sizes of several to several hundred nanometers. The nano-formulation of PSs renders high water solubility of PSs, and more importantly, it could fulfill tumor-targeted PDT effect by taking advantage of the enhance permeability and retention (EPR) effect. EPR effect is a unique phenomenon regarding the behaviors of macromolecules according to the abnormal anatomical and pathophysiological natures of tumor blood vasculature [6–11]. Compared to normal vasculature, tumor vasculature shows a large gap between the endothelial cells and exhibits high vascular permeability, as well as defected lymphatic functions, by which macromolecules with molecular weight higher than 40–50 kDa, or molecular size larger than 5–10 nm, will accumulate selectively and remain in tumor tissues for prolonged period of time, whereas they will not penetrate normal blood vessels, thus showing significantly less distribution in normal tissues compared to low molecular weight agents. The EPR effect was first discovered by Maeda and Matsumura in 1986 [6], and now it has been become a well-understood rationale for the design and development of anticancer nanomedicine [7–11]. In our laboratory, on the basis of the EPR effect, we have developed many macromolecular anticancer agents by using biocompatible polymers including polyethylene glycol (PEG), styrene maleic acid copolymer (SMA), and poly(N-(2-hydroxypropyl) methacrylamide) copolymer (HPMA) [7–19]. Polymer-modified PSs were also investigated, including PEG-conjugated zinc protoporphyrin (ZnPP) (PEG-ZnPP) [19,20], SMA micelles of ZnPP (SMA-ZnPP) [16–18], HPMA-conjugated ZnPP (HPMA-ZnPP) [12,14], and HPMA-conjugated pyropheophorbide a (P-PyF) [15], all of which showed tumor-targeting properties and potent PDT effect with high tumor selectivity. Along this line, in this study, we challenged a polymeric micellar formation of a clinically used PDT drug, temoporfin (mTHPC), using SMA copolymer.

mTHPC is the most potent second-generation PS [21], and it is approved in the European Union as a PDT drug for the treatment of squamous cell carcinoma of the head and neck [4]. As with other PSs, administration of mTHPC results in patients becoming highly sensitive to light, which lasts 7 to 15 days, and therefore appropriate light exposure precautions are necessary during this period [4]. mTHPC is water-insoluble and its standard formulation is dissolved in organic solvents, i.e., ethanol, which largely hampers its application. Accordingly, liposomal formulations of mTHPC have been developed showing high water-solubility as well as potent PDT effect [21–24], suggesting the benefit of nano-design for mTHPC.

Besides liposomal formulation, polymer micelle is another well-accepted nano-platform, in which amphiphilic polymers are utilized to form micelles in aqueous solutions by self-assembly where hydrophobic drugs are encapsulated in the core of micelles [25,26]. SMA is one such amphiphilic copolymer, containing hydrophobic styrene motif and hydrophilic maleic acid motif. We have successfully developed several SMA micelles of anticancer agents including doxorubicin, pirarubicin, and ZnPP, all of which showed high water solubility and tumor-targeting properties [18,27,28]. In this context, we report here a SMA micelle encapsulating mTHPC (SMA@mTHPC), which showed increased water solubility, potent PDT effect, and superior safety profile compared to native mTHPC.

2. Materials and Methods

2.1. Chemicals

Poly(styrene-co-maleic anhydride) (an SMA copolymer), with a mean molecular weight of 1600 Da, and mTHPC were purchased from Sigma Chemical Co. (St. Louis, MO, USA). 3-(4,5-Dimethyl-2-thiazolyl)-2,5-diphenyl-2H-tetrazolium bromide (MTT) and 1-ethyl-3-(3-dimethylaminopropyl) carbodiimide hydrochloride (WSC) were purchased from Wako Pure Chemical Industries Ltd. (Osaka, Japan). 2,2,6,6-Tetramethyl-4-piperidone (4-oxo-TEMP) was purchased from Tokyo Chemical Industry (Tokyo, Japan). Other reagents of reagent grade and solvents were purchased from Wako Pure Chemical Industries Ltd. and used without further purification.

2.2. Synthesis of SMA@mTHPC

2.2.1. Hydrolysis and Purification of SMA

The maleic anhydride residue of the SMA copolymer was hydrolyzed to the water-soluble maleic acid form by addition of 1 N NaOH at 50 mg/mL. The solution was heated at 50 °C during stirring for 24 h until a clear solution was obtained. Then, the pH of the solution was adjusted to 7.0 with 1 N HCl, followed by dialysis using a dialysis bag with molecular cut-off of 8000 Da (Wako), and then freeze-drying.

2.2.2. Preparation of SMA@mTHPC Micelles

SMA@mTHPC micelles were prepared by a similar protocol to that described earlier by us for SMA-ZhPP micelles [18], with some modifications. In brief, hydrolyzed SMA (100 mg) was dissolved in 20 mL deionized water and the pH was adjusted to 5.0 by 1 N HCl, to which 11 mg of mTHPC dissolved in 1 mL DMSO was added dropwise. One hundred milligrams of WSC was then added, and the reaction mixture was stirred at room temperature for 30 min. Then, the pH of reaction solution was adjusted to 11.0 by 1 N NaOH, with further stirring for 1 h. Finally, the pH or the reactant was adjusted to 7.4 by 1N HCl, followed by dialysis against deionized water at 4 °C for 3 days with 3-change of water, and then freeze-drying, in order to obtain the brown powder of SMA@mTHPC (91 mg).

2.3. Characterization of P-PyF

2.3.1. Measurement of Particle Size of P-PyF

SMA@mTHPC was dissolved in 0.01 M phosphate-buffered 0.15 M saline (PBS; pH 7.4) at 2.5 mg/mL and was filtered through a 0.2 µm filter. The particle size was measured by dynamic light scattering (ELS-Z2; Otsuka Photal Electronics Co. Ltd., Osaka, Japan).

2.3.2. Fluorescence Spectroscopy

Fluorescence spectra of SMA@mTHPC, dissolved in different solutions or solvents, were recorded on a spectrophotometer (FP6600, Jasco Corp.,Tokyo, Japan). The sample solution was excited at 420 nm (corresponding to the maximum absorbance of mTHPC), and emission from 600 to 800 nm was recorded. A standard curve for free mTHPC in DMSO was plotted as a reference for quantification of the release of mTHPC from SMA@mTHPC as describe below.

2.3.3. UV–VIS Spectroscopy

UV–VIS spectra of SMA@mTHPC were recorded on a spectrophotometer (V730, Jasco Corp.). mTHPC content was quantified on the basis of analysis of UV–VIS absorption of SMA@mTHPC that was dissolved in DMSO at 420 nm. A standard curve for free mTHPC in DMSO was plotted (inset of Figure S1) as a reference for calculating the loading of mTHPC in SMA@mTHPC.

2.3.4. Release Rate of mTHPC from the SMA@mTHPC Micelles

The release of mTHPC from SMA@mTHPC micelles was measured by a dialysis method. In brief, 5 mg of SMA@mTHPC micelles was dissolved in 1 mL deionized water and placed in sealed dialysis bags (Mw cut-off 8000 Da, Wako). The dialysis bags were submerged in 50 mL tubes (Falcon, BD labware, Franklin Lakes, NJ) containing 25 mL of 0.2 M sodium phosphate buffers of different pH values (i.e., pH 5.5, pH 6.5, and pH 7.4). The dialysis tubes were then incubated at 37 °C in the dark with reciprocal shaking at 1 Hz. The mTHPC released from the dialysis bags were collected at scheduled time intervals and its amount was quantified by recording fluorescence intensity after 10-time dilution by DMSO by using the standard curve of mTHPC.

2.4. Detection of $^1O_2$ Generation by Electron Spin Resonance (ESR) Spectroscopy

SMA@mTHPC was dissolved in PBS at 400 µg/mL (40 µg/mL mTHPC equivalent) with/without 0.1% Tween 20, to which 20 mM 4-oxo-TEMP (spin trapping agent) was added. Samples in a flat quartz cell (Labotec, Tokyo, Japan) were irradiated (25 mW/cm^2) for the indicated times, by using xenon light source (MAX-303; Asahi Spectra Co. Ltd., Tokyo, Japan) at 400–700 nm. The ESR spectrometer was usually set at a microwave power of 1.0 mW, amplitude of 100 kHz, and field modulation width of 0.1 mT.

2.5. In Vitro Cytotoxicity Assay

Mouse colon cancer C26 cells and African green monkey kidney cells (CCL-81) were maintained in RPMI-1640 medium (Wako), supplemented with 10% fetal calf serum (Nichirei Biosciences Inc., Tokyo, Japan) under 5% CO_2/air at 37 °C. Cells were seeded in 96-well plates at 5000 cells per well and preincubated for 24 h. SMA@mTHPC was then added at different concentrations, followed by irradiation with fluorescent blue light that had peak emission at 420 nm (1.0 J/cm^2) (TL-D; Philips, Eindhoven, the Netherlands) at 24 h after addition of SMA@mTHPC. After further 24 h of culture, the MTT assay was carried out to quantify viable cells. In some experiments, the dark cytotoxicity of SMA@mTHPC without light irradiation was carried out, in which MTT assay was performed at 48 h after SMA@mTHPC administration.

2.6. Intracellular Uptake of SMA@mTHPC

C26 cells were seeded in 12-well plates at 3×10^5 cells per well and preincubated for 24 h. Free mTHPC or SMA@mTHPC was then added at 2 µg/mL. After the desired time, the cells were harvested and collected. After being washed thrice with PBS, the internalized mTHPC were extracted by using ethanol under sonication (30 W, 30 s, UP50H homogenizer, Hielscher Ultrasonics GmbH, Teltow, Germany) on ice, and the supernatant subsequently obtained after centrifugation (13,000 rpm, 15 min) was subjected to fluorescence spectroscopy (excitation at 420 nm, emission at 590 nm). The amount of mTHPC was then calculated by using the standard curve of mTHPC (Figure S2). In some experiments, the culture medium of pH 5.5 was used to investigate the uptake of SMA@mTHPC in different pH conditions.

2.7. In Vivo Tissue Distribution of SMA@mTHPC

Male ddY mice used in this study were 6 weeks old and obtained from SLC Inc., Shizuoka, Japan. Mouse sarcoma S180 cells (2×10^6 cells) that had been grown in peritoneal cavity of ddY mice as ascitic form were implanted subcutaneously (s.c.) in the dorsal skin of ddY mice in order to establish a mouse S180 solid tumor model. All animals were maintained under standard conditions and fed water and murine chow ad libitum. All animal experiments were approved by the Animal Ethics Committees of Sojo University (no. 2020-P-009, approved on 1 April 2020) and were carried out according to the Guidelines of the Laboratory Protocol of Animal Handling, Sojo University.

At 10–12 days after tumor inoculation when the diameters of the tumor reached approximately 10 mm, 5 mg/kg (mTHPC equivalent) of SMA@mTHPC dissolved in physiological saline was injected intravenously (i.v.). At 24 h after injection, the mice were sacrificed. After perfusion with physiological saline, tumors as well as normal tissues, e.g., liver, spleen, and kidney etc., were then dissected and weighed, and DMSO (1 mL/100 mg of tissue) was added. Tissues were then homogenized and after centrifugation (12,000 × g, 25 °C, 10 min), and mTHPC extracted in the supernatant was quantified by fluorescence intensity (Ex. at 420 nm, Em. at 590 nm) by using a standard curve of mTHPC (Figure S2).

In some experiments, the collected tumors as well as normal tissues (i.e., the liver) were subjected to ex vivo imaging using IVIS XR (Caliper Life Science, Hopkinton, MA, USA).

2.8. Comparison of the In Vivo Toxicity of SMA@mTHPC with Native mTHPC

The mouse S180 tumor model described above was used in this study. At 7–10 days after tumor inoculation when the diameters of tumors reached approximately 8–10 mm, SMA@mTHPC dissolved in physiological saline was injected intraperitoneally (i.p.) at a concentration of 10 mg/kg (mTHPC equivalent). Native mTHPC that was dissolved in DMSO was administered i.p. at the same concentration (10 mg/kg). To some of the mice receiving SMA@mTHPC or mTHPC, irradiation to the tumor area was carried out by xenon light (MAX-303; Asahi Spectra) at 400–700 nm for 5 min (27 J/cm^2) at 24 h after injection of SMA@mTHPC or mTHPC. The conditions and survival of the mice were monitored regularly.

In a separate study, SMA@mTHPC or mTHPC was injected i.v. at 20 mg/kg, in which mTHPC was first dissolved in DMSO and further diluted 10 times by physiological saline to indicated concentration.

2.9. In Vivo Antitumor Activity of SMA@mTHPC

The mouse S180 tumor model described above was used in this study. At 7–10 days after tumor inoculation when the diameters of tumors reached approximately 8–10 mm, SMA@mTHPC or mTHPC (10 mg/kg, mTHPC equivalent) was administered i.v. At 24 and 48 h after injection, the tumor was irradiated by xenon light (MAX-303; Asahi Spectra) at 400–700 nm for 5 min (27 J/cm^2). Our previous studies verified that xenon light source is an efficient tool for PDT that could cover most of the absorptions of PS with high intensity and low cost [14,15]. The width (W) and length (L) of the tumors, as well as the body weight of mice, were measured every 2–3 days during the study period, and tumor volume (mm^3) was calculated as $(W^2 \times L)/2$. The survival rate of animals was also recorded.

2.10. Statistical Analyses

All data were expressed as means ± SD. Data were analyzed by using ANOVA followed by the Bonferroni *t*-test. A difference was considered statistically significant when $p < 0.05$.

3. Results

3.1. Synthesis and Characterization of P-PyF

As shown in Figure 1A, SMA@mTHPC micelles form by self-assembly with the hydrophobic core encapsulating mTHPC and hydrophilic outer phase of maleic acid. SMA@mTHPC shows good water-solubility, and a clear solution was found at 20 mg/mL in PBS without precipitate after centrifugation (12,000 rpm, 1 min) (Figure S3). In aqueous solution, it exhibits a molecular size of 98 nm (Figure 1B), indicating the formation of micelles.

The UV–VIS spectrum of SMA@mTHPC in DMSO was similar to that of native mTHPC (Figure S1), but a decreased and shifted spectrum was found when it was dissolved in PBS (Figure 2A), suggesting the formation change in different solvents, i.e., micelles was formed in PBS, but the micelles were disrupted in organic solvent DMSO resulting in the similar UV–VIS spectrum to free mTHPC. This finding also in part supported the micelle formation of SMA@mTHPC in aqueous solutions. By using the standard curve (concentration vs. UV–VIS absorption) of mTHPC, the mTHPC loading in SMA@mTHPC was calculated as 10% (Figure S1).

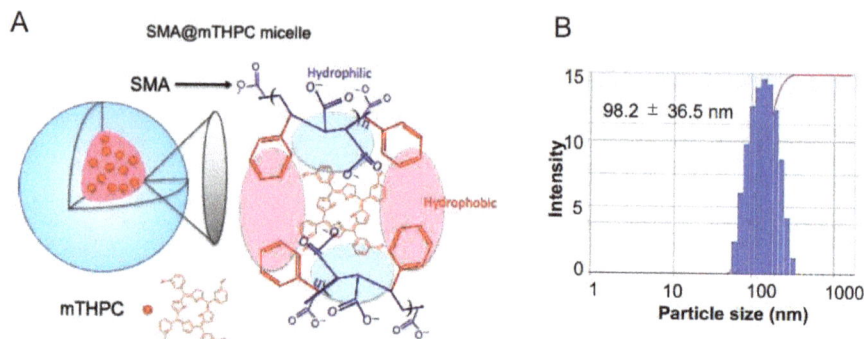

Figure 1. (**A**) Diagrammatic illustration of the micelle structure of SMA@mTHPC and (**B**) the hydrodynamic size of SMA@mTHPC in aqueous solution determined by dynamic light scatter (DLS).

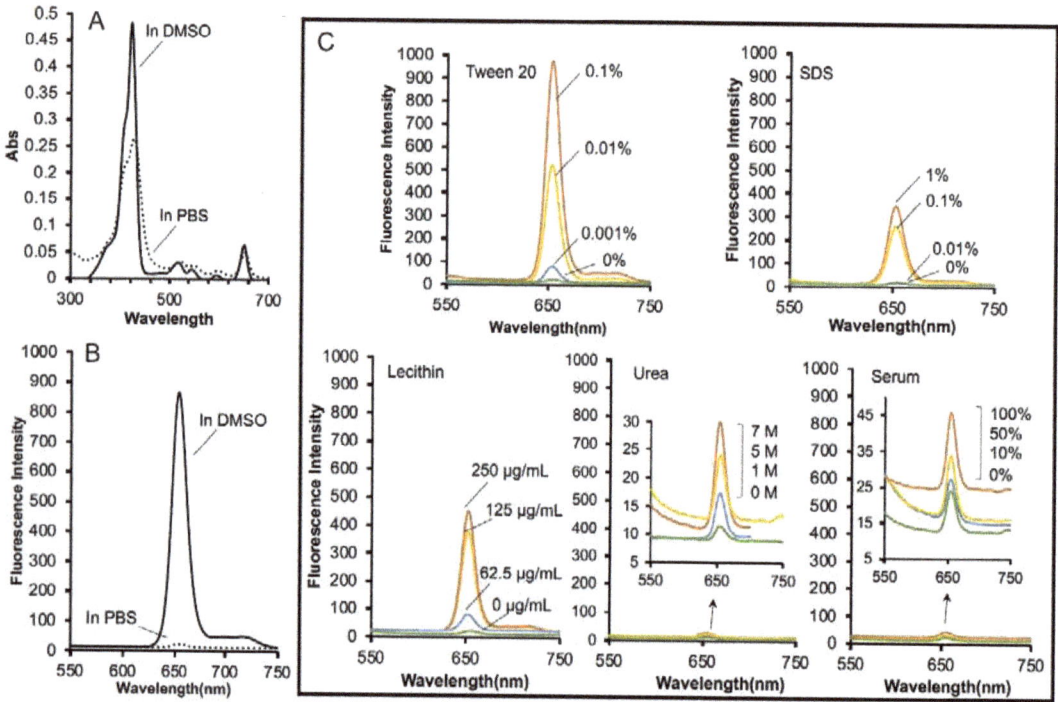

Figure 2. Characterization of the micelle formation of SMA@mTHPC. The UV–VIS spectra (**A**) and fluorescence spectra (**B**) of SMA@mTHPC in PBS as well as in DMSO were measured. The fluorescence spectra of SMA@mTHPC in the presence of detergent (Tween 20, SDS), the cell membrane component (lecithin), urea, and serum are shown in (**C**). See text for details.

The micelle formation of SMA@mTHPC in aqueous solution was further confirmed by detection of fluorescence. When mTHPC is encapsulated in the core of polymer micelle, aggregation of mTHPC molecules will occur, resulting in intense intermolecular π–π stacking interactions, consequently leading to fluorescence quenching, i.e., the decrease of fluorescence intensity [29]. As shown in Figure 2B, strong fluorescence was observed from SMA@mTHPC when it was dissolved in DMSO, in which the micelle formation was completely disrupted; however, the fluorescence of SMA@mTHPC in PBS was markedly quenched and was almost indetectable. Fluorescence quenching could also be liberated in the presence of Tween 20 and sodium dodecyl sulfate (SDS), which are surfactants disrupting the micelle self-assembly (Figure 2C), but urea did not affect fluorescence quenching (Figure 2C). These findings suggested hydrophobic interactions, but not hydrogen bond, may be involved in the micelle formation of SMA@mTHPC. More importantly, improvement of fluorescence was also observed in the presence of lecithin, the major component of cell membrane, but no increase of fluorescence was found in the presence of serum (Figure 2C), which indicated that SMA@mTHPC could behave as micelles stably in circulation; however, when it is taken up by cells, micelles will be disrupted to release free mTHPC rapidly.

3.2. Release of Free mTHPC from SMA@mTHPC

Release of free drug is a key issue for polymeric micellar drugs to fulfill their pharmacological effects. We thus investigated the release profiles of SMA@mTHPC in different conditions. In buffer solution of neutral pH (7.4), a constant release of free mTHPC, i.e., ≈20% per day, was observed (Figure 3).

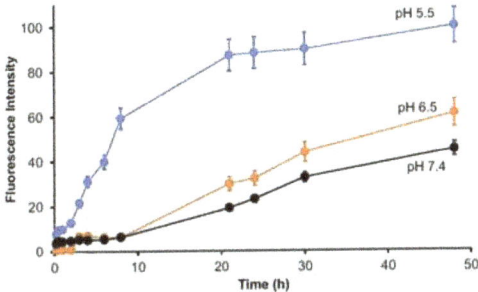

Figure 3. Release profile of SMA@mTHPC. SMA@mTHPC was dissolved in sodium phosphate buffer of different pH values and sealed in dialysis bags. After the indicated incubation time at 37 °C, the mTHPC released from the dialysis bags were measured and quantified by recording fluorescence intensity. A constant in vitro release rate of ≈20% per day was observed at neutral pH (7.4), whereas higher release was found at weak acidic pH (6.5, 5.5). Data are mean ± SD, n = 4. See text for details.

The release of mTHPC was largely increased at acidic pH; the release rate reached 50% after 48 h incubation at pH 6.5, and it further reached 90–100% at pH 5.5 (Figure 3). Given that tumors always show slight acidic pH (6.0–7.0) [30], tumor-specific release of free mTHPC could be anticipated for SMA@mTHPC.

3.3. Generation of $^1O_2$ from SMA@mTHPC under Light Irradiation

To elucidate the efficacy of SMA@mTHPC to produce $^1O_2$, we measured the $^1O_2$ generation using ESR. As shown in Figure 4, the $^1O_2$ generation from SMA@mTHPC was found negligible or very little in PBS; however, strong signal of $^1O_2$ was detected in an irradiation-dependent manner when Tween 20 was added into the solution (Figure 4). These findings were consistent with results of fluorescence quenching shown in Figure 2C, indicating that the micelle formation of SMA@mTHPC in aqueous solution also suppressed the generation of $^1O_2$, with disruption of micelle being necessary for SMA@mTHPC to achieve PDT effect.

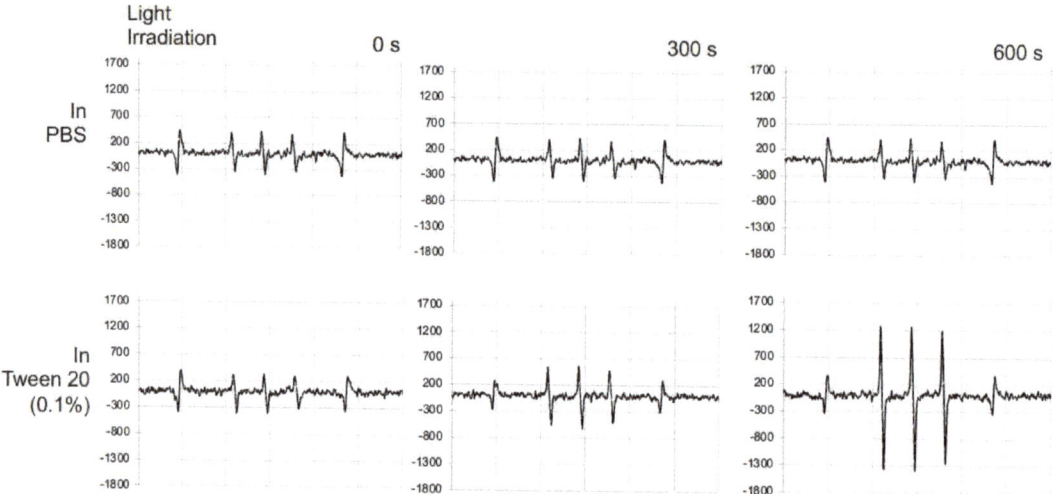

Figure 4. ESR measurement for singlet oxygen ($^1O_2$) generation from SMA@mTHPC. SMA@mTHPC was dissolved in PBS in the absence or presence of 0.1% Tween 20, and light irradiation (25 mW/cm^2) was carried out using xenon light of 400–700 nm, for the indicated times. $^1O_2$ generated was captured by 4-oxo-TEMP, and triplet 4-oxo-TEMPO signal due to $^1O_2$ was detected by ESR spectra. See text for details.

3.4. In Vitro Cytotoxicity of SMA@mTHPC

On the basis of the findings of $^1O_2$ generation described in Figure 4, we investigated the PDT effect of SMA@mTHPC in vitro by using a fluorescence blue light source that fits to the maximal absorbance of mTHPC.

As shown in Figure 5A, in cultured C26 colon cancer cells, SMA@mTHPC alone (no light irradiation) induced the cell death with an IC$_{50}$ of 2 µg/mL that was slightly lower than the cytotoxicity of free mTHPC (IC$_{50}$ of 1 µg/mL). However, after irradiation using blue light source (1.0 J/cm^2), cytotoxicities of both free mTHPC and SMA@mTHPC were remarkably increased (more than 100-fold), and the IC$_{50}$ of PDT using SMA@mTHPC and free mTHPC were 0.015 µg/mL and 0.0005 µg/mL, respectively (Figure 5A). Moreover, in normal cells (CCL-81), the cytotoxicity of SMA@mTHPC was largely lowered, and a 10-time higher IC$_{50}$ was observed both with light irradiation (IC$_{50}$ of 0.15 µg/mL) and without irradiation (IC$_{50}$ of 20 µg/mL) (Figure 5B).

3.5. Intracellular Uptake of SMA@mTHPC

As shown in Figure 6, free mTHPC was rapidly taken up by cancer cells, and almost 10% of the applied drugs were internalized within 4 h. In contrast, SMA@mTHPC showed a 10-time lower intracellular uptake than free mTHPC; however, at pH 5.5, the internalization of SMA@mTHPC was significantly increased (Figure 6). These findings are parallel with the results of release profiles (Figure 3), again suggesting the release of free mTHPC is a key factor for the therapeutic effect of SMA@mTHPC.

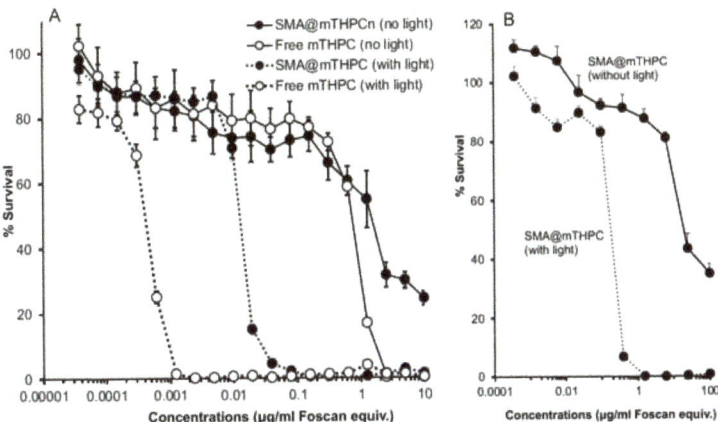

Figure 5. In vitro dark cytotoxicity and photocytotoxicity (PDT) of SMA@mTHPC in mouse colon cancer C26 cells (**A**) and African green monkey kidney cells (CCL-81) (**B**). Cells (5000/well) were seeded in a 96-well plate; after 24 h pre-incubation, different concentrations of SMA@mTHPC were added, and after further 24 h incubation, the viability of cells was measured by MTT assay. Photocytotoxicity was examined by irradiating the cells with light (blue light of 420 nm, 1 J/cm^2) at 24 h after addition of SMA@mTHPC. Data are mean ± SD, n = 6–8. See text for details.

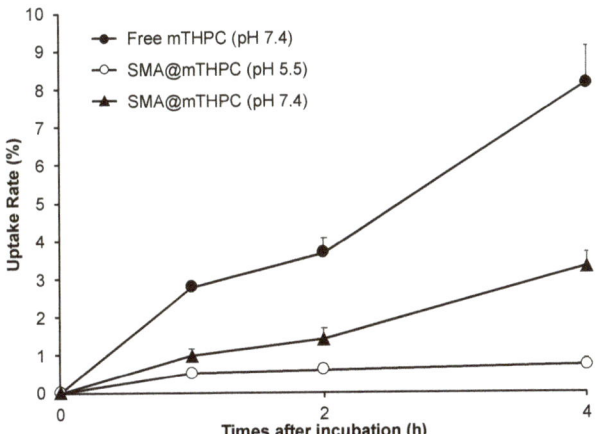

Figure 6. Intracellular uptake of SMA@mTHPC and free mTHPC in mouse colon cancer C26 cells. C26 cells were incubated with SMA@mTHPC or free mTHPC using media of different pH values (7.4 or 5.5). After indicated time, cells were collected, and the internalized mTHPC was quantified by measuring fluorescence intensity. Data are mean ± SD, n = 3. See text for details.

3.6. Tissue Distribution of SMA@mTHPC and In Vivo Imaging

For investigating the body distribution of SMA@mTHPC, we first carried out in vivo imaging in a S180 transplanted tumor model by taking advantage of the fluorescence property of mTHPC. As shown in Figure 7A, we found a relatively high accumulation of SMA@mTHPC in tumor at 24 h after i.v. injection, which was higher than those in most normal tissues including the muscle, colon, and heart. Compared to the tumor, higher accumulation in the liver, which is rich in the reticuloendothelial system that captures macromolecules, was observed (Figure 7A); however, in vivo imaging showed a much lower fluorescence in the liver than that in the tumor (Figure 7B). Moreover, relatively high accumulation was also observed in the kidney, which indicates the gradual release of free mTHPC in circulation. Similar distribution was also found for free mTHPC after i.v. injection, although it had to be dissolved in organic solvent (i.e., DMSO), which suggests that mTHPC may bind to serum proteins, thus behaving as large molecules similar to Evans blue, as described in many previous studies in the literature [6,31].

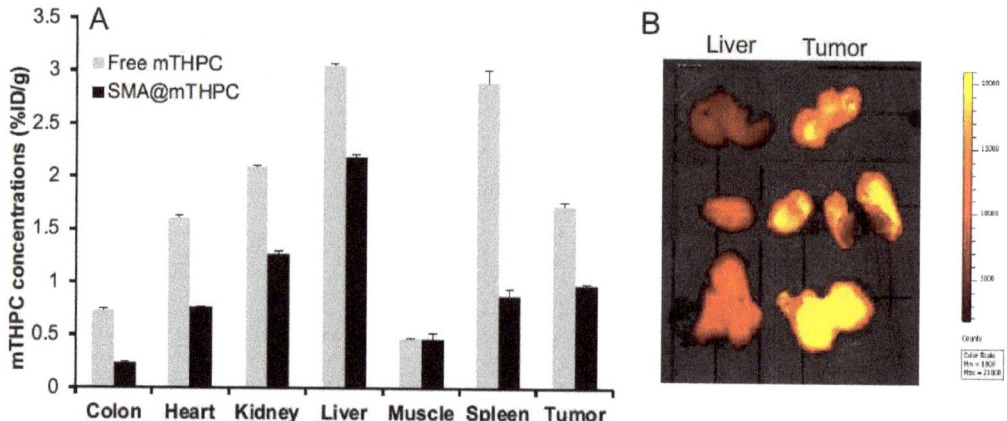

Figure 7. In vivo tissue distribution of SMA@mTHPC at 24 h after i.v. injection in sarcoma S180 tumor-bearing mice. In the S180 solid tumor model, SMA@mTHPC (5 mg/kg mTHPC equivalent) or free mTHPC (5 mg/kg) was i.v. injected when the tumor grew to the size of about 10 mm in diameter; the mice were then killed and indicated tissues were collected, and the amount of SMA@mTHPC in each tissue was quantified by detecting the fluorescence of mTHPC (**A**). In a separate experiment, the tumor and liver of SMA@mTHPC-treated mice were resected and applied to in vivo imaging using IVIS (**B**). See text for details. Data are mean ± SD, n = 3–6.

3.7. In Vivo Antitumor PDT Effect of SMA@mTHPC

To investigate the therapeutic (PDT) potential of SMA@mTHPC, we performed in vivo experiments using mouse sarcoma S180 solid tumor model. Treatment was carried out when the tumor grew to about 1 cm in diameter; SMA@mTHPC was first injected i.v., and then light irradiation was performed using xenon light source with a broadband light of 400–700 nm (90 mW/cm^2, 5 min [27 J/cm^2]) at 24 and 48 h after injection when SMA@mTHPC accumulated in the tumor preferentially with low accumulation in normal tissues.

The results, as indicated in Figure 8A, showed a significant suppression of tumor growth by the treatment, and similar therapeutic effects were achieved by using either SMA@mTHPC or free mTHPC (Figure 8A). However, during the treatment, we found a significant loss of body weight in free mTHPC-treated mice, in which one mouse died after 3 days of treatment (Figure 8B), whereas PDT using SMA@mTHPC did not show any apparent side effect during the period of observation, and the body weights of mice increased normally similar to control mice without treatment (the difference of body weight between SMA@mTHPC and control is considered mostly due to the difference of tumor weight) (Figure 8B). Free mTHPC-treated mice showed reddish and blackish coloration in the skin around the tumor (Figure S4), indicating severe inflammation in the skin, whereas no apparent changes were found in SMA@mTHPC-treated mice. These findings suggested the superior safety of SMA@mTHPC.

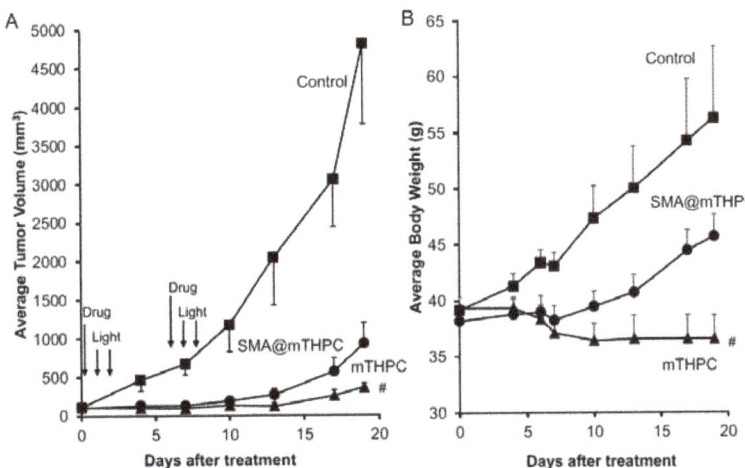

Figure 8. In vivo PDT effect of SMA@mTHPC in S180 solid tumor. A xenon light source was used (MAX-303; Asahi Spectra). Indicated concentrations of SMA@mTHPC were injected i.v. when tumor diameters reached 8–10 mm. After 24 and 48 h, light irradiation (90 mW/cm^2, 5 min, 27 J/cm^2) was carried out. Tumor volume (**A**) and body weight (**B**) were measured every 2 or 3 days. Arrows indicate the application of SMA@mTHPC or mTHPC, and light irradiation. Data are means ± SD; n = 4–8. # one mouse died during the treatment using mTHPC. See text for details.

In addition, light irradiation alone or SMA@mTHPC/mTHPC alone without light irradiation did not exhibit apparent tumor growth suppression (Figure S5), indicating that the therapeutic effect was mostly the outcome of PDT.

3.8. Decreased Toxicity of SMA@mTHPC Compared to Free mTHPC

Given that SMA@mTHPC exhibited a better safety profile than free mTHPC, as indicated in Figure 8B, we further investigated and compared the toxicity profile of SMA@mTHPC with that of free mTHPC by using different doses and administration routes.

First, we administered the drugs to S180 tumor-bearing mice by i.p. route because i.v. route is not a common route for organic solution of mTHPC, and we found 10 mg/kg of SMA@mTHPC did not show any apparent side effects and all mice survived up to 16 days after the treatment, either with light irradiation or without light irradiation (Figure 9A); however, administration of free mTHPC (10 mg/kg, mTHPC equivalent) showed severe toxicity, one out of four mice died even without light irradiation, and all mice died after light irradiation within 1 week after treatment (Figure 9A). Then, we confirmed the toxicity profiles of SMA@mTHPC/free mTHPC alone without light irradiation (but the mice were subjected to ambient light), by i.v. route in which free mTHPC was first dissolved in DMSO at a high concentration and then diluted to experimental concentration by PBS. As shown in Figure 9B, at the dose of 20 mg/kg (mTHPC equivalent), no apparent side effect (body weight loss) was observed for SMA@mTHPC, and all mice survived for up to 28 days after administration. In contrast, administration of free mTHPC induced a remarkable loss of body weight (Figure 9B); the mice were very weak during the experiment period, and one mouse died 9 days after injection. These finding further indicated the superior safety profile of SMA@mTHPC to free mTHPC for PDT.

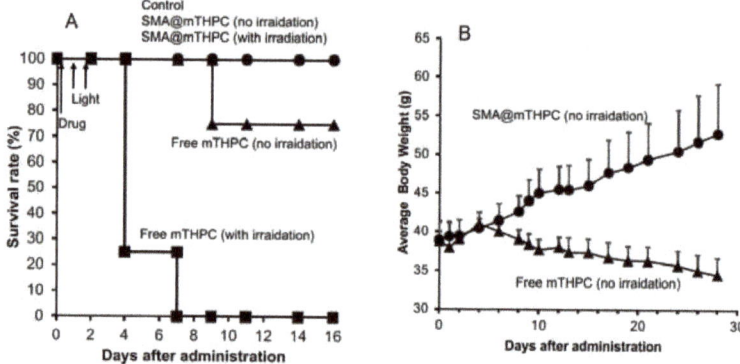

Figure 9. Toxicity profiles of SMA@mTHPC and free mTHPC as indicated by survival rate and body weight change in S180 tumor-bearing mice. (**A**) SMA@mTHPC or free mTHPC was injected i.p. at a concentration of 10 mg/kg (mTHPC equivalent), and in some mice, light irradiation was carried out as described in Figure 7, where the survival rate was recorded. In a separate study, SMA@mTHPC or free mTHPC was injected i.v. at a concentration of 20 mg/kg (mTHPC equivalent) with light irradiation, and the body weight change (**B**) was measured and calculated. Data are means ± SD; n = 4–8. See text for details.

4. Discussion

In the present study, we developed a polymeric micelle of PDT drug mTHPC, SMA@mTHPC, which showed potent therapeutic effect and high safety. SMA@mTHPC micelle was formed by self-assembly in aqueous solution through hydrophobic interaction between mTHPC and hydrophobic moiety of SMA (Figure 1A), with a hydrodynamic size of 98 nm (Figure 1B). As the micelle formation in physiological solution, SMA@mTHPC showed prolonged circulation time and tumor-targeted accumulation based on the EPR effect (Figure 7). SMA@mTHPC micelle is relatively stable in circulation, which ensured its safety because generation of $^1O_2$ and fluorescence will be quenched in micellar state (Figures 2 and 4). However, the micellar state will be disrupted in the tumor environment and during internalization, resulting in the appearance of strong fluorescence (Figure 7) and generation of $^1O_2$ (Figure 4). Consequently, potent antitumor PDT effect was achieved with little damage to the host (Figures 8 and 9).

Stability is one important issue for micellar drugs, as unstable micelles will release free drugs in circulation before accumulating in tumors, thus behaving similarly to free small molecular drugs. However, a too stable micelle is also not preferable, because release of active drugs from a micelle that is too slow and too little will largely affect the therapeutic effect. Accordingly, an ideal micelle drug is stable in circulation to achieve EPR effect-based tumor accumulation but rapidly release active drugs in tumor tissues to fulfill the antitumor effect, i.e., tumor environment-responsive nanomedicine. In this context, SMA@mTHPC showed a relatively high stability in physiological solution and in the presence of serum, as evidenced by almost completely fluorescence quenching (Figure 2B,C), as well as no or very little generation of $^1O_2$ (Figure 4). In vivo imaging also showed relatively low fluorescence intensity in the liver (Figure 7B), although the amount of SMA@mTHPC was relatively high (Figure 7A), which further supported this notion. More importantly and interestingly, tumor showed a strong fluorescence intensity, although tumor concentration was lower than that in the liver (Figure 7). These findings suggested that the micelles are disrupted in tumor tissues, and release of free mTHPC thus exhibits strong fluorescence. The release profile of SMA@mTHPC also indicated the tumor environment responsive behavior of SMA@mTHPC, for which more release occurred at weak acidic pH (6.5) that is seen in most solid tumors [30] than neutral pH (7.4) (Figure 3). Further, when SMA@mTHPC is taken up by tumor cells, in the lysosomal compartment (pH 5.0–5.5), extensive and rapid release of free mTHPC will occur, as indicated by the release profile (Figure 3) and enhanced intracellular uptake (Figure 6) at pH 5.5. It has been reported that SMA-modified nano-drugs showed marked intracellular uptake at acidic pH than at neutral pH because of the higher lipophilicity of maleyl carboxylic at acidic pH (HOOC-COO−) [32,33]. Taken together, the acidic pH of tumor tissue will trigger the release of mTHPC from SMA@mTHPC, as well as intracellular uptake of SMA@mTHPC, which further enhance the release cascade, consequently resulting in the extensive release in tumor tissue.

Benefiting from the tumor environment-responsive behavior as described above, SMA@mTHPC showed a remarkable antitumor PDT effect that was similar to the effect of free mTHPC (Figure 7). More importantly, it ensured the high safety of this treatment. Firstly, as a micellar nano-drug, it accumulated in tumor tissue at a relatively high concentration, whereas it distributes less in most normal tissues (Figure 6). Furthermore, in normal tissues such as the liver and blood, it maintains a stably micellar formation, and thus the generation of $^1O_2$ is suppressed; consequently, no or very few side effects were observed (Figures 8B and 9). In contrast, although free mTHPC showed a strong antitumor PDT effect, severe side effects including the death of host mice appeared (Figures 8 and 9), and the toxicity of free mTHPC could also be seen even under ambient light (without light irradiation using therapeutic xenon light source) (Figure 9). Indiscriminate tissue distribution and photoexcitation/generation of $^1O_2$ are the major causes of the toxicity of free mTHPC. In this regard, micellar modification of mTHPC not only decreases the distribution in most normal tissues, but also lowers the photosensitivity in normal tissues, resulting superior safety profiles. These findings, together with the high water-solubility of SMA@mTHPC, strongly suggest the advantages and applicability of SMA@mTHPC, which warrants further investigations.

Compared with free mTHPC, SMA@mTHPC showed lower cytotoxicity both under light irradiation (photocytoxicity) and without light exposure (dark cytotoxicity) (Figure 5). We considered that the reason is mostly that the micelle formation lowers the photosensitivity of mTHPC as described above. This result is also associated to the decreased toxicity of SMA@mTHPC. Moreover, regarding the dark cytoxicitiy of SMA@mTHPC and mTHPC, it may be partly due to the ambient light during incubation; however, mTHPC itself may also has inherent cytotoxicity, although the mechanism is not elucidated. Therefore, further studies are needed to clarify this issue.

Regarding the tissue distribution of SMA@mTHPC, besides the relatively high tumor accumulation, SMA@mTHPC also accumulates at high levels in the liver (Figure 7A). However, the fluorescence imaging exhibited a relatively low signal (Figure 7B). This finding is most probably due to the micellar stability in the liver as the polymer stays in a blood-like environment. The high concentrations of heme in the liver that may absorb light near the absorption band of mTHPC may also suppress the fluorescence of mTHPC. Taken together, these findings again support environment-responsive behavior of SMA@mTHPC: it is stable as a micelle in circulation and normal tissues such as those in the liver, thus showing very little toxicity and adverse effects (Figures 7 and 8), whereas micelle formation is destroyed in the tumor environment, thus exhibiting remarkable tumor imaging potential (Figure 7) as well as antitumor PDT effect (Figure 8). As for free mTHPC, we also found a relative tumor concentration that was similar to SMA@mTHPC (Figure 6). This was probably due to its binding property to circulation proteins such as albumin, as seen in Evans blue, the commonly used agent to indicate EPR effect that is known to bind to albumin and thus behave as a macromolecule. Similar behaviors have also been observed in some anticancer drugs such as paclitaxel and gemcitabine [34,35]. Thus, in circulation, mTHPC may behave as a macromolecule (albumin complex) showing prolonged retention, which was slightly higher than that of SMA@mTHPC (Figure 7). However, this complex formation of mTHPC is not well organized and the fluorescence and phototoxicity of mTHPC could not be efficiently suppressed by this formation; thus, although mTHPC showed a potent antitumor PDT effect, its long circulation time due to its protein binding, in contrast, induced severe side effects (Figures 8B and 9).

Taken together, these findings suggested SMA@mTHPC could become a candidate drug for PDT, which not only shows potent therapeutic effect, but more importantly exhibits high safety profiles, and thus we anticipate its application in the future.

Supplementary Materials: The following are available online at https://www.mdpi.com/article/10.3390/biomedicines9101493/s1, Figure S1: UV–VIS spectra of SMA@mTHPC and free mTHPC, Figure S2: Standard curve of mTHPC in DMSO as measured by fluorescence (Ex420nm/Em590nm), Figure S3: Pictures of SMA@mTHPC solution in PBS, Figure S4: Pictures of mice after free mTHPC treatment and SMA@mTHPC treatment, Figure S5: In vivo antitumor effect of irradiation alone (without SMA@mTHPC) and SMA@mTHPC alone (without light irradiation).

Author Contributions: Conceptualization, J.F.; methodology, J.F., S.G. and R.I.; software, J.F., S.G. and R.I.; validation, J.F. and S.G.; formal analysis, J.F. and S.G.; investigation, S.G., R.I., H.N., R.Y., N.Y., N.W., Y.Y. and N.N.; resources, J.F., J.-R.Z. and K.Y.; data curation, J.F.; writing—original draft preparation, J.F. and S.G.; writing—review and editing, J.F.; visualization, J.F. and S.G.; supervision, J.F., J.-R.Z. and K.Y.; project administration, J.F.; funding acquisition, J.F. All authors have read and agreed to the published version of the manuscript.

Funding: This work was supported by the research fund from Sojo University to J. Fang. and partly by a Grant-in-Aid for Scientific Research on Scientific Research (C) (JSPS KAKENHI grant numbers 19K09806 and 19K07743) to J. Fang.

Institutional Review Board Statement: All animal experiments were carried out according to the Guidelines of the Laboratory Protocol of Animal Handling, Sojo University, and approved by the Animal Ethics Committee of Sojo University (no. 2020-P-009, approved on 1 April 2020).

Data Availability Statement: The data presented in this study are available on request from the corresponding author.

Conflicts of Interest: The authors declare no conflict of interest.

References

1. McBride, G. Studies expand potential uses of photodynamic therapy. *J. Natl. Cancer Inst.* **2002**, *94*, 1740–1742. [CrossRef]
2. Wilson, B.C. Photodynamic therapy for cancer: Principles. *Can. J. Gastroenterol.* **2002**, *16*, 393–396. [CrossRef] [PubMed]
3. Dolmans, D.E.; Fukumura, D. Photodynamic therapy for cancer. *Nat. Rev. Cancer* **2003**, *3*, 380–387. [CrossRef]
4. O'Connor, W.; Gallagher, A. Byrne, Porphyrin and nonporphyrin photosensitizers in oncology: Preclinical and clinical advances in photodynamic therapy. *Photochem. Photobiol.* **2009**, *85*, 1053–1074. [CrossRef]
5. Fang, J.; Seki, T. Therapeutic strategies by modulating oxygen stress in cancer and inflammation. *Adv. Drug Deliv. Rev.* **2009**, *61*, 290–302. [CrossRef]
6. Matsumura, Y.; Maeda, H. A new concept for macromolecular therapeutics in cancer chemotherapy: Mechanism of tumoritropic accumulation of proteins and the antitumor agent SMANCS. *Cancer Res.* **1986**, *46*, 6387–6392. [PubMed]
7. Torchilin, V. Tumor delivery of macromolecular drugs based on the EPR effect. *Adv. Drug Deliv. Rev.* **2011**, *63*, 131–135. [CrossRef] [PubMed]
8. Fang, J.; Nakamura, H. The EPR effect: Unique features of tumor blood vessels for drug delivery, factors involved, and limitations and augmentation of the effect. *Adv. Drug Deliv. Rev.* **2011**, *63*, 136–151. [CrossRef]
9. Maeda, H. Toward a full understanding of the EPR effect in primary and metastatic tumors as well as issues related to its heterogeneity. *Adv. Drug Deliv. Rev.* **2015**, *91*, 3–6. [CrossRef] [PubMed]
10. Fang, J.; Islam, W. Exploiting the dynamics of the EPR effect and strategies to improve the therapeutic effects of nanomedicines by using EPR effect enhancers. *Adv. Drug Deliv. Rev.* **2020**, *157*, 142–160. [CrossRef]
11. Islam, R.; Maeda, H. Factors affecting the dynamics and heterogeneity of the EPR effect: Pathophysiological and pathoanatomic features, drug formulations and physicochemical factors. *Expert Opin. Drug Deliv.* **2021**, 1–14. [CrossRef]
12. Nakamura, H.; Liao, L. Micelles of zinc protoporphyrin conjugated to N-(2-hydroxypropyl) me- thacrylamide (HPMA) copolymer for imaging and light-induced antitumor effects in vivo. *J. Control Release* **2013**, *165*, 191–198. [CrossRef]
13. Islam, W.; Matsumoto, Y. Polymer-conjugated glucosamine complexed with boric acid shows tumor-selective accumulation and simultaneous inhibition of glycolysis. *Biomaterials* **2021**, *269*, 120631. [CrossRef] [PubMed]
14. Fang, J.; Liao, L. Photodynamic therapy and imaging based on tumor-targeted nanoprobe, polymer-conjugated zinc protoporphyrin. *Future Sci. OA* **2015**, *1*, 3. [CrossRef] [PubMed]
15. Fang, J.; Islam, W. N-(2-hydroxypropyl) methacrylamide polymer conjugated pyropheophorbide-a, a promising tumor-targeted theranostic probe for photodynamic therapy and imaging. *Eur. J. Pharm. Biopharm.* **2018**, *130*, 165–176. [CrossRef]
16. Fang, J.; Tsukigawa, K. Styrene-maleic acid-copolymer conjugated zinc protoporphyrin as a candidate drug for tumor-targeted therapy and imaging. *J. Drug Target* **2016**, *24*, 399–407. [CrossRef]

17. Iyer, A.K.; Greish, K. Polymeric micelles of zinc protoporphyrin for tumor targeted delivery based on EPR effect and singlet oxygen generation. *J. Drug Target* **2007**, *15*, 496–506. [CrossRef]
18. Iyer, A.K.; Greish, K. High-loading nanosized micelles of copoly (styrene-maleic acid)-zinc protoporphyrin for targeted delivery of a potent heme oxygenase inhibitor. *Biomaterials* **2007**, *28*, 1871–1881. [CrossRef]
19. Fang, J.; Sawa, T. In vivo antitumor activity of pegylated zinc protoporphyrin: Targeted inhibition of heme oxygenase in solid tumor. *Cancer Res* **2003**, *63*, 3567–3574. [PubMed]
20. Sahoo, S.K.; Sawa, T. Pegylated zinc protoporphyrin: A water-soluble heme oxygenase inhibitor with tumor-targeting capacity. *Bioconjug. Chem.* **2002**, *13*, 1031–1038. [CrossRef]
21. Dragicevic-Curic, N.; Scheglmann, D. Development of different temoporfin-loaded invasomes-novel nanocarriers of temoporfin: Characterization, stability and in vitro skin penetration studies. *Colloids Surf. B Biointerfaces* **2009**, *70*, 198–206. [CrossRef] [PubMed]
22. Dragicevic-Curic, N.; Fahr, A. Liposomes in topical photodynamic therapy. *Expert Opin. Drug Deliv.* **2012**, *9*, 1015–1032. [CrossRef] [PubMed]
23. Yakavets, I.; Francois, A. Effect of stroma on the behavior of temoporfin-loaded lipid nanovesicles inside the stroma-rich head and neck carcinoma spheroids. *J. Nanobiotechnology* **2021**, *19*, 3. [CrossRef]
24. Yakavets, I.; Millard, M. Current state of the nanoscale delivery systems for temoporfin-based photodynamic therapy: Advanced delivery strategies. *J. Control Release* **2019**, *304*, 268–287. [CrossRef]
25. Cabral, H.; Miyata, K. Block Copolymer Micelles in Nanomedicine Applications. *Chem. Rev.* **2018**, *118*, 6844–6892. [CrossRef]
26. Cabral, H.; Kataoka, K. Progress of drug-loaded polymeric micelles into clinical studies. *J. Control Release* **2014**, *190*, 465–476. [CrossRef] [PubMed]
27. Greish, K.; Sawa, T. SMA-doxorubicin, a new polymeric micellar drug for effective targeting to solid tumours. *J. Control Release* **2004**, *97*, 219–230. [CrossRef]
28. Greish, K.; Nagamitsu, A. Copoly (styrene-maleic acid)-pirarubicin micelles: High tumor-targeting efficiency with little toxicity. *Bioconjug. Chem.* **2005**, *16*, 230–236. [CrossRef]
29. Li, Q.; Li, Z. The Strong Light-Emission Materials in the Aggregated State: What Happens from a Single Molecule to the Collective Group. *Adv. Sci. (Weinh)* **2017**, *4*. [CrossRef]
30. Racker, E. Bioenergetics and the problem of tumor growth. *Am. Sci.* **1972**, *60*, 56–63.
31. Fang, J.; Qin, H. Carbon monoxide, generated by heme oxygenase -1, mediates the enhanced permeability and retention effect in solid tumors. *Cancer Sci.* **2012**, *103*, 535–541. [CrossRef] [PubMed]
32. Oda, T.; Maeda, H. Binding to and internalization by cultured cells of neocarzinostatin and enhancement of its actions by conjugation with lipophilic styrene-maleic acid copolymer1. *Cancer Res.* **1987**, *47*, 3206–3211.
33. Maeda, H.; Islam, W. Overcoming barriers for tumor-targeted drug delivery: The power of macromolecular anticancer drugs with the EPR effect and the modulation of vascular physiology. In *Polymer-Protein Conjugates: From Pegylation and Beyond*, 1st ed.; Pasut, G., Zalipsky, S., Eds.; Elsevier: Amsterdam, The Netherlands, 2020; pp. 41–58.
34. Qi, H.; Wang, Y. The different interactions of two anticancer drugs with bovine serum albumin based on multi-spectrum method combined with molecular dynamics simulations. *Spectrochim. Acta A Mol. Biomol. Spectrosc.* **2021**, *259*. [CrossRef] [PubMed]
35. Ali, M.S.; Muthukumaran, J. Experimental and computational investigation on the binding of anticancer drug gemcitabine with bovine serum albumin. *J. Biomol. Struct. Dyn.* **2021**, *17*, 1–14.

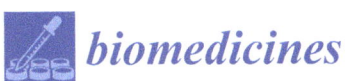

Article

Photodynamic Effects with 5-Aminolevulinic Acid on Cytokines and Exosomes in Human Peripheral Blood Mononuclear Cells

Kristian Espeland [1,2,3,*,†], Andrius Kleinauskas [2,†], Petras Juzenas [2], Andreas Brech [3,4], Sagar Darvekar [2], Vlada Vasovic [2], Trond Warloe [2], Eidi Christensen [2,5,6], Jørgen Jahnsen [1,3] and Qian Peng [2,7,*]

1. Department of Gastroenterology, Akershus University Hospital, N-1478 Lorenskog, Norway; jorgen.jahnsen@medisin.uio.no
2. Department of Pathology, Norwegian Radium Hospital, Oslo University Hospital, N-0310 Oslo, Norway; andrius.kleinauskas@rr-research.no (A.K.); petras.juzenas@rr-research.no (P.J.); sagar.darvekar@rr-research.no (S.D.); Vlada.Vasovic@rr-research.no (V.V.); trond.warloe@gmail.com (T.W.); eidi.christensen@ntnu.no (E.C.)
3. Institute of Clinical of Medicine, Faculty of Medicine, University of Oslo, N-0372 Oslo, Norway; abrech@rr-research.no
4. Department of Molecular Cell Biology, Institute for Cancer Research, Norwegian Radium Hospital, Oslo University Hospital, N-0372 Oslo, Norway
5. Department of Clinical and Molecular Medicine, Norwegian University of Science and Technology, N-7030 Trondheim, Norway
6. Department of Dermatology, St. Olavs Hospital, Trondheim University Hospital, N-7030 Trondheim, Norway
7. Department of Optical Science and Engineering, School of Information Science and Technology, Fudan University, Shanghai 200433, China

* Correspondence: eskris@ahus.no (K.E.); qian.peng@rr-research.no (Q.P.)
† These authors contributed equally to the work as first-authors.

Abstract: Photodynamic therapy (PDT) with 5-aminolevulinic acid (ALA), a precursor to the potent photosensitizer, protoporphyrin IX (PpIX), is an established modality for several malignant and premalignant diseases. This treatment is based on the light-activated PpIX in targeted lesions. Although numerous studies have confirmed the necrosis and apoptosis involved in the mechanism of action of this modality, little information is available for the change of exosome levels after treatment. We report from the first study on the effects of ALA-PDT on cytokines and exosomes of human healthy peripheral blood mononuclear cells (PBMCs). The treatment reduced the cytokines and exosomes studied, although there was variation among individual PBMC samples. This reduction is consistent with PDT-mediated survivals of subsets of PBMCs. More specifically, the ALA-PDT treatment apparently decreased all pro-inflammatory cytokines included, suggesting that this treatment may provide a strong anti-inflammatory effect. In addition, the treatment has decreased the levels of different types of exosomes, the HLA-DRDPDQ exosome in particular, which plays an important role in the rejection of organ transplantation as well as autoimmune diseases. These results may suggest future therapeutic strategies of ALA-PDT.

Keywords: 5-aminolevulinic acid (ALA); photodynamic therapy (PDT); photodynamic diagnosis; protoporphyrin IX (PpIX); peripheral blood mononuclear cells (PBMCs); cytokine; exosome; electron microscopy; flow cytometry

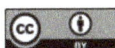

1. Introduction

Photodynamic therapy (PDT), an established treatment modality for several malignant and pre-malignant diseases, uses a combination of a lesion-localizing photosensitizing agent with light irradiation to induce photochemical and photobiological reactions in the presence of oxygen. These reactions lead to irreversible photodamage to the lesion. During this dynamic process, the absorbed light energy by the photosensitizer can be transferred to molecular oxygen to generate reactive oxygen species (ROS), including singlet oxygen ($^1O_2$). These species react further with cellular components to cause apoptosis and/or necrosis [1,2].

PDT with chemically synthesized sensitizers, has a major side-effect of skin phototoxicity, limiting clinical PDT to a great extent. Thus, considerable interest has been directed towards developing a PDT regimen with an endogenous potent photosensitizer, protoporphyrin IX (PpIX). 5-aminolevulinic acid (ALA), a naturally occurring amino acid formed from glycine and succinyl CoA, is a precursor to PpIX in the heme biosynthesis pathway. By adding exogenous ALA, the naturally occurring PpIX may accumulate in cells [3,4]. This intracellular PpIX accumulation has been exploited for its application in photodiagnosis and PDT [5]. Clinically, systemic administration of ALA is used for the PpIX fluorescence-guided surgical resection of glioma [6]; while topically applied ALA-PDT has already been approved by United States Food and Drug Administration (FDA) and European Medicines Agency (EMA) for actinic keratosis and basal cell carcinoma of the skin [4].

Cytokines are a family of small proteins that are involved in growth and activities of blood cells including immune cells. They are largely produced by immune cells such as macrophages, T-cells, B-cells, and non-immune cells including endothelial cells and fibroblasts. Once released, they signal and modulate the immune system.

Exosomes, with a diameter of about 50–150 nm, are extracellular lipid bilayer vesicles with an endosomal origin of cells. They carry nucleic acids, proteins, lipids, and other bioactive molecules. Exosomes can be secreted by healthy and diseased cells through different pathways [7]. They can merge with cells and are involved in signaling between cells, but it is still not clear how exosomes communicate with cells and which roles they play in a biological system [8,9]. It is known that PDT can lead to release of exosomes from tumor cells [10,11]. Further, Zhao et al. have shown that ALA-PDT-derived exosomes specifically enhanced anti-tumor immunity in squamous cell carcinoma cells [12].

Recently, the use of ALA-PDT has extended to treat hematological malignant cells [13] and autoimmune disease [14]. However, the mechanism of action on killing diseased and normal cells in the blood is far from understood. In this report, we have studied the photodynamic effects on cytokines and exosomes of human normal peripheral blood mononuclear cells (PBMCs) with ALA.

2. Materials and Methods

2.1. Chemicals

5-Aminolevulinic acid (ALA) was obtained from Sigma Aldrich (St. Louis, MO, USA). A fresh stock solution of ALA was prepared in Phosphate Buffered Saline (PBS) (VWR Life Science, Solon, OH, USA) to a concentration of 1 M and kept at 4 °C. This was further diluted to reach a concentration of 3 mM for each experiment. All chemicals used were of the highest purity commercially available.

2.2. Isolation and Culture of PBMCs

The human buffy coat samples from 4 anonymous healthy donors (Regional Committee for Medical Research Ethics, REK-S 03280) were obtained from the Blood Bank, Oslo University Hospital, Norway. The isolation of PBMCs from the buffy coats was done using the Lymphoprep density gradient solution (Axis-Shield, Oslo, Norway) in SepMate™ (Stemcell Technologies, Cambridge, UK) 50 mL tubes. Fifteen mL of Lymphoprep were pipetted to the SepMate™ tube. The buffy coats were diluted with an equal volume of RPMI-1640 growth medium (Gibco, Grand Island, NY, USA) containing 2% fetal bovine serum (FBS) (Biological Industries Israel Beit-Haemek Ltd., Kibbutz Beit-Haemek, Israel) and layered carefully above the density gradient solution. The tubes were centrifuged at $1200 \times g$ for 10 min at room temperature with the brake on. The top layer was poured off for maximally 2 s to a new falcon tube and washed twice with the growth medium with 2% FBS, firstly at $300 \times g$ for 15 min and secondly at $300 \times g$ for 10 min. The isolated PBMCs were then gradually frosted using a CoolCell™ (Corning Incorporated, Corning, NY, USA) and stored at −80 °C before use.

PBMCs had been defrosted and incubated in RPMI-1640 growth medium with 10% exosome-depleted FBS(Gibco), 100 units/mL penicillin (Gibco), 10 µg/mL streptomycin (Gibco), and 2 mM L-glutamine(Gibco) at 37 °C in a humidified atmosphere with 5% CO_2 for 24 h before experiments were performed.

2.3. Incubation with ALA and ALA Induced PpIX Production in PBMCs

The incubated PBMCs were changed with fresh medium and one mL of 2×10^6 cells/mL was added per well in a 24-well plate. The cells were then incubated with ALA at the concentration of 3 mM for 4 h in the dark at 37 °C. This ALA dose was chosen because of a therapeutic effect of ALA-PDT on PBMCs in our previous study [15]. Intracellular ALA-induced PpIX in the PBMC subsets was measured with flow cytometry (as described in Section 2.6) using a 405 nm violet laser for the excitation and a 660/20 BP emission filter for the detection of PpIX geometric mean fluorescence intensity.

2.4. Light Source

The Light Emitting Diode (LED) lamp of PhotoCure Aktilite CL 128 (Galderma SA, Lausanne, Switzerland) was used at the wavelength of 630 nm with a fluence rate of 100 mW/cm^2 for 30 min giving a total light dose of 180 J/cm^2.

2.5. PDT Treatment of PBMCs

Four hours after ALA incubation the cells were irradiated by the LED lamp at room temperature. After light exposure, the cells continued to be incubated for another 48 h in the dark at 37 °C with the same ALA-containing medium to keep cytokines and exosomes. The cells incubated with ALA alone were also included as controls. The survivals of PBMC subsets were measured with flow cytometry as described in Section 2.6.

2.6. Flow Cytometry Analysis

After incubation with ALA alone or ALA plus light, the cells were centrifuged and the supernatants were kept at −80 °C for the isolation, labelling, and measurements of cytokines and exosomes as described in Section 2.7. The cells were then incubated in PBS (2% FBS) with an antibody concentration of 2 µL/mL and AnnexinV concentration of 50 µL/mL. The cells were washed with PBS (2% FBS), centrifuged, and the supernatants removed. The amounts of ALA-induced PpIX (1 h antibody incubation) and cell viabilities (1.5 h antibody incubation) in the individual subsets of PBMCs were measured with 4 antibody/dye combination methods: (1) CD3-FITC (Invitrogen, Carlbad, CA, USA), CD19-PE (ImmunoTools GmbH, Friesoythe, Germany), Fixable viability dye-eF450 (Invitrogen), AnnexinV-AF647 (Life Technologies, Eugene, OR, USA); (2) CD3-FITC, CD56-APC-eF780 (Invitrogen), Fixable viability dye-eF450, AnnexinV-PE (Invitrogen); (3) CD4-FITC (eBioscience, San Diego, CA, USA), CD8-PE (Invitrogen), Fixable viability dye-eF450, AnnexinV-AF647; (4) CD11c-FITC (ImmunoTools), CD14-PE/Cy7 (Invitrogen), Fixable viability dye-eF450, Annexin V-AF647. The measurements were done using a Cytoflex S cytometer (Beckman Coulter Life Sciences, Indianapolis, IN, USA) with the Cytexpert software (Version 2.1, Beckman Coulter); and the analyses were performed using FlowJo software (Version 10, Treestar, Ashland, OR, USA).

2.7. Isolation, Labelling, and Measurement of Cytokines and Exosomes

Isolation and labelling of cytokines and exosomes are based on the Exosome Isolation Kit CD63 (Magnetic Exosome Isolation Beads) and MACSPlex Exosome Kit (MACSPlex Exosome Capture Beads, MACSPlex Exosome Detection Reagent CD63 and 3 Buffer Solutions) (both kits from MACS Miltenyi Biotech GmbH, Bergisch Gladbach, Germany). On day 1, after thawing 900 µL of a clean supernatant sample (containing both cytokines and exosomes) were transferred to an Eppendorf tube (Eppendorf AG, Hamburg, Germany).

Fifty µL of Magnetic Exosome Isolation Beads were added to the sample and the mixture was put on a shaker (Vortex T Genie-2, Scientific Industries, Bohemia, NY, USA) at Vortex speed 3 for 8 h at room temperature and stored overnight in a refrigerator at 4 °C before magnetic isolation of exosomes.

On day 2, a proposed µ-column (same manufacturer) was placed in a magnetic µMACS separator that was attached to a MACS multistand (same manufacturer). The µ-column was added with 100 µL of the Equilibration Buffer (same manufacturer) followed by washing with 100 µL of the Isolation Buffer for three times. The magnetically isolated sample from day 1 was then added to go through the µ-column for cytokine collection first (with no need of magnetic bead's help). Subsequently, the µ-column was washed four times using 200 µL of the Isolation Buffer. After washing, the µ-column was moved away from the magnetic separator and immediately flushed into a clean Eppendorf tube with 100 µL of the Isolation Buffer by using a plunger (Figure 1). For labelling of the exosomes, 15 µL of the MACSPlex Exosome Capture Beads were added to the same sample and mixed carefully. A control sample without exosomes was also included using the same Capture Beads. The sample was then put on the shaker for 1 h and stored overnight in a refrigerator at 4 °C.

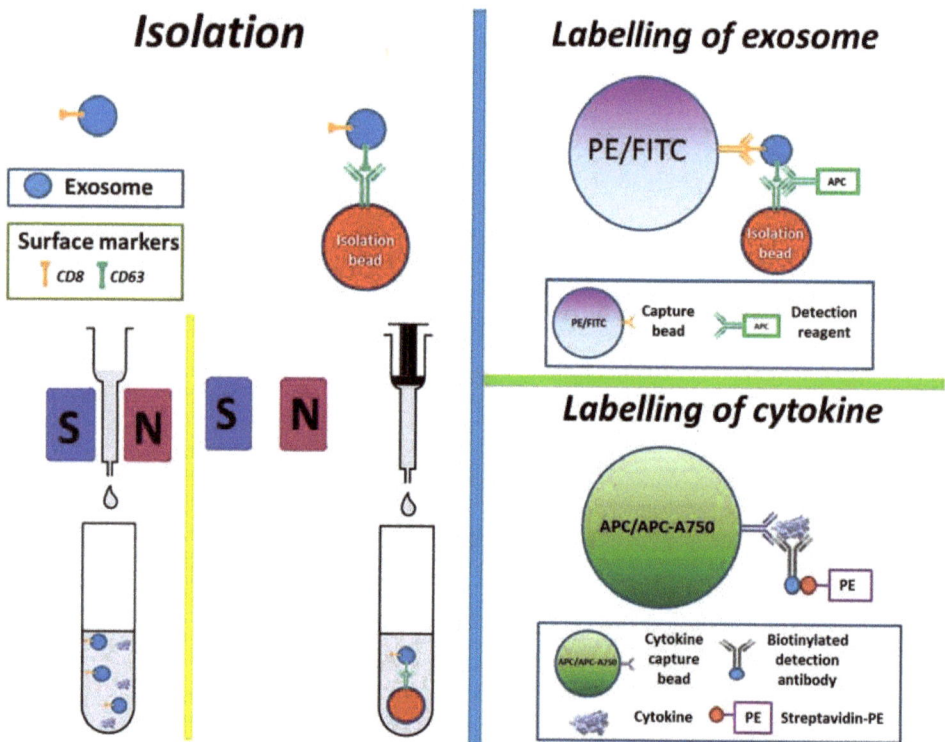

Figure 1. A simplified graphic description of the procedure for isolation and labelling of exosomes. FITC = Fluorescein isothiocyanate, APC = allophycocyanin, PE = phycoerythrin, S = south (on magnet), N = north (on magnet).

On day 3, the sample was put on the shaker at Vortex speed 3 for 5 h. One mL of the MACSPlex Buffer was added to the sample and centrifuged at 12,000 rpm for 10 min. The supernatant was removed and 5 µL of the MACSPlex Exosome Detection Reagent CD63 (for detection of surface markers of exosomes) was added before a 3 h incubation on the shaker (Figure 1). The sample was then washed twice by adding 1 mL of the MACSPlex Buffer, centrifuged at 12,000 rpm for 10 min, and the supernatant removed again.

Cytokines were labelled using Bio-plex Pro human Cytokine Grp 1 panel 27-Plex kit (Bio-Rad Laboratories, Inc., Hercules, CA, USA) (Figure 1). This was done by firstly mixing 50 µL of a sample with 50 µL of a bead solution in an Eppendorf tube. The bead solution was made by dilution of 2 µL beads in 50 µL assay buffer. After mixing, this was incubated for 30 min and washed by adding 1 mL of wash buffer (diluted 10 times in distilled water), centrifuged at 10,000 rpm for 5 min, and the supernatant removed. Then, 20 µL of detection antibody solution (2 µL detection antibody in 50 µL detection antibody diluent) was added and the sample was incubated for 30 min and washed as mentioned above before the supernatant was aspirated. Twenty µL of streptavidin—PE solution (1 µL streptavidin-PE in 100 µL detection antibody diluent) was then added and incubated for 10 min. The same wash step was repeated, and supernatant removed. Finally, 50 µL of the assay buffer were added per sample.

The cytokine and exosome samples were measured with the Cytoflex S cytometer as described in Section 2.6.

2.8. Electron Microscopy of Exosomes

Samples were deposited on glow-discharged formvar/carbon-coated mesh grids (100 mesh) and negatively stained with 2% uranyl acetate for 2 min. The observation of grids was done in a JEOL-JEM 1230 at 80 kV and images were acquired with a Morada camera (Olympus, Hamburg, Germany) using the iTem software.

2.9. Statistical Analyses

The results of the study are plotted and presented as maximum, minimum, and average values to see the spread.

3. Results

3.1. ALA-Induced PpIX Production in PBMCs

Figure 2 shows the PpIX production in the subpopulations of PBMCs from four different donors after ALA incubation at a concentration of 3 mM in the dark for 4 h.

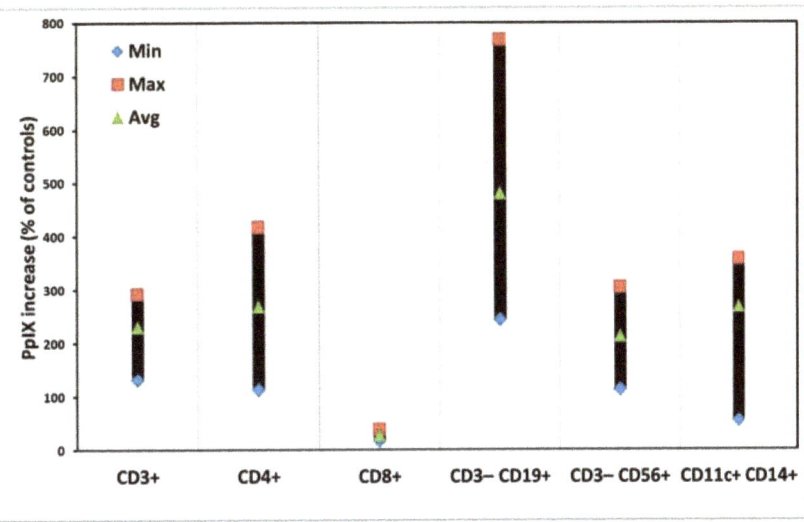

Figure 2. Intracellular amounts of PpIX in individual subsets of PBMCs after ALA incubation for 4 h. The data are presented as minimal, maximal, and average values.

Most subsets of PBMCs produced PpIX from ALA with average amounts of 200% to 300% of the control samples without ALA. However, $CD8^+$ T cells produced little ALA-induced PpIX, while $CD3^- CD19^+$ B cells had a higher average amount of PpIX with a big variation in the samples from four different donors (Table S1 in Supplementary Materials).

3.2. Dark Toxicity of PBMCs with ALA Alone

No apparent dark toxicities on various subpopulations of PBMCs were seen (Figure 3), although there are some variations among samples from donors. In the case of $CD3^- CD56^+$ of Natural Killer (NK) cells, however, there was a killing effect with ALA alone (Figure 3, Table S2 in Supplementary Materials).

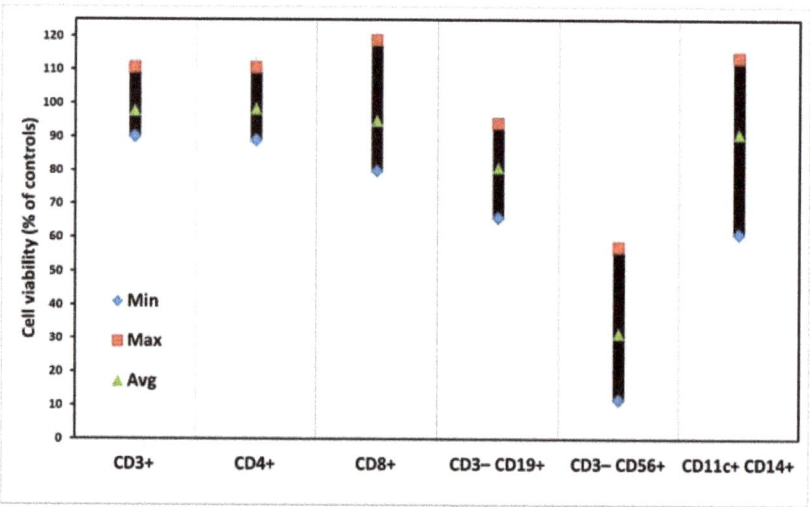

Figure 3. Dark toxicity of cells in individual subsets of PBMCs after ALA incubation for 52 h. The data are presented as minimal, maximal, and average values.

Generally, ALA alone at the concentration of 3 mM for a 4-h incubation does not cause any cytotoxicity. In this study, since the cells were incubated with ALA for 4 h followed by another 48 h to keep cytokines and exosomes, such a relatively long ALA incubation might result in some toxicity on certain subsets of PBMCs.

3.3. PDT of PBMCs with ALA

Figure 4 demonstrates clear photodynamic killing effects on subsets of PBMCs with ALA. In the subpopulations of T cells ($CD3^+$, $CD4^+$, and $CD8^+$) much smaller killing effects than those in the $CD3^- CD19^+$ B cells, $CD3^- CD56^+$ NK cells, and $CD11c^+ CD14^+$ dendritic cells were seen.

There are big variations of the PDT killing effects on the subpopulations of T cells among various samples (Table S3 in Supplementary Materials).

3.4. Effects of ALA-PDT on Cytokines of PBMCs

Many cytokines of PBMCs were affected after ALA-induced PDT. As shown in Figure 5, the data are presented from high to low levels of log decrease.

The log decrease is a $log_2(ALAi - PDTi)$, where ALAi is the cytokine fluorescence intensity in the control group with ALA alone and PDTi is the cytokine fluorescence intensity in the PDT group with ALA plus light. ALA-PDT led to various effects on different cytokines. For example, ALA-PDT clearly reduced the amount of MIP-1 alpha, whereas little effect was seen on the IL-12(p70). There are variations of the PDT effects on the levels of cytokines, particularly in the cases of IL-6, IFN-gamma, and IL-1ra (Table S4 in Supplementary Materials).

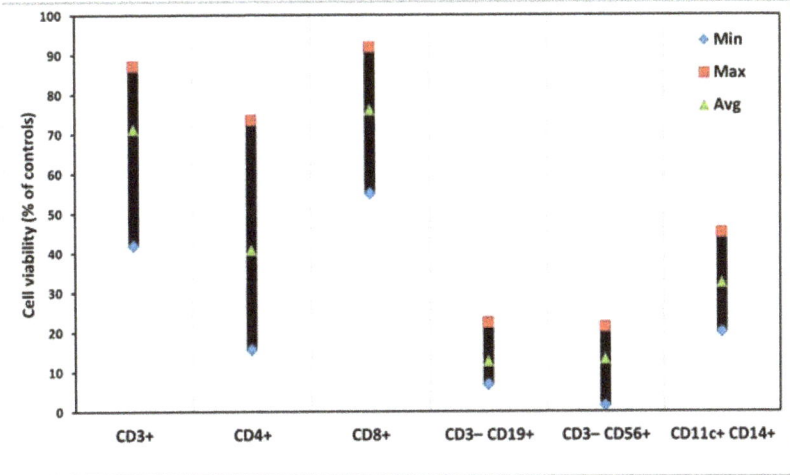

Figure 4. Photodynamic effects on cells in individual subsets of PBMC with ALA. The cells were incubated with ALA at a concentration of 3 mM for 4 h, followed by light exposure at a dose of 180 J/cm^2. The cells then continued to be cultured for another 48 h before the measurements of cell viabilities. The data are presented as minimal, maximal, and average values.

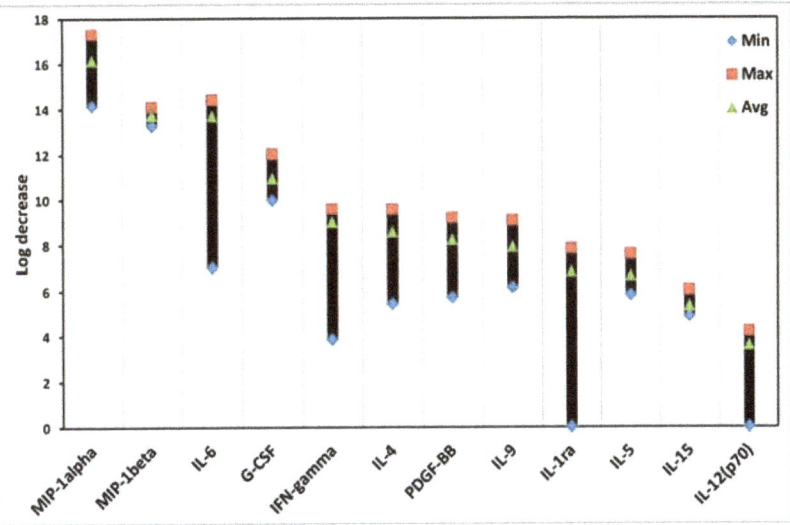

Figure 5. Photodynamic effects on cytokines of PBMCs with ALA. The PDT treatment was the same as that in Figure 4. The data are presented as minimal, maximal, and average log decrease values. The log decrease is a $\log_2(ALA_i - PDT_i)$, where ALA_i is a cytokine fluorescence intensity in the control group with ALA alone and PDT_i is a cytokine fluorescence intensity in the PDT group with ALA plus light. The higher log decrease value, the lower level of a cytokine.

3.5. Effects of ALA-PDT on Exosomes of PBMCs

ALA-PDT also affected various types of exosomes from PBMCs. Figure 6 presents the data from high to low levels of log decrease. The log decrease is a $\log_2(ALAi - PDTi)$, where ALAi is the fluorescence intensity of an exosome surface marker in the control group with ALA alone and PDTi is the fluorescence intensity of an exosome surface marker in the PDT group with ALA plus light. The higher log decrease value is, the lower level of an exosome is. ALA-PDT changed the amounts of different exosomes of PBMCs. For example, ALA-PDT decreased more the amount of CD29 exosomes than CD133-1 exosomes. There are relatively big variations of the PDT effects on the amounts of exosomes, particularly in the exosomes with the surface markers of HLA-ABC, CD69, and CD133-1 (Table S5 in Supplementary Materials).

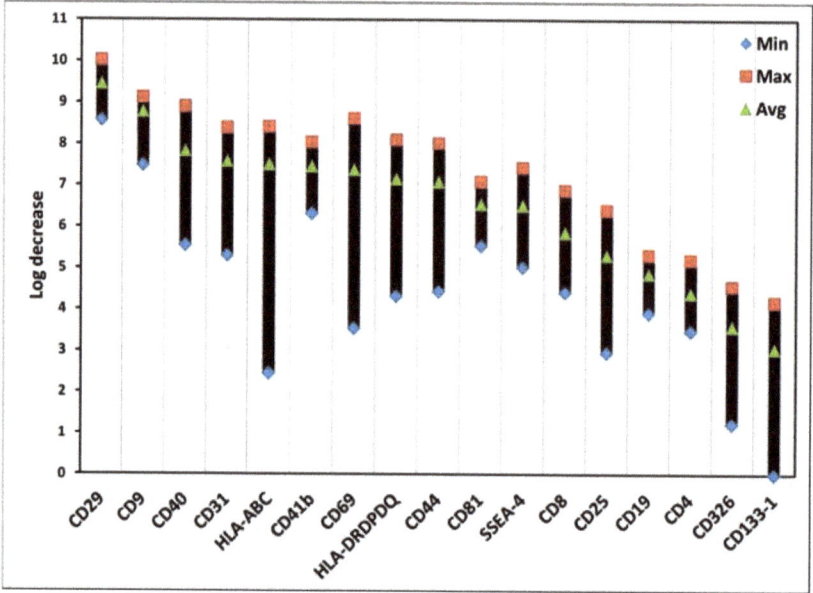

Figure 6. Photodynamic effects on exosomes of PBMCs with ALA. The PDT treatment was the same as that in Figure 4. The data are presented as minimal, maximal, and average log decrease values. The log decrease is a $\log_2(ALAi - PDTi)$, where ALAi is a surface marker fluorescence intensity of an exosome in the control group with ALA alone and PDTi is a surface marker fluorescence intensity of an exosome in the PDT group with ALA plus light. The higher log decrease value, the lower level of a surface marker fluorescence intensity of an exosome.

3.6. Effects of Light Alone on Subsets, Exosomes, and Cytokines of PBMCs

Light alone did not affect the cell survivals of subsets of PBMCs. No effects of light alone on the cytokine levels were seen, except for a minor decrease in IFNγ. The effects on the exosomes were also not found after the treatment with light alone, except a slightly stimulatory response of the CD133-1.

3.7. Electron Microscopy of Exosomes

Typical images of exosomes made by electron microscopy are shown in the Figure 7. The size of the exosomes in this study was confirmed to be around 85 nm.

Exosomes appeared to have a spherical shape with a typical central inflation caused by samples preparation and drying. These morphological data clearly demonstrate the exosomal identity of samples isolated using a combination of flow cytometry and magnetic beads.

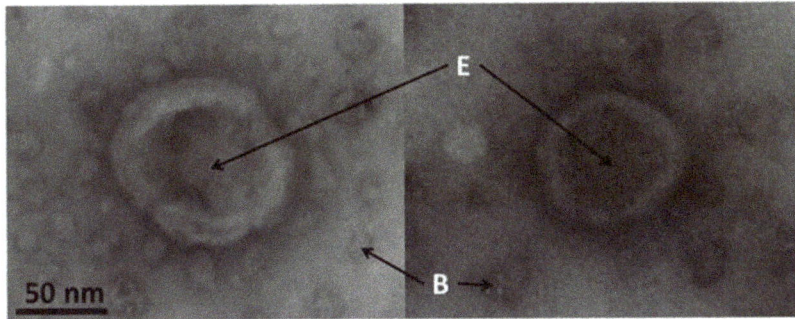

Figure 7. Typical images of exosomes made by electron microscopy. E: exosomes; B: magnetic beads. Detailed information on the preparation of the samples is found in Section 2.8. Scale bar = 50 nm.

4. Discussion

PDT with ALA is a clinically established modality for the treatment of malignant and premalignant diseases [1,16]. Although numerous reports have confirmed the mechanism of PDT action involved in the killing of the diseased cells via necrosis and apoptosis [17–19], no information so far is available for the effects of ALA-PDT on the exosomes of human PBMCs. To understand and explore the potential of exosomes has recently become an urgent issue for the improvement of the clinical ALA-PDT efficacy.

Generally, there are variations of ALA-induced PpIX production and PDT killing effects in the samples from different donors (Figures 2 and 4). The reasons for such individual variations are not known, although we have noticed a similar situation in our other studies [20]. This might be due to the fact that the PBMC samples were taken from various donors with different genders and ages. Light alone did not affect the survivals of all subsets of PBMCs. ALA alone caused no cytotoxicity of PBMCs either, except CD3$^-$CD56$^+$ NK cells (Figure 3). Since NK cells generally appear to be more fragile to any treatments, the reason for the ALA dark toxicity on the NK cells could be due to a relatively long cell culture in vitro with ALA for a total of 52 h. The CD8$^+$ T cells with a low ALA-PpIX production were killed much less than other subsets of PBMCs after light exposure; while the CD3$^-$CD19$^+$ B cells were killed more with a high ALA-PpIX production after light irradiation (Figures 2 and 4).

In physiological and pathological conditions, almost all types of cells release exosomes. Such exosomes contain biological and genetic molecules and carry them to other cells for cell communication and epigenetic regulation. Several techniques have been established to isolate exosomes. They include ultracentrifugation techniques (sequential ultracentrifugation and gradient ultracentrifugation), size-based isolation (ultrafiltration and size-exclusion chromatography), polymer precipitation, etc. These techniques are still under optimization. In the present study, we employed an immunoaffinity capture technique with specific binding between exosome markers and immobilized antibodies (ligands) measured with flow cytometry. The technique has several advantages over other methods including easy use, separation of exosomes from different origins, and high purity of exosomes with no chemical contamination [21]. In addition, we used electron microscopy to morphologically confirm the exosomes measured with flow cytometry (Figure 7).

ALA-PDT reduced the levels of most cytokines studied (Figure 5), although with different degrees of such reduction in various cytokines. Since almost all cytokines included in this study are pro-inflammatory, except IL-1ra that is anti-inflammatory (Table 1), these consistent results may suggest that ALA-PDT of PBMCs results in a strong anti-inflammatory effect.

Table 1. Effects of ALA-PDT on cytokines [1].

Cytokine	PDT Effect (Avg.)	Cell Type	Possible Biological Function
MIP-1alpha (macrophage inflammatory protein-1 alpha)	16.1	Macrophage	Pro-inflammation
MIP-1beta (macrophage inflammatory protein-1beta)	13.7	Macrophage	Pro-inflammation
IL-6 (interleukin-6)	13.7	Macrophage	Pro-inflammation
G-CSF (granulocyte colony stimulating factor)	10.9	Macrophage and other cells	Growth stimulation of white blood cells
IFN-gamma (interferon gamma)	9	T-cell and NK cell	Pro-inflammation and worsen autoimmune diseases
IL-4 (interleukin-4)	8.6	Mast cell, T-cell, granulocyte	Pro-inflammation
PDGF-BB (platelet-derived growth factor-BB)	8.2	Platelet, macrophage, and other cells	Wound healing and repair blood vessel
IL-9 (interleukin-9)	7.9	$CD4^+$ T cell	Pro-inflammation
IL-1ra (interleukin-1 receptor antagonist)	6.8	Macrophage and other cells	Anti-inflammation
IL-5 (interleukin-5)	6.7	T cell, granulocyte, and other cells	Pro-inflammation
IL-15 (interleukin-15)	5.4	Macrophage	Pro-inflammation
IL-12(p70) (interleukin 12p70)	3.6	Macrophage	Pro-inflammation

[1] Note: Since the types of cells and possible biological functions of the cytokines studied are complicated with different types of cells and multi-functions, the table only lists main cell types and functions of the cytokines.

This may also be true for the level of IFN-gamma, a well-known cytokine for pro-autoimmune diseases, which was clearly reduced after ALA-PDT (Table 1). This finding makes one tempting to speculate if ALA-PDT might have the potential for reducing the cytokine storm in COVID-19 cases [22].

ALA-PDT also decreased the amounts of all exosomes of PBMCs (Figure 6, Table 2). It is not clear if such decreased amounts of exosomes were due to a direct destruction of PDT effect, PDT-mediated damage to those parent cells making them unable to produce exosomes, or both.

However, the amount of $CD4^+$ exosomes is higher than $CD8^+$ exosomes after ALA-PDT (Table 2), even though $CD4^+$ cells produced more ALA-induced PpIX and killed more than $CD8^+$ cells. The reason for is not known, but our previous studies have confirmed that ALA-PDT could induce apoptosis of leukemia and lymphoma with the formation of apoptotic bodies [17–19].

It is interesting to note that both CD40 and CD19 as surface markers for B cells were apparently decreased, probably because the $CD3^-CD19^+$ B cells produced a high amount of PpIX from ALA (Figure 2) and were killed more after light exposure (Figure 4). A reduced amount of CD69 exosomes was also seen after PDT treatment (Table 2). Such exosomes are believed to activate and proliferate lymphocytes [23].

CD25 is an activating marker for lymphocytes and macrophage, particularly for T cells. Interestingly, the amount of CD25 exosomes was not affected very much as expected by ALA-PDT probably due to few activated T cells in the PBMC samples from healthy donors.

HLA-DRDPDQ is the surface marker for antigen-presenting cells (APC). Since APC is heavily involved in presenting the MHC class II molecules to $CD4^+$ T cells for the rejection of organ transplantation [24–28], the decrease in the amount of the APC-derived exosomes may indicate that such a reduction of HLA-DRDPDQ exosomes by ALA-PDT may have an impact on reducing such organ rejection. Similarly, a reduced amount of HLA-ABC exosomes, which are involved in presenting the MHC class I molecules to $CD8^+$ T cells, was seen. Such a finding suggests that ALA-PDT of PBMCs may reduce the MHC class I molecule-mediated cytotoxic $CD8^+$ immunity.

Both CD133-1 [29] and SSEA-4 [30] are markers for stem cells with lower reduction of exosomes after PDT. This could be due to the fact that stem cells normally are resting with a low energy demand, so that the rate of heme synthesis is minimal, through which a low amount of ALA-PpIX is produced. As a result, PDT with ALA has a minimal destructive effect on these cells.

Table 2. Effects of ALA-PDT on exosomes [1].

Surface Marker	PDT Effect (Avg.)	Cell Type	Possible Biological Function
CD29	9.4	White blood cells	Cell adhesion
CD9	8.8	Lymphocyte, macrophage	Platelet activation and aggregation and cell adhesion and migration
CD40	7.8	B-cell, macrophage	Cell proliferation and signal transduction
CD31	7.6	White blood cells	Cell adhesion, activation, and migration
HLA-ABC	7.5	Nucleated cells	MHC class I molecules presented to $CD8^+$ T cells
CD41b	7.4	Stem cell, platelet	Cell adhesion and platelet aggregation
CD69	7.4	White blood cells	Lymphocyte activation and proliferation
HLA-DRDPDQ	7.1	Antigen-presenting cell	MHC class II molecules presented to $CD4^+$ T cells
CD44	7.1	White blood cells	Cell adhesion
CD81	6.5	White blood cells but granulocyte	Cell adhesion
SSEA-4	6.5	Embryonic stem cell	Pluripotent stem cell marker
CD8	5.9	T cell	Cytotoxic T cell marker
CD25	5.3	Lymphocyte and macrophage	Lymphocyte activation
CD19	4.9	B cell	B cell marker
CD4	4.4	T cell	Helper T cell marker
CD326	3.6	T cell, dendritic cell, epithelial cell	Epithelial cell marker unknown functions on immune cells
CD133-1	3.1	Stem cell and endothelial cell	Stem cell marker

[1] Note: Since the cell types and possible biological functions of the exosomes studied are complicated with multi-cell types and multi-functions, the table only lists main cell types and functions of the exosomes.

CD9 and CD41b exosomes are involved in platelet activation and aggregation and were also used as markers for rejection of heart transplantation [31]. After ALA-PDT, the amount of the exosomes was reduced, suggesting a favorable response to this treatment.

Cell adhesion molecule are cell surface proteins. They help cells to bind other cells to maintain cells/tissue functional. They also play important roles in cell growth and death, contact inhibition, etc. ALA-PDT also decreased several exosomes that are involved in cell adhesion, including CD29, CD9, CD31, CD41b, CD44, and CD81 exosomes. The biological implications of such a PDT effect are not known and warrant further investigation.

5. Conclusions

This is the first report to study the effects of ALA-PDT on cytokines and exosomes of human healthy PBMCs. ALA-PDT reduced all cytokines and exosomes studied, although there was variation among individual PBMC samples. This reduction is consistent with ALA-PDT-mediated survivals of subsets of PBMCs. More specifically, the ALA-PDT treatment apparently decreased all pro-inflammatory cytokines included, suggesting that this treatment provides a strong anti-inflammatory effect. In addition, the treatment has decreased the levels of different types of exosomes with a particular interest in the HLA-DRDPDQ exosome, which plays an important role in presenting the MHC class II molecules to $CD4^+$ T cells for rejection of organ transplantation and autoimmune diseases [24–28].

Supplementary Materials: The following supporting information can be downloaded at: https://www.mdpi.com/article/10.3390/biomedicines10020232/s1, Table S1: Intracellular PpIX in individual subsets of PBMCs after ALA incubation for 4 h, Table S2: ALA dark toxicity in subsets of PBMCs after ALA incubation for 4 h, Table S3: Killing effects on individual subsets of PBMCs after PDT with ALA. Table S4: PDT effect on cytokines with ALA, Table S5: PDT effect on exosomes with ALA.

Author Contributions: Conceptualization, K.E., A.K., J.J. and Q.P.; Methodology, A.K., K.E., P.J., A.B., S.D., V.V. and Q.P.; Formal analysis, A.K., K.E., P.J. and Q.P.; Investigation, A.K., K.E., P.J. and A.B.; Writing original draft: K.E. and Q.P.; Writing, review, and editing: K.E., E.C., T.W., J.J. and Q.P.; Supervision, E.C., J.J. and Q.P.; Project administration, J.J. and Q.P.; Funding acquisition, Q.P. All authors have read and agreed to the published version of the manuscript.

Funding: The South-Eastern Norway Regional Health Authority (Project numbers: 2016092, 2017058, 2020069), The Norwegian Cancer Society (Project number: 190397) and the Norwegian Radium Hospital Research Foundation (Project number: SE1701).

Institutional Review Board Statement: Peripheral blood mononuclear cells from anonymous healthy donors at The Blood Bank in Oslo were collected after informed consent according to the guidelines of the Declaration of Helsinki and approved by the Regional Committee for Medical Research Ethics (REK S-03280).

Informed Consent Statement: Informed consent was obtained from all subjects involved in the study.

Data Availability Statement: The data presented in this study are available in the Supplementary Materials.

Acknowledgments: We are grateful to the Jeanette and Søren Bothners legat, (Oslo, Norway) and the Radiumhospitalets Legater (Oslo, Norway) for their financing the purchase of a Cytoflex S flow cytometer, and to Morten Oksvold for constructive discussions.

Conflicts of Interest: The authors have no conflict of interest to declare. The funders had no role in the design of the study; in the collection, analyses, or interpretation of data; in the writing of the manuscript, or in the decision to publish the results.

References

1. Dougherty, T.J.; Gomer, C.J.; Henderson, B.W.; Jori, G.; Kessel, D.; Korbelik, M.; Moan, J.; Peng, Q. Photodynamic therapy. *J. Nat. Cancer Inst.* **1998**, *90*, 889–905. [CrossRef] [PubMed]
2. van Straten, D.; Mashayekhi, V.; de Bruijn, H.S.; Oliveira, S.; Robinson, D.J. Oncologic Photodynamic Therapy: Basic Principles, Current Clinical Status and Future Directions. *Cancers* **2017**, *9*, 19. [CrossRef] [PubMed]
3. Peng, Q.; Warloe, T.; Berg, K.; Moan, J.; Kongshaug, M.; Giercksky, K.E.; Nesland, J.M. 5-Aminolevulinic acid-based photodynamic therapy. Clinical research and future challenges. *Cancer* **1997**, *79*, 2282–2308. [CrossRef]
4. Peng, Q.; Berg, K.; Moan, J.; Kongshaug, M.; Nesland, J.M. 5-Aminolevulinic acid-based photodynamic therapy: Principles and experimental research. *Photochem. Photobiol.* **1997**, *65*, 235–251. [CrossRef] [PubMed]
5. Peng, Q.; Juzeniene, A.; Chen, J.; Svaasand, L.O.; Warloe, T.; Giercksky, K.E.; Moan, J. Lasers in medicine. *Rep. Prog. Phys.* **2008**, *71*, 056701. [CrossRef]
6. Stummer, W.; Pichlmeier, U.; Meinel, T.; Wiestler, O.D.; Zanella, F.; Reulen, H.J. Fluorescence-guided surgery with 5-aminolevulinic acid for resection of malignant glioma: A randomised controlled multicentre phase III trial. *Lancet Oncol.* **2006**, *7*, 392–401. [CrossRef]
7. Mosquera-Heredia, M.I.; Morales, L.C.; Vidal, O.M.; Barceló, E.; Silvera-Redondo, C.; Vélez, J.I.; Garavito-Galofre, P. Exosomes: Potential Disease Biomarkers and New Therapeutic Targets. *Biomedicines* **2021**, *9*, 1061. [CrossRef]
8. Kalluri, R.; LeBleu, V.S. The biology, function, and biomedical applications of exosomes. *Science* **2020**, *367*, 6977. [CrossRef]
9. Yang, D.; Zhang, W.; Zhang, H.; Zhang, F.; Chen, L.; Ma, L.; Larcher, L.M.; Chen, S.; Liu, N.; Zhao, Q.; et al. Progress, opportunity, and perspective on exosome isolation-efforts for efficient exosome-based theranostics. *Theranostics* **2020**, *10*, 3684–3707. [CrossRef]
10. Mkhobongo, B.; Chandran, R.; Abrahamse, H. The Role of Melanoma Cell-Derived Exosomes (MTEX) and Photodynamic Therapy (PDT) within a Tumor Microenvironment. *Int. J. Mol. Sci.* **2021**, *22*, 9726. [CrossRef]
11. Jiang, Y.; Xu, C.; Leung, W.; Lin, M.; Cai, X.; Guo, H.; Zhang, J.; Yang, F. Role of Exosomes in Photodynamic Anticancer Therapy. *Curr. Med. Chem.* **2020**, *27*, 6815–6824. [CrossRef] [PubMed]
12. Zhao, Z.; Zhang, H.; Zeng, Q.; Wang, P.; Zhang, G.; Ji, J.; Li, M.; Shen, S.; Wang, X. Exosomes from 5-aminolevulinic acid photodynamic therapy-treated squamous carcinoma cells promote dendritic cell maturation. *Photodiagn. Photodyn. Ther.* **2020**, *30*, 101746. [CrossRef] [PubMed]
13. Sando, Y.; Matsuoka, K.-I.; Sumii, Y.; Kondo, T.; Ikegawa, S.; Sugiura, H.; Nakamura, M.; Iwamoto, M.; Meguri, Y.; Asada, N.; et al. 5-aminolevulinic acid-mediated photodynamic therapy can target aggressive adult T cell leukemia/lymphoma resistant to conventional chemotherapy. *Sci. Rep.* **2020**, *10*, 17237. [CrossRef]
14. Christensen, E.; Foss, O.A.; Quist-Paulsen, P.; Staur, I.; Pettersen, F.; Holien, T.; Juzenas, P.; Peng, Q. Application of Photodynamic Therapy with 5-Aminolevulinic Acid to Extracorporeal Photopheresis in the Treatment of Patients with Chronic Graft-versus-Host Disease: A First-in-Human Study. *Pharmaceutics* **2021**, *13*, 1558. [CrossRef] [PubMed]

15. Darvekar, S.; Juzenas, P.; Oksvold, M.; Kleinauskas, A.; Holien, T.; Christensen, E.; Stokke, T.; Sioud, M.; Peng, Q. Selective Killing of Activated T Cells by 5-Aminolevulinic Acid Mediated Photodynamic Effect: Potential Improvement of Extracorporeal Photopheresis. *Cancers* **2020**, *12*, 377. [CrossRef]
16. Casas, A. Clinical uses of 5-aminolaevulinic acid in photodynamic treatment and photodetection of cancer: A review. *Cancer Lett.* **2020**, *490*, 165–173. [CrossRef] [PubMed]
17. Furre, I.E.; Møller, M.T.; Shahzidi, S.; Nesland, J.M.; Peng, Q. Involvement of both caspase-dependent and -independent pathways in apoptotic induction by hexaminolevulinate-mediated photodynamic therapy in human lymphoma cells. *Apoptosis* **2006**, *11*, 2031–2042. [CrossRef] [PubMed]
18. Furre, I.E.; Shahzidi, S.; Luksiene, Z.; Møller, M.T.N.; Borgen, E.; Morgan, J.; Tkacz-Stachowska, K.; Nesland, J.M.; Peng, Q. Targeting PBR by hexaminolevulinate-mediated photodynamic therapy induces apoptosis through translocation of apoptosis-inducing factor in human leukemia cells. *Cancer Res.* **2005**, *65*, 11051–11060. [CrossRef]
19. Shahzidi, S.; Čunderlíková, B.; Więdłocha, A.; Zhen, Y.; Vasovič, V.; Nesland, J.M.; Peng, Q. Simultaneously targeting mitochondria and endoplasmic reticulum by photodynamic therapy induces apoptosis in human lymphoma cells. *Photochem. Photobiol. Sci.* **2011**, *10*, 1773–1782. [CrossRef]
20. Holien, T.; Gederaas, O.A.; Darvekar, S.R.; Christensen, E.; Peng, Q. Comparison between 8-methoxypsoralen and 5-aminolevulinic acid in killing T cells of photopheresis patients ex vivo. *Lasers Surg. Med.* **2018**, *50*, 469–475. [CrossRef]
21. Zhang, Y.; Bi, J.; Huang, J.; Tang, Y.; Du, S.; Li, P. Exosome: A Review of Its Classification, Isolation Techniques, Storage, Diagnostic and Targeted Therapy Applications. *Int. J. Nanomed.* **2020**, *15*, 6917–6934. [CrossRef] [PubMed]
22. Ragab, D.; Salah Eldin, H.; Taeimah, M.; Khattab, R.; Salem, R. The COVID-19 Cytokine Storm; What We Know so Far. *Front. Immunol.* **2020**, *11*, 1446. [CrossRef] [PubMed]
23. Gorabi, A.M.; Hajighasemi, S.; Kiaie, N.; Gheibi-Hayat, S.M.; Jamialahmadi, T.; Johnston, T.P.; Sahebkar, A. The pivotal role of CD69 in autoimmunity. *J. Autoimmun.* **2020**, *111*, 102453. [CrossRef] [PubMed]
24. Marino, J.; Paster, J.; Benichou, G. Allorecognition by T Lymphocytes and Allograft Rejection. *Front. Immunol.* **2016**, *7*, 582. [CrossRef]
25. Timrott, K.; Beetz, O.; Oldhafer, F.; Klempnauer, J.; Vondran, F.W.R.; Jäger, M.D. The importance of MHC class II in allogeneic bone marrow transplantation and chimerism-based solid organ tolerance in a rat model. *PLoS ONE* **2020**, *15*, e0233497. [CrossRef]
26. Khaddour, K.; Hana, C.K.; Mewawalla, P. *Hematopoietic Stem Cell Transplantation*; StatPearls Publishing: Treasure Island, FL, USA, 2021.
27. Howell, W.M.; Carter, V.; Clark, B. The HLA system: Immunobiology, HLA typing, antibody screening and crossmatching techniques. *J. Clin. Pathol.* **2010**, *63*, 387. [CrossRef]
28. Leeaphorn, N.; Pena, J.; Thamcharoen, N.; Khankin, E.; Pavlakis, M.; Cardarelli, F. HLA-DQ Mismatching and Kidney Transplant Outcomes. *Clin. J. Am. Soc. Nephrol.* **2018**, *13*, 763–771. [CrossRef]
29. Barzegar Behrooz, A.; Syahir, A.; Ahmad, S. CD133: Beyond a cancer stem cell biomarker. *J. Drug Target.* **2019**, *27*, 257–269. [CrossRef]
30. Trusler, O.; Huang, Z.; Goodwin, J.; Laslett, A.L. Cell surface markers for the identification and study of human naive pluripotent stem cells. *Stem Cell Res.* **2018**, *26*, 36–43. [CrossRef]
31. Castellani, C.; Burrello, J.; Fedrigo, M.; Burrello, A.; Bolis, S.; Di Silvestre, D.; Tona, F.; Bottio, T.; Biemmi, V.; Toscano, G.; et al. Circulating extracellular vesicles as non-invasive biomarker of rejection in heart transplant. *J. Heart Lung Transplant.* **2020**, *39*, 1136–1148. [CrossRef]

MDPI
St. Alban-Anlage 66
4052 Basel
Switzerland
Tel. +41 61 683 77 34
Fax +41 61 302 89 18
www.mdpi.com

MDPI Books Editorial Office
E-mail: books@mdpi.com
www.mdpi.com/books

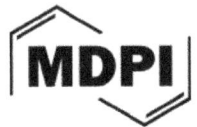

www.ingramcontent.com/pod-product-compliance
Lightning Source LLC
LaVergne TN
LVHW070211100526
838202LV00015B/2035